Principles and Practice of
IMMUNOTOXICOLOGY

Principles and Practice of
IMMUNOTOXICOLOGY

Edited by

KLARA MILLER
PhD, FRCPath
British Industrial Biological Research Association
Carshalton, Surrey

JOHN L. TURK
MD, DSc
Professor, Department of Pathology
Royal College of Surgeons of England
London

STEPHEN NICKLIN
PhD
British Industrial Biological Research Association
Carshalton, Surrey

Foreword by

JACK H. DEAN
PhD, Dip. ABT
Centre Director and Vice President
Drug Safety Assessment
Sterling Research Group
Sterling–Winthrop
Northumberland

OXFORD
BLACKWELL SCIENTIFIC PUBLICATIONS
LONDON EDINBURGH BOSTON
MELBOURNE PARIS BERLIN VIENNA

© 1992 by
Blackwell Scientific Publications
Editorial Offices:
Osney Mead, Oxford OX2 0EL
25 John Street, London WC1N 2BL
23 Ainslie Place, Edinburgh EH3 6AJ
3 Cambridge Center, Cambridge
  Massachusetts 02142, USA
54 University Street, Carlton
  Victoria 3053, Australia

Other Editorial Offices:
Librairie Arnette SA
2, rue Casimir-Delavigne
75006 Paris
France

Blackwell Wissenschafts-Verlag
Meinekestrasse 4
D-1000 Berlin 15
Germany

Blackwell MZV
Feldgasse 13
A-1238 Wien
Austria

First published 1992

Set by Times Graphics, Singapore
Printed in Great Britain at
The Alden Press, Oxford
and bound by
Hartnolls Ltd, Bodmin, Cornwall

DISTRIBUTORS

Marston Book Services Ltd
PO Box 87
Oxford OX2 0DT
(*Orders:* Tel: 0865 791155
       Fax: 0865 791927
       Telex: 837515)

USA
Blackwell Scientific Publications, Inc.
3 Cambridge Center
Cambridge, MA 02142
(*Orders:* Tel: 800 759-6102)

Canada
Times Mirror Professional Publishing, Ltd
5240 Finch Avenue East
Scarborough, Ontario M1S 5A2
(*Orders:* Tel: 416 298-1588)

Australia
Blackwell Scientific Publications
(Australia) Pty Ltd
54 University Street
Carlton, Victoria 3053
(*Orders:* Tel: 03 347-0300)

British Library
Cataloguing in Publication Data

Principles and practice of
immunotoxicology
   1. Humans. Immune reactions.
   Effects of toxic chemicals
   I. Miller, Klara   II. Turk, John
   III. Nicklin, Stephen
   616.0795

   ISBN 0-632-02563-8

Contents

List of Contributors

DAVID E. BICE PhD, *Inhalation Toxicology Research Institute, Lovelace Biomedical and Environmental Research Institute, Albuquerque, New Mexico, USA*

JANET M. DEWDNEY PhD, *Director, Biotechnology (Europe), SmithKline Beecham, Great Burgh, Surrey, UK*

ROBERT G. EDWARDS *SmithKline Beecham, Great Burgh, Surrey, UK*

ERNST GLEICHMANN MD, *Professor, Division of Immunology, Medical Institute of Environmental Hygiene, Heinrich Heine University of Düsseldorf, Düsseldorf, Germany*

HELGA GLEICHMANN MD, *Professor, Diabetes Research Institute, Heinrich Heine University of Düsseldorf, Düsseldorf, Germany*

WILLIAM F. GREENLEE PhD, *Professor and Head, Department of Pharmacology and Toxicology, School of Pharmacy and Pharmacological Sciences, Robert E. Heine Building, Purdue University, West Lafeyette, IN 47907, USA*

ANNE S. HAMBLIN PhD, *Senior Lecturer, Immunology Department, United Medical and Dental Schools of Guy's and St Thomas' Hospitals, St Thomas' Campus, London SE1 7EH, UK*

MERYL H. KAROL, PhD, *Professor, Department of Environmental and Occupational Health, Graduate School of Public Health, University of Pittsburgh, Pittsburgh, PA 15261, USA*

IAN KIMBER PhD, *ICI Central Toxicology Laboratory, Alderley Park, Macclesfield, Cheshire SK10 4TJ, UK*

MAGDA A.M. KRAJNC-FRANKEN PhD, *Laboratory for Pathology, National Institute of Public Health and Environmental Protection, 3720–BA, Bilthoven, The Netherlands*

BRIAN E. LEONARD MD, *Professor, Pharmacology Department, University College, Galway, Ireland*

NOEL R. LING MD, *Reader, Department of Immunology, University of Birmingham, Birmingham, UK*

HENK VAN LOVEREN PhD, *Laboratory for Pathology, National Institute of Public Health and Environmental Protection, 3720–BA, Bilthoven, The Netherlands*

CLIVE MEREDITH PhD, *Gene Expression Group, Immunotoxicology Department, British Industrial Biological Research Association, Woodmansterne Road, Carshalton, Surrey SM5 4DS, UK*

HANS F. MERK MD, *Professor, Department of Dermatology, Clinical and Experimental Division, University of Cologne, J. Stelzmannstrasse 9, D-5000 Köln 41, Germany*

KLARA MILLER PhD, FRCPath, *British Industrial Biological Research Association, Woodmansterne Road, Carshalton, Surrey SM5 4DS, UK*

MICHAEL J. MURRAY PhD, *Procter and Gamble Company, Miami Valley Laboratories, Cincinnati, OH 45239, USA*

STEPHEN NICKLIN PhD, *Department of Immunotoxicology, British Industrial Biological Research Association, Woodmansterne Road, Carshalton, Surrey SM5 4DS, UK*

A. K. PRASAD PhD, *Immunobiology Division, Industrial Toxicology Research Centre, PO Box 80, M.G. Marg, Lucknow-226 001, UP, India*

P.K. RAY PhD, DSc, *Head of Immunobiology Division, and Director, Industrial Toxicology Research Centre, PO Box 80, M.G. Marg, Lucknow-226 001, UP, India*

HENK-JAN SCHUURMAN PhD, *Division for Histochemistry and Electron Microscopy, Department of Pathology and Internal Medicine, University Hospital, 3508 GA Utrecht, The Netherlands*

JACOB SHOHAM MD, PhD, *Professor, Department of Life Sciences, Bar-Ilan University, Ramat-Gan 52900, Israel*

TEE-PING LEE PhD, *Department of Medicine, Veterans Administration Medical Centre, 3495 Bailey Avenue, Buffalo, New York 14215, USA*

PETER T. THOMAS PhD, *IIT Research Institute, 10 West 35th Street, Chicago, IL 60616, USA*

JOHN L. TURK MD, DSc, *Professor, Department of Pathology, Royal College of Surgeons of England, London, UK*

JOSEPH G. VOS DVM, PhD, *Laboratory for Pathology, National Institute of Public Health and Environmental Protection, 3720–BA, Bilthoven, The Netherlands*

ROEL A. DE **WEGER** PhD, *Division for Histochemistry and Electron Microscopy, Department of Pathology, University Hospital, 3508 GA Utrecht, The Netherlands*

KIMBER L. WHITE JR PhD, *Department of Pharmacology and Toxicology and Department of Biostatistics, Medical College of Virginia, Virginia Commonwealth University, Richmond, VA 23298, USA*

DANIEL WIERDA PhD, *Research Scientist, Lilly Research Laboratories, Eli Lilly and Company, Greenfield, IN 46140, USA*

Foreword

This volume provides the opportunity for the reader to be introduced to many of the 'newer stars' in the emerging field of immunotoxicology. Many chapters in this volume were prepared by selected young workers in the field which should give the reader a contemporary perspective of the form of this subdiscipline which 'bridges' toxicology and immunology. The growth of interests in immunotoxicology indicates recognition in the field of toxicology that the immune system can be an occasional target for toxic effects of drug and non-drug chemicals, as has been shown for the more classical target organ systems such as liver, lung, kidney, gastrointestinal, reproductive and neurological systems which have been routinely evaluated during pre-clinical or pre-release evaluation. Drug and non-drug interactions with the immune system can be expressed as changes in the histomorphology or function of its cellular constituents or be an allergic or autoimmune response to a novel antigen(s) resulting from this interaction. These interactions can either be expressed subclinically and within the physiological reserve or be below the response level of the system so that no adverse effect results.

This book, like most books trying to define an emerging field of science, firstly provides two sections (I and II) describing the basic science underpinning this hybrid discipline to include its cellular constituents, their pharmacological responses, homeostatic controls, and currently accepted concepts about this organ system. These sections also include the influence of external factors (e.g. nutrition and psychoneurological influences) as well as xenobiotics on immune responses. These sections are well integrated and should allow the reader a quick understanding of the basic biology underpinning the discipline.

The next section (III) includes four chapters describing examples of effects in humans, both immune parameter changes and allergy, following exposure to several classes of environmentally relevant chemicals. Section IV is methodologically oriented with chapters describing approaches to the evaluation of hypersensitivity changes, histomorphometric changes, changes in immune function assays, and finally molecular biology and cell culture approaches. This is an exciting and challenging volume which should be appreciated by a broad spectrum of readers.

The principal purpose of determining if the immune system is a potential target during pre-clinical or pre-release evaluation of a new substance is because of the pivotal role the immune system performs in maintaining health and protecting against opportunistic microbial agents, and to reduce the potential of a sensitizer being introduced into the product which might result in an allergic event. The simple message is that not all changes in immune parameters should be interpreted to be indicative of disease potential since the immune system has a significant physiological reserve, that biologically significant change depends on the degree of change or function(s) altered, and that species variation is a cardinal feature of toxicology. The data generated on potential immunotoxicity when indicated during a routine subacute toxicity evaluation of a new drug or chemical entity should improve human risk assessment.

As can be seen in this volume, the data developed to date by investigators in this field have primarily involved experimental animal systems to develop or validate testing methods and approaches or to understand mechanisms underlying immune changes observed in animal species. Evidence for chemical-induced immunotoxicity documented in well-controlled human studies with resultant immunologic disease other than environmental allergic or drug-induced autoimmunity is limited. Defining human populations with accidental or occupational exposure and related immune changes as described in rodents continues to be a critical issue for the discipline of immunotoxicology. The tier testing approaches which have proved so valuable in the rodent models and which have been used to select methods predictive of host-resistant changes are not ready to be applied broadly to predict disease potential and susceptibility to cancer in human cohorts following putative chemical exposures. There is no scientific basis for the speculation that any change in an immune function parameter or assay in humans should be interpreted to signify environmental chemical exposure as has been claimed in certain lawsuits in the USA. What is needed is the selection and validation of appropriate methods to use in epidemiological studies where exposure to an immunotoxic agent is suspect.

JACK H. DEAN
Centre Director and Vice President
Drug Safety Assessment
Sterling Research Group
Sterling–Winthrop
Northumberland

Part I
The basis of the
immune system

1
Cells of the immune system

NOEL R. LING

Introduction

The cells responsible for generating and sustaining an immune response are to be found in greatest numbers in peripheral lymphoid tissues (lymph nodes, spleen and collections of lymphoid cells chiefly associated with the respiratory and alimentary tracts). The commonest cell in these tissues is the lymphocyte, for long an enigma as far as function was concerned, but a cell which has been intensively studied since it became recognized as the cell type responsible for the remarkable specificity of immune responses. Lymphocytes do not, however, function in isolation and there are many other contributing cells, such as those concerned with the capture of antigen and its presentation to lymphocytes during the initiation of the response and others, such as neutrophils, eosinophils, mast cells,

monocytes and macrophages, concerned with the execution of the various effector stages of the response. Immune responses have evolved chiefly as a defence against infections with micro-organisms and are part of a diverse range of defence mechanisms which include the enhanced blood flow and local accumulation of leucocytes seen in inflammation and the exudation of mucus and wave movement of cilia on mucous surfaces. These all link in with immunological defences, the various facets of which are themselves interdependent, as has been recognized since Almoth Wright demonstrated that the agents of humoral immunity, antibody and complement, also have opsonic properties in inducing ingestion of bacteria by phagocytes. As our knowledge of the subpopulations of cells involved, their surface receptors and factor production has increased, the role of cell–cell interactions has become more and more evident and yet more difficult to unravel in isolated cell systems.

Lymphocytes

Most of the lymphocytes found in blood and lymph are small round cells with a pachychromatic nucleus surrounded by a thin rim of cytoplasm which contains a small number of mitochondria, some ribosomes and a poorly developed Golgi (Figs 1.1 & 1.2). The small lymphocyte looks what it is, a cell designed to move around for long periods of time with metabolic activity kept at the minimum required for this task, with most genes switched off and DNA tightly packed, but with the capacity to change to an active state once the surface receptors

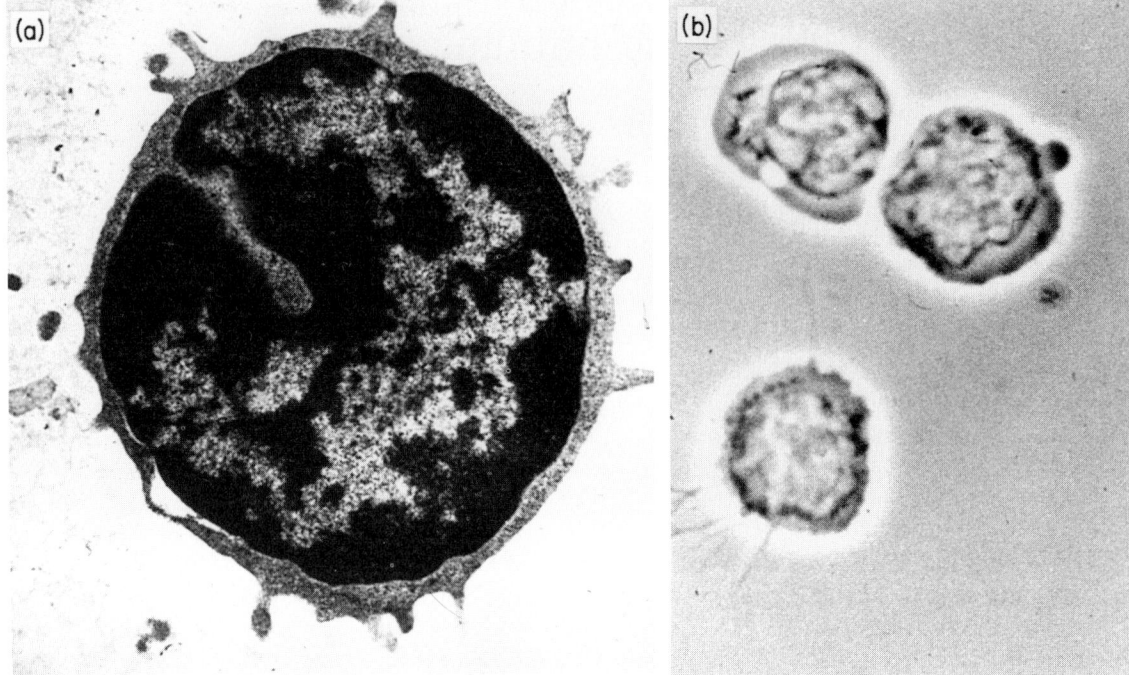

Fig. 1.1(a). Small lymphocyte from human blood. Electron micrograph showing areas of dense and light chromatin in the nucleus and no clearly visible organelles in the thin rim of cytoplasm. (b) Small lymphocytes from human blood observed under phase-contrast. Microprojectives are clearly seen on some cells.

have received the appropriate signal. When this is encountered the resting form of the cell changes into a large blast form with loose, light-staining chromatin, prominent nucleoli in the enlarged nucleus and a cytoplasm containing abundant polyribosomes, increased numbers of mitochondria and an enlarged active Golgi (Fig. 1.3). Most of the lymphocytes present in blood and lymph and peripheral lymphoid tissues are small and medium lymphocytes. Activated lymphocytes tend to migrate out of the circulation to sites of inflammation or remain sequestered at sites of antigen localization, although some activated lymphocytes are frequently found in the circulation during a vigorous immune response.

Lymphocytes are by nature migrating cells. When added to cultures of fibroblasts or epithelial cells, lymphocytes attach to their surface and crawl over them. Periods of attachment alternate with periods of free-swimming [1]. Lymphocyte motility is greatly increased by activation and in cultures of blood mononuclear cells containing a foreign antigen or a mitogenic lectin, blastogenic activation is associated

with clustering around macrophages [1]. Comparable cell-attachment phenomena occur in tissues *in vivo*, e.g. in the localized migration of lymphocytes along the enterocytes of the villi of gut surfaces and in the way that lymphocytes squeeze between the heightened endothelial cells in the paracortex in migration from the blood into a lymph node (Fig. 1.4). It is indeed the curious preference of lymphocytes for this migratory route which is the basis for the characteristic recirculatory pathway of lymphocytes which is quite different from the route taken by monocytes or neutrophils.

Since lymphocytes attach to autologous as well as to foreign cells the attachment phenomenon is not solely immunological in nature but it is heightened in immunological reactions and is an essential component of them. This is particularly evident in the early stages of a response in the clustering of lymphocytes around interdigitating cells or macrophages in lymphoid tissues following the capture of antigen [2], but it is also a feature of the late effector stages, e.g. during the rejection of homografts. The

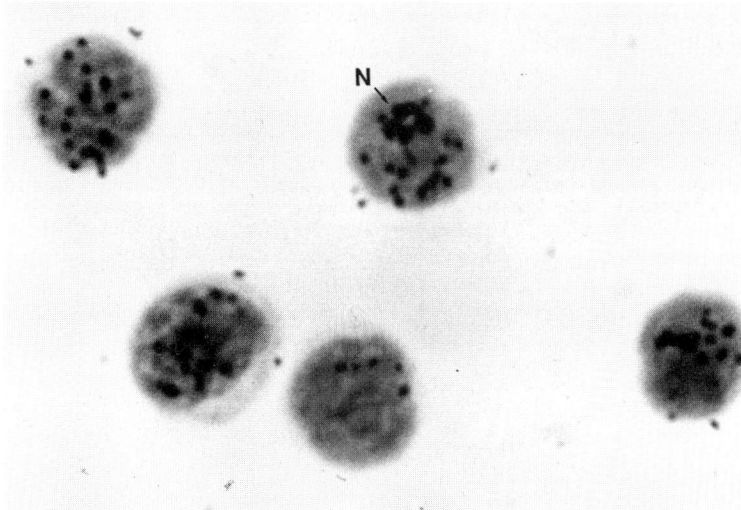

Fig. 1.2. Small lymphocytes from human blood. Autoradiograph after exposure of cells to ^{3}H-uridine for 2 h. All lymphocytes show labelled nuclear RNA but to a variable extent. N = cell showing nucleolar localization of label.

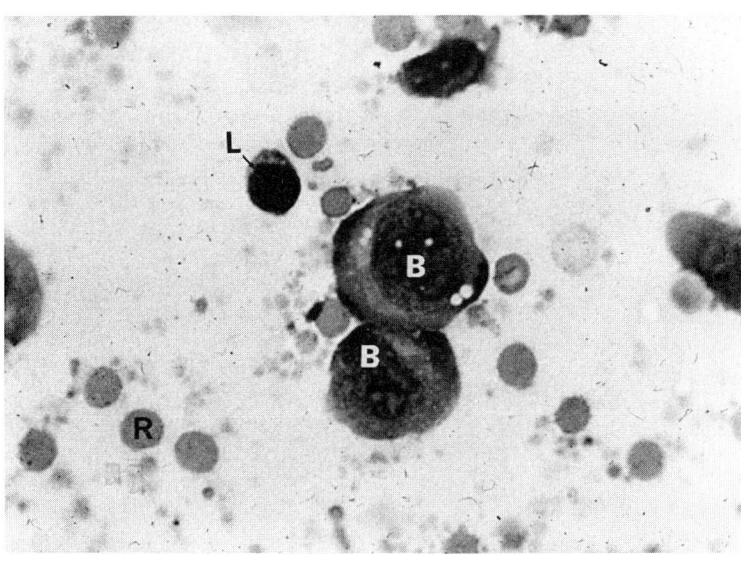

Fig. 1.3. Activated human lymphocytes from a 4-day culture of blood mononuclear cells with staphylococcal filtrate. B = blast cells; L = small lymphocyte; R = red cells.

cell–cell interactions may include direct transfer of proteins (e.g. lysosomal enzymes can be transferred from a lymphocyte to the cell to which it is attached).

Lymphocytes are functionally heterogeneous and consist of two main populations, T and B, which develop along distinct differentiation pathways and utilize different recognition and effector mechanisms. B lymphocytes bear surface immunoglobulin and are the direct precursors of antibody-secreting cells. T lymphocytes co-operate with B cells in antibody production and, more generally, regulate immune responses. Some T lymphocytes, when activated, can act as effector cells which are directly cytotoxic to virus-infected, aberrant or foreign cells. The generation of B lymphocytes takes place in the bone marrow whereas T lymphocytes are generated in the thymus from precursors arising from the division of stem cells which have migrated from the bone marrow to the thymus. These virgin T and B cells which have emerged from the primary tissue, and the progeny of T and B cells which have undergone a proliferative response to antigen constitute the population in the peripheral lymphoid

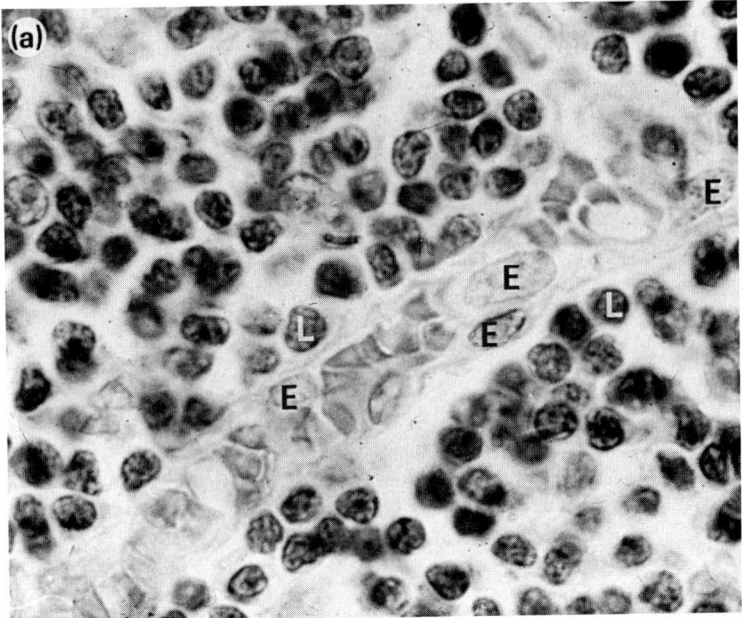

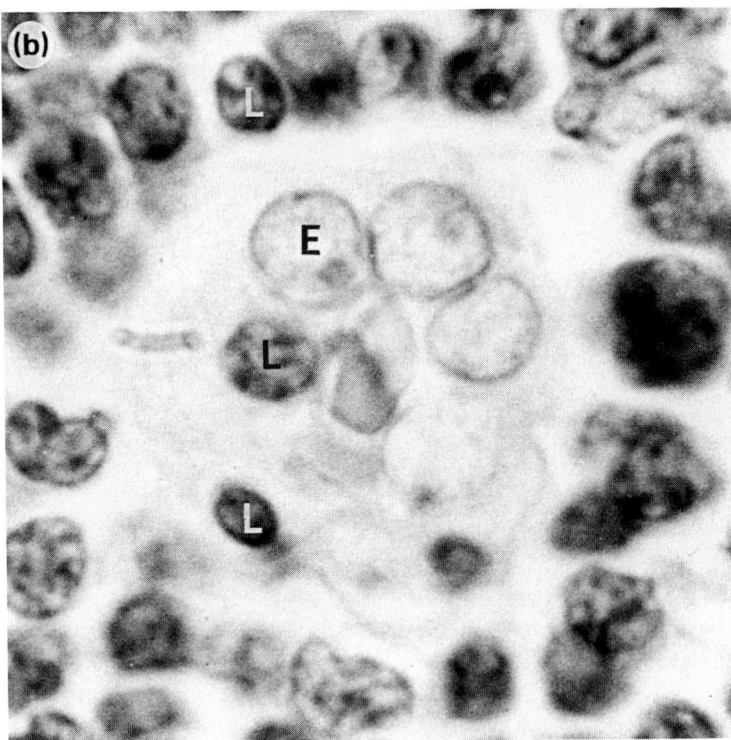

Fig. 1.4. Post-capillary venules, human lymph node. (a) longitudinal section; (b) transverse section. L = lymphocyte; E = endothelial cell.

tissues. Recirculation of lymphocytes through these tissues via blood and lymph ensures an efficient interchange of antigen-reactive cells in the substantial peripheral lymphocyte pool.

T lymphocytes

About 80% of the lymphocytes in human blood and 60% of lymphocytes in peripheral lymphoid tissues are of T lineage. Most of these cells bear the mature T cell marker T3 (CD3). The T3 complex, which comprises four proteins (designated T3-γ, T3-δ, T3-ε and T3-ζ), is linked to the T cell antigen receptor (TCR) in a surface structure which is the site of signal transduction following encounter of the T cell with suitably presented antigen [3]. In most CD3$^+$ T cells the TCR consists of disulphide-linked α and β chains (TCR2) which have variable and constant domains encoded in different gene segments joined through rearrangements during T-cell ontogeny in the thymus. However, when marker tests were performed with a monoclonal antibody to a non-polymorphic determinant on the α/β chains it was found that a small part of the CD3$^+$ population lacked α/β. This population (1–2% of the T cells) has a different TCR (TCR1) in which two different chains (γ and δ) are linked to CD3 complex. This population is detectable with a monoclonal antibody to a non-polymorphic determinant on the γ chain [4]. The antigen recognition repertoires of the two populations is extensive but in the α/β population is primarily dependent on V-region segments whereas with the γ/δ population junctional diversity plays a major part in generating diversity [5]. The proportions of TCR1$^+$ and TCR2$^+$ cells are approximately the same in blood, thymus medulla and peripheral lymphoid tissues, i.e. there is no tissue tropism [5].

Most peripheral T cells bear either the T4 (CD4) or T8 (CD8) antigen, although there are a few double negatives and double positives. Cells bearing CD4 are concerned with activation of B cells and macrophages and recognize antigen in association with the major histocompatibility complex (MHC) class II molecules, whereas cells bearing CD8 recognize antigen in association with MHC class I molecules. Cells within the CD4$^+$CD3$^+$ population will provide help for specific antibody responses but it is now known that this is not true of all CD4$^+$CD3$^+$

cells [6–9]. Studies with cloned CD4$^+$ cells have shown that some clones will provide help for specific antibody production, whereas others have a different role. In the mouse a functional distinction has been made between T4 helper cells and T4 inflammatory cells. The T4 inflammatory cells have cytotoxic and suppressive activity and are involved in delayed hypersensitivity reactions [6–9]. Although it is clear that there are CD4$^+$ subsets in mouse and human, there is no clear parallel between the subsets demonstrated in the two species. In the mouse two subsets called T_H1 and T_H2 both express only the 170/190 kDa isoform of the leucocyte common antigen (LCA). Whereas T_H1 cells produce interleukin 2 (IL-2), lymphotoxin and γ-interferon, the T_H2 subset produces IL-4 [6–9]. In humans one CD4$^+$ subset expresses a 200–220 kDa form of the LCA and the other a 150/190 kDa isoform. Both subsets produce IL-2 and γ-interferon.

Helper T cells are thought to have evolved primarily as a component of antibody-based surveillance mechanisms against extracellular pathogens, whereas T4 cells associated with inflammatory and hypersensitivity reactions are concerned with defence against intracellular pathogens, particularly those that reside in vesicles inside macrophages, such as mycobacteria. One role of the T cells at these sites might be to induce a suicidal response of the infected cell, thereby producing a lethal intracellular environment for a period prior to the apoptic death of the host cell and providing maximal opportunity for killing of the intracellular organism before its release.

A different T cell population, composed of CD3$^+$CD8$^+$ cells (T8 population) is thought to have evolved principally to combat virus-infected cells by a direct cell–cell cytotoxic mechanism. CD8$^+$ T cells also have the capacity to act as suppressor cells [3]. Compared with T4, the T8 antigen is better represented on TCR1 cells, although most TCR1 cells are negative for both T4 and T8 antigens [5].

The first clear stage in the differentiation of T-lineage cells is the arrival of a stem cell in the thymus via the blood, although there is evidence that the immigrant cells have already undergone some division and differentiation before migration to the thymus. The cells which contain terminal deoxynucleotidyl transferase (TdT) and express MHC class II antigen and a T-cell marker have been classified as prothymocytes [10]. Lineage commitment of progenitor cells is not, however, absolute but is a progressive and sequential process [11]. Within the thymus the earliest pro-T cell is CD4⁻CD8⁻ but expresses a 40 kDa molecule (CD7) which is also found on T-lineage acute lymphocytic leukaemia cells [12]. Although surface CD3 is found only on mature T cells, cytoplasmic CD3 γ chain appears very early, preceding the CD2 (T11) antigen [12]. The CD7 antigen is also present on multipotent stem-cell leukaemias and on immature TdT⁺ acute myelogenous leukaemia cells but is otherwise T-lineage-specific [13]. Considerable mitotic activity occurs in the cortex of thymic lobules, which histologically are seen to be populated almost exclusively by small and medium lymphocytes and fewer lymphoblasts (Figs 1.5 & 1.6). Cortical thymocytes have long been known to lack immunobiological activity and we now know that this is due to lack of surface structures found on mature T cells (such as the T3–TCR complex).

A diagram of the phenotypic changes accompanying maturation is shown in Fig. 1.7. Dual positive (CD4⁺CD8⁺) cells which arise in the thymic cortex from CD4⁻CD8⁻ precursors produce a TCR and give rise to separate CD4⁺ or CD8⁺ cells which are exported. The epithelial cells, fibroblasts, dendritic cells and macrophages of the thymus provide a micro-environment essential for differentiation to occur. Stem cells from mouse foetal liver are able to proliferate in culture but rearrangement of V regions of TCR genes and expression of a functional TCR will only occur if the stem cells are explanted into a thymic rudiment [14]. Part of the considerable death rate of cortical thymocytes is probably due to some cells failing to rearrange TCR genes effectively but there is also evidence that some clonal abortion of cells recognizing self MHC antigens (and possibly self antigens from other tissues brought into the thymus on dendritic cells) occurs. The relatively small numbers of thymocytes in the thymic medulla are phenotypically and functionally similar to peripheral T lymphocytes. It does not follow that they are finished cells on the way out to the periphery; some medullary thymocytes (in the mouse) remain resident in the thymus for long periods [15].

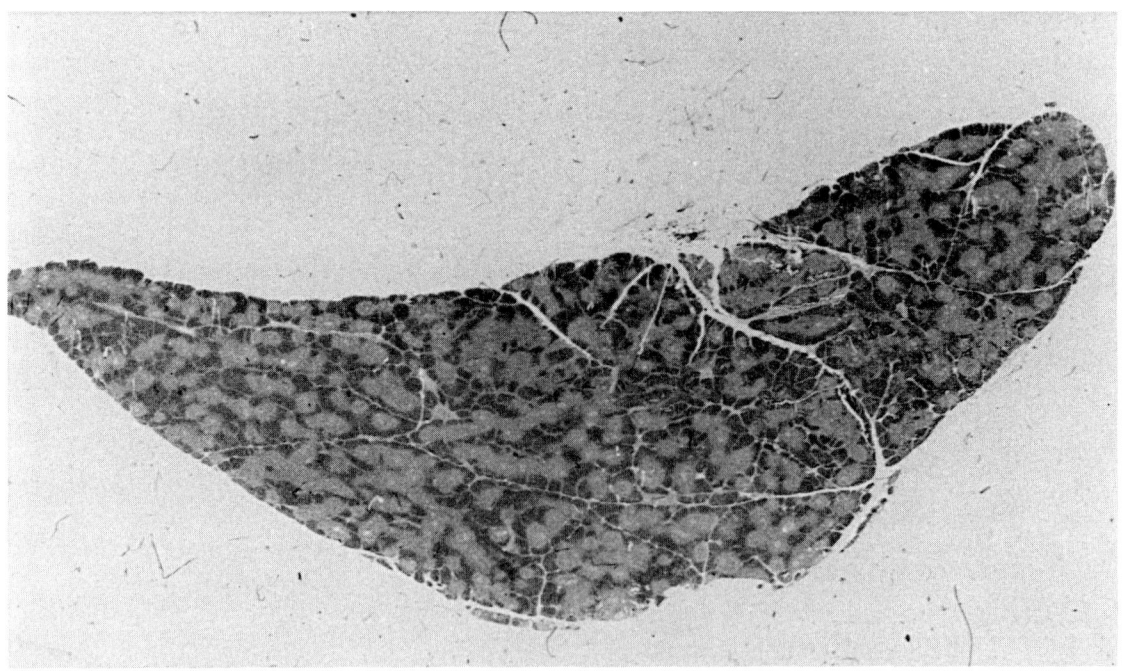

Fig. 1.5. Lobe of human thymus. Cortical areas of lobules are darkly stained; medullary areas are lightly stained.

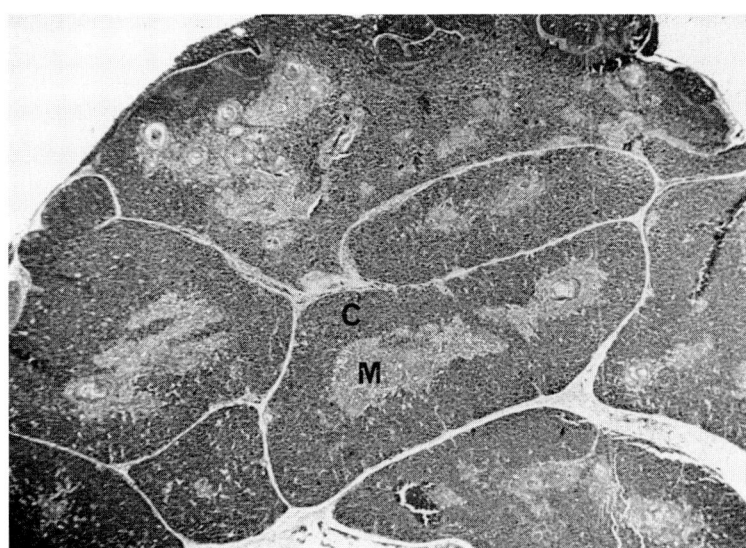

Fig. 1.6. Guinea pig thymus. C = cortex; M = medulla.

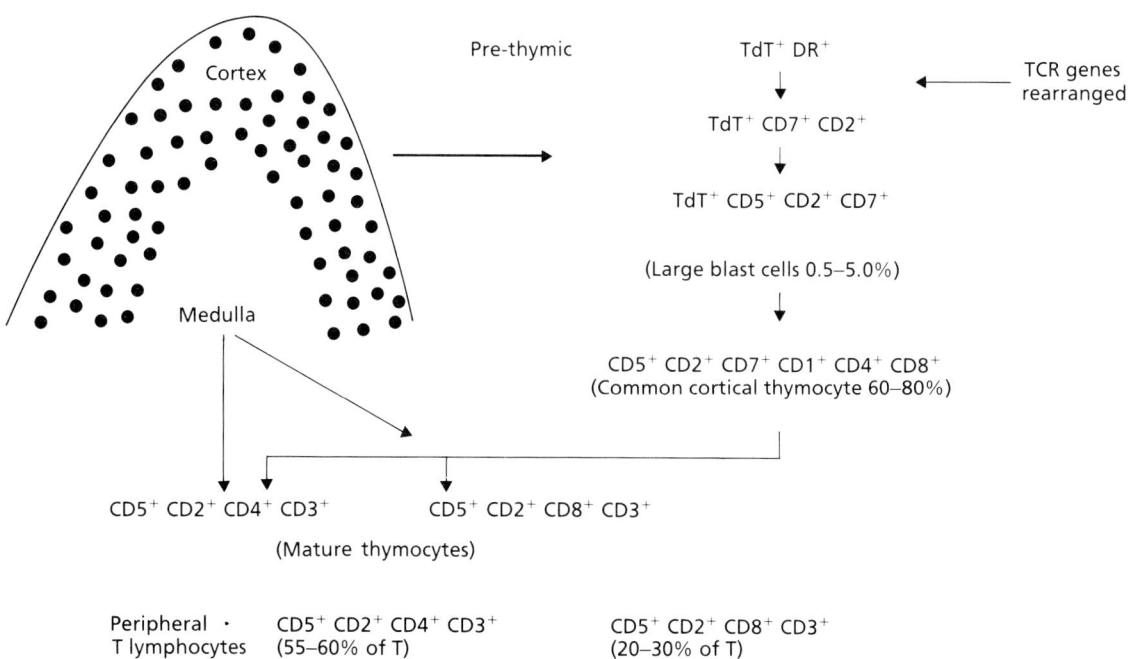

Fig. 1.7. Some common human T-cell differentiation markers. TdT is an intracellular marker; all other markers shown are detected as surface antigens. The CD3 marker is not found on the surface until the complete 20–25 kDa glycoprotein is formed, although mRNA for CD3 δ and ε chains is present from a very early stage. CD7 is the Fcμ receptor. CD2 = T11; CD5 = T1; CD1 = T6.

B lymphocytes

B lymphocytes in peripheral lymphoid tissues recognize antigens by their surface immunoglobulin and the resultant cell activation and cell–cell interactions constitute the initial stages of an antibody response. The cells secreting the antibody found in the serum during immune responses are generated by antigen-driven clonal expansion and differentiation of the appropriate B cells. The stageposts of the B-series differentiation pathway are the stem cell, the B cell and the plasma cell. The stem cell to B cell stage takes place in the primary tissue, is antigen-independent and the developing cells are not competent to respond to antigen until the B-cell stage is reached. The stages from the B cell to antibody-secreting cell take place in peripheral lymphoid tissues.

The primary compartment in which new B cells are produced from stem cells is the bone marrow and it is during this stage that recognition diversity is principally generated. The first phenotypic change accompanying differentiation of stem-cell progeny along the B pathway is the appearance of a characteristic B-lineage glycoprotein (CD19) on the surface. Subtle, but as yet unidentified, signals produced by stromal and possibly some of the haemopoietic cells themselves in the bone marrow environment induce rearrangements of heavy chain and subsequently κ and λ light chain V-region genes. The first immunoglobulin molecule detectable is free μ chain in the cytoplasm and pre-B cells were originally defined as sIg$^-$, cyto μ^+ cells. Once light chain is also produced, whole immunoglobulin M (IgM) is detectable on the cell surface; the appearance of surface IgD soon follows and most B cells leaving the marrow for peripheral tissues express both IgM and IgD of identical specificity. Only about 5–10% of the lymphocytes in human blood are B cells. Most of these B cells express IgM and IgD but some cells bearing IgG and IgA are also found. In adult blood only a single isotype is detectable, whereas IgG- or IgA-expressing cells in foetal spleen also express IgM or IgM and IgD. The role of sIgD is still unknown; it is not essential for activation or isotype-switching. There are species variations in the proportion of T and B lymphocytes in blood and in the properties of B cells. About half of the lympho-cytes in rabbit blood are B cells and rabbit lympho-cytes are much more easily triggered into DNA synthesis by anti-immunoglobulin.

Most newly formed B cells reach the peripheral tissues where their survival depends on activation by encounter with antigen. This is most likely to occur at sites where antigen-capturing cells such as dendritic cells have removed antigen from blood or lymph and retained it on their surface. Since both B and T cells, during recirculation, pass from blood into lymphatic tissue near sites where dendritic cells are numerous there is opportunity for B cells bearing surface antibody directed against one of the epitopes on the antigen to become selectively removed from the circulation and attracted to the antigen presented to it. B cells recirculate through the peripheral lymphoid tissues in a similar manner to that described for T cells but they do so more slowly and migrate to particular B-cell areas [16]. After entry into a node by migrating through the high endothelium of venules in the paracortical region, B cells migrate to follicles and remain there for varying periods of time before leaving the node via efferent lymphatics. Newly formed B cells do not readily gain access to follicles [17]. There is a massive production of new B cells daily (approximately 10^8 day^{-1} in the mouse, which is equivalent to about one-fifth of the total peripheral B-cell pool). Clearly most of the cells will die, otherwise there would be a progressive increase in peripheral B-cell numbers. The rate of B lymphopoiesis may increase slightly after immunization but not in an antigen-specific manner, i.e. there is no feedback to the primary compartment. The existence of non-specific stimulating effects from immunization is also apparent from the fact that mice reared under germ-free conditions show reduced numbers of peripheral B cells. Production of polyspecific B-cell stimulants, such as endotoxins, by gut bacteria could partly account for this phenomenon. Newly formed B cells have to overcome a syngeneic barrier before they penetrate into the established circulating pool [17]. If the pool is drained off or depleted by cell destruction this has the effect of creating more 'B space' and a high proportion of newly formed B cells become long-lived virgin B cells, whereas few unstimulated new B cells normally survive. Another form of regulation must occur after antigen stimulation since the size of peripheral B-cell clones is tightly regulated and does not expand to fill a depleted B-cell pool [17].

As far as B cells are concerned the first phase of the immune response occurs when antigen is encountered on the surface of interdigitating cells in extrafollicular areas of secondary lymphoid tissues. Both newly formed and established B cells have the opportunity of responding to the antigen concerned. Antibody-secreting cells and memory B cells will arise from activated virgin and established B cells [17]. In a second phase which takes place after antibody has formed (i.e. late primary or secondary response) antigen is bound in the form of immune complexes which are taken up by and held on the surface of follicular dendritic cells (FDCs). During the long periods of antigen display on FDC there is a drive towards dominance of clones producing higher-affinity antibody through hypermutation mechanisms acting on immunoglobulin V-region genes and subsequent selection [18].

Most antigens are proteins or compounds complexed with protein. B cells responding to these so-called thymus-dependent antigens do so in co-operation with T cells which recognize epitopes on the protein. The mitotically activated B cells typically generate subclones, each making antibody of one of the immunoglobulin classes. Thus the various progeny of a single activated B cell may make antibody of IgG, IgA, IgM, IgD and IgE classes. Although numerous soluble factors are involved a full response to thymus-dependent protein antigen requires direct cell–cell interaction of antigen-presenting cell, B cell and T helper cell. A different population of B cells responds to so-called thymus-independent antigens (TI-1 and TI-2) without involvement of T cells with a predominant IgM response (in humans mainly IgM and IgG2; in mice IgM > IgG3 > IgG1 > IgG2b < IgG2a). Macrophages and dendritic cells capable of presenting TI carbohydrate antigens of bacterial origin in rats are found in marginal zones of spleen and in parts of the subcapsular sinuses of lymph nodes. These are sites of activation of TI B cells. The $\mu^+\delta^-$ cells in marginal zones responding to TI antigens remain in this zone and show little tendency to migrate [17].

As well as bearing structures enabling them to respond to antigen and growth factors such as IL-2, peripheral B cells bear receptors for Fc of IgG, IgM, IgA and IgE and complement (CR1 and CR2) and thus are able to bind immune complexes other than via antigen (Fig. 1.8). The functional role of these receptors on the B cell is not fully understood. Attachment of antibody to IgGFc receptors has a suppressive action on the B cell [19]. The chief function of the receptors, however, appears to be the transport of immune complexes. One site to which transport may occur has been shown to be the germinal centre where the complexes are unloaded on to FDC [20, 21]. Twenty-four hours after injection of colloidal gold particles, particles were found

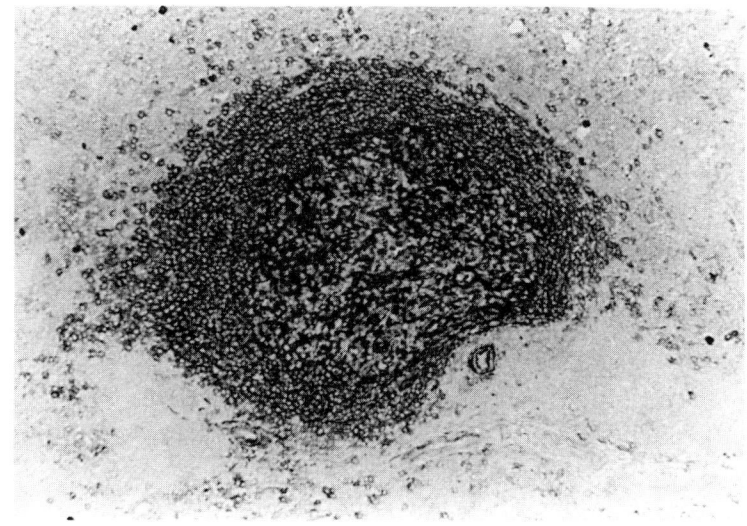

Fig. 1.8. Human spleen stained with a CD21 monoclonal antibody by indirect immunoperoxidase. This antibody recognizes the receptor for C3*d* (CR2) and EBV. The characteristic strong staining of follicular dendritic cells in the germinal centre is clearly seen. B lymphocytes in the follicular mantle and in the marginal zone outside it are also stained. Reproduced with permission from Ling NR *et al.* B-cell antigens: new and previously defined clusters. In: McMichael AJ, ed. *Leucocyte Typing III.* Oxford: Oxford University Press, 1987: 302–35.

on cytoplasmic extensions of FDC and *in vitro* experiments confirmed that immune complexes could be transferred from B cells to FDC [21].

The stages between the B cell and the plasma cell are complex (Fig. 1.9 & 1.10). The clonal expansion of antigen-responding B cells during a primary response gives rise to memory cells and (if the stimulus is adequate) to differentiation of a portion of the activated B cells to plasma cells [22]. In the late stages of a vigorous primary response and in secondary and tertiary responses structures called germinal centres appear and are the site of important changes in activated B cells. Unstimulated recirculating B lymphocytes gather into collections of cells in the cortex of a lymph node; these areas are called *primary* follicles. In nodes subjected to ongoing stimulation by antigens (e.g. during hyperimmunization or from persistent antigen entry from a mucosal surface as in the case of mesenteric nodes) *secondary*

follicles are also seen. Secondary follicles consist of a pale (germinal) centre surrounded by a mantle of small B lymphocytes. Most of the lymphoblasts within the centre are of B lineage but have cleaved nuclei and multiple nucleoli and are morphologically different from B lymphoblasts. They are called centroblasts. They are a mitotically activated B population and are found in the dark zone of the germinal centre. Their progeny, centrocytes, are found in the light zone of the centre. Somatic mutation within genes coding for V regions of immunoglobulin chains occurs at a high rate in centroblasts. Subsequent intimate contact with antigen (Ag), present in the form of immune complexes on the surface of FDCs within the centre, results in preferential activation and survival of those mutated B cells expressing antibody with the highest affinity for antigen. The germinal centre is also the site where isotype-switching occurs. The features of the

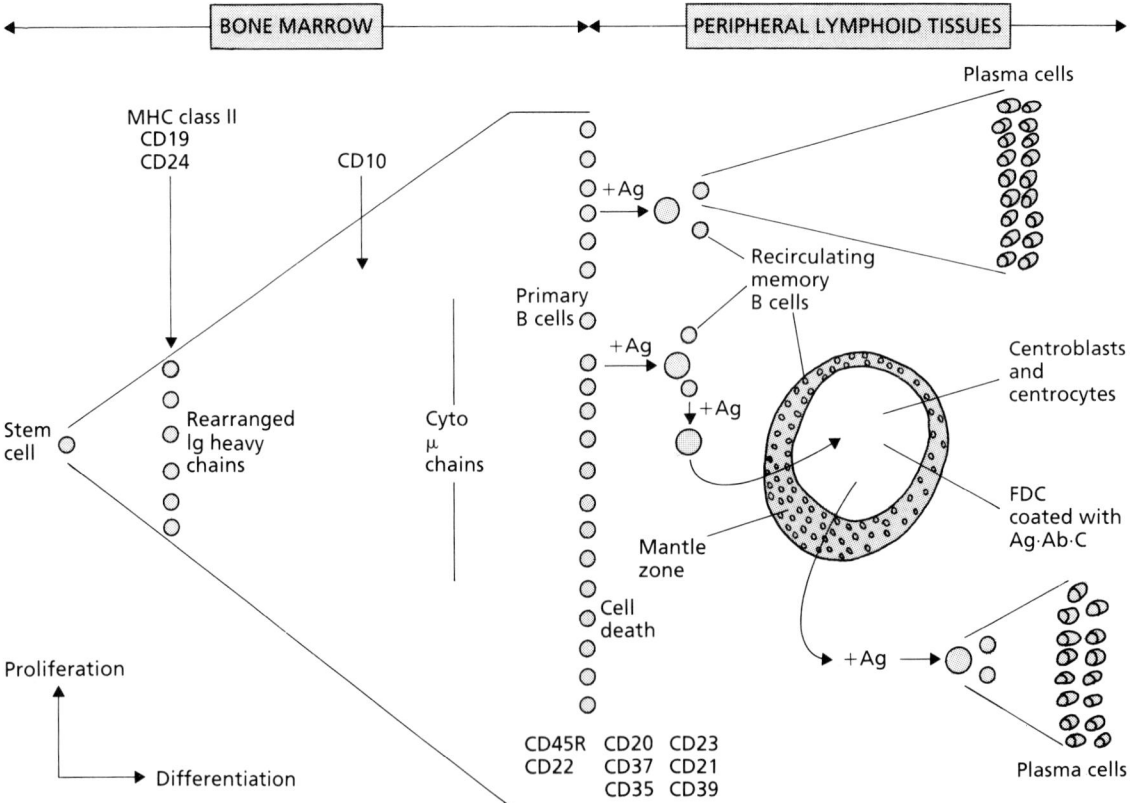

Fig. 1.9. Stages of B-cell differentiation. The antigens found on human B-lineage cells at the various stages are identified by CD number. For further details see [22].

micro-environment in the germinal centre which confer these changes on the sequestered B cells are not understood but it is known that FDCs, T cells and macrophages all contribute. Surviving centrocytes leave the germinal centre and after a further encounter with antigen outside the follicles complete their differentiation to plasma cells. The relative contributions of primary and memory B cells in an immune response to a T-dependent antigen have been studied in rats [17]. Primary B cells are recruited only in the first few days following immunization, after which the response is sustained by long-lived cells belonging to memory clones.

Plasma cells have lost most identifiable B-series antigens; this is to be expected as their limited specialized role as sessile antibody-secreting cells does not require the capacity to bind to Fc or complement components or to respond to growth and differentiation factors operative in clonal expansion. Myeloma cells and probably some normal immunoglobulin-secreting cells do respond to B-cell stimulatory factor (BSF-2/IL-6) [23] (discussed in Chapter 2). Plasma cells are found in medullary cords of lymph nodes, in the red pulp of spleen near to the marginal zone, beneath mucous surfaces and in nasopharyngeal lymphoid tissue. They are also found in large numbers in the bone marrow, so that this tissue contains cells at the end of B differentiation as well as the pre-antigen stages. Plasma cells in the medullary cords and splenic red pulp become labelled when ^{3}H-thymidine is injected into rats whereas bone marrow plasma cells are true end cells [17]. Plasma cells in the bone marrow typically produce IgG (all subclasses, but one plasma cell produces only one subclass) or IgA monomer, whereas the cells found in the lamina propria of the gut secrete dimeric IgA which is converted to secretory IgA when secretory component (produced by epithelia) is picked up on passage of the antibody through the mucosal surface or from the liver or gall bladder on transport through the internal lymphatic route. IgM producers are common in the spleen whereas IgD producers, although generally rare, are relatively common in the tonsil. Thus, at the final secretory stage of differentiation, or shortly before it, B-lineage cells home to characteristic sites which are different to those where B or T lymphocytes migrate. Some immunoglobulin-secreting cells, while resembling plasma cells in possessing the highly developed rough endoplasmic reticulum typical of protein-secreting cells, are morphologically closer to lymphocytes when examined under the light microscope and are called lymphoplasmacytoid cells. The main features of the B differentiation pathways are shown in Fig. 1.8.

Subpopulations of B cells (other than the thymus-independent B cells) have been identified, mainly on the basis of surface marker phenotype, but their relation to functional differences is unclear. There is currently much interest in CD5$^+$ cells. A small

Fig. 1.10. Human spleen stained for IgD by indirect immunoperoxidase. The B lymphocytes in the follicular mantle are the only cells clearly stained. The B cells within the germinal centre (G) and in the marginal zone (M) show little expression of IgD. Reproduced with permission from Ling NR *et al.* B-cell antigens: new and previously defined clusters. In: McMichael AJ, ed. *Leucocyte Typing III*. Oxford: Oxford University Press, 1987: 302–35.

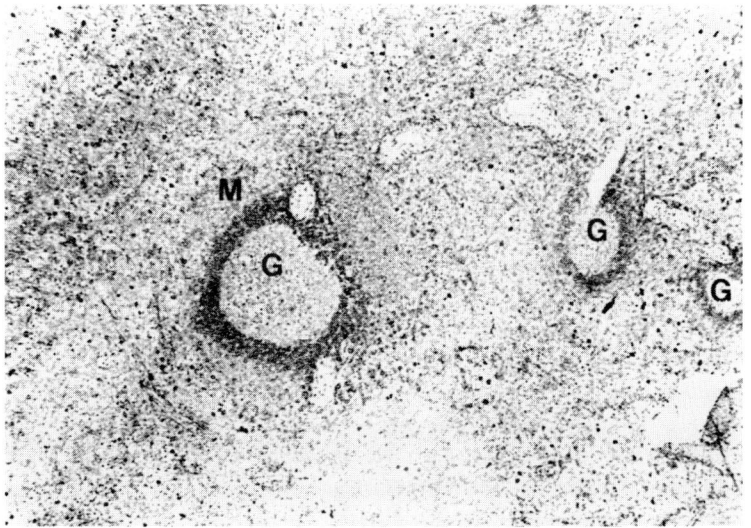

proportion of circulating B cells in the adult bear this antigen. Larger numbers are found in cord blood and the abnormal B lymphocytes found in the blood in chronic lymphocytic leukaemia frequently express the antigen strongly. CD5 is not detectable on newly formed B lymphocytes in the bone marrow, suggesting that it is not a marker of immaturity. It may identify a functionally distinct subpopulation but this has yet to be proven. A monocytoid B subpopulation has been described which is present at sites where there is immediate contact with antigen; these B cells show a high degree of epithelial tropism [24]. Cells previously described as immature histiocytes are now suspected as belonging to the B-cell series [25]. No normal equivalent of the distinctive malignant B cell responsible for hairy cell leukaemia has yet been identified.

Macrophages

Macrophages are defined as phagocytic mononuclear cells and are a very heterogeneous group of cells. They include the phagocytic cells scattered throughout connective tissue (histiocytes) and Kupffer's cells of the liver. Osteoclasts, the multinucleate giant cells which ingest effete bone, are now known to be closely related to macrophages. Bone marrow reconstitution experiments have shown that osteoclasts are derived from a marrow precursor via a blood-borne monocyte [26]. One of the two cell types of which synovial membranes are composed is of the macrophage family and similar cells are present in synovial fluid [27]. Within the central nervous system, the entire glial cell population is now thought to be made up of cells related to macrophages. In addition to microglial cells (phagocytic mononuclear cells probably derived from monocytes), the cells of the macroglial family (astrocytes, oligodendrocytes and ependymal cells), which provide a controlled metabolic environment for neurons, are also macrophage-related and respond to products of activated macrophages and T cells.

Macrophages are especially common in the spleen and bone marrow, in the lamina propria of both small and large intestine and in the alveolar walls of the lung. They tend to gather around vascular spaces and beneath epithelia. The mononuclear phagocytes in the blood (monocytes) are continuously generated from stem cells in the bone marrow at the rate of approximately 7×10^6 cells kg^{-1} h^{-1}. They remain circulating in the blood with a half-life of about 8–12 h before migrating into the tissues and there undergoing further differentiation to macrophages. The major source of macrophages is the haemopoietic tissue of the marrow [28] but tissue macrophages are also capable of proliferation when suitably stimulated. Some macrophages remain highly localized in a tissue with a long lifespan. They may be dispersed or in aggregates and in granulomatous inflammatory tissue may form multinucleate giant cells. Others may move to a different site. In some sites, such as the peritoneal cavity, and in the respiratory tract, they may remain free in suspension and are a common source of macrophages for *in vitro* experiments. Alveolar macrophages which have ingested particles may pass up the bronchial tree and be spat out. Likewise, particle-laden Kupffer's cells may enter the blood, reach the pulmonary capillaries and leave via the bronchial tree.

Macrophages lining the lymph channels may be visualized by their capacity to trap injected colloidal dyes or Indian ink. Locally injected dyes entering a lymph node via afferent lymphatics are extensively trapped in macrophages lining the medullary sinuses and the marginal (subcapsular) sinus with very little localization in the cortex. Other macrophages in sequestered sites not in the main stream of lymph flowing through lymphatic tissue (such as the macrophages in germinal centres) are also not labelled. Even within a single region of a lymphoid tissue there are phenotypic differences between macrophages at different sites. In Peyer's patches the large, acid phosphatase-positive macrophages in germinal centres are phenotypically distinguishable from macrophages in the lamina propria [29].

The role of opsonization in enhancing the removal of particulate antigens has long been a matter of argument. Even in the total absence of natural antibody some degree of fixation of complement on the surface via the alternative pathway is likely to occur. There is no doubt that both the nature of the antigen and the level of opsonization influence the site of localization of antigen. Macrophages within the blood sinusoids of the marginal zone in the spleen avidly take up large polysaccharides such as hydroxyethyl starch or polysucrose, a property not shown by red pulp macrophages or FDCs or inter-digitating cells [17]. The initial fate of an antigen is influenced more by its physical state than by its immunogenicity. Plastic and silica or carbon particles are as rapidly removed as foreign cells.

Collectively, macrophages recognize a great range of antigens, not only those of external origin. Their surveillance role includes the removal of effete red cells through glycolipid and phospholipid recognition systems. Macrophages have effector functions other than those dependent on phagocytosis; they also have trophic and antigen-presenting functions.

Attachment of particles to the surface of monocytes and their ingestion are two distinct processes. Ingestion requires attachment over a large surface area and operates by a 'zipper' mechanism which is more readily triggered by engaging receptors for FcIgG than for complement components. The stages in the phagocytosis of a micro-organism are usually described as: (i) attachment; (ii) endocytosis; (iii) formation of phagosome in the cytoplasm; (iv) fusion of phagosome with a lysosome yielding a phagolysosome; (v) killing and digestion of the organism; and (vi) exoplasmosis of degradation products at the cell surface. The lysosomal hydrolases include phosphatases, sulphatase, esterases, lipase, phospholipases, glycosidases and proteases. An oxidative destructive mechanism also operates in addition to attack by the lysosomal enzymes. A respiratory burst triggered by the ingestion gives rise to increased uptake of oxygen and greatly enhances metabolism of glucose in the pentose cycle with generation of hydrogen peroxide and superoxide yielding hydroxyl radicals and singlet oxygen. These toxic oxidizing agents are passed into the phagolysosome where they exert their damaging effect [30, 31].

Changes associated with the differentiation of monocytes to macrophages *in vitro* include the following:

1 A morphological change from the rounded appearance of freshly attached monocytes to a population of spreadout cells which may be of spiky, triangular, round or spindle-shaped morphology.

2 Increase in *N*-acetylglucosaminidase content and increased release of the enzyme when the cells are subjected to a phagocytic stimulus.

3 A gradual disappearance of peroxidase-positive granules. *In vivo*, the monocyte to macrophage maturation takes place in quite different environments in different tissues. Environmental factors are sufficient to account for the extreme heterogeneity of macrophages in different locations, but some specific homing of monocyte subpopulations cannot be excluded [32].

Mature macrophages have secretory activity. Products secreted include enzymes such as collagenase, arginase, lysozyme (particularly from alveolar macrophages), a range of hydrolases, growth-regulating factors such as IL-1 and several important plasma proteins such as α_2-macroglobulin and complement components. Fibronectin, an important adhesion molecule which sticks to denatured collagen, is also secreted. Macrophages from different sites show considerable differences in secretion patterns and in numbers of organelles such as mitochondria and lysosomes. They also show differences in energy source. Alveolar macrophages and monocytes depend mainly on aerobic pathways whereas peritoneal macrophages rely on glycolysis [33].

Macrophages which are maximally functional in any assay (anti-microbial, tumoricidal or antigen-presenting assays) are referred to as activated macrophages. Activated macrophages spread more extensively on glass or plastic and have a higher density of Fc receptors. Macrophages which have been activated by the products of an antigen-specific lymphocyte activation are non-specifically more effective in ingesting and killing a wide range of bacteria.

Although a large number of agents (tumour necrosis factor, interleukins, etc.) are thought to have some macrophage-activating effect, two of the most potent agents which have been thoroughly studied are γ-interferon and lipopolysaccharide (LPS). Gamma-interferon is regarded as a priming signal leading to increased expression of MHC class II (important in antigen presentation), the high-affinity IgGFc receptor (FcγR1) and the adhesion molecule, LFA-1 (Table 1.1). Expression of the transferrin receptor (a marker strongly expressed on proliferating cells) is reduced. LPS provides a different kind of stimulus and functions as a second signal which pushes macrophages to a fully activated stage with secretion of neutral proteases and lysosomal hydrolases. As described earlier, activation, even when induced by immunospecific activation of lympho-

Table 1.1 Leucocyte integrin family*

Name of antigen	Name and size (kDa) of chains		Cells expressing	Binding substance
	α	β		
LFA-1	190 (CD11a)	95 (CD18)	All leucocytes	ICAM-1 (CD54)
Mac-1 (CR3)	165 (CD116)	95 (CD18)	Monocytes, macrophages, granulocytes, NK cells	C3bi
p150/95 (CR4)	150 (CD11c)	95 (CD18)	Monocytes, macrophages, granulocytes	C3bi

*Sometimes called the LFA family or the CD11/CD18 family.

cytes, causes macrophages to exhibit a broad-ranging enhancement of effector activity but not to an equivalent effect on all micro-organisms. Activation increases the ability of macrophages to kill ingested *Toxoplasma* or *Listeria* micro-organisms but does not increase their capacity to destroy staphylococci [31].

Lymphoid dendritic cells

As the name implies, these are cells of dendritic morphology found in lymphoid tissue. They belong to a family of irregularly shaped cells with active processes or dendrites, sometimes taking the form of bulbous pseudopods or 'veils'. The nucleus is usually irregular in shape and the cytoplasm contains mitochondria, a well developed smooth endoplasmic reticulum but little rough endoplasmic reticulum [34]. Dendritic or interdigitating cells are found in T areas of spleen, lymph nodes, Peyer's patches and in the medullary region of the thymus; 'veiled' cells are found in peripheral lymph and drift into nodes via the afferent lymphatics but are virtually absent from efferent and central lymph. Langerhans cells, which also belong to the dendritic family [2], are found in the epidermis of skin and stratified epithelia of other surfaces such as tonsil. In addition, there are dendritic cells in the interstitial tissues of non-lymphoid organs.

All these cell types have properties in common which distinguish them from macrophages and FDCs. They have low buoyant density and are poorly endocytic. They are not phagocytic, have weak pinocytotic activity and few lysosomes or endocytic vesicles. They stain weakly, if at all, for acid phosphatase, peroxidase, non-specific esterase and adenosine triphosphatase. They do not proliferate in culture, do not express Fc receptors, but express MHC class I and II antigens (very strongly) (Fig. 1.11). They do not produce IL-1.

In *in vitro* cultures veiled cells are non-phagocytic, do not adhere readily to glass or plastic and are potent antigen-presenting cells and stimulator cells in mixed lymphocyte reaction [35,36]. Similar cells studied *in vivo* in sheep do apparently show some phagocytic activity [37], but as far as function is concerned, the essential point is that substantial amounts of antigen are retained on the cell surface.

Bone marrow origin of dendritic cells and their relation to macrophages. Surface markers

Dendritic cells isolated from human tonsil cell suspensions depleted of T and B cells and monocytes do not express CD3, CD20, CD24 or macrophage antigens but stain strongly for MHC class II antigens [2]. The cells are large (15–20 μm) and show

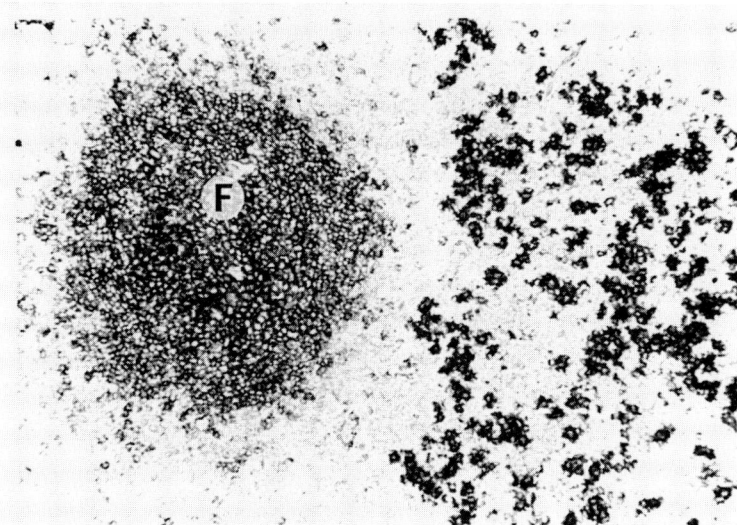

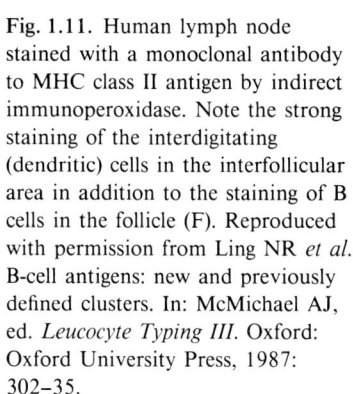

Fig. 1.11. Human lymph node stained with a monoclonal antibody to MHC class II antigen by indirect immunoperoxidase. Note the strong staining of the interdigitating (dendritic) cells in the interfollicular area in addition to the staining of B cells in the follicle (F). Reproduced with permission from Ling NR *et al.* B-cell antigens: new and previously defined clusters. In: McMichael AJ, ed. *Leucocyte Typing III.* Oxford: Oxford University Press, 1987: 302–35.

dendritic processes. Under the electron microscope numerous mitochondria, free ribosomes, little rough endoplasmic reticulum and a large Golgi apparatus could be seen. Lysosomes and peroxidase are absent and the cells are not phagocytic. The cells express the LCA (CD45) but lack IgGFc and complement receptors, transferrin receptor and natural killer (NK) markers. Thus they are quite distinct from lymphocytes and macrophages. Blood dendritic cells are also phenotypically distinguishable from monocytes [35]. Data from recent leucocyte workshops have also indicated that dendritic cells share few antigens with monocytes or macrophages [38]. Langerhans cells from tonsillar epithelium share only the leucocyte integrin antigen CD11c and some unclassified macrophage antigens (Table 1.1). On epidermal Langerhans cells no macrophage antigens are detectable. Strangely, Langerhans cells express CD1 (T6), an antigen which in the T-cell series is found only on thymocytes. Osteoclasts, which are now acknowledged as members of the macrophage family, share CD13 and some other antigens with macrophages [38]. Like macrophages and osteoclasts, dendritic cells express CD45, confirming their origin from bone marrow leucocytes, in contrast to FDCs which do not express this antigen. The blood-borne precursor of tissue dendritic cells is thought to be a monocyte but if this is true they must have undergone substantial phenotypic alteration at the terminal stage.

The three types of Fcγ receptor (namely FcγRI, FcγRII and FcγRIII) are all present on the monocyte/macrophage series. These receptors have now been defined antigenically with monoclonal antibodies as well as functionally. FcγRI is the only FcγR which binds IgG monomer with high affinity. It is present on monocytes, macrophages and activated neutrophils. FcγRII (CD32) is a 40 kDa glycoprotein with very low affinity for IgG monomer, but which binds immune complexes and opsonized particles. It is present on monocytes, macrophages, eosinophils, neutrophils, platelets and B cells. Another low-affinity receptor, FcγRIII (CD16) is a 55–70 kDa glycoprotein present on neutrophils and macrophages but virtually absent from monocytes and eosinophils. It is the only Fc receptor on killer (K) and NK cells.

Follicular dendritic cells

An alternative name for FDCs is dendritic reticulum cells (DRCs). They have been recognized since the time of Maximow as non-phagocytic cells with long processes found in lymphoid tissue. FDCs are found only in B-cell follicles in peripheral lymphoid tissues. In the germinal centres of secondary follicles their cytoplasmic processes form a dense network with processes extending into the mantle zone. FDCs bind antigen–antibody–complement complexes very strongly and retain them on their surface for long periods, thereby presenting antigens to lymphocytes (mainly B lymphocytes) sequestered within the centre. The origin of FDCs and their relation to other cell types is unknown, but there is evidence from mouse reconstitution experiments that they are not derived from bone marrow precursors [39]. FDCs are readily seen in tissue sections stained with antibodies to complement, IgM or IgG or with FDC-specific monoclonal antibodies [40]. In the electron microscope desmosome-like junctions have been seen. A curious feature of FDCs is that they share many surface antigens with leucocytes, especially B cells, even though they are not of bone marrow origin. There is an obvious possibility that FDC may take up soluble forms of antigens shed by B cells, or that they may acquire them directly from the B-cell surface during intimate cell–cell contact. The likelihood that intimate FDC–B cell interactions occur follows from the recent confirmation that immune complexes taken up by B cells at extrafollicular sites are actively transported into the germinal centre where they are transferred to FDC [21].

Recently, studies on isolated FDCs have been performed to distinguish intrinsic from acquired surface antigens [41, 42]. The FDCs were obtained from washed tonsil dispersions incubated with collagenase or collagenase plus a protease, which would be likely to remove most of the passively bound protein. The isolated cultured FDCs remained positive for CD19, CD21 (CR2, C3dR, EBVR), CD35 (C3bR, CR1) and CD23. Thus, it is possible that these antigens, normally found only on cells of haemopoietic origin, are actively produced by FDC. As yet the question is an open one. The active transfer of complex-bound antigen to FDCs in the interior of germinal centres is also a curious and unexplained phenomenon but is compatible with the recent finding that in the short term, antigen is localized at extrafollicular sites and does not reach germinal centre sites until antibody is generated and complexes formed [17].

Antigen recognition by lymphocytes and the antigen-presenting role of macrophages and dendritic cells

In immune responses T and B lymphocytes respond to antigen on an accessory cell rather than to free antigen. The presented antigen may be unmodified but attached to the surface of a dendritic cell or an immune complex on a follicular dendritic cell, or it may be a peptide fragment of a protein antigen produced by ingestion and partial digestion in a macrophage with subsequent presentation of the processed antigen on the surface in conjunction with an MHC antigen. What B cells recognize in an immune response can be assessed by examining the fine specificity of the antibodies appearing in the serum during the response, since these antibodies have been produced by clones derived from the antigen-activated B cells. The capacity of virgin or memory B cells to bind a radioactively labelled antigen or antigen fragment can also be tested. T cells do not bind free antigen and need secondary bonds involving T4, T8, MHC antigens and leucocyte adhesion molecules to achieve firm and sustained attachment to the antigen-presenting cell. The antigen-induced proliferation of T cells during the response generates antigen-specific memory T cells. Accordingly the specificity of T-cell responses (and the presence of T memory cells in blood and lymphoid tissues at various times after antigen priming) may be tested by measuring DNA synthesis induced by culture with antigen *in vitro* in cultures containing adequate numbers of accessory cells. Tests of this kind indicate that immune serum contains antibodies which bind to whole antigen in preference to antigen fragments. Antibodies to conformational determinants are present, indicating that unmodified antigen is recognized [43]. T cells appear to respond to peptide fragments but also recognize unmodified antigen, including conformational determinants. The *in vitro* tests also indicate that antigen-specific T cells persist for a very long time and account for T-cell memory. Tests based on polyclonal stimulation of peripheral T plus B lymphocytes and measurement of antibody produced after 7 days of culture have shown that B memory cells may also persist for long periods. With both T and B populations memory is affected by antigen persistence (e.g. a latent infection in the case of a virus) and the location of the memory cells is affected by the site of antigen retention.

Many cell types other than macrophages, dendritic cells and B cells are able to present antigen effectively. This is correlated with the appearance of MHC class II antigen on the surface which may occur with epithelial cells as a result of stimulation by γ-interferon; T cells also express class II strongly after activation by antigen or a lectin.

K, NK and NK-like cytotoxic cells

K cells are cells of lymphocyte morphology from non-immunized donors which are able to lyse suitable target cells which have been sensitized with a minute amount of IgG antibody [28,33]. This is called an antibody-dependent cellular cytotoxicity (ADCC) reaction. Cell attachment occurs via low-affinity Fc receptors (CD16) present on the K cells. Complement is not involved. An apparently different reaction, also obtained with lymphocytes from non-immunized donors or from lymphoid tissues of normal mice, but not requiring antibody coating of the target cells, has been recognized for some years [44]. The cells responsible were named NK cells. Although the reaction is not immuno-specific there is considerable variation in the ease of killing of various types of target cells. Cells of certain T-cell lines and the erythromyeloid line K562 are particularly susceptible. In both humans and mice, NK activity was recognized at an early stage to be contained in a population of non-adherent, non-immunoglobulin-bearing lymphocytes, apparently not of thymus origin. Cells with NK activity are present in foetal liver and cord blood. Athymic rodents have high levels of NK cell activity.

NK cells were originally discovered and, until recently, defined solely by a functional test and it has become clear that NK or NK-like activity is not restricted to cells of a single lineage. This is not surprising when it is recalled that the first clear demonstration of *in vitro* lymphocyte-mediated cytotoxicity was with unfractionated blood lymphocytes activated with phytohaemagglutinin or other polyspecific stimulant [45]. The killing was not immunospecific but only a limited number of target cells (within or across species) tested were susceptible [44], as was later observed for NK cells.

Activation of blood lymphocytes by culture with cells of an autologous B-lymphoblastoid cell line (B-LCL) also produced effector cells capable of

killing a broad range of targets in addition to the autologous B-LCL cells [46]. An important difference from NK killing was that activated, but not resting, lymphocytes showed cytolytic activity in these systems. Recently, structural and marker studies have clarified the picture. True NK cells are large granular lymphocytes which lack CD3 and a T-cell receptor and these are not T cells. They express CD16, CD45 and other leucocyte antigens but do not possess a distinct specific marker. The markers HNK-1 (CD57, present on a subset of T cells, some B cells and weakly on monocytes and myeloma cells) and NKH-1 (CD56, present on monocytes and neuroectodermal cells), although useful in detecting NK cells, are also found on other cell types. NK cells mediate cytolytic reactions not involving MHC class I or class II antigens on the target cells. Some T lymphocytes bearing TCR1 or TCR2 show NK-like activity after stimulation. After incubation with IL-2 both NK and T cells show greatly enhanced killer activity. The term lymphokine-activated killer (LAK) cells has been suggested as appropriate for these cells [47, 48]. In retrospect it is seen that the non-specific cytotoxicity shown by stimulated unfractionated lymphocytes in early experiments was attributable to a mixed bag of cells showing NK, NK-like and LAK activities.

NK and K cells are related and are thought to be of bone marrow origin, although potential progenitors have not been identified, nor has the nature of the recognition receptor. The direct cell–cell lysis test used to identify NK cells does not necessarily reflect their true function, which may include defence against virus infections. NK cells secrete a variety of lymphokines, including interferon, when appropriately stimulated.

Neutrophils

Neutrophils play a vital role in defence against a large group of micro-organisms which are susceptible to its powerful intracellular killing mechanisms following phagocytosis. They function entirely as effector cells and have no recognition role. Their armoury is contained in cytoplasmic granules, of which two major types have been identified [49]. The so-called primary (azurophilic) granules contain lysosomal enzymes including neutral proteases (such as elastase and collagenase), acid proteases and other acid hydrolases such as acid phosphatase, β-glucuronidase, myeloperoxidase and cationic proteins. Secondary (poorly staining) granules which appear later in development as the promyelocytes mature to a myelocyte in the bone marrow contain lactoferrin and lysozyme. There are also vesicles containing alkaline phosphatase. The surfaces of neutrophils are rich in complement (CR1 and CR3) and Fc receptors which make the cell very efficient in attaching to opsonized particles and ingesting them. Migration of neutrophils to a site of infection is enhanced by generation of chemotactic factors, including C5a. As the neutrophil moves into a site the leading edge of the pseudopod is free of granules and the trailing edge has retraction fibrils that attach to tissue. Attachment is followed by a circumferential flow of phagocytic membrane around the opsonized particle, 'zipping up' the particle into what becomes a phagosome. Since the energy for the ingestion comes from glycolysis, ingestion can take place even in the anaerobic conditions at the centre of an abscess. The destruction of susceptible micro-organisms within neutrophils is intimately associated with the process of degranulation, i.e. the release of the granule contents into phagosomes. Killing is brought about inside phagosomes by the oxidative mechanisms initiated by the respiratory burst which leads to superoxide and H_2O_2 production and by the low pH. Other oxygen-independent mechanisms (not requiring a respiratory burst) include those involving cationic proteins, lactoferrin and lysozyme. The type-2 granules containing lactoferrin and lysozyme are very motile and fuse with the phagosome before entry of the lysosomal enzymes, which enter when fusion of the phagosome with an azurophilic granule occurs. Exoplasmosis occurs later, leading to the expulsion of inert particles and enzymes. A release of hydrolytic enzymes may occur even without ingestion of particles. This is demonstrable *in vitro* when neutrophils crawl over a prepared surface (e.g. a plastic dish coated with aggregated IgG), a phenomenon known as frustrated phagocytosis [49]. There are many other activities of neutrophils, partly consequent on the degranulation process, which are important at sites of inflammation. These include release of active peptides such as bradykinin, an arteriolar smooth muscle relaxant, thromboplastin-like activity associated with lysosomal membranes and dissolution of fibrin through release of plasmin activators.

Eosinophils

Another type of granulocyte, the eosinophil, has long been known to be associated with allergic reactions and parasite infections but its role in immunological defence was until recently unclear. There is now abundant evidence that it is important as an effector cell in parasitism [50, 51]. Eosinophils are produced in the bone marrow, have only a brief existence in the blood and then migrate into tissues, notably the submucosa and lamina propria of the gastrointestinal tract, particularly the large intestine. Eosinophils are less phagocytic than neutrophils and the size and content of their granules are different. A large part of the total granule protein (55% in guinea pig eosinophils) consists of a protein called the major basic protein (MBP). This protein binds to heparin and is toxic to a variety of cells. MBP is in the core of the granule. A different protein of molecular weight 21 000, which is very basic and contains zinc, the eosinophilic cationic protein (ECP), is localized to the granule matrix. It consists of a single polypeptide chain with an isoelectric point >11. ECP is a potent toxin for *Schistosoma mansoni*. ECP is related to another protein, eosinophil-derived neurotoxin (EDN) and both are homologous to ribonuclease. Another eosinophil-associated enzyme is eosinophil peroxidase (EPO) which is present in the granule matrix and is distinct from neutrophil myeloperoxidase. It acts in a similar manner in facilitating the killing of micro-organisms in the presence of H_2O_2 and halide; it also induces mast cell degranulation and histamine release. Eosinophils contain a metalloprotein able to degrade types I and III collagen. They also contain a variety of other enzymes including acetylcholinesterase, adenosine triphosphatase, catalase, alkaline phosphatase and phospholipases, but no elastase or neutral proteinase.

The induction mechanisms which bring about the differences in the composition of the granules of eosinophils and neutrophils have not been identified. Cells of the promyeloid leukaemic cell line HL-60, which can be induced to differentiate to macrophages in the presence of phorbol ester and to neutrophils in the presence of dimethylsulphoxide, will differentiate along the eosinophil pathway if cultured for 7 days at pH 7.6–7.8 [51]. After this time 80–85% of the cells have been found to contain MBP. For isolation of eosinophils from blood, the high density of the main fraction of these cells (1.088) has been regularly exploited. However, it has been shown that some eosinophils are present in a lower-density fraction (1.075–1.077) and these cells have somewhat different properties (such as higher numbers of IgGFc and complement receptors) and activities (e.g. they possess IgE-dependent cytotoxicity for schistosomes) [48]. Eosinophils survive very well in human leucocyte cultures (for 7 days or more), in contrast to neutrophils. Isolated eosinophils, however, do not survive well and there is evidence that activated lymphocytes provide essential survival factors.

The functional significance of eosinophils has only recently begun to be understood. The observed association of eosinophils with mast cells in allergic reactions led to a down-regulation hypothesis in which eosinophils modulated mast cell responses to allergens. The presence of histaminase (to inactivate histamine), aryl sulphatase (to combat slow-reacting substances) and a phospholipase D (acting on a platelet-activating factor) in eosinophil granules was compatible with this view. This role is now considered to be of less importance than the effector role of eosinophils against large invading organisms such as parasites [50]. It is likely that eosinophils are involved in inflammatory reactions of many different kinds. Spry [50] lists the following differences between eosinophils and neutrophils: (i) eosinophils are mainly perivascular cells, whereas neutrophils defend intravascular sites; (ii) eosinophils respond to IgG, IgE and complement components, whereas neutrophils do not respond to IgE stimulation; (iii) eosinophils secrete whereas neutrophils ingest; (iv) eosinophils mostly take part in acute and chronic hypersensitivity reactions and are often found close to other cells, whereas neutrophils are common in areas of acute necrosis; and (v) eosinophils are mainly associated with allergic parasitic and chronic inflammatory responses, whereas neutrophils are primarily found in acute bacterial infections, ischaemic lesions and reactions to damaged cells and tissues.

Mast cells and basophils

These are two related but distinct types of cell with basophilic granules in the cytoplasm which are important in inflammatory and allergic reactions. Mast cells are widely distributed in connective tissue. They are mainly located alongside small blood vessels and are particularly abundant in the skin and gastrointestinal tract (especially the mucosa of the small intestine). Basophils make up a small proportion (about 1%) of blood leucocytes. Their early differentiation is closer to that of eosinophils than to neutrophils.

Mast cells have Fcε receptors on their surface by which they bind IgE with antigen-binding sites of the antibody displayed. Upon encounter with the appropriate antigen or allergen, degranulation is triggered with release of a range of soluble mediators acting locally or systemically. Depending on the site of the reaction, the response may include contraction of smooth muscle in bronchial walls with resulting bronchial constriction, increase in mucus and other secretions, and dilatation of small blood vessels causing redness and oedema. The active substances released include histamine (rapid action, short-lived), leukotrienes and prostaglandins (of slow and prolonged action), heparin, platelet-activating factors and factors chemotactic for neutrophils and eosinophils.

Basophils also bind IgE antibody and the triggering by contact with divalent antigen and consequences of release of granule contents are similar to those described for mast cells. However, they have been shown by marker tests and other criteria to be a different cell type. Like basophils, mast cells are of haemopoietic origin and express the LCA (CD45) but no other haemopoietic marker defined by a large panel of monoclonal antibodies [52]. In contrast to basophils they do not express the CD16 and CD13 antigens. On SDS-PAGE analysis the surface glycoproteins of basophils show a pattern similar to that of the promonocyte line U937 or the promyeloid line HL-60, whereas the pattern obtained from mast cells is strikingly different [52]. Also, many human sera contain antibodies which bind to mast cells but not to basophils [53]. The maturation of mast cells from precursors appears to require environmental factors provided by T cells. Mast cell precursors have been shown to be present in lymphoid tissues and during maturation may take up IgE produced locally by plasma cells in, for example, a mesenteric node before migrating to a mucosal surface [54].

References

1 Ling NR. *Lymphocyte Stimulation*. Amsterdam: North-Holland, 1968:25.

2 Austyn JM. Lymphoid dendritic cells. *Immunol* 1987; 62:161–70.

3 Schlossman SF, Morimoto C, Streuli M, Anderson P, Rudd C. Surface structures defining functional T-cell subsets. In: *Proceedings of the IVth International Workshop on Human Leucocyte Differentiation Antigens*. Oxford: Oxford University Press, 1989: 1070–3.

4 Borst J, van Dongen JJM, Bolhuis RLH, Peters PJ, Hafler DA, de Vries E, van de Griend RJ. Distinct molecular forms of human T cell receptor $\gamma\delta$ detected on viable T cells by a monoclonal antibody. *J Exp Med* 1988; 167:1625–44.

5 Groh V, Porcelli S, Fabbi M, Lanier LL, Picker LJ, Anderson T, Warnke RA, Bhan AK, Stroninger JL, Brenner MB. Human lymphocytes bearing T cell receptor γ/δ are phenotypically diverse and evenly distributed throughout the lymphoid system. *J Exp Med* 1989; 169:1277–94.

6 Janeway CA, Carding S, Jones B, Murray J, Portoles P, Rasmussen R, Rojo J, Saizawa K, West J, Bottomly K. CD4$^+$ T cells: specificity and function. *Immunol Rev* 1988; 101:39–80.

7 Bottomly K. A functional dichotomy in CD4$^+$ T lymphocytes. *Immunol Today* 1988; 9:268–74.

8 Rudd CE, Morimoto C, Wong LL, Schlossman SF. The subdivision of the T4 (CD4) subset on the basis of the differential expression of L-C/T200 antigens. *J Exp Med 1987; 166:1758–73.*

9 Butterfield K, Fathman CG, Budd RC. A subset of memory CD4$^+$ helper T lymphocytes identified by expression of Pgp-1. *J Exp Med* 1989; 169:1461–6.

10 Van Dongen JJM, Hodijkaas H, Comans–Bitter M, Hählen K, de Klein A, van Zanen GE, van T Veer MB, Abels J, Brenner R. Human bone marrow cells positive for terminal deoxynucleotidyl transferase (TdT), HLA–DR and a T cell marker may represent prothymocytes. *J Immunol* 1985; 135:3144–50.

11 Brown G, Bunce CM, Lord J, McConnell F. The development of cell lineages: a sequential model. *Differentiation* 1988; 39:83–9.

12 Haynes BF, Denning SM, Singer KH, Kurtzberg J. Ontogeny of T cell precursors: a model for the initial stages of human T cell development. *Immunol Today* 1989; 10:87–90.

13 Kurtzberg J, Waldmann TA, Davey MP, Bigner SH, Moore JO, Hershfield MS, Haynes BF. CD7$^+$CD4$^-$CD8$^-$ Acute leukaemia: a syndrome of malignant pluripotent lymphohaematopoietic cells. *Blood* 1989; 73:381–90.

14 Williams GT, Kingston R, Owen MJ, Jenkinson EJ, Owen JJT. A single micromanipulated stem cell gives rise to multiple T cell receptor gene rearrangements in the thymus *in vitro*. *Nature* 1986; 324:63–4.

15 Elliott EV. The persistent PHA-responsive population in the mouse thymus 1. Characterisation of the population. *Immunol* 1977; 32:383–94.

16 Ford WL. Lymphocyte migration and immune responses. *Prog Allergy* 1975; 19:1–59.

17 MacLennan ICM, Gray D. Antigen-driven selection of virgin and memory B cells. *Immunol Rev* 1986; 91:61–86.

18 Ling NR, Hardie D, Lowe J, Johnson GD, Khan M, MacLennan ICM. A phenotypic study of cells from Burkitt lymphoma and EBV-B-lymphoblastoid lines and their relationship to cells in normal lymphoid tissues. *Int J Cancer* 1989; 43:112–18.

19 Hanumi K, Gray P, Suzuki T. Fcγ-mediated suppression of γ-interferon-induced Ia antigen on a murine macrophage-like cell line (P338D). *J Immunol* 1984; 133:2852–6.

20 Brown JC, Harris G, Papamichail M, Slijivic VS, Holborow EJ. The localisation of aggregated human γ-globulin in the spleens of normal mice. *Immunol* 1973; 24:955–68.

21 Heinen E, Braun M, Coulie PG, van Snick J, Moeremans M, Cormann M, Kinet-Doel C, Simar LJ. Transfer of immune complexes from lymphocytes to follicular dendritic cells. *Eur J Immunol* 1986; 16:167–72.

22 Ling NR. The relationship of B-lymphocyte surface marker phenotype to cell differentiation. In: Bird G, Calvert J, eds. *B Lymphocytes in Human Disease*. Oxford: Oxford University Press, 1988; 174–92.

23 Jackson N, Lowe J, Ball J, Bromidge E, Ling NR, Larkins S, Griffith MJ, Franklin IM. Two new IgA plasma cell leukaemia cell lines (JJN1 and JJN2) which proliferate in response to B cell stimulation factor 2. *Clin Exp Immunol* 1989; 75:93–9.

24 Fend F, Huber H, Thaler J, Gattringer C, Denz H, Nachbaur D, Stauder R, Lechleitner M, Miller–Hermelink HK. Reactivity of intrathymic medullary B cells with monoclonal antibodies of the workshop B panel. *Tissue Antigens* 1989; 33:184.

25 Nachbaur D, Ford F, Denz H, Thaler J, Stauder R, Lechleitner M, Gattringer C, Huber H. Reactivity of immature sinus histiocytes in lymph node toxoplasmo-

sis and infectious mononucleosis with B cell panel antibodies. *Tissue Antigens* 1989; 33:187.

26 Loutit JF, Nisbet NW, Marshall MJ, Vaughan JM. Versatile stem cells in bone marrow. *Lancet* 1982; ii:1090–3.

27 Williamson N, James K, Ling NR, Holt LP. Synovial cells. A study of the morphology and an examination of protein synthesis of synovial cells. *Ann Rheum Dis* 1966; 25:534–46.

28 Van Furth R. Origin and kinetics of mononuclear phagocytes. In: Van Furth R, ed. *Mononuclear Phagocytes, Functional Aspects*. Boston: Nijhoff, 1980:1–10.

29 Mahida YR, Patel S, Jewell DP. Mononuclear phagocyte system of human Peyer's patches: an immunohistochemical study using monoclonal antibodies. *Clin Exp Immunol* 1989; 75:82–6.

30 Adams DO, Hamilton TA. The cell biology of macrophage activation. *Ann Rev Immunol* 1984; 2:283–318.

31 Adams DO. Molecular interactions in macrophage activation. *Immunol Today* 1989; 10:33–5.

32 Dimitriu–Bona A, Burmester GR, Waters SJ, Winchester RJ. Human mononuclear phagocyte differentiation antigens. Patterns of antigenic expression on the surface of human monocytes and macrophages defined by monoclonal antibodies. *J Immunol* 1983; 130:145–52.

33 Russell S. Stimulate the phagocytes. *Immunol Today* 1986; 7:347–9.

34 Hart DNJ, Mackenzie J. Isolation and characterisation of human tonsil dendritic cells. *J Exp Med* 1988; 168:157–70.

35 Knight S, Farrant J, Bryant A, Edwards AJ, Burman S, Lever A, Clarke J, Webster ADB. Non-adherent low density cells from human peripheral blood contain dendritic cells and monocytes, both with veiled morphology. *Immunol* 1986; 57:595–603.

36 Balfour B, Drexhage HA, Kamperdijk EWA, Hoefsmit ECM. Antigen-presenting cells, including Langerhans cells, veiled cells and interdigitating cells. *CIBA Foundation Symposium* 1981; 84:281–3.

37 Miyasaka M, Trnka Z. Lymphocyte migration and differentiation in a large animal: the sheep. *Immunol Rev* 1986; 91:87–114.

38 Radzun HJ, Hogg N. Summary of myeloid workshop M4: mononuclear phagocytes. In: McMichael A, ed. *Leucocyte Typing III*. Oxford: Oxford University Press, 1987:664.

39 Humphrey JH, Grennan D, Sundaram V. The origins of follicular dendritic cells in the mouse and the mechanism of trapping of immune complexes on them. *Eur J Immunol* 1984; 14:859–64.

40 Johnson GD, Hardie D, Ling NR, MacLennan ICM. Human follicular dendritic cells (FDC): a study with monoclonal antibodies. *Clin Exp Immunol* 1986; 64:205–13.

41 Petrasch S, Schmitz J, Perez–Alvarez C, Brittinger G. Reactivity of monoclonal antibodies of the B cell panel with isolated follicular dendritic cells. *Tissue Antigen* 1989; 33:137.

42 Schriever F, Freedman AS, Messner E, Nadler LM. Isolation and phenotypic characterisation of follicular dendritic cells from human tonsil. *Tissue Antigens* 1989; 33:138.

43 Ling NR, Elliott D, Lowe J. Modulation of the murine immune response to human IgG by complexing with monoclonal antibodies 1. Antibody responses to determinants on the constant region of light chains and gamma chains. *Immunol* 1987; 62:1–6.

44 Perlmann P, Holm G. Cytotoxic effects of lymphoid cells *in vitro*. *Adv Immunol* 1969; 11: 117–95.

45 Holm G, Perlmann P, Werner B. Phytohaemagglutinin induced cytotoxic action of normal lymphoid cells on cells in tissue culture. *Nature* 1964; 203:841–3.

46 Steel CM, Hardy DA, Ling NR, Lauder IJ. The interaction of normal lymphocytes and cells from lymphoid cell lines VI. Line directed cytotoxic specificity of lymphocytes activated by autochthonous or allogeneic LCL cells. *Immunol* 1974; 26:1013–23.

47 Jondal M. The human NK cell—a short overview and an hypothesis on NK recognition. *Clin Exp Immunol* 1987; 70:255–62.

48 Kimber I. Natural killer cells. *Med Lab Sci* 1985; 42:60–77.

49 Goldstein IM. Polymorphonuclear leukocyte lysosomes and immune tissue injury. *Prog Allergy* 1976; 20:301–40.

50 Spry CJF. Eosinophils. A comprehensive review and guide to the scientific and medical literature. Part I. *Cellular Biology of Eosinophils*. Oxford: Oxford University Press, 1988:3–130.

51 Gleich GJ, Adolphson CR. The eosinophilic leukocyte: structure and function. *Adv Immunol* 1986; 39:177–253.

52 Rimmer EF, Horton MA. Mast cells form a unique haemopoietic lineage. In: McMichael A, ed. *Leucocyte Typing III*. Oxford: Oxford University Press, 1987:729–31.

53 Rizzetto M, Doniach D. Human antibodies to mast cells. *Clin Exp Immunol* 1973; 14:327–34.

54 Gillon J. Where do mucosal mast cells acquire IgE? *Immunol Today* 1981; 2:80–1.

2

Regulation of the immune system by pharmacological and biological mediators

ANNE S. HAMBLIN

Introduction

The immune response to antigen is regulated by a variety of products of both cells of the immune system and cells of the microenvironment of the immune system. These mediators are responsible for both the amplification and the limitation of the immune response. Their uncontrolled production may lead to damaging immune reactions, such as hypersensitivity or chronic inflammation, and their underproduction may lead to immunodeficiency. It follows that drugs or toxic agents which act on the mediators themselves, or cells that produce them, may cause aberrant immune responses.

There are many molecules involved in immune regulation including cytokines, interferons, other peptide hormones, complement components, prostaglandins and leukotrienes, free radicals, histamine and serotonin, platelet-activating factor (PAF) and many more. The network formed by these molecules in co-ordinating immune responses is complex, closely intertwined and is still being revealed, as will be evident from the discussions below. As well as being produced by, and acting on, cells of the immune system many of the molecules may also be produced by, and act on, cells outside the immune system. In this way they connect the immune system with other physiological systems of the body. Here are described the structure and functions of various soluble immune mediators which have been reported as having a role in immune responses.

Cytokines

Cytokines are polypeptides which are major regulators both of the normal adaptive immune response and the innate inflammatory response. They have attracted considerable attention for the parts they may play in the development of acute and chronic inflammation and malignancy, and for their potential role as therapeutic agents for stimulation of the immune response.

Terminology and background

The terminology which has been applied to various cytokines has changed with the development of knowledge on the subject.

In the earliest studies, there was particular interest in how the interaction of sensitized lymphocytes with the sensitizing antigen led to immune responsiveness. The term *lymphokine* was introduced in 1969 [1] to describe 'cell-free soluble factors generated by the interaction of sensitized lymphocytes with specific antigen and expressed without reference to the immunological specificity'. It was designed to emphasize the apparent lymphocytic origin of the biological activities found in the tissue-culture supernatants of sensitized lymphocytes interacting with sensitizing antigens. The culture supernatants influenced the *in vivo* and *in vitro* behaviour of the cells implicated in immune response in such a way that it was concluded that they contained the factors which were the intercellular messages important in both cellular and humoral immunity. Preliminary biochemical evidence suggested that these factors derived from lymphocytes were proteins, and not immunoglobulins.

It soon became clear that within any single culture supernatant a very large number of biological activities was demonstrable by bioassay, suggesting that either immune responses were influenced by many different factors, or that a single factor had many different activities [2]. Lists of factors sometimes reached more than 100 [2]. It proved extremely difficult to separate the biological activities of lymphokines in such a way that a single biological activity could be unequivocally ascribed to a single protein. Furthermore, when attention focused on the cells producing the biological activities, it was shown that not only lymphocytes but also mononuclear phagocytes and cells outside the immune system could be the source of biological activities relevant to the functioning of the immune system.

At this point, it was felt that the term *lymphokine* should be restricted to factors produced by lymphocytes; that the term *monokine* should be used for factors produced by mononuclear phagocytes, and *cytokine* should be employed either for factors produced by cells other than lymphocytes and mononuclear phagocytes [3], or as an umbrella term for all the soluble factors. Further confusion in nomenclature was introduced in 1979 by the term *interleukin* (between leucocytes) which was inaugurated to 'free nomenclature from the constraints associated with definitions by single bioassays' [4]. Biochemical separation techniques had improved in such a way that it was possible to show that factors, defined by a number of different bioassays, were in fact the same molecular entity. For example, the factor derived from monocytes causing lymphocyte activation, which had previously been known as lymphocyte-activating factor (LAF), appeared to be the same as that which was previously known as mitogenic protein (MP), T-cell-replacing factor III (TRF-III), B cell-activating factor (BAF) and B cell differentiation factor (BDF), and was renamed *interleukin 1* (IL-1) [4]. The main alternative names for the cytokines are shown in Table 2.1.

Whilst the nomenclature was being revised a number of technical developments rapidly led to clarification of the nature of soluble protein factors involved in immune responses [5]. In particular, the availability of recombinant cytokines and of anti-cytokine monoclonal antibodies revolutionized the scope of cytokine research. Dissection of the genomic structure and location and of the protein structure of cytokines has been possible. Genetic engineering has provided large amounts of homogeneous material with which to work, so that it is now possible to state categorically that immune responses are mediated by many different cytokines and that a single cytokine has many different biological activities, thus substantiating the suspicions which already were being held in the 1960s. Molecular techniques may be used to look at the expression of genes for cytokines in individual cells and tissues. Monoclonal antibodies may be used to purify cytokines, which are often produced from natural sources in combinations which are otherwise difficult to separate, and for their specific bioassay [6].

Table 2.1 Cytokines and their major synonyms

Cytokine	Abbreviation	Major synonyms
Interleukin-1	IL-1	Endogenous pyrogen (EP) Lymphocyte-activating factor (LAF) Haematopoietin 1 (HP1)
Interleukin-2	IL-2	T cell growth factor (TCGF)
Interleukin-3	IL-3	Multipotential colony-stimulating factor (multi CSF) Mast cell growth factor (MCGF) Haemopoietic cell growth factor (HCGF)
Interleukin-4	IL-4	B cell stimulation factor 1 (BSF-1) B cell growth factor (BCGF-1) B cell differentiation factor-γ (BCDF-γ)
Interleukin-5	IL-5	T cell-replacing factor (TRF) B cell growth factor (BCGF-II) Eosinophil differentiation factor (EDF)
Interleukin-6	IL-6	Interferon β_2 (IFN β_2) B cell-stimulating factor 2 (BSF2) Hybridoma growth factor (HGF) B cell differentiation factor (BCDF) 26 kDa protein
Interleukin-7	IL-7	Lymphopoietin 1 Pre-B cell growth factor
Interleukin-8	IL-8	Monocyte-derived neutrophil chemotactic factor (MDNCF)
Granulocyte–macrophage colony-stimulating factor	GM-CSF	Colony-stimulating factor α Pluripoietin
Macrophage colony-stimulating factor	M-CSF	Colony-stimulating factor 1 (CSF-1)
Granulocyte colony-stimulating factor	G-CSF	Colony-stimulating factor β (CSF-β)
Tumour necrosis factor	TNF	Cachectin, tumour necrosis factor α (TNFα)
Lymphotoxin	LT	Tumour necrosis factor β (TNFβ)

It must be noted that the terminology has not kept pace with the rapid expansion of biological knowledge. The terms *cytokine, lymphokine* and *interleukin* are often used interchangeably and precise definitions of any one are not available. The term *interleukin* was intended for immunoregulatory factors produced by cells of the immune system, and for which the nucleotide sequence was known [7]. Eight factors have been called interleukin (IL-1–8). However, there are a number of interleukins which are within the general definition but which have retained their original title, e.g. tumour necrosis factor (TNF), the colony-stimulating factors (CSFs) and interferon-γ (IFN-γ). In view of their pleiotropic biological action (see below) the term *cytokine* rather than *interleukin* seems more appropriate and will be used in this text. No doubt some revision of the terminology will eventually emerge.

General molecular and biochemical properties

Cytokines are encoded within genes for which there is only one copy per haploid cell, and which consist typically of 3–4 introns and 4–5 exons (Table 2.2). They are located on a number of different chromosomes but it is of interest that several [IL-3, IL-4, IL-5, granulocyte–macrophage colony-stimulating factor (GM-CSF) and macrophage colony-stimulating factor (M-CSF)] are clustered on the short arm of chromosome 5 [9] and that TNF and lymphotoxin (LT) are encoded within the major histocompatibility complex (MHC) [12].

Table 2.2 Genomic structure and location of human cytokines

Name	Exon number	Chromosome	References
IL-2	4	4q	[8]
IL-3	5	5q23–5q31	[9,10]
IL-4	4	5q23–5q31	[9]
IL-5	4	5q23–5q31	[9]
IL-6	5	7p21–7p24	[11]
TNF	4	6p23–6q12	[12]
LT	4	6	[12]
GM-CSF	4	5q23–5q31	[9,10]
G-CSF	5	17q21–17q22	[13]
M-CSF	10	5q 33.1	[9]

For abbreviations see Table 2.1.

The biochemical structure of the cytokines is shown in Table 2.3. The cDNAs for cytokines predict mature proteins of 100–200 amino acids, and these primary structures have usually been confirmed by sequence analysis of the mature protein. Most cDNAs predict a clearly defined hydrophobic signal sequence which is cleaved from the protein before it leaves the cell. However, for some, e.g. TNF and IL-1, this signal sequence is not readily identifiable.

Many cytokines contain cysteine residues which are involved in intramolecular disulphide bonding. The importance of these molecular bonds for retention of biological activity can be demonstrated by site-directed mutagenesis, or mercaptoethanol treatment. Many cytokines are also glycosylated (usually *N* but sometimes *O* glycosylation), although the biological role of the glycosylation is not clear. Most recombinant cytokines prepared in *Escherichia coli*, which does not glycosylate proteins, have the same biological properties as the natural glycosylated equivalent, and the half-life of recombinant proteins injected *in vivo* is often the same as the natural glycosylated protein. It is difficult to believe that glycosylation is not important for cytokine stability *in vivo*, localization, or clearance, or indeed target specificity but this remains to be determined. Location of glycosylation points in the tertiary structure of cytokines as they are determined may enable a better prediction of their role.

Analysis of the nucleotide sequences and primary protein structure of cytokines has permitted comparison of the structure of genes and proteins of the same and different cytokines within and between species [29]. Such comparisons are useful for analysis of the phylogeny of cytokine genes as well as definition, if it exists, of a lymphokine supergene family. Whilst the interleukins do not overall show similarities in structure, there are interleukins which share sequence homology, suggesting their common . origin from primordial genes. Thus the genes encoding IL-2, IL-4, IL-5 and GM-CSF appear to be phylogenetically related by intron/exon organization and the position of cysteine residues [29].

The tertiary structure of three cytokines, IL-2 [36] IL-1β [37] and TNF [38], has been determined. Each has a different structural motif, and thus the biolog-

Table 2.3 Biochemical structure of human cytokines

Name	Molecular weight mature protein (kDa)	cDNA	Amino acids in mature protein	Glycosylation (type *N* or *O*)	Number of cysteine residues	References
IL-1α	15–17	271	~154	No	0	[14,15]
IL-1β	15–17	269	~153	No	0	[14,15]
IL-2	14–16	153	133	Yes (*O*)	2	[16]
IL-3	15–25	152	133	Yes (*N*)	2	[17–19]
IL-4	20	153	129	Yes (*N*)	6	[20–22]
IL-5	20–45	134	129–133	Yes (*N*)	2	[22,23]
IL-6	27	212	185	Yes (*N*)	4	[11,24]
IL-7	25 (m)*	173	148	Yes (*N*)	6	[25–27]
IL-8	8	99	72	No	4	[28]
GM-CSF	15–35	144	127	Yes (*N*)	4	[29,30]
G-CSF	18–25	207	174–177	Yes (*O*)	5	[29]
M-CSF	60–100	224	(158–233) $\times$ 2			[29,31,32]
TNFα	17	233	157	No	2	[33,34]
LT	25	205	171	Yes (*O*)	0	[35]

For abbreviations see Table 2.1. *m = mouse.

ical activities they may have in common are not reflected in their structure.

General biological properties

There are a number of general biological effects of cytokines which are important for understanding and interpreting their roles. A single cytokine can affect a number of different cell types; it is said to be pleiotropic [5,39,40]. Many of the studies demonstrating this have been undertaken *in vitro* and, whilst there is no doubt that the reports accurately reflect the observed effects, some caution is needed in transferring the observations to implications for biological activity *in vivo*. It is necessary to ask whether the doses used *in vitro* reflect the levels that might be seen *in vivo*, and whether the cytokine might be expected to be generated *in vivo* close to the type of target cell used *in vitro*, and under what circumstances. Putting caution aside, one is left with evidence that most cytokines are capable of a wide variety of effects on very different target cells.

Cytokines are secreted polypeptides which exhibit both autocrine and paracrine effects [39,40]. Thus, several cytokines in turn act on the cells that secreted them (autocrine effect). For example, IL-1 and IL-2 are produced by macrophages [41] and T

cells [42] respectively, and can bind to their receptors on the cells that secreted them, producing more cytokine secretion. Many cytokines act on neighbouring cells, inducing the production of other cytokines (paracrine effects), an action presumably of great importance in the amplification of the immune response. This biological action has important implications for the interpretation of both *in vivo* and *in vitro* experiments on cytokines; any effect seen may not necessarily be directly ascribed to the cytokine under investigation, since it may induce a second cytokine which produces the biological effect. Such effects may be unravelled by the appropriate use of cytokine-specific antibodies [6]. Thus IL-1-induced thymocyte proliferation may be inhibited by antibodies to IL-6, suggesting that thymocyte proliferative activity is mediated via IL-1 induction of IL-6 [43].

A further important biological feature of cytokines is their ability to act synergistically with each other and with other stimulants [5]. This frequently means that minute levels of cytokines, which on their own are ineffective, in combination may produce pronounced biological effects. For example, IL-2 and IL-4 synergize, causing proliferation of T cell clones [44].

Cytokines are produced by many different cells (Table 2.4). Lymphocytes, particularly CD4-positive

Table 2.4 Cell sources and targets of cytokines

Cytokine	Source	Target
IL-1α and β	Diverse, including endothelial cells; epithelial cells; monocytes/ macrophages; large granular lymphocytes B cells	Diverse, including haematopoietic and non-haematopoietic cells
IL-2	T cells	T cells; B cells; natural killer cells; (macrophages)
IL-3	T cells	Multipotential stem cells; mast cells; granulocytes; monocytes/macrophages; eosinophils; megakaryocytes
IL-4	T cells Mast cells	B cells; T cells; mast cells; haematopoietic/progenitor cells; monocytes/macrophages; thymocytes
IL-5	T cells	Eosinophils; B cells
IL-6	Diverse, including fibroblasts; endothelial cells; epithelial cells; T cells; monocytes/ macrophages	B cells; fibroblasts; hepatocytes; thymocytes; T cells, haematopoietic progenitor cells
IL-7	? Stromal cells	Pre-B cells; thymocytes
IL-8	Monocytes/macrophages	Neutrophils
GM-CSF	T cells; endothelial cells; fibroblasts; monocytes/macrophages	Multipotential stem cells; monocyte/macrophages; neutrophils; eosinophils
M-CSF	Fibroblast; monocyte/macrophages; endothelial cells	Multipotential stem cells; monocytes/macrophages
G-CSF	Monocytes/macrophages; fibroblasts; endothelial cells	Multipotential stem cells; neutrophils
TNF	Diverse, including monocyte/macrophages; T cells; B cells; natural killer cells	Diverse, including tumour cells; transformed cell lines; fibroblasts; neutrophils; adipocytes; endothelial cells; chondrocytes; hepatocytes; monocyte/macrophages
LT	T cells	

For abbreviations see Table 2.1

T cells, are a predominant source of many. In the mouse there is evidence from *in vitro* work for two types of CD4-positive T cells, referred to as TH_1 and TH_2 cells, which each produce a different spectrum of cytokines [6]. The TH_1 cells produce IFN-γ and IL-2, the cytokines associated with delayed-type hypersensitivity and induction of macrophage cytotoxicity, whereas the TH_2 cells produce IL-4, IL-5 and IL-6—cytokines associated with providing help for antibody production by B cells [45,46]. It is noteworthy that in spite of intense efforts to date no similar subsets have been described in humans.

A further dominant source of cytokines is mononuclear phagocytes. These cells produce IL-1 and TNF, some of the most pleiotropic cytokines. However, it should be noted that these same cytokines may be produced by many cell types (Table 2.4). Here again, it is worth remembering that demonstration of production of a cytokine *in vitro* by a cell may not be taken as evidence that the cell necessarily produces the cytokine *in vivo*. Progress on this front relies on demonstration that the genes for cytokines are activated in histological tissue, by using *in situ* hybridization, and confirmation that the protein is produced there by immunocytochemical methods.

Individual cytokines have biological activities relevant to roles in normal immune responses or in stress/inflammation responses, or in both of these [5,7,40,47]. IL-1 and IL-2 are important in interactions between antigen-presenting cells and T cells which initiate primary and secondary immune responses to antigen [48,49]. IL-3 and the CSFs are important in the development of myeloid haemopoietic cells from pluripotent stem cells in response to stress, and it is assumed—although not established — that they play a role in normal haemopoiesis [50–52]. These same cytokines also play a role in the activation of mature cells during normal immune or inflammatory stimulation. IL-7 is a growth factor for early lymphoid cells of B and T lineage [27]. IL-4 and IL-5 and IL-6 are essential for the development of humoral immune responses by B cells [24,53]. Two of these same cytokines, IL-1 and IL-6, [24,54], as well as TNF and IL-8, have biological actions which are relevant to an important role in inflammation [28,33], and IL-4 and IL-5 have potent effects on eosinophils and mast cells/basophils, compatible with a role in allergic disease and inflammation [21,54].

It is probable that in many normal situations cytokines are released by, and act on, cells in close contact. In such a way detrimental 'bystander' effects of cytokines would be limited. In contrast, acute or chronic inflammation may be accompanied by their release into the circulation and systemic action. The fever induction and acute-phase protein release stimulated by IL-1, TNF and IL-6 suggest their action at a site remote from their synthesis, and the observation that cytokines, such as IL-6, are found in the serum of patients suffering with febrile illness [56] implies this is their route of transmission.

Structure and functions of individual cytokines

In the following sections, the properties of the individual cytokines whose genes have been cloned are described.

Interleukin-1

In 1972 Gery *et al.* described a factor which was derived from activation of adherent human leucocytes (monocytes) which promoted the proliferation of mouse thymocytes [57]. It later became apparent that the same biochemical entity was responsible for a number of biological effects and was synonymous with other factors detected by bioassays (Table 2.1; [5,54]). In 1979, the factor was renamed interleukin-1 [4].

IL-1 is a non-glycosylated polypeptide produced particularly by monocytes and macrophages. For these cells lipopolysaccharide (LPS) is a potent inducer of IL-1, but it can also be induced by itself (autocrine action) and by TNF, LT and GM-CSF [58]. Many other cell types are capable of IL-1 synthesis (Table 2.4; [41]).

cDNA cloning has shown that IL-1 consists of two species named IL-1α and IL-1β with isoelectric points (pI) of 5 and 6.8 [14,15]. Whilst the major species produced on activation of mononuclear phagocytes is IL-1β the reverse is true for keratinocytes. The two types of IL-1 have 26% homology at the amino acid level, but appear to bind to the same widely distributed high-affinity receptor, which has been cloned [7,59]. IL-1 is synthesized as a biologically inactive precursor molecule of 31 kDa, which is subsequently processed to give 15–17 kDa mature protein. Biologically active subfragments of these molecules have been described [60] and peptides, synthesized so that they correspond to different regions of the whole IL-1β molecule, show different biological activities [61]. Using such technology, the inflammatory properties and immunomodulatory properties of IL-1 have been assigned to different regions of the whole molecule [60,61].

IL-1 has a very large array of biological activities on different target cells involved in both immune and inflammatory responses [54]. The biological activities of IL-1 are listed in Table 2.5. Engagement of the MHC-antigen fragment complex on the antigen-presenting cell with the T cell receptor leads to clonal expansion of the T cells. Evidence suggests that antigen-presenting cell must also produce IL-1, which presumably binds to a receptor on the T cell [62,63]. However, IL-1 may have an enhancing rather than obligatory role in T-cell proliferation [49]. It is not clear whether the IL-1 may be soluble or whether it must be in special membrane-bound form to exert this effect on T cells [64]. The proliferation of cloned TH_2 cells is enhanced by the presence of IL-1 whilst that of TH_1 cells is unaffected, suggesting that different T cells may have different requirements for IL-1 in their proliferation [65,66]. The presence of IL-1 could thus favour the antibody synthetic TH_2-type of responses, rather than the cell-mediated TH_1 type of responses.

Table 2.5 Biological activities of interleukin-1

Augments IL-2 production and expression of IL-2 receptor by T cells
Pro-inflammatory
Induces fever and slow-wave sleep
Induces prostaglandin E_2 production by fibroblasts
Induces collagenase production by fibroblasts
Stimulates fibroblast growth
Activates B cells
Induces synthesis of acute-phase proteins
Stimulates bone resorption
Augments natural killer cell activity
Primes stem cells to become responsive to colony-stimulating factors

---

The actions of IL-1 listed in Table 2.5 are indicative of the important role which the molecule is believed to play in inflammation [41,54]. These many diverse activities of IL-1, when limited, can be appreciated as beneficial to the host. For example, IL-1 acts on the brain to initiate fever, which has been shown to enhance the activity of T and B lymphocytes [67], and stimulates hepatocytes to produce acute-phase proteins which assist in the clearance of micro-organisms by the reticuloendothelial system [68]. However, uncontrolled excessive IL-1 production is suspected of playing a major role in chronic inflammatory diseases such as rheumatoid arthritis. Whilst it is believed that in the antigen-driven immune response macrophages are the principal source of IL-1, the other cellular sources of IL-1 are considered extremely important in inflammation.

Other important roles for IL-1 include priming stem cells to become responsive to colony-stimulating factors [69] and accessory growth factor activity for B cells [70].

Interleukin-2

This cytokine, originally described as T cell growth factor (TCGF) [71], has an important role in the clonal expansion of T cells. The primary structure of human IL-2 was determined in 1983 [16] and the tertiary structure in 1987 [36]. It is synthesized predominantly by CD4-positive T cells, activated by either antigen or mitogen [42]. Production of IL-2 is controlled at the level of transcription; the level of secreted IL-2 corresponds to the level of message within the cell. Withdrawal of the stimulus to the cell results in shutdown of transcription and then to cessation of IL-2 release [72]. The liberated IL-2 may act on the cell that released it or neighbouring T cells, to stimulate their proliferation. Stimulation of growth of CD4- or CD8-positive T cells [73] and natural killer (NK) cells [74] is brought about by binding of IL-2 to its receptor. Proliferation is instigated by the binding of IL-2 to a high-affinity receptor made up of two non-covalent linked 75 kDa (β) and 55 kDa (α) chains [75–77]. The 75 kDa chain has a large intracellular component and provides the signal for cell growth, whilst binding is facilitated by the 55 kDa molecule. Following binding, the ligand, IL-2, and its receptor are internalized; the half-life for the event is 20–30 min.

Receptor expression parallels activation. Resting T cells express few IL-2 receptors. Following binding of antigen or mitogen to the cell surface, the IL-2 receptor message is synthesized and IL-2 receptors appear at the cell surface. Following internalization and with cessation of the activation signal the receptors are no longer synthesized and the cells revert to their inactive state [48,77,78].

IL-2 receptors of low affinity (55 kDa) are found on other cells such as B cells and mononuclear phagocytes. The 75 kDa molecule can be induced on B cells by *Staphylococcus aureus* Cowan I and on mononuclear phagocytes by LPS and IFN-α [79]. The expression of these IL-2 receptors presumably reflects the observation that under some conditions B cells can be shown to undergo differentiation in the presence of IL-2 [80]. Apart from one observation that macrophages increase their tumour-directed cytotoxicity in the presence of IL-2 [81], little is known about the biological significance of IL-2 receptors on macrophages.

Incubation of the resting peripheral blood lymphocytes with IL-2 results in augmentation of NK and the generation of lymphokine-activated killer (LAK) cells [82]—an observation which has led to the use of IL-2 in cancer immunotherapy [83]. The proliferation of these cells seems to be particularly mediated through the IL-2 receptor β chain [75,84].

Interleukin-3

IL-3 supports the proliferation of early haematopoietic stem cells which are capable of becoming committed to differentiation along a variety of lineages, and supports the terminal differentiation of several myeloid lineages [50–52,85]. When injected into mice, IL-3 induces splenomegaly with increases in eosinophils, neutrophils, mast cells and macrophages [86–88]. IL-3 is produced by activated T cells [18] as well as by a number of cell lines [89,90]. IL-3 supports the growth of mast cells [91] and potentiates the activities of eosinophils [92], basophils [93] and monocytes [94].

The structures of human [17], rat and mouse [19] IL-3 have been deduced from sequencing cDNA or genomic clones. There appears to be little sequence homology between IL-3 from different species and, consistent with this, there is little cross-species bioreactivity [18]. In spite of this, the biological functions of IL-3 appear to have been conserved in evolution. The IL-3 receptor has not been cloned, although there is information on the binding characteristics of the protein for the receptor [18].

Interleukin-4

Concordant with some of its original names (Table 2.1), IL-4 causes activation, proliferation and differentiation of B cells [95–97]. It is also a growth factor for T cells [98] and mast cells [20] and influences a large number of haematopoietic stem cells. Thus, IL-4 induces resting B cells to increase their expression of class II MHC and low-affinity receptors for the Fc portion of immunoglobulin E (IgE) (activation); co-stimulates B cells in the presence of anti-immunoglobulin (proliferation) and induces the production of IgG_1 and IgE antibodies (differentiation) [21]. It is therefore of importance in enhancing the capacity of B cells to present antigen to T cells and the production of certain immunoglobulin isotypes, namely IgG_1 and IgE. In this latter respect, it may be the only cytokine which can regulate IgE production [99,100].

IL-4 stimulates the growth of mature CD4- and CD8-positive T cells [6,22] but appears to act in a different fashion from IL-2 [6,21]. It induces the proliferation of $CD4^-8^-$, $CD4^+8^-$ and $CD4^-8^+$ thymocytes in combination with phorbol ester, suggesting it may have a role in T-cell ontogeny [101], and it may induce CD8 expression on $CD4^+$ human T-cell clones [102]. Murine IL-4 is a growth factor for mast cells of the connective tissue and mucosal type [103] and acts on immature erythroid, myelomonocytic and megakaryocytic precursors [104]. It has been recorded as having negative effects by inhibiting the generation of IL-2-activated killer cells [105] and human B-cell proliferation to IL-2 [106].

The structure of the IL-4 genome and protein is summarized in Tables 2.2 and 2.3. IL-4 shows some homology with GM-CSF and IFN-γ, suggesting a phylogenetic relationship. Human and mouse proteins share approximately 50% amino acid homology [22].

There seems to be a single high-affinity receptor present in low numbers on most cells studied. In the mouse the receptor has a molecular weight of 65 kDa; in humans it is 140 kDa [21].

Interleukin-5

This cytokine was first identified as a factor which could replace the T-cell help in assays for differentiating B lymphocytes into immunoglobulin-secreting cells after antigen stimulation [107]. It is now clear that IL-5 has further effects on B cells [96] and also on eosinophils [23,108]. Murine IL-5 causes proliferation and IgM secretion by a mouse B lymphoma (BCL1), induces proliferation and secretion of IgM and IgG by activated mouse B cells and enhances IgA production by mouse B cells [55]. Whilst some reports suggest that human IL-5 does not have similar effects on human B cells to that seen on mouse B cells [109], other reports suggest that it does [22,96].

IL-5 is a potent differentiation factor for eosinophil precursors and also enhances the cytotoxic activity of the mature cells [23]. In this respect mouse IL-5 is active on human cells [110] and vice versa [109].

The structure of the IL-5 genome and protein is summarized in Tables 2.2 and 2.3. The biologically active protein appears to be a homodimer, with a similar structure and 67% amino acid homology in humans and mice [22,111].

The nature and expression of the IL-5 receptor have yet to be fully elucidated [55].

Interleukin-6

This cytokine was originally shown to stimulate antibody secretion from activated normal, or Epstein–Barr virus-transformed human B cells without stimulating proliferation [11], earning it the title B cell differentiation factor (BCDF) and B cell-stimulating factor-2 (BSF-2). It is now clear that IL-6 has a wide variety of biological activities [24]. IL-6 has been shown to support the growth of human hybridomas and plasmacytomas [112] and to have weak antiviral activity [113]. IL-6 also acts on normal bone marrow precursors to stimulate granulocyte and macrophage colony formation [114] and

acts as a co-stimulator in the proliferation of human and mouse T cells [115,116]. It causes differentiation of cytotoxic T cells [116,117] and stimulates hepatocytes to synthesize acute-phase proteins [118].

IL-6 was first shown to be derived from activated T cells or T-cell lines, but subsequently also to be produced by macrophages, endothelial cells and fibroblasts [53]. IL-6 is a multifunctional cytokine with many biological activities similar to those of IL-1. It seems that it is produced during tissue injury and infection and plays an important role in homeostasis. Production of IL-6 is induced by other cytokines such as IL-1, TNF and platelet-derived growth factor (PDGF) [119,120]. It has been shown that some of the biological activity attributable to IL-1 may be in fact due to its paracrine induction of IL-6 [121], underlining the difficulty in attributing biological effects to a particular cytokine, and the interdependence of the cytokine network.

The genomic and protein structure of IL-6 is shown in Tables 2.2 and 2.3. There is 41% amino acid homology between mouse and human proteins, which are each active on cells from the other species.

IL-6 receptors are expressed on hepatocytes, activated B and T cells, resting T cells and myeloma cells; high- and low-affinity receptors have been described [53]. A single cDNA clone encoding both high- and low-affinity receptors has been isolated [122].

Interleukin-7

IL-7 is a growth factor for early lymphoid cells of both B and T lineages without effect on myeloid cells, thereby distinguishing it from the colony-stimulating factors [27]. IL-7 supports the growth of human and mouse bone-marrow-enriched B cells. It causes proliferation of pre-B cells, which have heavy and light chain genes in germ-line configuration, and pre-B cells which have rearranged genes and express cytoplasmic immunoglobulin heavy chains, but not mature B cells. It does not cause differentiation of B cells.

IL-7 is mitogenic for resting adult thymocytes and is comitogenic in the presence of the phytohaemagglutin and concanavalin A plant lectins (PHA/ConA). Although similar to IL-2 and IL-4 in its actions, IL-7 bioactivity is not inhibited by antibodies to IL-2 and IL-4, and IL-7 does not increase the specific message for these cytokines. IL-7 stimulates the proliferation of the least mature CD4$^-$, CD8$^-$ population of thymocytes. The thymus has a high level of message, probably in the stroma, suggesting a role for IL-7 in thymocyte differentiation [26]. IL-7 is comitogenic for mature T cells in the presence of ConA.

Murine IL-7 has a 25-amino-acid leader sequence followed by 129 amino acids, predicting a protein of 14.9 kDa molecular weight. It has potential N glycosylation sites at amino acid 69 and 90 and six cysteine residues [25,26]. Loss of biological activity when the molecule is treated with 2-mercaptoethanol suggests these are important. Human and murine IL-7 share 60% homology at the amino acid level with preservation of the six cysteines. Human IL-7 however has a 19-amino-acid insert at residues 96–114, due to an additional exon in the human genome.

Interleukin-8

IL-8 is an 8 kDa non-glycosylated protein which is structurally and functionally related to a number of proteins, such as macrophage inflammatory proteins 1 and 2. It is a chemotactic factor for neutrophils [28] and therefore probably plays an important role in inflammation. Monocyte IL-8 secretion is induced by IL-1 and TNF, suggesting again that these cytokines may exert some of their reported biological activities via another intermediary cytokine.

Granulocyte–macrophage colony-stimulating factor

GM-CSF stimulates the formation of granulocyte, macrophage, mixed granulocyte–macrophage and eosinophil colonies from pluripotent stem cells and is believed to be important in the development of these cells within the bone marrow, particularly in response to stress [30,50–52,85,123]. The factor is produced by activated T cells, fibroblasts and endothelial cells stimulated with IL-1, TNF-α and LPS and monocytes and macrophages stimulated with IL-1 and LPS [29,124,125]. Apart from its function as a stimulator of haematopoiesis, GM-CSF has a wide variety of effects on mature macrophages, monocytes, neutrophils and eosinophils [123,126]. In particular, it enhances their tumoricidal and

microbicidal activities [127,128].

The GM-CSF gene is located close to the IL-3 gene on chromosome 5 [9,10] and encodes a single polypeptide chain (Table 2.2). The mature protein is glycosylated and contains disulphide bonds which are essential for biological activity (Table 2.3).

Granulocyte colony-stimulating factor

G-CSF stimulates the formation of granulocyte colonies from bone marrow pluripotent stem cells [50–52,85]. It is made by monocytes and macrophages stimulated with IL-3, LPS, M-CSF and IFN-γ, endothelial cells and fibroblasts stimulated with IL-1, as well as a number of melanoma and carcinoma cell lines [29]. It also influences mature neutrophils by enhancing their tumorilysis properties and their production of superoxide anions [29]. The human gene, located on chromosome 17 [13] like that for GM-CSF, encodes a single polypeptide chain which is glycosylated and contains disulphide bonds [129].

Macrophage colony-stimulating factor

M-CSF stimulates the formation of macrophage colonies from bone marrow pluripotent stem cells [50–52,85]. It is produced by monocytes stimulated with IL-1, IFN-γ, GM-CSF and LPS [29,130], endothelial cells stimulated with IL-1 and TNF, fibroblasts stimulated with IL-1 as well as various T and B cell lines [29]. It also affects the biological activity of mature macrophages and monocytes in a variety of ways, including induction of other cytokines (IL-1, G-CSF and IFN-γ), stimulation of tumorilysis and stimulation of intracellular killing [131].

The M-CSF gene is extremely complicated. It consists of 10 exons which can encode at least seven species of mRNA by alternate splicing events [31,131]. Two mRNA species predominate—a 4.5 kb message encoding a 554 amino acid precursor and a 1.64 kb message encoding a 256 amino acid precursor [132,133]. The protein sequence predicts an N-terminal signal sequence, a hydrophobic transmembrane region and a cytoplasmic tail at the C-terminal end. M-CSF is assembled as dimers transported to the surface and the soluble factor released from the cell surface consists of two 158–223 amino acid chains.

All three CSFs (GM-CSF, G-CSF and M-CSF) bind to individual specific receptors and there is no cross-reactivity between them.

Lymphotoxin and tumour necrosis factor

LT is released by activated T lymphocytes; it is cytotoxic and cytostatic for some tumour cell lines and causes haemorrhagic necroses of certain tumours *in vivo* [134,135]. TNF was first detected in the sera of mice injected with bacille Calmette-Guérin and subsequently challenged with endotoxin. It was shown capable of causing necrosis of some tumours *in vivo* and of being cytostatic for cell lines *in vitro* [33]. It is now clear that the principal actions of these two cytokines are inflammatory. By their actions on many different cells, they lead to physiological changes important in acute and chronic inflammation. These two cytokines share only limited (30%) amino acid sequence homology [33,35] but they bind to the same receptor [136] and have similar *in vivo* and *in vitro* biological activities. However, their cell of origin and the stimuli required to produce them are quite different. TNF is largely produced by activated macrophages and LT by activated lymphocytes. Whilst there are no reports of LT production by macrophages there are reports of TNF production by lymphocytes, NK cells and some tumour cells [33].

Particular interest in TNF arises from evidence that it mediates endotoxin shock [137–139] and that chronic exposure to TNF is responsible for the cachexia or wasting [140] associated with a number of diseases, including advanced malignancy [141] and parasitic infections [142].

The documented biological properties of TNF and LT overlap considerably with those of IL-1. This may be because these two cytokines evoke similar responses in cells. Alternatively, since TNF is known to induce macrophages to produce IL-1, the biological consequences of TNF induction may occur via IL-1.

The TNF and LT genes are separated by only 1100 base pairs and reside within the MHC on chromosome 6 in humans and 17 in mice [12,143].

TNF is synthesized as a biologically inactive prohormone of 233 amino acids in the human which is cleaved, possibly at the cell surface, to yield a 157 amino acid mature non-glycosylated protein of 17 kDa molecular weight which is the biologically active molecule [33]. The LT gene encodes a 205 amino acid sequence protein, of which the first 34 are a signal sequence [35]. The mature 171 amino acid protein is *N*-glycosylated and has a molecular weight of 25 kDa. The proteins are synthesized *de novo* on activation of the cells.

The receptor shared by TNF and LT is widely distributed, although its structure, and the signal evoked by receptor/ligand interaction, is poorly understood.

Interferons

The term *interferon* referred originally to a factor produced by cells in response to viral infection, which protected other cells from infection by the same, or other, viruses [144]. There are three main species of interferons: IFN-α, IFN-β and IFN-γ. The latter two are encoded by single genes on chromosome 9 and 12 respectively in humans, whilst the former is encoded by at least 23 different genes on chromosome 9. They have between 165 and 187 amino acids and the native proteins have molecular weights of 17–25 kDa [145–147]. Interferons induce a great many biological effects on cells by up- or down-regulating the expression of various genes. They do this by acting on regulatory genes upstream from the coding regions [148].

All three species of interferons are cytostatic and can induce an antiviral state. They confer treated cells with resistance to infection by either DNA or RNA viruses by inhibiting various stages of the viral life-cycle. In addition all three species induce expression of class I MHC antigens along with β_2-microglobulin, have anti-tumour activity *in vivo*, and induce fever. IFN-α is produced by peripheral blood mononuclear cells in response to viruses, bacteria or double-stranded RNA. IFN-β is produced by fibroblasts and epithelial cells in response to similar stimuli. IFN-γ is produced particularly by T lymphocytes upon stimulation with antigens, mitogens or alloantigens. It can be produced by CD4- or CD8-positive T lymphocytes, although the former are the major producers [149]. Interferons form an important link within the cytokine network and their production may be stimulated by other cytokines, such as IL-1, IL-2, TNF and the CSFs [147].

There are two distinct interferon receptors, one shared by IFN-α and IFN-β, thought to be of 110–130 kDa, and one used by IFN-γ which has been cloned [150].

Of paramount importance in regulation of the immune response is the ability of all interferons to induce cell-surface antigen expression, particularly that of class I MHC antigens, and of IFN-γ to induce class II MHC antigen expression. The ability to enhance the expression of existing class I MHC antigens or to induce the *de novo* expression of class II antigens renders these cytokines able to make cells more open to attack by class I MHC-restricted cytotoxic T cells, or able to act as class II-restricted antigen-presenting cells.

IFN-γ is a potent macrophage-activating factor [151] and stimulates T-cell growth and B-cell differentiation. IFN-γ inhibits both the expression of low-affinity Fcε receptor on B cells and the production of IgE by B cells. IFN-γ and IFN-α are both able to enhance the cytotoxic activities of NK and LAK cells. IFN-γ synergizes with LT and TNF in their anti-proliferative activity.

The potent ability of IFN-γ to stimulate immune responses has led to its use as an immunological adjuvant [152] and immunomodulatory drug [145]. The anti-proliferative activity of IFN-α has led to its use in the treatment of malignant disease [146].

Thymic hormones

The thymus is the organ where immature T cells develop and acquire the ability to recognize self MHC antigens and to develop tolerance [153]. These functions are acquired by the interaction of the developing thymocytes with the microenvironment of the thymus. Both cell–cell contacts and soluble factors influence thymocytes and are responsible for a sequence of changes in which immature thymocytes become mature T cells, expressing the T-cell receptor, the surface antigens CD3 and CD4 or CD8. The soluble factors which have been reported to influence thymocytes include cytokines, already

described, and other polypeptides, referred to as thymic hormones (see Chapter 1).

Two types of evidence suggest that the thymocytes are influenced by cytokines. The first is the demonstration that environmental cells of the thymus produce cytokines or express mRNA for cytokines. Thus, thymic epithelial cells produce IL-1 [154] and IL-6 and IL-7 mRNAs are expressed in thymic stromal cells [24,26]. The second type of evidence is derived from the experimental addition of cytokines to isolated thymocytes. Immature thymocytes become more mature in phenotype in the presence of IL-1 and phorbol ester [155] and combinations of IL-1 and IL-2 can activate thymocytes [156], although IL-2 alone has no effect in spite of the fact that immature thymocytes express receptors for IL-2 [157]. The addition of IL-4 has also been shown to activate thymocytes and change their surface phenotype (see above and [21]). IL-7 is mitogenic for thymocytes [27,158]. These fragmentary pieces of evidence suggest that cytokines play an important role in thymocyte development, although the sequence in which they act and their exact roles remain to be defined.

The thymic epithelium also produces a number of other polypeptides with immunopharmacological properties. These peptides, referred to as thymic hormones, stimulate T-cell functions in T-cell-deficient rodents and humans [159]. Their physiological functions include the induction of differentiation antigens on thymocytes and the enhancement or induction of the helper or suppressor functions of mature T cells.

Several polypeptides have been extracted from the thymus [159]. Thymosin fraction V (TF-V) was originally prepared from calf thymus [160] and has been used as the starting point for purification of a number of components. The TF-V mixture contains a number of polypeptides which have been purified, including thymosin β_1 (which is the same as ubiquitin [161]) and thymosin β_4 [162], both of which have immunological activity, as well as a number of others which do not. These two molecules have yet to be proven to be truly hormonal products, particularly since they are not unique to the thymus. Of the many biological activities associated with these extracts only a few have been well enough characterized to suggest an important biological role. Only thymopoietin and thymulin are produced exclusively by the thymic epithelium. These induce mature T-cell markers on precursors and stimulate various mature T-cell functions. Their biological activities are demonstrable in extracted pure native proteins or synthesized peptides. The major chemical and biological characteristics of the most investigated thymic peptides are briefly described below.

Thymosin α_1

This is a 28 amino acid peptide with a molecular weight of 3108 [160]. There is some suggestive evidence that thymosin α_1 is a proteolytic degradation product of a larger 113 amino acid prothymosin precursor molecule, of which α_1 forms the NH_2 terminus [163]. Its biological activities include stimulation of murine lymphocyte mitogenic responses and antibody production, induction of lymphokine secretion, augmentation of the number of mouse Thy 1^+, Lyt 1,2,3-positive cells and modification of terminal deoxynucleotidyl transferase (TdT) expression.

Thymopoietin

Thymopoietin is a 49 amino acid peptide with a molecular weight of 5562 which has been isolated from bovine thymus [164]. It has been shown to induce the expression of various mature T-cell antigens on thymocytes *in vitro* [165], to enhance the rejection of 3LL carcinoma, to prevent the development of autoimmunity in mice and to enhance the generation of cytotoxic T cells. The complete amino acid sequence of human thymopoietin has been determined [166] and the biological activity has been shown to reside in a pentapeptide known as thymopentin at residues 32–36 with the sequence Arg-Lys-Asp-Val-Tyr [167].

Thymulin, previously facteur thymique serique (FTS)

This is a nonapeptide, initially from porcine serum [168] but subsequently from the sera of other species, including humans. The peptide, which has a molecular weight of 847 and the sequence Glu-Ala-Lys-Ser-Glu-Gly-Gly-Ser-Asn, depends on the binding of zinc for its biological activity. The active complex with zinc therefore has a molecular weight of 922. Analogues of thymulin have been synthesized and the biological activity is found in the 7 terminal amino acids.

Thymulin is produced exclusively by the thymic epithelium and circulates in the serum. It binds to receptors on T cells, enhancing their various functions. At high levels it seems to stimulate the biological activity of suppressor T cells whilst at lower levels it can affect either T helper or suppressor cells.

Thymic humoral factor

This is a low-molecular-weight peptide originally prepared from crude thymic extract dialysate [169]. It has a molecular weight of less than 3000. It regulates the proliferation, differentiation and maturation of T helper and suppressor cells [170] and restores the competence of lymphoid cells from neonatally thymectomized mice, enabling them to participate in mixed lymphocyte reactions, to kill tumour cells and to respond to T-cell mitogens.

Other peptide regulatory factors

There have been many peptide regulatory factors identified which have important roles outside the immune system. These factors have now stimulated immunological interest because they may also be produced by or influence cells of the immune system, may be induced by cytokines or may induce cytokine secretion. In this way they may be seen as part of a larger network of cellular communication, which includes the immune system [40].

Transforming growth factor-β (TGF-β)

TGF-β is a 25 kDa disulphide-linked homodimer originally found in transformed fibroblasts. It is a member of a family of glycoproteins important in embryonic development and tissue repair [171–173]. Polypeptide chains are synthesized as inactive precursors of 360–588 amino acids with bioactive domains of 100–134 amino acids. These form hetero- or homodimers which are secreted by, and act on, a wide variety of cell types. They have been shown both to stimulate and to suppress cytokine production [158,174].

Platelet-derived growth factor

PDGF is a 30 kDa molecule consisting of two polypeptide chains of molecular weight 16 and 14 kDa which may be associated as hetero- or homodimers. PDGF is important in phases of normal cell growth, in wound repair, and in inflammatory reactions associated with fibroblast proliferation [175]. Whilst, as its name implies, it was originally isolated from human platelets, it is now clear that the molecule can be synthesized by many types of cells, including activated macrophages and endothelial cells [176]. Again, originally considered a mitogen only for connective tissue cells, it has now been shown to induce the growth of many cell types which may include blood leucocytes [177]. IL-1 can induce fibroblasts or smooth muscle cells to synthesize PDGF which then acts in an autocrine fashion and TGF-β can induce PDGF production [176].

Cyclo-oxygenase and lipoxygenase products

The pathways for prostaglandins and leukotrienes are shown in Fig. 2.1. Arachidonic acid oxygenation involves two principal enzyme pathways—the cyclo-oxygenase pathway, producing prostaglandins (PGs) [178] and the lipoxygenase pathway, which produces leukotrienes [179,180]. Their vasodilatory and hyperalgesic action are believed to contribute to the erythema, oedema and pain which characterize the inflammatory response. Their release following cytokine interaction with target cells may well mediate the biological effects of cytokines. For example, PGE_2 is a potent pyrogenic agent, and its production is thought to account for the fever induced by IL-1 and associated with its endogenous pyrogen activity [181]. Their local synthesis may modify antigen-driven immune responses. For example, at high concentrations PGE_2 is a potent inhibitor of lymphocyte activation [182], whilst at low concentrations it may stimulate immune responses. They may

act as intracellular mediators of cellular immune activation [179].

Cyclo-oxygenase products

The cyclo-oxygenase products of arachidonic acid include the PGs and thromboxanes [178]. Cyclo-oxygenase is widely distributed in mammalian cells, in all cells but erythrocytes, and cyclo-oxygenase products are synthesized in response to many inflammatory stimuli. In most situations the predominant product is PGE_2 although $PGF_{2\alpha}$, PGD_2, 6-keto $PGF_{1\alpha}$ and thromboxane B_2 have also been reported.

Evidence that PGs are important inflammatory mediators comes from the detection of prostaglandins in inflamed tissues, and the correlation between the inhibition of PGE_2 synthesis and the anti-inflammatory effects of non-steroidal anti-inflammatory drugs (NSAIDS) such as aspirin [183].

PGE_2 and PGI_2 are the most important PGs in inflammation causing vasodilation [184]. PGE_1, E_2, $F_{2\alpha}$, D_2 and I_2 may potentiate histamine, PAF and bradykinin-induced skin oedema [185]. PGD_2 causes inflammation of the skin, the histology of which reveals neutrophil infiltration [186] and causes histamine release from human basophils [187]. PDG_2 and thromboxane A_2 are chemokinetic for neutrophils [188].

Lipoxygenase products

Arachidonic acid may be oxygenated by specific lipoxygenases leading to the formation of leukotrienes, lipoxins and several hydroxyacids [179]. The leukotrienes are lipoxygenase-derivatives with at least three conjugated double bonds and include leukotriene B, C, D and E [180]. The 5-lipoxygenase pathway products seem to be particularly important in allergy and in inflammation. They are made by monocytes, neutrophils, basophils and mast cells. Any organ undergoing an inflammatory response can be shown to synthesize these products. They are produced by cells in response to both immunological and non-immunological stimuli (Table 2.6). Leukotriene B_4 is produced rapidly by mast cells, basophils, neutrophils, monocytes and perhaps lymphocytes *in vivo*. It is a major mediator of leucocyte

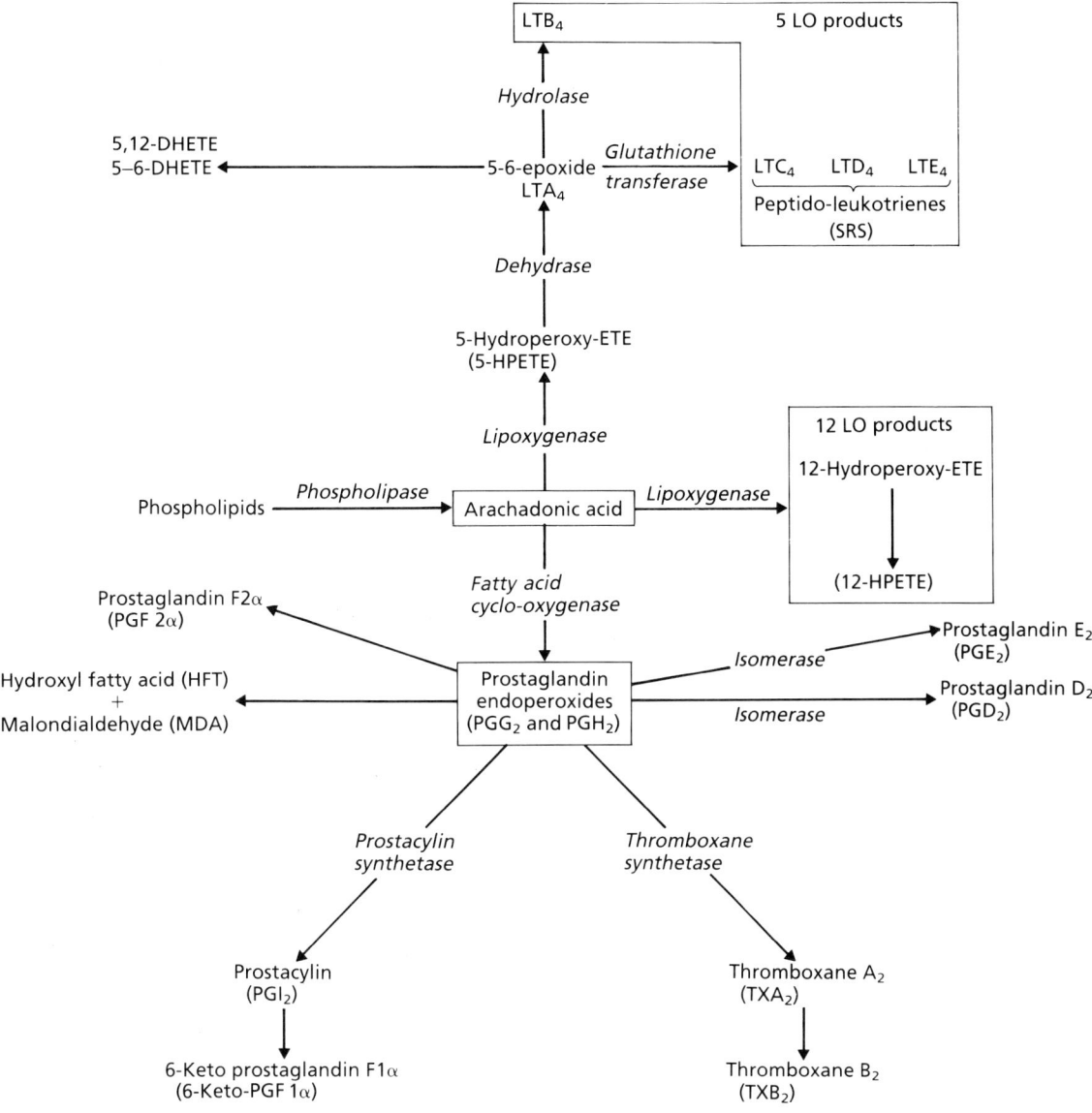

Fig. 2.1. The lipoxygenase and cyclo-oxygenase pathways. After [178, 179].

activation, causing lysosomal enzyme release, non-directed migration and chemotaxis and particularly leucocyte aggregation [189]. It is also a potent inhibitor of lymphocyte transformation, inhibiting DNA synthesis in CD4-positive T cells [190].

5-Lipoxygenase products, including leukotriene B_4, also seem to act as mediators within the cells from which they originate. They seem to be important in intracellular signalling and response to inter-leukins. Thus, in cell lines that respond either to IL-1 or to IL-2, each interleukin stimulates lipoxygenation of arachidonic acid in that target cell [191]. Participation of lipoxygenase activity seems to be required for both induction of IL-2 and IL-1 production and for regulation of proliferation and secretion of IFN-γ by IL-2 [191]. IL-1 and IL-2, as well as T-cell mitogens such as phorbol myristate acetate (PMA), may both stimulate the lipoxygenase

Immunological	Non-immunological
Micro-organisms + immunoglobulins and complement	Calcium ionophore A-23187
Phagocyte stimuli	Formyl methionyl leucyl phenylalanine (FMLP)
Aggregated immunoglobulins	Cobra venom
Multivalent anti-receptor antibodies	Serum-activated zymosan
	Purified complement components
	Lectins

Table 2.6 Stimuli of 5-lipoxygenase product formation [178]

pathway which may then be involved in the signal transduction process regulating secretion and proliferation. It is noteworthy that lipoxygenase inhibitors inhibit lymphocyte mitogenesis [192].

The slow-reacting substances are leukotrienes C, D and E. They produce slowly evolving sustained contractile responses in airway and gastrointestinal smooth muscle. Leukotriene C_4 is produced first and is usually converted rapidly to leukotriene D_4 and less rapidly to leukotriene E_4. In humans, antigen stimulates the formations of slow-reacting substances in tissues sensitized with IgE and possibly IgG_4. The major source of slow-reacting substances is considered to be mast cells [193] but macrophages may also contribute [194]. Their main biological activity is their spasmogenic action on smooth muscle and amplification of other anaphylactic stimuli [195]. Of additional immunological interest is their ability to stimulate myeloid colony formation [196].

Platelet-activating factor

This is a phospholipid mediator formed from membrane phospholipids by stimulation of inflammatory cells such as neutrophils, platelets, macrophages, eosinophils and vascular endothelial cells [197,198]. Amongst the many immunological stimulants reported to cause cells to synthesize PAF are included GM-CSF, TNF, IFN-γ and IL-1 [199–201]. Phospholipase A_2 stimulates the formation of PAF from membrane phospholipids upon cell stimulation. PAF is not stored but is synthesized rapidly within a few minutes on demand [202]. PAF activates eosino-

phils, neutrophils, macrophages and platelets, and, in view of its rapid release, would affect cells before protein cytokines like TNF and IFN-γ which are synthesized more slowly (within hours). It has been reported to induce many effects on cells, related to inflammation (Table 2.7). It has been particularly implicated as having a role in bronchial asthma (as discussed in Chapter 12) since it causes acute bronchoconstriction, bronchopulmonary hyperreactivity, platelet, eosinophil and macrophage activation, and recruitment of these cells into the airways [203]. On any one of these cells, PAF has been reported as causing a variety of effects, for example, PAF-stimulated macrophage/monocyte chemotaxis [204], aggregation [205], superoxide production [206], prostaglandin biosynthesis [207], cytotoxicity for tumour cells [208] and IL-1 production [209].

Table 2.7 Platelet-activating factor actions on inflammatory cell

Action	Cells
Activation	Platelets, eosinophils, macrophages
Aggregation	Platelets, neutrophils, monocytes
Release of lipoxygenase and cyclo-oxygenase products	Platelets, neutrophils, monocytes, eosinophils
Chemotaxis	Neutrophils, eosinophils
Dermal infiltration	Neutrophils and mononuclear cells

Free oxygen radicals

Free radicals are chemical species with one or more unpaired electrons in their outer orbit. Their production is essential to normal metabolism but unimpaired production may result in inflammation [210]. Production of superoxide anion radical ($O_2.^-$) in the respiratory burst leads to the production of hydrogen peroxide (H_2O_2) and the hydroxyl radical. The respiratory burst is produced by neutrophils, monocytes and macrophages, mast cells and eosinophils. Oxygen radicals have been reported to have various toxic effects on cells, including inhibition of certain enzymes, damage to DNA, lipid peroxidation and protein oxidation.

The physiological function of respiratory burst oxidants is destruction of invading micro-organisms, including bacteria, fungi, unicellular parasites and metazoa which are killed either intra- or extracellularly. The phagocyte is designed to restrict oxidant production to a small region like the membrane in contact with the target. However, leakage of free radicals into the microenvironment may cause damage. Such products have thus been implicated in the acute alveolar damage and pulmonary oedema seen in adult respiratory distress syndrome as well as in chronic lung disease [211].

Histamine and serotonin

Histamine and serotonin are naturally occurring amines stored within the body which play a major role in inflammation. Serotonin is important in rodents (but probably not in humans) where it causes oedema following mast cell degranulation. Histamine is stored preformed in cytoplasmic granules of mast cells and basophils, and may form 5–10% of the content of human mast cell granules. It is secreted by these cells following stimulation with a number of agents, but particularly following cross-linking of Fc receptor for IgE by IgE/antigen complexes [212] in sensitized individuals. It therefore plays a major role in the pathology of type I hypersensitivity and in particular of asthma [203]. It induces acute inflammation by causing vasodilation, increased microvascular permeability and oedema. It is also chemotactic to inflammatory cells such as eosinophils and neutrophils and stimulates T suppressor function [213].

It produces its effects by acting on specific receptors on target cells which studies with selective agonists and antagonists reveal are of three types— H_1, H_2 and H_3. H_1 receptors have been localized to airway epithelial cells, macrophages and alveolar cells in guinea pig lung, whereas the location of H_2 and H_3 receptors is not clear.

Conclusions

Soluble products are released when cells are stimulated by immunological, mechanical or chemical challenge. They act both separately and together to alter the function of the secreting cells, other neighbouring cells or distant cells. Their activities are compatible with roles in inflammatory/immune responses. Inflammatory changes frequently form part of the normal immune response and, when limited, may be regarded as beneficial. However, prolonged immunological or traumatic challenge may lead to damaging acute or chronic inflammation.

The nature of the response to cell stimulation will in part depend on the mix of mediators generated and their quantity. The cellular response of secretion of soluble factors may be immediate, when the substances are already preformed within the cell or can be rapidly synthesized. In these cases the response to stimulation may be generated within minutes or seconds and would constitute an immediate defence mechanism. Secretion of other products may occur much later, particularly if *de novo* protein synthesis is required. Most of the cytokines and interferons are only synthesized when the genes for them are activated following cell stimulation; they are not stored preformed in cells. As such, they will be secreted some hours after cell stimulation and constitute a less immediate response. In contrast the prostaglandins and leukotrienes, free radicals, complement components and histamine are produced rapidly by immediate synthesis or from storage granules and can exert their effects within minutes.

The balance determining whether secreted soluble factors produce a satisfactory limited immune response or tissue-damaging reaction also depends on homeostatic mechanisms. Continued cellular stimulation may result in continued production of mediators, which then induces a chain of responses which unchecked could be damaging. Frequently the local or limited availability of the initial stimulus is restricting and compartmentalization of a response to a particular anatomical location may further control events. A short half-life of soluble factors is evidence that most are rapidly deactivated by a variety of different processes, thereby ensuring their unavailability for bioactivity.

In summary, there is a very great number of soluble cell products which can regulate the activity of the immune system. They interact in a complex fashion to produce a beneficial effect which is limited by a variety of homeostatic mechanisms. Interference with such homeostasis may lead to the release of inappropriate levels or combinations of factors, which may ultimately result in an inappropriate immune response.

Note added in proof

There are now 11 interleukins; IL-9 (p 40, mast cell growth factor, mast cell enhancing activity, T-cell growth factor); IL-10 (cytokine synthesis factor, CS1F); and IL-11 (plasmacytoma stimulator activity).

References

1 Dumonde DC, Wolstencroft RA, Panayi GS, Matthew M, Morley J, Howson WT. "Lymphokines": non-antibody mediators of cellular immunity generated by lymphocyte activation. *Nature* 1969; 224:38–42.

2 Waksman BH. Overview: biology of the lymphokines. In: Cohen S, Pick E, Oppenheim JJ, eds. *Biology of the Lymphokines.* New York: Academic Press, 1979:585–616.

3 Cohen S. Current state of studies of mediators of cellular immunology. *Cell Immunol* 1977; 33:233–44.

4 Aarden LA, Brunner TK, Cerottini J-C *et al.* Revised nomenclature for antigen non-specific T-cell proliferation and helper factors. *J Immunol* 1979; 123: 2928–9.

5 Hamblin AS. In: Male D, Rickwood D, eds. *Lymphokines.* Oxford: IRL Press, 1988.

6 Mosmann TR, Coffman RL. TH$_1$ and TH$_2$ cells; different patterns of lymphokine secretion lead to different functional properties. *Annu Rev Immunol* 1989; 7:145–73.

7 Meager M. *Cytokines.* Buckingham: Open University Press, 1990.

8 Holbrook NJ, Smith KA, Fornace AJ, Comeau C,

Wiskocil RL, Crabtree GR. T cell growth factor: complete nucleotide sequence and organization of the gene in normal and malignant cells. *Proc Natl Acad Sci USA* 1984; 81:1634–8.

9 Van Leeuwen BH, Martinson ME, Webb GC, Young IG. Molecular organisation of the cytokine gene cluster involving human IL-3, IL-4, IL-5 and GM-CSF genes on chromosome 5. *Blood* 1989; 73:1142–8.

10 Yang Y-C, Kovacic S, Kriz R, Wolf S, Clark SC, Wellerns TE, Nieuhuis A, Epstein N. The human genes for GM-CSF and IL-3 are closely linked in tandem on chromosome 5. *Blood* 1988; 71:958–61.

11 Hirano I, Yasukawa K, Harada H, Taga T, Watanabe Y, Matsuda T, Kashiwamura S, Nakajima K, Koyama K, Iwamatsu A, Tsunasawa S, Sakiyama F, Matsui H, Takahara Y, Taniguchi T, Kishimoto T. Complementary DNA for a novel human interleukin (BSF-2) that induces B lymphocytes to produce immunoglobulin. *Nature* 1986; 324:73–6.

12 Spies T, Morton CC, Nedospasov SA, Fiers W, Pious D, Strominger JL. Genes for the tumor necrosis factors α and β are linked to the human major histocompatibility complex. *Proc Natl Acad Sci USA* 1986; 83:8699–702.

13 Kanada N, Fukushige S. Human gene coding G-CSF is assigned to the q21-q22 region of chromosome 17. *Somatic Cell Mol Genet* 1987; 13:679–84.

14 Lomedico PT, Gubler U, Mizel SB. Cloning and expression of murine, human and rabbit interleukin 1 genes. *Lymphokines* 1987; 13:139–50.

15 March CJ, Mosley B, Larsen A, Cerretti DP, Braedt G, Price V, Gillis S, Henney CS, Kronheim SR, Grabstein K, Conlon PJ, Hopp TP, Cosman D. Cloning, sequence and expression of two distinct human interleukin 1 complementary DNAs. *Nature* 1985; 315:641–7.

16 Taniguchi T, Matsui H, Fujita T, Takaoka C, Kashima N, Yoshimoto R, Hamuro J. Structure and expression of a cloned cDNA for human interleukin 2. *Nature* 1983; 302:305–10.

17 Yang YC, Ciarletta AB, Temple PA, Chung MP, Kovacic S, Witek-Giannotti JS, Leary AC, Kriz R, Donahue RE, Wong GG, Clark SC. Human IL-3 (multi-CSF) identification by expression cloning of a novel hematopoietic growth factor related to murine IL-3. *Cell* 1986; 47:3–10.

18 Ihle JN. The molecular and cellular biology of interleukin 3. In: Cruse JM, Lewis RE, eds. *The Year in Immunology 1988. Immunoregulatory Cytokines and Cell Growth.* Basel: Karger, 1989:59–102.

19 Fung MC, Hapel AJ, Ymer S, Cohen DR, Johnson RM, Campbell HD, Young IG. Molecular cloning of cDNA for murine interleukin-3. *Nature* 1984; 307:233–7.

20 Lee F, Yokota T, Otsuka T, Meyerson P, Villaret D, Coffman R, Mosmann T, Renwick D, Roehm N, Smith C, Zlotnik A, Arai K. Isolation and characterization of a mouse interleukin cDNA clone that expresses B-cell stimulatory factor 1 activities and T-cell and mast-cell stimulating activities. *Proc Natl Acad Sci USA* 1986; 83:2061–5.

21 Ohara J. Interleukin 4: molecular structure and biochemical characteristics, biological function and receptor expression. In: Cruse JM, Lewis RE, eds. *The Year in Immunology 1988. Immunoregulatory Cytokines and Cell Growth.* Basel: Karger, 1989:126–59.

22 Yokota T, Arai N, De Vries J, Spits H, Banchereau J, Zlotnik A, Rennick D, Howard M, Takebe Y, Miyatake S, Lee F, Arai KE. Molecular biology of interleukin 4 and interleukin 5 genes and biology of their products that stimulate B cells, T cells and haemopoietic cells. *Immunol Rev* 1988; 102:137–87.

23 Sanderson CJ, Campbell HD, Young IG. Molecular and cellular biology of eosinophil differentiation factor (interleukin-5) and its effects on human and mouse B cells. *Immunol Rev* 1988; 102:29–47.

24 van Snick J. Interleukin 6: an overview. *Ann Rev Immunol* 1990, 8: 253–78.

25 Namen AE, Schmierer AE, March CJ, Overell RW, Park LS, Urdal DL, Mochizuki DY. B cell precursor growth promoting activity; purification and characterization of a growth factor active on lymphocyte precursors. *J Exp Med* 1988; 167:988–1002.

26 Namen AE, Lupton S, Hjerrild K, Wignall J, Mochizuki DY, Schmierer A, Mosley B, March CJ, Urdal D, Gillis S, Cosman D, Goodwin RG. Stimulation of B cell progenitors by cloned murine interleukin-7. *Nature* 1988; 333:571–3.

27 Henney CS. Interleukin 7: effects on early events in lymphopoiesis. *Immunol Today* 1989; 10:170–3.

28 Matsushima K, Morishita K, Yoshimura T, Lavu S, Kobayashi Y, Lew W, Appella E, Kung HF, Leonard EJ, Oppenheim JJ. Molecular cloning of a human monocyte-derived neutrophil chemotactic factor (MDNCF) and the induction of MDNCF mRNA by interleukin 1 and tumour necrosis factor. *J Exp Med* 1988; 167:1883–93.

29 Ralph P, Warren MK. Molecular biology, cell biology and clinical future of myeloid growth factors. In: Cruse JM, Lewis RE, eds. *The Year in Immunology 1988; Immunoregulatory Cytokines and Cell Growth.* Basel: Karger, 1989:103–25.

30 Metcalf D. The molecular biology and functions of GM-CSF. *Blood* 1986; 67:257–67.

31 Ladner M, Martin GA. Human CSF-1. Gene structure and alternative splicing of mRNA precursors. *Eur Mol Biol Org J* 1987; 6:2693–8.

32 Wong GG, Temple PA, Leary AC *et al.* Human CSF-1. Molecular cloning and expression of a 4kb cDNA encoding the hematopoietin and determination of the complete amino acid sequence of human urinary protein. *Science* 1987; 235:1504–8.

33 Beutler B, Cerami A. The biology of cachectin/TNF—a primary mediator of the host response. *Annu Rev Immunol* 1989; 7:625–55.

34 Tavernier J, Fransen L, Marmenout A, van der Heydon J, Ruysschaert M-K, van Vliet A, Bauden R, Fiers W. Isolation and expression of the genes coding for mouse and human tumor necrosis factor (TNF) and biological properties of recombinant TNF. *Lymphokines* 1987; 13:181–98.

35 Gray PW. Molecular characterisation of human lymphotoxin. *Lymphokines* 1987; 13:199–208.

36 Brandhuber BJ, Boone T, Kenney WC, McKay DB. Three dimensional structure of interleukin-2. *Science* 1987; 238:1707–9.

37 Priestle JP, Schar HP, Grutter MG. Crystal structure of the cytokine interleukin – 1β. *EMBO J* 1988; 7:339–43.

38 Jones EY, Stuart DI, Walker NPC. Structure of tumour necrosis factor. *Nature* 1989; 338:225–8.

39 Hamblin AS, Brennan F. Cytokines. *Trends in Pharmacol* 1989; 10.

40 Green AR. Peptide regulatory factors: multifunctional mediators of cellular growth and differentiation. *Lancet* 1989; i:705–7.

41 Dinarello CA. Interleukin 1. *Dig Dis Sci* 1988; 33:255–355.

42 Watson J, Mochizuki D. Interleukin 2: a class of T cell growth factors. *Immunol Rev* 1980; 51:257–78.

43 Helle M, Boeije L, Aarden LA. Interleukin-6 is an intermediate in interleukin-1 induced thymocyte proliferation. *J Immunol* 1989; 142: 4335–8.

44 Stone-Wolf DS, Yip Y-K, Kelker HC, Lee J, Henriksen-De Stefano D, Rubin BY, Rinderknecht E, Aggarwal BB, Vilcek J. Interrelationship of human interferon gamma with lymphotoxin and monocyte cytotoxin. *J Exp Med* 1984; 159:828–43.

45 Mossmann TR, Cherwinski H, Bond MW, Giedlin MA, Coffman RL. Two types of murine helper T cell clone I. Definition according to profiles of lymphokine activities and secreted proteins. *J Immunol* 1986; 136:2348–57.

46 Cherwinski HM, Schumacher JH, Brown KD, Mosmann TR. Two types of mouse helper T cell clone III. Further differences in lymphokine synthesis between Th$_1$ and Th$_2$ clones revealed by RNA hybridization, functionally monospecific bioassays and monoclonal antibodies. *J Exp Med* 1987; 166:1229–44.

47 O'Garra A. Interleukins and the immune system 2. *Lancet* 1989; i:1003–5.

48 Smith KA. Interleukin 2; inception, impact and im-

plications. *Science* 1988; 240:1169–76.

49 Mizel S. Interleukin 1 and T-cell activation. *Immunol Today* 1987; 8:330–2.

50 Clarke SC, Kamen R. The human hematopoietic colony-stimulating factors. *Science* 1987; 236:1229–37.

51 Metcalf D. Haemopoietic growth factors 1. *Lancet* 1989; i: 825–7.

52 Sieff CA. Hematopoietic growth factors. *J Clin Invest* 1987; 79:1549–57.

53 Kishimoto T, Hirano T. Molecular regulation of B lymphocyte responses. *Annu Rev Immunol* 1988; 6:485–512.

54 Oppenheim JJ, Kovacs EJ, Matsushima K, Durum SK. There is more than one interleukin I. *Immunol Today* 1986; 7:45–56.

55 Harriman GR, Strober W. The immunobiology of interleukin 5. In: Cruse JM, Lewis RE, eds. *The Year in Immunology 1988; Immunoregulatory Cytokines and Cell Growth.* Basel: Karger, 1989:160–77.

56 Ueno Y, Takano N, Kanegane T, Yokoi T, Yachie A, Miyawaki T, Taniguchi N. The acute phase nature of interleukin 6: studies in Kawasaki disease and other febrile illnesses. *Clin Exp Immunol* 1989; 76:337–42.

57 Gery IR, Gershon RK, Waksman BH. Potentiation of the lymphocyte response to mitogens I. The responding cell. *J Exp Med* 1972; 136:143–52.

58 di Giovine FS, Duff GW. Interleukin 1: the first interleukin. *Immunol Today* 1990; II:13–20.

59 Sims JE, March CJ, Cosman D, Widmer MB, MacDonald HR, McMahan C, Grubin CE, Wignall JM, Jackson JL, Call SM, Friend D, Alpert AR, Gillis S, Urdal DL, Dower SK. cDNA expression cloning of the IL-1 receptor, a member of the immunoglobulin superfamily. *Science* 1988; 241:585-9.

60 Auron PE, Warner SJC, Webb AC, Cannon JG, Bernheim HA, McAdam KJPW, Rosenwasser LJ, Lopreste G, Mucci SF, Dinarello CA. Studies on the molecular nature of human interleukin 1. *J Immunol* 1987; 138:1447–56.

61 Boraschi D, Nencioni L, Villa L, Censini S, Bossu P, Ghiara P, Presentini R, Perin F, Frasco D, Doria G, Forni G, Musso T, Giovarelli M, Ghezzi P, Bertini R, Besedovsky HO, Del Rey A, Sipe JD, Antoni G, Silvestri S, Tagliabue A. *In vivo* stimulation and restoration of the immune response by the non-inflammatory fragment 163–171 of human interleukin-1β. *J Exp Med* 1988; 168:675–86.

62 Scala G, Oppenheim JJ. Antigen presentation by human monocytes: evidence for stimulant processing and requirement for interleukin 1. *J Immunol* 1983; 131:1160–6.

63 Kurt-Jones EA, Virgin HW, Unanue ER. Relationship of macrophage Ia and membrane IL-1 expression to antigen presentation. *J Immunol* 1985; 135:3652–4.

64 Kurt-Jones EA, Beller DI, Mizel SB, Unanue ER. Identification of a membrane associated IL-1. *Proc Natl Acad Sci (USA)* 1985; 82:1204–8.

65 Rock KL, Haber SI, Liano D, Benacerraf B, Abbas AK. Antigen presentation by hapten specific B lymphocytes III. Analysis of the immunoglobulin dependent pathway of antigen presentation to IL-1 dependent T lymphocytes. *Eur J Immunol* 1986; 16:1407–12.

66 Kurt-Jones EA, Hamberg S, Ohara J, Paul WE, Abbas AK. Heterogeneity of helper/inducer T lymphocytes I. Lymphokine production and lymphokine responsiveness. *J Exp Med* 1987; 166:1774–87.

67 Jampel HD, Duff GW, Gershon RK, Atkins E, Durum SK. Fever and immunoregulation III. Hyperthermia augments the primary *in vitro* humoral immune response. *J Exp Med* 1983; 157:1229–38.

68 Pepys MB, Baltz M. Acute phase proteins with special reference to C-reactive protein and related proteins (pentaxins) and serum amyloid A protein. *Adv Immunol* 1983; 34:141–212.

69 Mochizuki DY, Eisenmann JR, Conlon PJ, Larsen AD, Tushinski RJ. Interleukin 1 regulates haematopoietic activity, a role previously ascribed to haemopoietin I. *Proc Natl Acad Sci (USA)* 1987; 84:5267–71.

70 Howard M, Paul WE. Regulation of B-cell growth differentiation by soluble factors. *Annu Rev Immunol* 1983; 1:307–33.

71 Morgan DA, Ruscetti FW, Gallo R. Selective *in vitro* growth of T lymphocytes from normal human bone marrows. *Science* 1976; 193:1007–8.

72 Kaempfer R, Efrat S, Marsh S. Regulation of human interleukin 2 gene expression. *Lymphokines* 1987; 13:59–72.

73 Watson J. Continuous proliferation of murine antigen-specific helper T lymphocytes in culture. *J Exp Med* 1979; 150:1510–19.

74 Heberman R, Ortaldo J. Natural killer cells; their role in defenses against disease. *Science* 1981; 214:24–9.

75 Tsudo M, Kozak RW, Goldman CK, Waldman TA. Demonstration of a non-Tac peptide that binds interleukin 2: a potential participant in a multichain interleukin 2 receptor complex. *Proc Natl Acad Sci (USA)* 1986; 83:9694–8.

76 Teshigawara K, Wang HM, Kato K, Smith KA. Interleukin 2 high affinity receptor expression requires two distinct binding proteins. *J Exp Med* 1987; 165:223–38.

77 Smith K. The interleukin 2 receptor. *Adv Immunol* 1988; 42:165–79.

78 Cantrell DA, Smith KA. Transient expression of interleukin 2 receptors. Consequences for T-cell

growth. *J Exp Med* 1983; 158:1895–911.

79 Sharon M, Siegel JP, Tosato G, Yodoi J, Gerrard TL, Leonard WJ. The human interleukin 2 receptor beta chain (p70). Direct identification, partial purification and patterns of expression on peripheral blood mononuclear cells. *J Exp Med* 1988; 167:1265–70.

80 Leibson HJ, Marrack P, Kappler JW. B cell helper factors I. Requirement for both interleukin 2 and another 40 000 mol. wt. factor. *J Exp Med* 1981; 154:1681–93.

81 Malkowsky M, Loveland B, North M, Asherson GL, Gao L, Ward P, Fiers W. Recombinant interleukin-2 directly augments the cytotoxicity of human monocytes. *Nature* 1987; 325:262–5.

82 Grimm EA, Mazumder A, Zhang HZ, Rosenberg SA. Lymphokine activated killer cell phenomenon; lysis of natural killer resistant fresh solid tumour cells by interleukin 2-activated autologous human peripheral blood lymphocytes. *J Exp Med* 1982; 155:1823–41.

83 Rosenberg SA, Lotze MT, Muul LM, Leitman S, Chang AE, Ettinghausen SE, Matory YL, Skibber JM, Shiloni E, Vetto JT, Seipp CA, Simpson C, Reichert CM. Observations on the systemic administration of autologous lymphokine activated killer cells and recombinant interleukin 2 to patients with metastatic carcinoma. *N Engl J Med* 1985; 313:1485–97.

84 Siegel JP, Sharon M, Smith PL, Leonard WJ. The IL-2 receptor beta chain (p70): role in mediating signals for LAK, NK and proliferative activities. *Science* 1987; 238:75–80.

85 Metcalf D. The molecular control of cell division, differentiation commitment and maturation in haemopoietic cells. *Nature* 1989; 339:27–30.

86 Kindler V, Thorens B, Kossodo S de, Allet B, Eliason JF, Thatcher D, Farber N, Vassalli P. Stimulation of haematopoiesis *in vivo* by recombinant bacterial murine interleukin 3. *Proc Natl Acad Sci USA* 1986; 83:1001–5.

87 Metcalf D, Begley CG, Johnson GR, Nicola NA, Lopez AF, Williamson DJ. Effects of purified bacterially synthesized murine multi-CSF (IL-3) on haematopoiesis in normal adult mice. *Blood* 1986; 68:46–57.

88 Kimoto M, Kindler V, Higaki M, Ody C, Izui S, Vassalli P. Recombinant murine IL-3 fails to stimulate T or B lymphopoiesis *in vivo*, but enhances immune responses to T cell-dependent antigens. *J Immunol* 1988; 140:1889–94.

89 Prystowsky MB, Ely JM, Beller DI, Eisenberg L, Goldman J, Goldman M, Goldwasser E, Ihle J, Quintans J, Remold H, Vogel SN, Fitch FW. Alloreactive cloned T cell lines VI. Multiple lymphokine activities secreted by cytolytic cloned T lymphocytes. *J Immunol* 1982; 129:2337–44.

90 Lee JC, Hapel AJ, Ihle JN. Constitutive production of a unique lymphokine (IL-3) by the WEH1-3 cell line. *J Immunol* 1982; 128:2393–8.

91 Razin E, Ihle JN, Selden D, Mencia-Huerta JM, Katz HR, Le Blanc PA, Hein A, Caulfield JP, Austen KF, Stevens RL. Interleukin 3. A differentiation and growth factor for the mouse mast cell that contains chondroitin sulphate E proteoglycan. *J Immunol* 1984; 132:1479–86.

92 Lopez AF, To LB, Yang Y-C, Gamble JR, Shannon MF, Burns GF, Dyson PG, Juttner CA, Clark SC, Vadas MA. Stimulation of proliferation, differentiation and function of human cells by primate interleukin 3. *Proc Natl Acad Sci USA* 1987; 84:2761–5.

93 Hauck-Frendscho M, Aria N, Aria KI, Beeza ML, Finn A, Kaplan AP. Human recombinant granulocyte-macrophage colony stimulating factor and interleukin 3 cause basophil histamine release. *J Clin Invest* 1988; 82:17–25.

94 Cannistra SA, Vellenga E, Groshek P, Rambaldi A, Griffin JD. Human granulocyte-monocyte colony stimulating factor and interleukin 3 stimulate monocyte cytotoxicity through a tumor necrosis factor-dependent mechanism. *Blood* 1988; 71:672–6.

95 Howard M, Farrar J, Hilfiker M, Johnson B, Takatsu K, Hamaoka T, Paul WE. Identification of a T-cell derived B-cell growth factor distinct from interleukin-2. *J Exp Med* 1982; 155:914–23.

96 Coffman RL, Seymour BW, Lebman DA, Hiraki DD, Christiansen JA, Shrader B, Cherwinski HM, Savelkoul HF, Finkelman FD, Bond MW, Mosmann TR. The role of helper T cell products in mouse B cell differentiation and isotype regulation. *Immunol Rev* 1988; 102:5–28.

97 Snapper CM, Finkelman FD, Paul WE. Regulation of IgG and IgE production by interleukin 4. *Immunol Rev* 1988; 102:29–56.

98 Hu-Li J, Shevach EM, Mizuguchi J, Ohara J, Mosmann T, Paul WE. B cell stimulatory factor-1 (interleukin 4) is a potent costimulant for normal resting T lymphocytes. *J Exp Med* 1987; 165:157–72.

99 Finkelman FP, Katona I, Urban J, Snapper CM, Ohara J, Paul WE. Suppression of *in vivo* polyclonal IgE responses by monoclonal antibody to the lymphokine BSF-1. *Proc Natl Acad Sci USA* 1986; 83:9675–83.

100 Coffman RL, Ohara J, Bond MW, Carty J, Zlotnik A, Paul WE. B cell stimulatory factor-1 enhances the IgE response of lipopolysaccharide-activated B-cells. *J Immunol* 1986; 136:4538–41.

101 Zlotnick A, Ransom J, Frank G, Fisher M, Howard M. Interleukin 4 is a growth factor for activated thymocytes: possible role in T-cell ontogeny. *Proc Natl Acad Sci USA* 1987; 84:3856–60.

102 Paliard X, de Waal Malefijt R, De Vries J, Spits H. Interleukin-4 mediates CD8 induction on human CD4⁺ T cell clones. *Nature* 1988; 335:642–4.

103 Hamaguchi Y, Kanakura Y, Fujita J, Takeda S, Nakano T, Tarui S, Honjo T, Kitamura Y. Interleukin 4 as an essential factor for *in vitro* clonal growth of murine connective tissue-type mast cells. *J Exp Med* 1987; 165;268–73.

104 Peschel C, Paul WE, Ohara J, Green I. Effects of B cell stimulating factor 1/interleukin 4 on haematopoietic progenitor cells. *Blood* 1987; 70:254–63.

105 Spits H, Yssel H, Paliard X, Kastelein R, Figdor C, de Vries JE. IL-4 inhibits IL-2 mediated induction of human lymphokine activated killer cells, but not the generation of antigen-specific cytotoxic T lymphocytes in mixed lymphocyte cultures. *J Immunol* 1988; 141:29–36.

106 Jellinek DF, Lipsky PE. Inhibitory influence of IL-4 on B cell responsiveness. *J Immunol* 1988; 141:164–73.

107 Schimpl A, Wecker E. Replacement of T cell function by a T cell product. *Nature* 1972; 237:15–19.

108 Sanderson CJ, O'Garra A, Warren DJ, Klaus GGB. Eosinophil differentiation factor also has B-cell growth factor activity; proposed name interleukin 4. *Proc Natl Acad Sci USA* 1986; 83:437–40.

109 Clutterbuck E, Shields JG, Gordon J, Smith SH, Boyd A, Callard RE, Campbell HD, Young IG, Sanderson CJ. Recombinant human interleukin 5 is an eosinophil differentiation factor but has no activity in standard human B cell growth factor assays. *Eur J Immunol* 1987; 17:1743–50.

110 Lopez AF, Begley CG, Williamson DJ, Warren DJ, Vadas MA, Sanderson CJ. Murine eosinophil differentiation factor. An eosinophil-specific colony-stimulating factor with activity for human cells. *J Exp Med* 1986; 163:1085–99.

111 Campbell HD, Tucker WQJ, Hort Y, Martinson ME, Mayo G, Clutterbuck EJ, Sanderson CJ, Young IG. Molecular cloning, nucleotide sequence and expression of the gene encoding human eosinophil differentiation factor (interleukin 5). *Proc Natl Acad Sci USA* 1987; 84:6629–33.

112 Van Damme J, Opdenakker G, Simpson RJ, Rubira MR, Cayphas S, Vink A, Billiau A, van Snick J. Identification of the human 26-KD protein interferon β_2 (IFN β_2), as a B cell hybridoma/plasmacytoma growth factor induced by interleukin 1 and tumour necrosis factor. *J Exp Med* 1987; 165:914–19.

113 Zilberstein A, Ruggieri R, Korn JH, Revel M. Structure and expression of cDNA and genes for human interferon-beta-2, a distinct species inducible by growth stimulatory cytokines. *EMBO J* 1986; 5:2519–37.

114 Wong CG, Witek-Giannotti JS, Temple PA, Kriz R, Ferenz C, Hewick RM, Clark SC, Ikebuchi K, Ogawa M. Stimulation of murine haemopoietic colony formation by human IL-6. *J Immunol* 1988; 140:3040–4.

115 Garman RD, Jacobs KA, Clark SC, Raulet DH. B cell stimulatory factor 2 (β_2 interferon) functions as a second signal for interleukin-2 production by mature murine T cells. *Proc Natl Acad Sci USA* 1987; 84:7629–33.

116 Uyttenhove C, Coulie PG, Van Snick J. T cell growth and differentiation induced by interleukin-HP 1/IL-6, the murine hybridoma/plasmacytoma growth factor. *J Exp Med* 1988; 167:1417–27.

117 Takui Y, Wong GC, Clark SC, Burakoff SJ, Herrmann SH. B cell stimulatory factor-2 is involved in the differentiation of cytotoxic T lymphocytes. *J Immunol* 1988; 140:508–12.

118 Gauldie J, Richards C, Harnish D, Landsdorp P, Baumann H. Interferon β_2/B-cell stimulatory factor type 2 shares identity with monocyte-derived hepatocyte-stimulating factor and regulates the major acute phase protein response in liver cells. *Proc Natl Acad Sci USA* 1987; 84:7251–5.

119 Kohase M, May LT, Tamm I, Vilcek J, Sehgal PB. A cytokine network in human, diploid fibroblasts: interaction of β-interferons, tumour necrosis factor, platelet-derived growth factor, and interleukin-1. *Mol Cell Biol* 1987; 7:273–80.

120 Content L, De Wit L, Poupart P, Opdenakker G, Van Damme J, Billiau A. Induction of a 26-KDa-protein mRNA in human cells treated with an interleukin-1-related, leukocyte-derived factor. *Eur J Biochem* 1985; 152:253–7.

121 Helle M, Brakenhoff JPJ, De Groot ER, Aarden LA. Interleukin 6 is involved in interleukin-1 induced activities. *Eur J Immunol* 1988; 18:957–9.

122 Yamasaki K, Taga T, Hirata Y, Yawata H, Kawanishi Y, Sead B, Taniguchi T, Hirano T, Kishimoto T. Cloning and expression of the human interleukin-6 (BSF-2/IFN β-2) receptor. *Science* 1988; 241:825–8.

123 Metcalf D, Begley CG, Johnson GR, Nicola NA, Vadas MA, Lopez AF, Williamson DJ, Wong GG, Clark SC, Wang EA. Biologic properties *in vitro* of a recombinant human granulocyte-macrophage colony stimulating factor. *Blood* 1986; 67:37–45.

124 Thorens B, Mermod JJ, Vassalli P. Phagocytosis and inflammatory stimuli induce GM-CSF mRNA in macrophages through post-transcriptional regulation. *Cell* 1986; 48:671–9.

125 Sieff CA, Tsai S, Faller DV. Interleukin 1 induces cultured human endothelial cell production of granulocyte-macrophage colony-stimulating factor. *J Clin Invest* 1987; 79:48–51.

126 Lopez AF, Williamson DJ, Gamble JR, Begley CG,

Harlan JM, Kelbanoff SJ, Waltersdorph A, Wong G, Clark SC, Vadas MA. Recombinant human granulocyte-macrophage colony-stimulating factor stimulates *in vitro* mature human neutrophil and eosinophil function, surface receptor expression and survival. *J Clin Invest* 1986; 78:1220–8.

127 Vadas MA, Nicola NA, Metcalf D. Activation of antibody-dependent cell-mediated cytotoxicity of human neutrophils and eosinophils by separate colony-stimulating factors. *J Immunol* 1983; 130:795–9.

128 Grabstein KH, Urdal DL, Tushinski RJ, Mochizuki DY, Price VL, Cantrell MA, Gillis S, Conlon PJ. Induction of macrophage tumoricidal activity by granulocyte macrophage colony-stimulating factor. *Science* 1986; 232:506–8.

129 Souza LM, Boone TC, Gabrilove JL, Lai PH, Zsebo KM, Murdock DC, Chazin VR, Bruszewski J, Lu H, Chen KK, Barendt J, Platzer E, Moore MAS, Mertelsmann R, Welte K. Recombinant human granulocyte colony stimulating factor: effects on normal and leukaemic myeloid cells. *Science* 1986; 232:61–5.

130 Rambaldi A, Young DC, Griffin JD. Expression of the M-CSF (CSF-1) gene by human monocytes. *Blood* 1987; 69:1409–15.

131 Ralph P, Warren MK, Ladner MB. Molecular and biological properties of human CSF-1. *Cold Spring Harbor Symp Q Biol* 1986; 51:679–83.

132 Arsdell JV, Warren MK, Coyne MY *et al.* Molecular cloning of a complementary DNA encoding human macrophage-specific colony-stimulating factor (CSF-I). *Science* 1985; 230:291–6.

133 Wong GG, Temple PA. Human CSF-1. Molecular cloning and expression of a 4Kb cDNA encoding the haematopoietin and determination of the complete amino acid sequence of the human urinary protein. *Science* 1987; 235:1504–8.

134 Paul NL, Ruddle NH. Lymphotoxin. *Annu Rev Immunol* 1988; 6:407–38.

135 Carswell EA, Old LJ, Kassel RL, Green S, Fiore N, Williamson B. An endotoxin-induced serum factor that causes necrosis of tumours. *Proc Natl Sci USA* 1975; 72: 3666–70.

136 Aggarwal BB, Eessalu TE, Hass PE. Characterisation of receptors for human necrosis factor and their regulation by gamma-interferon. *Nature* 1985; 318:665–7.

137 Tracey KJ, Vlassara H, Cerami A. Peptide regulatory factors; cachectin/tumour necrosis factor. *Lancet* 1989; i:1122–6.

138 Mannel DN, Falk W, Northoff H. Endotoxic activities of tumour necrosis factor independent of IL-1 secretion by macrophages/monocytes. *Lymphokine Res* 1987; 6:151–9.

139 Bauss F, Droege W, Mannel DN. Tumour necrosis factor mediates endotoxic effects in mice. *Infect Immunol* 1987; 55:1622–5.

140 Oliff A, Defeo-Jones D, Bayer M, Martinez D, Kiefer D, Vuocolo G, Wolfe A, Socher SH. Tumours secreting human TNF/cachectin induce cachexia in mice. *Cell* 1987; 50:555–63.

141 Balkwill F, Burke F, Talbot D, Tavernier J, Osborne R, Naylor S, Durbin H, Fiers W. Evidence for tumour necrosis factor/cachectin production in cancer. *Lancet* 1987; ii:1229–32.

142 Grau GE, Fajardo LF, Piguet PF, Allet B, Lambert PH, Vassalli P. Tumour necrosis factor (cachectin) as an essential mediator in murine cerebral malaria. *Science* 1987; 237:1210–12.

143 Semon D, Kawashima E, Jongeneel CV, Shakhov AN, Nedospasov SA. Nucleotide sequence of the murine TNF locus, including the TNF-α (tumour necrosis factor) and TNF-β (lymphotoxin) genes. *Nucleic Acids Res* 1987; 15:9083–4.

144 Issaacs A, Lindenmann J. Virus interference. The interferon. *Proc R Soc Lond* 1957; Series B: 259–67.

145 Balkwill FR. Peptide regulatory factors; interferons. *Lancet* 1989; i:1060–3.

146 Balkwill FR. *Cytokines in Cancer Therapy.* Oxford: Oxford University Press, 1989.

147 De Maeyer E, De Maeyer-Guignard J. *Interferons and Other Regulatory Cytokines.* Chichester: John Wiley, 1988.

148 Revel M, Chebath J. Interferon-activated genes. *Trends Biochem Sci* 1986; 11: 166–70.

149 Trinchieri G, Perussia B. Immune interferon: a pleiotropic lymphokine with multiple effects. *Immunol Today* 1985; 6:131–6.

150 Aguet M, Dembic Z, Merlin G. Molecular cloning and expression of the human interferon γ receptor. *Cell* 1988; 55:273–80.

151 Adams DO, Hamilton TA. Molecular transductional mechanisms by which IFN γ and other signals regulate macrophage development. *Immunol Rev* 1987; 97:5–27.

152 Playfair JHL, De Souza JB. Recombinant γ interferon is a potent adjuvant for a murine malaria vaccine in mice. *Clin Exp Immunol* 1987; 67:5–10.

153 Lamb J, Owen M. In: Male D, Rickwood D, eds. *Immune Recognition.* Oxford: IRL Press, 1988.

154 Le PT, Tuck DT, Dinarello CA, Haynes BF, Singer KH. Human thymic epithelial cells produce interleukin 1. *J Immunol* 1987; 138:2520–6.

155 De Vries JE, Vyth-Dreese FA, Figdor CG, Spits H, Leemans JM, Bont NS. Induction of phenotypic differentiation, interleukin 2 production and PHA-responsiveness of "immature" human thymocytes by interleukin 1 and phorbol ester. *J Immunol* 1983; 131:201–6.

156 Mannel DN, Mizel SB, Diamantstein T, Falk W. Induction of interleukin 2 responsiveness in thymocytes by synergistic action of interleukin 1 and interleukin 2. *J Immunol* 1985; 134:1241–9.

157 Fox DA, Hussey RE, Fitzgerald KA, Bensussan A, Daley JF, Schlossman S. Activation of human thymocytes via the 50Kd T11 sheep erythrocyte binding protein induces the expression of interleukin 2 receptors on both T3+ and T3– populations. *J Immunol* 1985; 134:330–5.

158 Chantry D, Turner M, Feldman M. IL-7 stimulates thymocyte growth; regulation by TGF β. *Eur J Immunol* 1989; 19:783–6.

159 Trainin N, Pecht M, Handzel ZT. Thymic hormones, inducers and regulators of T cell system. *Immunol Today* 1983; 4:16–21.

160 Goldstein AL, Low TLK, Mcadoo M, Mclure J, Thurman GB, Rossio JJ, Lai CY, Chang D, Wang SS, Harvey C, Ramel AH, Meienhoffer J. Thymosin α_1: isolation and sequence analysis of immunologically active thymic polypeptide. *Proc Natl Acad Sci USA* 1977; 74:725–9.

161 Schlesinger DH, Goldstein G, Niall HD. The complete amino acid sequence of ubiquitin, an adenylate cyclase stimulating polypeptide probably universal in living cells. *Biochem* 1975; 14:2214–18.

162 Schulof RS, Goldstein AL. Thymosins and other thymic hormones. In: Stewart JW, Stewart WE II, eds. *The Lymphokines, Biochemistry and Biological Activity.* New Jersey: Humana Press, 1981:397–402.

163 Haritos AA, Blacher R, Stein S, Caldarella J, Horecker BL. Primary structure of rat thymus prothymosin α. *Proc Natl Acad Sci USA* 1985; 82:343–5.

164 Goldstein G, Lau C. Thymopoietin and immunoregulation. In: Beer RF, Basselt EG, eds. *Polypeptide Hormones.* New York: Raven Press, 1980:459–65.

165 Komuro K, Boyse EA. Induction of lymphocytes from precursor cells *in vitro* by a product of a thymus. *J Exp Med* 1973; 139:193–207.

166 Audhya T, Schlesinger DH, Goldstein G. Isolation and complete amino acid sequence of human thymopoietin and splenin. *Biochemistry* 1987; 84:3545–9.

167 Goldstein G, Scheid MP, Boyse EA, Schlesinger DH, Van Vauwe J. A synthetic pentapeptide with biological activity characteristic of the thymic hormone thymopoietin. *Science* 1979; 204:1309–10.

168 Bach JF, Dardenne M, Pleau JM, Rosa J. Biochemical characterisation of a serum thymic factor. *Nature* 1976; 266:55–6.

169 Trainin N, Rolter V, Yakir Y, Leve R, Handzel ZT, Shahat B, Zaizov R. Biochemical and biological properties of THF in animal and human models. *Ann NY Acad Sci* 1979; 332:9–22.

170 Trainin N, Handzel ZT, Pecht M. Biological and clinical properties of THF. *Thymus* 1985; 7:137–50.

171 Massagué J. The TGF-β family of growth and differentiation factors. *Cell* 1987; 49:437–8.

172 Slack JMW. Peptide regulatory factors in embryonic development. *Lancet* 1989; i:1312–15.

173 Wahl SM, McCartney-Francis N, Mergenhagen SE. Inflammatory and immunomodulatory roles of TGF-β. *Immunol Today* 1989; 10:258–61.

174 Chantry D, Turner M, Abne E, Feldman M. Modulation of cytokine production by transforming growth factor-β. *J Immunol* 1989; 142:4295–300.

175 Ross R. Peptide regulatory factors: platelet derived growth factor. *Lancet* 1989; i:1179–82.

176 Ross R, Raines EW, Bowen-Pope DF. The biology of platelet-derived growth factor. *Cell* 1986; 46:155–9.

177 Deuel TF. Polypeptide growth factors: roles in normal and abnormal cell growth. *Annu Rev Cell Biol* 1987; 3:443–92.

178 Salmon JA, Higgs GA. Prostaglandins and leukotrienes as inflammatory mediators. *Br Med Bull* 1987; 43:285–96.

179 Parker CW. Lipid mediators produced through the lipoxygenase pathway. *Annu Rev Immunol* 1987; 5:65–84.

180 Piper PJ, Samhoun MN. Leukotrienes. *Br Med Bull* 1987; 43:297–311.

181 Bernheim HA, Gilbert TM, Stitt JT. Prostaglandin E levels in third ventricular cerebrospinal fluid of rabbits during fever and changes in body temperature. *J Physiol* 1980; 301:69–78.

182 Goodwin JS, Bankhurst AD, Messner RP. Suppression of human cell mitogenesis by prostaglandin. *J Exp Med* 1977; 146:1719–34.

183 Shen TY. Prostaglandin synthetase inhibitors I. In: Vane JR, Ferreira SH, eds. *Anti-Inflammatory Drugs.* Berlin: Springer-Verlag, 1979; 65: 305–47.

184 Williams TJ. Prostaglandin E_2, prostaglandin I_2 and the vascular changes of inflammation. *Br J. Pharmacol* 1979; 517–24.

185 Williams TJ, Morley J. Prostaglandins as potentiators of increased vascular permeability in inflammation. *Nature (Lond)* 1973; 246:215–17.

186 Soter NA, Lewis RA, Corey EJ, Austen KF. Local effects of synthetic leukotrienes (LTC4, LTD4, LTE4 and LTB4) in human skin. *J Invest Dermatol* 1983; 80:115–19.

187 Peters SP, Kagey-Sobotka A, MacGlashan DW, Lichtenstein LM. Effect of prostaglandin D_2 in modulating histamine from human basophils. *J Pharmacol Exp Ther* 1984; 228:400–6.

188 Goetzl EJ, Weller PF, Valone FH. Biochemical and functional basis of the regulatory and protective roles of the human eosinophil. In: Weissman G, Samuelson B, Paoletti R, eds. *Advances in Inflammation Re-*

search. New York: Raven Press, 1976:157–67.

189 Ford-Hutchinson AW, Bray MA, Doig MV, Shipley ME, Smith MJH. Leukotriene B$_4$, a potent chemokinetic and aggregating substance released from polymorphonuclear leukocytes. *Nature* 1981; 286:264–5.

190 Gualde N, Atluru D, Goodwin JS. Effect of lipoxygenase metabolites of arachidonic acid on proliferation of human T cells and T cell subsets. *J Immunol* 1985; 134:1125–9.

191 Farrar WL, Humes JL. The role of arachidonic acid metabolism in the activities of interleukin 1 and 2. *J Immunol* 1985; 135:1153–9.

192 Kelly JP, Parker CW. Effects of arachidonic acid and other unsaturated fatty acids on mitogenesis in human lymphocytes. *J Immunol* 1979; 122:1556–62.

193 Robin JL, Seldin DC, Austen KF, Lewis RA. Regulation of mediator release from mouse bone-marrow derived mast cells by glucocorticoids. *J Immunol* 1985; 135:2719–26.

194 Bonney RJ, Opas EE, Humes JL. Lipoxygenase pathways of macrophages. *Fed Proc* 1985; 44:2933–6.

195 Parker CW. The chemical nature of slow-reacting substances. In: Weissmann I, ed. *Advances in Inflammation Research.* vol 4. New York: Raven Press, 1982:1–24.

196 Ziboh VA, Wong T, Wu M-C, Yunis AA. Modulation of colony stimulating factor-induced murine myeloid colony formation by S peptide-lipoxygenase products. *Cancer Res* 1986; 46:600–3.

197 Braquet P, Shen TY, Touqui L, Vargaftig BB. Perspectives in platelet activating factor research. *Pharmacol Rev* 1987; 39:97–145.

198 Vargaftig BB, Braquet PG. PAF-acether today—relevance for acute experimental anaphylaxis. *Br Med Bull* 1987; 43:312–35.

199 Bussolino F, Breviario F, Tetta C, Aglietta M, Mantovani A, Dejana E. Interleukin 1 stimulates plateletactivating factor production in cultured human endothelial cells. *J Clin Invest* 1986; 77:2027–33.

200 Camussi G, Bussolino F, Salvidio G, Baglioni C. Tumour necrosis factor/cachectin stimulates peritoneal macrophages, polymorphonuclear neutrophils and vascular endothelial cells to synthesize and release platelet-activating factor. *J Exp Med* 1987; 166:1390–1404.

201 Wirthmueller U, De Weck AL, Dahinden CA. Platelet-activated-factor production in human neutrophils by sequential stimulation with granulocyte-macrophage colony-stimulating factor and the chemotactic factors CSA or formyl-methionyl-leucyl-phenylalanine. *J Immunol* 1989; 142:3213–18.

202 Tence M, Polonsky J, Le Couedic JP, Beuveniste J. Release, purification and characterisation of platelet activating factor (PAF). *Biochimie* 1980; 62:251–9.

203 Barnes PJ, Chung KF, Page CP. Inflammatory mediators and asthma. *Pharmacol Rev* 1988; 40:49–84.

204 Valone FH, Goetzl EJ. Specific binding by human polymorphonuclear leukocytes of the immunological mediator 1-0-hexadecyl/octadecyl-2-acetyl-sn-glycero 3 phosphocholine. *Immunol* 1983; 48:141–9.

205 Yasaka T, Boxer LA, Baehner RL. Monocyte aggregation and superoxide anion release in response to formyl-methionyl-leucyl-phenylalanine (FMLP) and platelet-activating factor (PAF). *J Immunol* 1982; 128:1939–44.

206 Hyashi H, Kudo I, Inoue H, Onozaki K, Tsushima S, Nomura H, Nojima S. Activation of guinea pig peritoneal macrophages by platelet activating factor (PAF) and its agonists. *J Biochem* 1985; 97:1737–45.

207 Barthelson RA, Valone FH, Debs R, Philip R. Synergy in interleukin 1 release by human monocytes stimulated with platelet activating factor plus gamma interferon or tumour necrosis factor. *FASEB J* 1988; 2:A 1228.

208 Valone FH, Philip R, Debs RJ. Enhanced human monocyte cytotoxicity by platelet activating factor. *Immunology* 1988; 64:715–18.

209 Salem P, Dulioust A, Deryckx S, Vivier E, Benveniste J, Thomas Y. PAF-acether (platelet activating factor) increases interleukin 1 secretion by human monocytes. *Fed Proc* 1987; 46:992.

210 Babior BM. Oxidants from phagocytes: agents of defense and destruction. *Blood* 1984; 64:959–66.

211 Sacks T, Moldow CF, Craddock PR, Bowers TK, Jacob HS. Oxygen radicals mediate endothelial cell damage by complement-stimulated granulocytes: an *in vitro* model of immune vascular damage. *J Clin Invest* 1978; 61:1161–7.

212 Friedman MM, Kaliner MA. Human mast cells as asthma. *Am Rev Resp Cir Dis* 1987; 135:1157–64.

213 Plaut M, Lichtenstein LM. Histamine and immune responses. In: Ganellin CR, Parsons ME, eds. *Pharmacology of Histamine Receptors.* Bristol: Wright, 1982:392–435.

3
Homeostatic mechanisms in the immune response

JOHN L. TURK

Introduction

Homeostatic mechanisms in the immune response may be found at a number of different levels between the presentation of antigen and the development of the immune reaction in the periphery. Many toxic substances can upset the delicate balance that exists at all levels; this may result in a decrease in responsiveness or an increased reaction. Examples of decrease are to be found with those substances that depress the immune response. Increased responsiveness may lead, among other effects, to severe allergic reactions.

Toxic effects on immune reactions may be the result of actions either centrally or peripherally. Central regulation of the immune response may be as a result of cell–cell interaction or due to the production of intercellular messenger molecules. Similar molecules induce inflammatory reactions in the periphery or activate cells that play a role in these reactions, or themselves produce other mediators.

Regulation of cell–cell interaction involving the participation of antibodies is in many cases antigen-specific. However, that involving soluble mediators and other pharmacological agents is mostly antigen-non-specific.

In specific homeostatic mechanisms we should discuss the role of antigen, antibody and immune complexes, specifically, the role of anti-idiotype antibodies and the network theory. Regulatory cells may be T cells, B cells, or macrophages. Of the non-specific factors that can influence the immune response we shall have to consider the role of the complement cascades. Eicosanoids, both prostaglandins and leukotrienes, have been shown to have a regulatory role. An important group of agents are the cytokines which may be of lymphocyte or macrophage origin. Finally, the effect of biological response modifiers should be considered. Biological response modifiers are agents that have been shown to modify the host's immune response in tumour immunology. As well as many of the agents described above such as cytokines and, particularly, interferon, they include other agents of biological origin, such as thymic hormones etc. [1] (Table 3.1).

Specific mechanisms

Control by antigen: immunological tolerance

The concept that the immune response could be regulated by antigen was introduced by Medawar and his colleagues [2]. They showed that antigen introduced into an animal at the time of immunological immaturity, that is, late foetal or early neonatal life,

Table 3.1 Mechanisms of regulation of the immune response

Genetic control by major
  histocompatibility complex
Inhibition of clonal proliferation by antigen
  (immunological tolerance)
Immunological enhancement by blocking antibody
Network formed by auto-anti-idiotypic antibodies
Helper T lymphocytes
Suppressor T lymphocytes
Suppressor B lymphocytes
Cytokines
Prostaglandins
Leukotrienes
Thymic hormones
Macrophages

would induce a state of specific immunological tolerance to that antigen. These experiments were performed with antigens of the major histocompatibility complex (MHC). It was later shown that tolerance to MHC antigens could be induced in adult animals if a 100-fold increase in the dose of antigen is given. High-dose tolerance can affect both T and B cells. Tolerance caused by repeated low doses of antigen affects T cells only. The mechanism of tolerance caused by antigen is poorly understood. It has been suggested that during development the lymphocyte goes through a phase when contact with specific antigen results in cell death or inactivation. This is referred to as clonal deletion or clonal inactivation. Clonal deletion or inactivation is difficult to prove as it is a negative concept. It is, therefore, used for those forms of unresponsiveness or regulation in which it cannot be shown that suppressor cells are involved. Chase [3] showed that a large dose of nitrobenzenes given orally makes an animal specifically unresponsive. Subsequently, it was shown that these animals contained suppressor T lymphocytes. However, if the animals made unresponsive by an intravenous injection were pretreated with cyclophosphamide (CY) before sensitization was attempted, the unresponsiveness was only partially broken [4]. This would indicate that the unresponsiveness was only partially due to suppressor cells and that there was another more permanent element, possibly clonal deletion. If the animals were made unresponsive by being fed nitrobenzenes they were only partially unresponsive and CY treatment restored their complete responsiveness, indicating that there was no additional clonal deletion (Fig. 3.1).

A state of unresponsiveness can be induced in adult animals more easily if the number of responder T cells is reduced. This may be done by treating the animal with anti-lymphocyte serum (ALS) and CY. CY acted to reduce the rate of elimination of ALS from the circulation. This prolongs the time during which there is a reduced number of specific lymphocytes exposed to antigen [5]. A course of ALS and CY need only be given for a period of 5 days, starting 2 days before the application of a skin allograft, to obtain indefinite graft survival.

Recently the development of cell cloning techniques has helped to define the role of antigen-induced clonal reduction as a means of regulation of the immune response. There is no doubt that B cells can become tolerant to a wide range of antigens presented at quite low concentration at the time when the receptors for these antigens are first appearing [6]. Less is known about T-cell anergy. However, there is some indication that a functional clonal deletion of T cells can be induced. A deficit in cytotoxic T-cell precursors can be demonstrated in which tolerance to major histocompatibility antigens had been demonstrated. The term

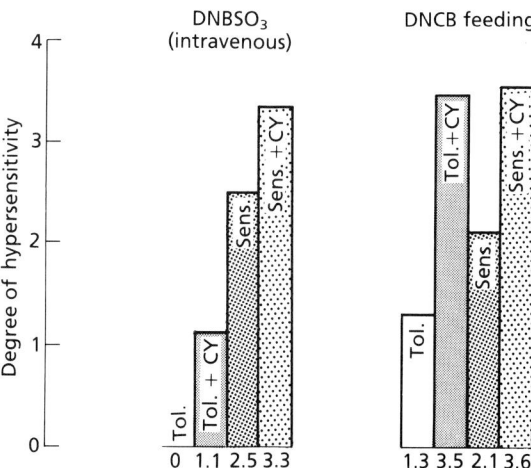

Fig. 3.1 Reversal of tolerance to I-chloro-2,
4-dinitrobenzene (DNCB) by cyclophosphamide (CY)
treatment.

clonal silence has been suggested rather than clonal abortion or clonal anergy. The term *clonal abortion* has been used to explain the situation found in B-cell tolerance.

A new approach to the analysis of the mechanism of immunological tolerance has been by the use of transgenic mice [7]. By this technique DNA containing gene material is injected into a fertilized egg *in vitro*. The egg is then allowed to develop in uterus of a pseudopregnant female. The gene selected may code for a foreign protein which is then synthesized by the foetus and is treated as a self-antigen. Transgenic mice can also be prepared that develop anti-self properties and thus autoimmunity. T-cell tolerance in transgenic mice may involve either clonal anergy or active suppression. Tolerance of B cells appears to result from the process of clonal anergy.

Control by antibody

The control of the immune response by specific antibody has been studied since the turn of the century [8]. Although it has been described mainly in transplanted tumour systems, terms such as *immunological enhancement* or *immunological facilitation* have been used in the past to refer to increased tumour growth under conditions where the immune response to the transplanted tumour has been reduced by antibody specific to the transplanted tumour. Further models of immunological control by specific antibody have been described using non-neoplastic allografted tissue such as skin or ovarian and endocrine grafts, and the system has been extended to include increased survival of kidney allografts. Other systems involving tissue antigens have included experimental allergic encephalomyelitis were specific antibodies may cause a reduction in the disease observed. Antibody control of the immune response to soluble antigen has also been described, particularly affecting cell-mediated immune response and delayed-type hypersensitivity reactions. There are many ways in which humoral antibody can interfere with the immune response. In the first place, during antigen recognition, antibody can block the specific epitopes, thus blocking the development of the immune response at its earliest stage. A central action has also been postulated

inhibiting clonal expansion directly. Finally, on the efferent side of the immune response, there may be secondary protection of the target by specific antibody.

The nature of the immunoglobulin involved has also been studied. It appears that the Fc fragment of the molecule is not involved, but the antibody-binding site of the molecule is particularly important. Although there are reports of specific effect from immunoglobulin M (IgM) and IgG$_2$ antibodies, a particular activity has been localized to the IgG$_1$ fraction of immunoglobulin in a number of systems. Enhancing antibody has also been found to be non-cytotoxic and non-complement-fixing. Antibody regulation of the immune response has been demonstrated in delayed-type hypersensitivity, IgM and IgG synthesis. It plays a role in infection with virus, fungi and protozoa, as well as bacteria, by protecting the organisms when multiplying and by having a desensitizing effect. Antibodies against tumour-specific transplantation antigens play a role in the establishment of development of tumours and allow tumour cells to sneak through the protective immune response.

Circulating immune complexes

The presence of immune complexes in the circulation has been postulated to control the immune response. Serum factors were capable of maintaining a reduced cell-mediated immune response. This was because the serum contained an antigen in a particular 'tolerogenic' state, which may be explained by its conjugation to antibody forming an immune complex [9].

Network theory: anti-idiotype antibodies

The idiotype is the individual antigen specificity of an antibody molecule. The antigen-binding site of the Fab part of the antibody is antigenic in its own right. Thus, it is possible to generate anti-idiotype antibodies that will recognize the specific amino acid sequence in the variable (V) region of the antigen-combining site of an antibody. These anti-idiotype antibodies will recognize similar antigen-binding sites on B cells programmed to produce the antibodies, or on T cells involved in a specific cell-mediated response against the same antigen. It is thus possible to state that the T cells in cell-mediated immunity carry, as part of their membrane, antigen-binding sites that are similar in structure and probably have the same amino acid sequence as is found in the region of the immunoglobulin antibodies directed against the same antigen.

Anti-idiotypic antibody (anti-id) can react with the idiotypic determinants of effector T lymphocytes. As a result, they can inhibit the proliferative response of sensitized lymphocytes to specific antibody. Anti-id can also stimulate T lymphocytes to express antigen-reactive receptor sites and be able to transfer delayed-type hypersensitivity reactions *in vivo*. Moreover, mice injected with low doses of anti-id antibody will develop a state of delayed-type hypersensitivity to the specific antigen.

The concept of an immunological network depends upon this dual capacity of the antibody molecule. The antigen-combining site can combine with antibody against its own antigenic determinant (idiotype) as well as antigen. A normal auto-anti-idiotype antibody will form as part of the immune response. Furthermore, idiotype-specific T suppressor cells will also be formed. Idiotype–anti-id interactions provide positive and/or negative immunoregulatory signals that will give a basic regulation of the immune response.

An antibody bearing an idiotype will induce an anti-idiotypic antibody which will suppress the production of the specific antibody and, at the same time, induce the production of a further antibody. The basic pattern is suppression, and through it, the maintenance of an equilibrium.

Studies of suppressive types of networks have been made using antibodies against dinitrophenyl (DNP) and trinitrophenyl (TNP) haptens. Myeloma proteins with the properties of antibodies against DNP and TNP have been used to immunize Balb/C mice who develop an auto-id antibody response. Mice with such antibodies have a reduced antibody response to DNP or TNP hapten and this can be shown to be due to a failure to develop specific plaque-forming B cells [10]. In other studies [11,12] a rapid decline in anti-TNP plaque-forming B cells was observed following immunization of AKR mice with TNP-ficoll. The response declines between the fourth and seventh day after immunization.

This phenomenon was postulated as being due to an anti-id antibody as the serum factor involved could be removed by anti-mouse Ig and AKR anti-TNP antibody immunoabsorbents. The decline of the anti-TNP antibody response was explained by the transient presence of cells which secrete anti-id antibodies that block the secretion of anti-TNP antibody-forming B cells. Specific anti-id antibodies given immediately before or just after immunization have been found to decrease significantly delayed hypersensitivity responses to pneumococcal vaccine [13]. Small doses stimulated the development of delayed hypersensitivity to the same determinant. Similar results were found by Sy *et al.* [14] using the response to the azobenzene arsonate hapten. In studies on contact sensitivity to dinitrofluorobenzene, which is a transient phenomenon in the mouse occurring on day 5 after sensitization and declining on day 8, Sy *et al.* [15] found an inhibitory factor in the serum that behaved as an anti-id autoantibody. This factor was removed by anti-mouse Ig immunosorbent and immune lymphoid cells, but not by dinitrophenylated keyhole limpet haemocyanin or anti-DNP antibody immunoabsorbent. It has been suggested that suppressor B cells, which are found to regulate T cell function in certain delayed hypersensitivity reactions [16], might also be producing similar anti-id autoantibodies.

Auto-anti-id plaque-forming cells have been demonstrated as well as serum anti-id autoantibodies during a conventional immune response. Anti-id antibody formation, however, needs T-cell participation. The nude mouse that lacks T cells has a slower fall-off of the immune response to TNP, indicating the probability that it does not make auto-anti-id antibodies. The normal slower fall-off of the immune response is restored to the nude mouse by a thymus graft [17].

Although the basic pattern of the idiotype network is suppression, anti-id antibodies can enhance the immune response under certain circumstances. This happens if the anti-id antibodies enhance the expression of silent or suppressed clones of B cells by eliminating idiotype-specific suppressor cells.

In the same way as anti-id antibodies are not produced in T-cell-deficient mice, one can surmise that the whole network of idiotype–anti-id will be destabilized by immunosuppressive agents. A critical level of such an agent may upset the gently balanced equilibrium whose basic effect is undertaken through suppression. This may result in an enhancement rather than a suppression of the immune response.

Regulatory T and B lymphocytes

Another major advance in our understanding of the immune response has been the realization that T lymphocytes are not just involved directly in cell-mediated immune reactions, but are also important in the regulation of almost all immune responses. The action of these cells is usually antigen-specific. However, many of the factors produced once the cells have interacted with antigen act non-specifically on cells involved in the immune reaction, whether they are T cells, B cells, or macrophages. The regulatory activity of T cells may play a positive or negative role. Thus we talk about helper T (T_H) cells or suppressor T (T_S) cells. T_H and T_S cells in the mouse belong to distinct subpopulations of T cells [17] that can be recognized by specific antigenic determinants. T_H cells in the mouse are Lyt 1^+23^-, while T_S cells are Lyt 1^-23^+. T_H cells are cyclophosphamide-insensitive, whereas T_S cells are a cyclophosphamide-sensitive population. In humans helper cells have also been shown to carry distinct antigens which are recognizable by specific monoclonal antibodies. T_H cells carry OKT$_4$ or Leu$_3$ antigens, whereas T_S cells are OKT$_8$ or Leu$_2$-positive. These antibodies detect CD markers on the surface of lymphocytes. The markers on T_H cells in both mice and humans are referred to as CD4 and the markers detected on T_S cells as CD8. These markers help to define specialized subsets of T cells. It should be remembered, however, that not all CD4 cells are T_H. This subset also contains effector cells of delayed hypersensitivity. Also, CD8 cells contain cytotoxic cells and those involved in host resistance to infection, as well as suppressor cells. In a number of acquired immunodeficiency states in humans, there is a reversal of the normal T_H:T_S ratio, related directly to the immunosuppressed state.

The first observation leading to an identification of T_H cells was the demonstration that normal thymus function was important for the full manifestation of a B-cell response. Identification of a specific population of T_H cells has led to the demonstration in a number of experiments of the release of soluble T helper factors. Progress in this field was slow until the use of T-cell-cloning techniques [19]. A number of reports on the soluble products of T_H cell clones indicate that these products may be a heterogeneous mixture of antigen-specific and MHC-restricted factors with molecular weight varying between 10 000 and 70 000. T_H cell function does not appear to play a role in the immune response to polysaccharide antigens, although it seems to be important in the response to antigens containing a protein moiety. Much of the work on T helper factors has been with influenza virus, as well as sheep erythrocytes as antigens in the mouse.

There is some controversy as to whether T_H cells always act through soluble T_H factor. This is particularly important with reference to cell-surface antigens, which matter most in various models of cancer. Mitchison [20] has suggested that there may be direct cell-to-cell instruction by means of a bridge between the T and B cell, consisting of antigen together with the Ia molecule, and believes that this may play an important role in the response to the MHC. There appears to be evidence also that the T_H cells show marked genetic restriction, which cannot be abrogated by the addition of appropriate macrophages.

The demonstration that the state of immunological tolerance could be transferred from one animal to another by lymphocytes [21] opened up the whole field of suppressor cells that can suppress or regulate the immune response. Initially most of the models studied were those of immunological tolerance, in which an animal was made unresponsive by a large dose of antigen generally given by the intravenous route. These suppressor cells were mainly T lymphocytes [22]. T_S cells in initial animal studies were found to be mainly antigen-specific. T_S cells in human and mouse lymphocyte cultures can be stimulated non-specifically by the plant mitogen concanavalin A (ConA). In mouse models a soluble immune response suppressor (SIRS) can be released from ConA-activated Lyt 2^+ T cells that non-specifically suppress the immune response of B cells to sheep erythrocytes *in vitro* [23]. The target of SIRS is the macrophage suppressor factor, which acts not only on normal proliferating B cells but also on proliferating neoplastic cells *in vitro* [24]. SIRS has been produced by a T-cell hybridoma and has been shown to be a single polypeptide chain of molecular weight 21 500.

Antigen-specific T_S has now been demonstrated in a wide range of immune responses, both T-cell-mediated and involving antibody production. These include many tumour models as well as chemical contact sensitivity [25–27]. In a number of these studies the precursors of these cells have been shown to be sensitive to CY. Treatment of animals with CY results, therefore, in an increase in the immune response and in the case of tumour-bearing animals, in an increase in the mean time to death.

A population of B lymphocytes regulates delayed hypersensitivity reactions in the guinea pig [28]. These suppressor cells are not destroyed by anti-T-cell serum that destroys the T cells that transfer delayed hypersensitivity in the guinea pig [29]. At the same time the suppressor cells may be removed by passage through a degalan bead column coated with specific anti-guinea pig immunoglobulin antibody prepared in the rabbit, indicating that they have surface Fc receptors [30]. These cells will specifically suppress the delayed hypersensitivity reactions in guinea pigs whose own suppressor cells have temporarily been destroyed by CY pretreatment. Other evidence for suppressor B lymphocytes has been provided during normal sensitization of the mouse with picryl chloride by Zembala *et al.* [31], using similar transfer studies.

The specificity of reaction of such B cells in the guinea pig [16] and the failure of transfer with serum from the same animals indicate a membrane-bound receptor that is probably an immunoglobulin. A recent suggestion is that this may turn out to be an auto-anti-id antibody. Another possibility is that this is an enhancing antibody with affinity for antigen stronger than the T-cell receptor that mediates the delayed hypersensitivity reaction. The effects of the toxic agent CY on immunoregulation are illustrated in Figs 3.2–3.4. This agent gives an enhanced delayed hypersensitivity response to a contact sensitizer such as 2,4-dinitrofluorobenzene if given before sensitization or around the time of sensitization. Figure 3.2 shows the effect of CY (300 mg kg^{-1}), given before or after contact sensitization with 2,4-dinitrofluorobenzene on skin reactivity at 24 and 48 h after epi-

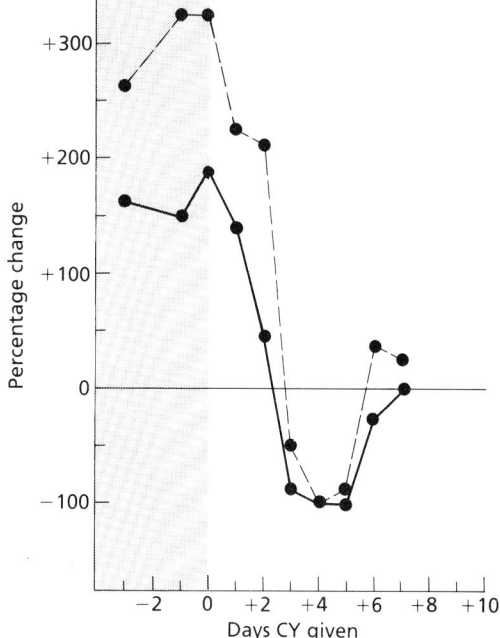

Fig. 3.2 Effect of cyclophosphamide (CY; 300 mg kg^{-1}) given before or after sensitization. Skin reactivity at 24 h,—; 48 h,---.

cutaneous application of the sensitizer. It can be seen that maximum potentiation is achieved when the drug is given between the 3rd day before immunization and the 1st day after. If the drug is given later, between the 3rd day after immunization and the 5th, the response is depressed. This is the time after immunization when T lymphocytes in the draining lymph node enter their maximum proliferative phase [32]. A study of the effect of this dose of CY on T-lymphocyte proliferation in the draining lymph node shows that T-cell proliferation is maximally depressed on days 4 and 5 after sensitization by CY given on days 2 and 3 respectively (Fig. 3.3). This indicates that effector T lymphocytes are maximally sensitive to CY during their proliferative phase. They appear to be most susceptible to CY given 48 h before the period of maximum DNA and RNA synthesis, when they can be visualized as large pyroninophilic cells in the paracortical area of the draining lymph node. If, however, CY is given 1 day before sensitization, there is a massive increase in T-cell proliferation 5 days after sensitization, indicating that these cells had been released from normal immunoregulatory control.

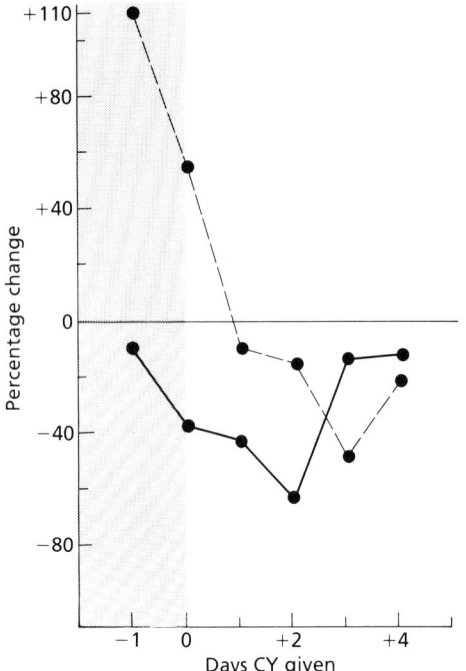

Fig. 3.3 Effect of cyclophosphamide (CY; 300 mg kg^{-1}) given before or after sensitization. T-lymphocyte proliferation in draining lymph node on day 4,—; day 5,---after sensitization.

The potentiating action of CY on the immune response has frequently been the first indication of a homeostatic immunoregulatory mechanism mediated through a separate population of suppressor cells. In many cases this can be substantiated by identifying a population of cells that can be transferred from normally sensitized animals and which are able to replace the suppressor cells depleted by the drug. Whether suppressor cells are T or B lymphocytes, CY will have a potentiating effect that depends on the relative rate of turnover of the precursors of these cells. The action of CY appears to be on rapidly dividing cells only. If the precursors of the cells regulating the response are slowly turning over, CY will not have an immunopotentiating effect (Fig. 3.4).

Ozer and colleagues [33] have studied the effect of 4-hydroperoxycyclophosphamide (4HC), an *in vitro* acting CY compound, on defined human immunoregulatory subsets in humans. ConA T-cell suppression of B-cell differentiation was completely abrogated by low doses of 4HC. The ConA-induced T-cell suppressors were found to be in the CD4 subset, indicating a presuppressor population. Suppressor precursors and differentiated suppressors for T-effector function were also restricted to the CD4 subset.

The role of macrophages in regulating the immune response

Macrophages play an important role in regulating the immune response (Table 3.2). These cells are as important in regulation as in antigen presentation. Allison [34] indicated a number of soluble products

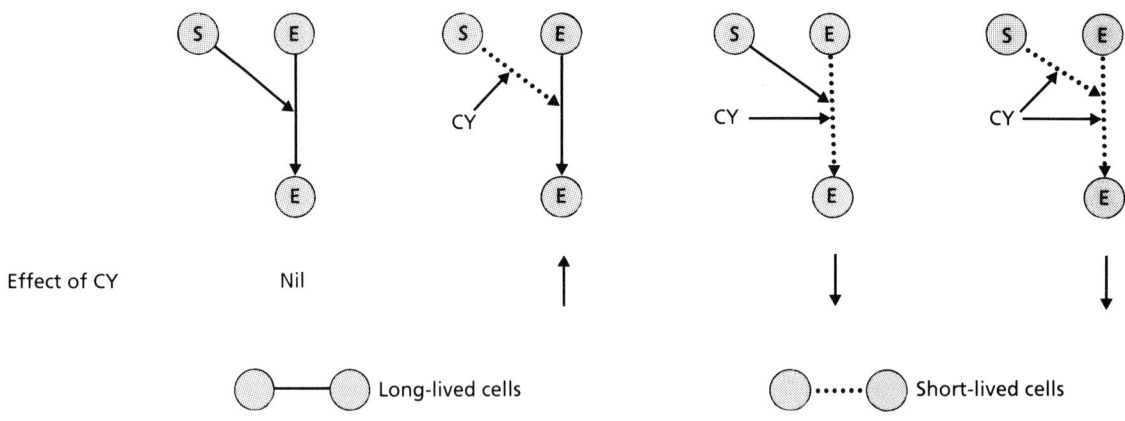

Fig. 3.4 Effect of cyclophosphamide (CY) on immunoregulation.

Table 3.2 Products of activated macrophages regulating lymphocyte responses

---

Thymidine
Arginase
Polyamine oxidase
Complement cleavage products (C3, C4, C2, factor B)
Leukotrienes
Prostaglandins
Cyclic adenosine monophosphate
Interferon (INF)
Interleukin 1 (IL-1)
Tumor necrosis factor (TNF)
B cell-differentiating factor
T cell-activating molecule
Thymic differentiating factor
Granulocyte–stimulating factor (GSF)
Granulocyte–macrophage colony-stimulating factor
  (GM-CSF)
Macrophage colony-stimulating factor (MCSF)

---

of activated macrophage origin that would act directly on T- or B-cell function to inhibit the response of these cells. These include thymidine, arginase, and polyamine oxidase. The role of complement has been emphasized in the studies of Klaus and Humphrey [35], who depleted thymectomized mice of circulating C3 by treatment with cobra venom factor primary immunization with dinitrophenylated keyhole limpet haemocyanin. This treatment abrogated the development of B-cell memory and appeared to involve impaired precursor proliferation following primary immunization. Lack of C3 also prevents uptake of antigen by dendritic cells.

The roles of prostaglandins, cyclic adenosine monophosphate, interferon and interleukin-1 have been discussed previously. Other factors such as B cell and thymic-differentiating factors and the T-cell-activating molecule [36] await further chemical characterization.

There are very few reports of the direct suppression of immunobiological reactivity by macrophages *in vivo*. However, purified peritoneal exudate macrophages injected intravenously into guinea pigs sensitized with DNP-bovine γ-globulin can non-specifically suppress delayed hypersensitivity reactions to this antigen [37].

Non-specific mechanisms—soluble factors

Complement

The complement system involves at least 14 serum proteins, the most important of which is the third component (C3) which is present in highest concentration in the serum $(1500\,\mu\mathrm{g\,ml}^{-1})$. Much of the biological activity of complement emanates from the activation of C3. There are two pathways to the activation of C3, both of which consist of a cascade of enzymes, each one activating the next. The two pathways are referred to as the classical pathway and the alternative pathway. The classical pathway is initiated by antigen–antibody complexes and there is a receptor for the CIq part of CI on the Fc portion of IgG_1 and IgG_3 and, to a lesser degree, IgG_2 and IgM in humans. The C42 complex acts as the C3 convertase capable of clearing C3. The alternative pathway is so called because it proceeds in the absence of antibody. It is initiated by polysaccharides and lipopolysaccharides which may be derived from infecting organisms. The alternative pathway does not involve C1, C4 or C2, but another series of proteins that are chemically distinct although functionally similar. These are factor B, factor D and properdin. The cleavage product of C3-C3b is also involved in the formation of the alternative pathway activator of C3 as well as the cleavage of C5. The cleavage product of C5-C5b is involved in the activation of C6 which, in turn, acts on C7. C7 acts on C8 and the activation of C8 on C9 is the end-product involved in cell lysis. C3a, C3b and C5a are active in biological processes, particularly inflammation. Regulation of the complement cascade is undertaken by a series of inhibitors that may intervene at a number of levels. Lack of inhibitors may cause a deficiency of a particular component due to a failure of regulation. Some of the control mechanisms are so much an integral part of the activation process that the paralysis of inactivation may constitute an initiating event.

The complement system interacts with coagulation, fibrinolytic and kinin systems. This is through the Hageman factor. Lipopolysaccharides activate the Hageman factor which is a key enzyme in clotting, fibrinolysis and kinin formation. Plasmin, the peptidase of the fibrinolytic system, is a potent complement activator. It acts on the classical pathway by cleaving C1. In addition, it cleaves C3 and factor B. Kallikrein, the main enzyme of the kinin system, cleaves C5. The complement system is involved in host defence against infection and the inflammatory reaction. The complement cascade may be activated by all infectious organisms either by the classical or by the alternative pathway. This cascade, taken to its final end-point, can undertake the lysis of bacteria and other organisms.

Complement is involved in the phagocytosis of organisms by polymorphonuclear leucocytes and macrophages which carry receptors for complement components on their surface. There are three types of receptor—CR1, CR2 and CR3—found on different cell types and reacting with different breakdown products of C3. Virus-infected cells are the target of complement-mediated elimination. The role of complement in the inflammatory reaction is twofold. Firstly, an increase in vascular permeability is produced by the anaphylatoxins (C3a, C5a and C4a) which may act independently of most cell degranulation and histamine release. The other main role of complement in inflammation is in leucocyte migration. It is now generally accepted that C5a is by far the most active and relevant component *in vivo*.

Much insight into the role of complement in the control of immune responses and reactions may be obtained from a study of the effect of deficiencies of complement components. Bacteraemia or recurrent infections occur if there is deficiency of C3 or its activities through the alternative pathway. Defects in the classical pathway components tend to be associated with immune complex disease, predominantly of the systemic lupus type. Deficiencies of C5–C8 weaken defences, particularly against

Neisseria sp. A hereditary defect in the C1-inhibitor (C1-INH) may give rise to a hereditary angioneurotic oedema. This may be due to deficiency in synthesis of C1-INH, inactive C1-INH or C1-INH complexed to albumin and thus being inactive. Acquired angioedema may occur from a spontaneous deficiency of C1-INH or a deficiency associated with underlying disease such as lymphoma or autoimmune haemolytic anaemia. Three cases have been associated with cyclosporin-A therapy [38]. C1-INH deficiency leads to an impaired inactivation of plasma kallikrein, an increased turnover of kininogen, delayed kallikrein activation and diminished activation of Hageman factor [39].

A number of aluminium and zirconium compounds that have been found to induce granuloma formation have been shown to activate complement (Table 3.3). These include kaolin, aluminium hydroxide and compounds used as anti-perspirants, aluminium chlorohydrate and zirconium aluminium glycinate. These compounds activated C3 as determined by two-dimensional electrophoresis (Fig. 3.5) and the production of anaphylatoxin. Activation occurred in the absence of Ca^{++} and Mg^{++} and therefore did not involve the classical or alternative pathways. However, activation could not take place if plasminogen had been removed on a lysine-sepharose column. Reconstitution with plasminogen allowed inactivation to take place, confirming the role of these compounds on plasmin-splitting of C3, possibly through the activation of Hageman factor [40,41].

Cytokines and macrophage factors

Details of these agents and the role they play in homeostatic mechanisms in the immune response

	Plasminogen-depleted serum	Plasminogen-depleted serum + plasminogen*
Buffer	5.6 ± 2.3	3.6 ± 2.1
Zymosan 2 mg ml^{-1}	57.7 ± 3.0	60.2 ± 5.9
ACH 10 mg ml^{-1}	0	36.4 ± 6.3
Al(OH)$_3$ 10 mg ml^{-1}	0	33.2 ± 4.6
ZAG 10 mg ml^{-1}	0	36.5 ± 1.7

Table 3.3 Conversion of complement 3 (C3) in human serum by aluminium chlorhydrate [ACH] aluminium hydroxide [Al(OH)$_3$] and zirconium aluminium glycinate (ZAG) in the presence or absence of plasminogen

*100 μg of plasminogen was added to 1.0 ml of plasminogen-depleted serum. Conversion of C3 was demonstrated by two-dimensional electrophoresis. Each value represents mean ± SE of four experiments.

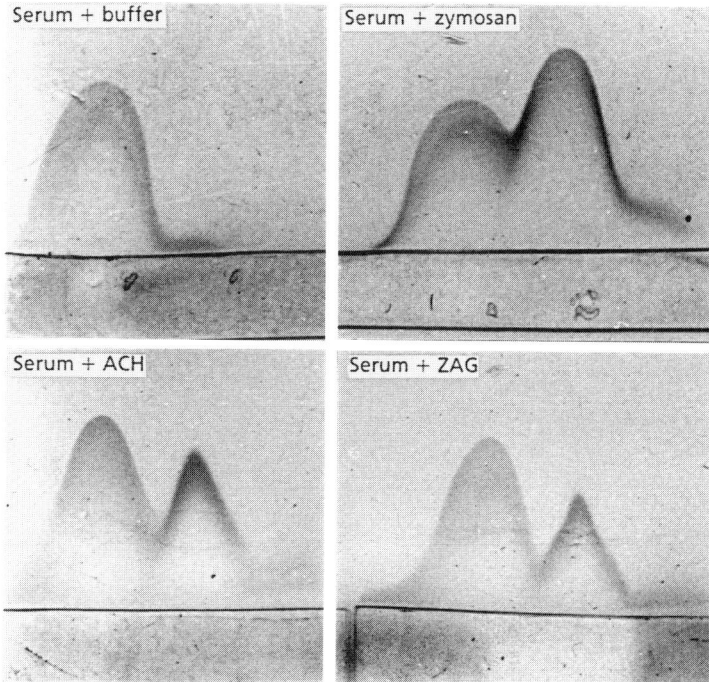

Fig. 3.5 Conversion of C3 demonstrated by two-dimensional electrophoresis.

have been discussed in Chapter 2. In this section emphasis will be placed on how the production of these agents can be destabilized by toxic substances *in vitro* and *in vivo*. A number of immunosuppressive agents will inhibit the production of the lymphokine interleukin-2 (IL-2) at a dose level that is not directly cytocidal to lymphocytes. These include vincristine, vinblastine and the two *in vitro* active analogues of cyclophosphamide—4 hydroperoxycyclophosphamide (4HC) and mafosfamide, as well as the anti-T cell antibiotic cyclosporin-A ($C_S A$) [42,43].

A recent development in the study of cell-mediated immunity has been to investigate the effect of anti-cancer agents on cytokine production. Two anti-cancer agents, bleomycin (BLM) and Adriamycin (ADR), have been studied extensively in our current programme. BLM was found to enhance contact sensitivity in guinea pigs to 2,4-dinitrofluorobenzene. To achieve this effect the drug was given in a single dose ($125 \, \text{mg} \, \text{kg}^{-1}$) on the day of or up to 3 days after sensitization. In addition, if BLM was given 2 or 3

days after sensitization it caused increased T-cell proliferation in lymph nodes draining the skin sensitization site. This suggested the possibility that the potentiating effect of BLM might be due to an effect on local IL-2 production [44]. ADR has been found to augment the generation of cytotoxic lymphocytes against mastocytoma cells in the mouse. It does this without affecting progenitor cytotoxic lymphocytes and without the elimination of suppressor cells. This suggested that this compound might also act by increasing cytokine production [45].

When BLM was added to spleen cells of Lewis rats or Balb/C mice in the presence of a suboptimal dose of ConA, interleukin-2 release was markedly increased. This effect was detected by assay on CTLL/16 cells, an IL-2-dependent cell line, and could be detected with a dose of BLM less than $1 \, \mu\text{g} \, \text{ml}^{-1}$ (Fig. 3.6). BLM was also tested for its ability to alter IL-1 production by peritoneal exudate macrophages using D10.b4.1 cells as target cells in the assay. The effect of BLM on IL-1 was less obvious than that on IL-2.

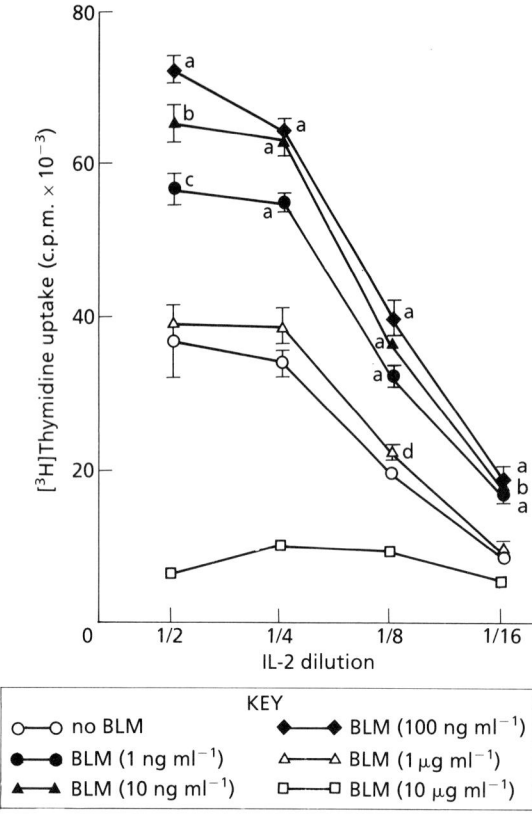

Fig. 3.6 Effect of bleomycin (BLM) on interleukin-2 (IL-2) production by rat splenocytes *in vitro*. 1 × 10⁶ rat splenocytes were incubated with ConA ($0.5 \mu g\,ml^{-1}$) and varying amounts of BLM. Supernatants were harvested after 24 h, dialysed to remove the drug and assayed for IL-2 activity against the IL-2-dependent cell line (CTLL 16). The results are given as mean c.p.m. of [³H]thymidine incorporation ± SD. A negative control of the cell line + medium alone gave 75 ± 14 c.p.m. a = $P <$ 0.001 as compared to the cultures without BLM; b = $P <$ 0.002 as compared to the cultures without BLM; c = $P < 0.005$ as compared to the cultures without BLM; d = $P < 0.01$ as compared to the cultures without BLM.

It therefore seemed unlikely that the increased production of IL-2 occurred as a direct result of an effect on IL-1 production, even though there is some alteration in the release of this monokine [46]. ADR had a similar effect to BLM down to a dose of $1\,ng\,ml^{-1}$. The effect on IL-1 production was even less than that of BLM although there was a statistically significant enhanced effect. The two derivatives

of CY active *in vitro*, 4HC and mafosfamide, were found markedly to inhibit IL-2 release, but had no effect on the release of IL-1 [42].

The effect of these agents given *in vivo* was also studied. Spleen cells from rats previously injected with BLM ($10\,mg\,kg^{-1}$) or ADR ($1\,mg\,kg^{-1}$) given 3 days previously were found to release higher levels of IL-2 than cells from untreated animals. The level of drug used did not change the proportions of CD4 or CD8 T-cell subsets. In contrast, CY ($200\,mg\,kg^{-1}$) given 3 days previously markedly reduced the level of IL-2 production. This, however, occurred in the presence of a marked reduction in the proportion of CD4 cells in the spleen and could have been the result of a reduction in the regulatory T-helper cell population [47].

Other cancer chemotherapeutic agents such as vincristine and vinblastine have also been studied for their effect on IL-2 and IL-1 production. Both these agents cause a reduction in IL-2 production *in vivo* as well as *in vitro*.

Lymphokines such as interferon-γ and tumour necrosis factor may be studied in a similar manner and their production shown to be susceptible to the effect of toxic agents *in vitro* and *in vivo*.

Thymic hormones

A number of preparations of the thymus have been produced since the role of the thymus in regulating the immune response was first discovered by Miller [48]. Some of these have been reviewed in Chapter 2.

Among other functions, thymic factors have been involved in the study of ageing [49]. Both thymopoietin and facteur thymique serique (FTS) levels in the serum decline with age. Immune deficiencies of old mice can be reversed by an injection of thymopoietin-fraction 5. FTS in high concentration can be shown to have a stimulatory effect on T suppressor cells similar to that described for thymosin, in that it can cause the suppression of dinitrofluorobenzene sensitivity and skin graft rejection. In humans, FTS has been shown under certain circumstances to depress the generation of T suppressor cells *in vitro*.

It has been suggested that these agents might be useful in reconstituting T-cell numbers or function *in vivo* in situations where T-cell function is deficient, as in acquired immune deficiency syndrome (AIDS) or in thymic-deprived mice. However, studies in athymic nude mice indicate that they are inactive in the absence of a functional thymic microenvironment or mature T cells [50]. Similarly, these agents appear to show little or no effect in patients with AIDS where this profound involution of the thymus involves a loss of Hassell's corpuscles.

References

1 Mihich E, Fefer A. (eds) *Biological Response Modifiers*: Subcommittee Report. NCI Monograph 63. Bethesda; Maryland: Department of Health and Human Services, Public Health Service, National Institute of Health, 1983.

2 Billingham RE, Brent L. Quantitative studies on tissue transplantation immunity. III. Actively acquired tolerance. *Philos Trans (B)* 1956; 239: 357–414.

3 Chase MW. Inhibition of experimental drug allergy by prior feeding of the sensitizing agent. *Proc Soc Exp Biol (NY)* 1946; 61:257.

4 Turk JL, Parker D, Polak L. Control mechanisms in delayed hypersensitivity. *Br Med Bull* 1976; 32:165–70.

5 Polak L, Frey JR, Turk JL. Antilymphocyte serum and cyclophosphamide in the induction of tolerance to skin allografts in guinea pigs. *Transplantation* 1972; 13:310–15.

6 Nossal GJV. Unifying concepts of tolerance and immune regulation. *Regulation of the Immune Response.* Basel: Karger, 1982:1–11.

7 Miller JFAP, Morahan G, Allison J. Immunological tolerance: new approaches using transgenic mice. *Immunol Today* 1989; 10:53–7.

8 Voisin GA. Immunological facilitation, a broadening of the concept of the enhancement phenomenon. *Prog Allergy* 1971; 15:328–485.

9 Hellström I, Hellström KE, Allison AC. Neonatally induced allograft tolerance may be mediated by serum-borne factors. *Nature* 1971; 230:49–50.

10 Granato D, Braun DG, Vasalli P. Induction of anti DNP antibodies: suppressive effect of circulating anti-idiotypic antibodies to mouse myeloma. *J Immunol* 1974; 113:417–20.

11 Schrater AF, Goidl A, Thorbecke GJ, Siskind GW. Production of auto-anti-idiotypic antibody during the normal immune response to TNP-Ficoll. I Occurrence in AKR/J and Balb/c mice of hapten augmentable anti-TNP plaque forming cells in recipients of immune spleen cells. *J Exp Med* 1979; 150:138–53.

12 Schrater AF, Goidl A, Thorbecke GJ, Siskind GW. Production of auto-anti-idiotypic antibody during the normal immune response to TNP-Ficoll. II Absence in nu/nu mice: evidence for T cell dependence of the anti-idiotypic antibody response. *J Exp Med* 1979; 150:808–17.

13 Julius MH, Augustin AA, Cosenza H. Recognition of a naturally occurring idiotype by autologous T-cells. *Nature* 1977; 265:251–3.

14 Sy MS, Brown AR, Benacerraf B, Green MI. Antigen and receptor driven regulatory mechanisms. III Induction of delayed-type hypersensitivity to σZ0 benzene-arsonate with anti-cross reactive idiotype antibodies. *J Exp Med* 1980; 151:896–909.

15 Sy MS, Bach BA, Dohi Y, Nisonoff A, Benacerraf B, Greene MI. Antigen and receptor driven regulatory mechanisms. I Induction of suppressor T cells with anti-idiotypic antibodies. *J Exp Med* 1979; 150:1216–28.

16 Katz SI, Parker D, Turk JL. B cell suppression of delayed hypersensitivity reactions. *Nature* 1974; 251:550–1.

17 Kelsoe G, Isaak D, Cerny J. Thymic requirement for cyclical idiotypic and reciprocal anti-idiotypic immune responses to a T-independent antigen. *J Exp Med* 1980; 151:289–300.

18 Cantor H, Boyse EA. Functional subclasses of T-lymphocytes bearing different types of Ly antigens. II Co-operation between subclasses of Ly⁺ cells in the generation of killer activity. *J Exp Med* 1975; 141:1376–89.

19 Fischer A, Beverley PCL, Feldmann M. Long-term human T-helper lines producing specific helper factor reactive to influenza virus. *Nature* 1981; 294:166–8.

20 Mitchison NA. Regulation of the immune response to cell surface antigens. In: Pernis B, Vogel HJ, eds. *Regulatory-T-Lymphocytes.* New York: Academic Press, 1980:147–58.

21 Gershon RK, Kondo K. Infectious immunological tolerance. *Immunol* 1971; 21:903–14.

22 Zembala M, Asherson GL. Depression of the T cell phenomenon of contact sensitivity by T cells from unresponsive mice. *Nature* 1973; 244:227–8.

23 Rich RR, Pierce CW. Biological expressions of lymphocyte activation. II Generation of a population of thymus derived suppressor lymphocytes. *J Exp Med* 1973; 137:649–59.

24 Aune TM, Pierce CW. Mechanism of action of soluble immune response suppressor (SIRS). In: Hadden JW, Chedid L, Dukor P, Spreafico F, Willoughby D, eds. *Advances in Immunopharmacology. vol 2.* Oxford: Pergamon Press, 1983:597–602.

25 Glaser M. Augmentation of specific immune response against a syngeneic SV40-induced sarcoma in mice by depletion of suppressor T cells with cyclophosphamide. *Cell Immunol* 1979; 48:339–45.

26 Glaser M. Regulation of specific cell-mediated cytotoxic response against SV40-induced tumor associated antigens by depletion of suppressor T cells with cyclophosphamide in mice. *J Exp Med* 1979; 149:774–9.

27 Schwartz A, Askenase PW, Gershon RK. Regulation of delayed hypersensitivity reactions by cyclophosphamide sensitive T cells. *J Immunol* 1978; 121:1573–7.

28 Turk JL, Parker D. Effect of cyclophosphamide on immunological control mechanisms. *Immunol Rev* 1982; 65:99–113.

29 Ota F, Parker D, Turk JL. Further evidence for non-T cell regulation of delayed hypersensitivity in the guinea pig. *Cell Immunol* 1979; 43:263–70.

30 Katz SI, Parker D, Sommer G, Turk JL. Suppressor cells in normal immunization as a basic homeostatic mechanism. *Nature* 1974; 248:612–14.

31 Zembala M, Asherson GL, Nowowlski T, Mahew B. Contact sensitivity to picryl chloride. The occurrence of B suppressor cells in the lymph nodes and spleen of immunized mice. *Cell Immunol* 1976; 25:266–78.

32 Turk JL, Stone SH. Implications of the cellular changes in lymph nodes during the development and inhibition of delayed type hypersensitivity. In: Amos B, Koprowski H, eds. *Cell-bound Antibodies.* Philadelphia: Wistar Institute Press, 1963:51–60.

33 Ozer H. Effect of alkylating agents in immunoregulatory mechanisms. In: Mihich E, Sakurai Y, eds. *Biological Responses in Cancer. Immunomodulation by Anticancer Drugs.* New York: Plenum, 1985.

34 Allison AC. Mechanism by which activated macrophages inhibit lymphocyte responses. *Immunol Rev* 1978; 40:3–27.

35 Klaus GB, Humphrey JH. The generation of memory cells. I. The role of C3 in the generation of B memory cells. *Immunology* 1977; 33:31–40.

36 Unanue EK. The regulation of lymphocyte functions by the macrophage. *Immunol Rev* 1978; 40:227–55.

37 Katayama I, Parker D, Turk JL. *In vivo* macrophage suppression of delayed hypersensitivity in the guinea pig. *Immunol* 1982; 47:709–16.

38 Isenberg DA, Snaith ML, Al-Khader AA, Cohen SL, Fischer C, Morrow WJW, Mobray J. Cyclosporin relieves arthralgia, causes angioedema. *N Engl J Med* 1980; 303:754.

39 Cullman W, Kovary PM, Muller N, Dick W. Complement, coagulation and fibrinolytic parameters in hereditary angioedema (HAE). *Clin Exp Immunol* 1982; 49:618–22.

40 Ogston D, Ogston CM, Ratnoff DD, Forbes CD. Studies on a complex mechanism for the activation of plasminogen by kaolin and by chloroform: the participation of the Hageman factor and additional cofactors. *J Clin Invest* 1969; 48:1786.

41 Ramanathan VD, Badenoch-Jones P, Turk JL. Complement activation by aluminium and zirconium compounds. *Immunol* 1979; 37:881–8.

42 Ahmed K, Hamied TA, Turk JL. Inhibition of release of interleukin-2 by vincristine and vinblastine. *Immunopharmacol Immunotoxicol* 1987; 9:391–407.

43 Hamied TA, Parker D, Turk JL. Effects of adriamycin, 4 hydroperoxycyclophosphamide and AstaZ 7557 (Mafosfamide) on the release of IL-2 and IL-1 *in vitro. Int J Immunopharmacol* 1987; 9:355–61.

44 Parker D, Turk JL. Potentiation of T-lymphocyte function by bleomycin. *Immunopharmacol* 1984; 7:109–13.

45 Ehrke MJ, Mihich E. Adriamycin and other anthracyclines. *Clinics in Immunol Allergy* 1984; 4:259–77.

46 Hamied TA, Parker D, Turk JL. Potentiation of release of IL-2 by bleomycin. *Immunopharmacol* 1986; 12:127–34.

47 Hamied TA, Turk JL. Enhancement of IL-2 release in rats by treatment with bleomycin and adriamycin *in vivo. Cancer Immunol Immunother* 1987; 25:245–9.

48 Miller JFAP. Immunological function of the thymus. *Lancet* 1961; ii:748–9.

49 Aiuti F, Wigzell H (eds) *Thymus, Thymic Hormones and T-Lymphocytes.* New York: Academic Press, 1980.

50 Hadden JW, Caspritz G, Zheng Q-Y, Chen H, Wolstencroft R, Hadden EW. Thymosin interleukins, isoprinosine and imuthiol do not reconstitute T cells in athymic nude mice. *Int J Immunopharmacol* 1989; 11:13–19.

Part II
Immunotoxicology: current concepts

4
Toxic consequences of chemical interactions with the immune system

MICHAEL J. MURRAY & PETER T. THOMAS

Introduction

The immune system is composed of a complex set of cellular and chemical components that are designed to protect the body against foreign pathogens while not responding adversely to self elements. Immunotoxicology is the discipline concerned with the study of the deleterious effects of chemical xenobiotics on the immune system. Adverse effects of chemicals on the immune system can range from immunosuppression and the associated increased risk of infection and tumour growth to immunoenhancement and the associated risk of developing autoimmune or allergic reactions. In this regard, the immune system may serve as a passive target for the chemical, or the chemical may serve as an antigenic stimulus (along or in combination with self components) to the immune system, with the ensuing immune response resulting in the adverse effect(s). In the former instance, immunosuppression has been the most frequently observed immunotoxic outcome; in the latter instance,

hypersensitivity responses are the immunotoxic manifestation. Many of the topics introduced in this chapter are expanded elsewhere in this book.

Immunotoxicity associated with hypersensitivity responses is dependent upon both the mechanism of hypersensitivity and the target organ involved. Four mechanistically distinct types of hypersensitivity responses exist and examples of chemicals whose exposure is associated with each type of response in humans can be identified. Hypersensitivity responses are either cell- or antibody-mediated. Cell-mediated hypersensitivity generally requires 24–48 h to develop following exposure in a previously sensitized individual (i.e. delayed response), while antibody-mediated hypersensitivity occurs within minutes of exposure (immediate response). Each requires an initial exposure to the chemical for sensitization, and a subsequent exposure to elicit clinical symptoms.

In considering environmental and occupational exposure to chemicals, the respiratory tract and the skin are the two primary routes of sensitization and the two principal target organs of toxicities. A substantial database exists in humans and laboratory animals on respiratory and skin (contact) sensitization. The use of therapeutic drugs in humans, however, has also been associated with hypersensitivities, some of which may be manifested as autoimmune-like responses. Autoimmune-like responses and auto-immunity *per se* will not be considered in this chapter. Although important, these areas are not yet specifically addressed in most immunotoxicity assessments. Several excellent references exist discussing autoimmunity and autoimmune responses [1].

In contrast to chemically mediated hypersensitivity, there is limited human information available on other immunotoxicities resulting from occupational or environmental exposure to chemicals. Even less is known concerning the relevance of those effects on human resistance to disease. However, there is compelling evidence in laboratory animals that many chemicals adversely alter the immune system, and chemically induced immunosuppression is often correlated with decreased host resistance to challenge with infectious agents or tumour cells. Significant immunosuppression in humans due to genetic, disease-related, or chemotherapy-induced defects in immunity nearly always results in decreased resistance to infections. Likewise, there is a broad base of data demonstrating enhanced tumour development in patients undergoing immunosuppressive drug therapy [2]. Thus, increased incidence and severity of infection and increased incidence of cancer are justifiable concerns following exposure to immunotoxic chemicals. Table 4.1 summarizes the types of chemicals which are associated with immune alterations in animals and humans following exposure.

From a human safety standpoint, defining the risk for developing adverse immune responses associated with chemical exposure is the primary purpose of immunotoxicity assessment. Managing that risk deals not only with the real risk associated with the agent of interest but often involves perceived risk as well. Potential consequences of immunosuppression (i.e. susceptibility to infection and the development of neoplasias) may be perceived by the public to present a greater risk than those associated with hypersensitivity, even though consequences of both types of immunotoxicity may be life-threatening. This perception has been magnified by the enormous amount of attention focused on the immune system by the acquired immune deficiency syndrome (AIDS) pandemic. Whether this degree of concern is justified, considering the scientific evidence for the ability of environmental or occupational exposure to xenobiotics to alter the immune system, is unclear. It is clear, however, that adverse hypersensitivity responses to many classes of chemicals occur quite frequently in humans and are of considerable importance from both an economic and occupational disease perspective.

A thorough discussion of the extensive human and animal database concerning occupational and environmental allergens is beyond the scope of this chapter. This chapter will allude to the diversity of these compounds and briefly consider animal and human testing methods, either predictive or diagnostic for human sensitizers. The focus will be on animal methods available for assessing non-hypersensitivity end-points of chemically induced immunotoxicity and the animal and human database supporting the immunotoxic potential of classes of chemicals to which humans are exposed. A discussion of animal and human hypersensitivity and other immunotoxicity data associated with one class of compounds, the pesticides, should provide perspective as to human risk associated with exposure to these compounds. In addition, this discussion will serve to identify some of the areas of uncertainty in immunotoxicity risk assessment.

Table 4.1 Overview of classes of chemicals associated with non-hypersensitivity related immunological alterations in rodents and humans (modified from [3])

	Immunological alterations	
Chemical class	Rodent*	Human†
Polyhalogenated aromatic hydrocarbons	+	+ /-
Polycyclic aromatic hydrocarbons	+	ND
Aromatic hydrocarbons	+	+ /-
Aromatic amines	+	+ /-
Air pollutants	+	+ /-
Pesticides	+	+ /-
Organotins	+	ND
Metals	+	ND

*Not all members of any class have been demonstrated to cause immunological alterations.
+ At least one chemical in the particular class has been shown to alter immune parameters in humans.
ND = not determined.

Methodologies used to assess immune function

Methods of assessing immune status must be sensitive and reproducible and should lend themselves to extrapolation for human immune competence. Although it may be judicious to test for subtle changes in immune status, statistically significant changes in immune parameters do not always translate to biologically relevant health effects. Thus, alterations must be positioned in terms of their likely health implications when considering risk.

Testing methods have been developed for immunotoxicity safety assessment dealing with immune suppression and contact hypersensitivity. Methods for evaluation of potential immune suppression by a chemical in experimental animals can be conveniently grouped. These methods are commonly used in conjunction with a subchronic exposure regimen to the test compound of interest. One group of methods focuses on evaluating relevant pathological, haematological and structural parameters associated with the immune system. These include such things as body and lymphoid organ weights, histopathology of lymphoid organs, and differential and total white blood cell counts. A second group of methods evaluates functional competence of immune cells. This can be accomplished using *in vitro* immune function assays and *in vivo* host resistance assays in which animals are challenged with infectious agents or tumour cells. While the *in vitro* assays are sensitive and especially useful for identifying specific functional defects among immune cell populations, the host resistance assays provide a more holistic evaluation of immune function in the animal and allow one to discern biologically relevant immunomodulation. This is of particular importance since experimental evidence suggests that a substantial resilience exists in the immune system to chemically mediated toxicity.

Several approaches for immunotoxicity assessment exclusive of hypersensitivity end-points have been proposed. These approaches generally combine methods described above into a tiered system of assays [4]. The first tier of assays provides a screening mechanism for identifying immunomodulatory compounds. The second tier provides added perspective as to the significance of effects observed in the first tier, as well as data useful in elucidating mechanisms of action of the compound.

With respect to predictive testing of chemicals capable of sensitizing humans, the guinea pig has been the classical animal model. Alternative methods including *in vitro* and/or murine models currently are under development. Table 4.2 summarizes

Table 4.2 Commonly used guinea pig skin sensitization test methods

Method	Induction route/challenge route	Adjuvant
Optimization test	ID/ID + EC*	Yes
Buehler test	EC*/EC*	No
Open epicutaneous test	EC/EC	No
Guinea pig maximization test	ID + EC*/EC*	Yes

ID = intradermal; EC = epicutaneous.
*Occluded.

commonly accepted guinea pig tests for contact sensitizers. Differences between methods involve the use of an adjuvant in conjunction with the test material, as well as variations in schedules and methods of application of the compound. There are also several methods used clinically to assess human contact sensitization potential of a chemical. One such test is the human repeat insult patch test (HRIPT). Although not used for predictive purposes, another human test, the diagnostic patch test, allows the identification of individuals previously sensitized to a particular contact sensitizer.

In contrast to contact sensitizers, few predictive animal models exist for chemicals capable of causing immediate hypersensitivity responses in humans. Those under development primarily utilize the guinea pig as a model and evaluate sensitization potential of low- and high-molecular-weight compounds where exposure is via the respiratory tract. Following an appropriate induction period, respiratory responses are monitored upon challenge with the test compound. Serum allergic antibody titres may also be determined. Clinical methods of testing for immediate hypersensitivity usually include either intradermal injection of a small amount of the suspect allergen, or the topical application of the material to the skin, which is subsequently scratched or pricked through the test chemical. Measuring allergen-specific serum immunoglobulin E (IgE) antibodies by a radioallergo-sorbent test is also a commonly used diagnostic method for immediate hypersensitivity in humans. Table 4.3 summarizes several classes and/or sources of chemicals either associated with or known to cause respiratory or skin (contact) sensitization. Also included are commonly

Table 4.3 Agents associated with or known to cause human respiratory or skin sensitization following occupational or environmental exposure

Type of hypersensitivity	Immunological mechanism	Clinical symptoms	Source of chemical/chemical*	
			Low mol. wt	High mol. wt
Respiratory	Antibody-mediated (predominantly IgE)	Asthma Rhinitis Urticaria	Di-isocyanates Anhydrides Wood dust Metals Fluxes Drugs Azodicarbonamide Formalin Paraphenylene diamine	Laboratory animals Insects Birds Plants Grains Biological enzymes Vegetables
Skin (contact)	Cell-mediated (predominantly mononuclear leucocytes)	Redness Oedema Induration Vesiculation	Clothing/textiles Cosmetics Foods Medicaments Metals Pesticides Plants Wood Plastics Preservatives/ anti-bacterials	Not applicable

*Not all members of the class/group have been associated with hypersensitivity responses. For a more complete listing, including references, see Chan-Yeung and Lam [5] for respiratory sensitizers and Cronin [6] for contact sensitizers.

observed adverse clinical responses associated with exposure in sensitized individuals.

Adverse effects of chemicals on the immune system (Table 4.4)

Halogenated aromatic hydrocarbons

Among the most extensively studied classes of chemicals in terms of their immunotoxic properties are the halogenated aromatic hydrocarbons. They are widespread environmental contaminants which persist in the environment and bioaccumulate in animal tissues. The class includes the polychlorinated biphenyls (PCBs) and polybrominated biphenyls (PBBs), the dibenzo-*p*-dioxins and dibenzofurans. Through both accidental, occupational and environmental exposure, considerable human information concerning the immunotoxic effects of some of these compounds also exists. Studies in laboratory animals implicate a number of isomers of the

halogenated aromatic hydrocarbons as carcinogens, teratogens, neurotoxins and immunotoxins [7].

PCBs have been used in numerous industrial applications, including plasticizers, dielectric fluids, pesticide extenders and as a heat-transfer medium in electrical transformers. Human exposure to PCBs has been documented following two separate incidents in which Chinese and Japanese people consumed rice contaminated with PCBs [8–10]. The clinical studies are described in Chapter 13.

PCB exposure in laboratory animals has commonly been associated with atrophy of both primary and secondary lymphoid organs. The thymus appears to be particularly sensitive to PCB exposure. Suppression of humoral immune responses, including reduced circulating immunoglobulin levels and antigen-specific antibody responses, appears to be a consistent observation in PCB-exposed animals [11–13]. Reported effects of PCBs on cellular immunity include depressed delayed-type hypersensitivity responses [11] and reduced natural killer cell activity

Table 4.4 Some environmentally important chemicals reported to affect the immune system

Class	Chemical	Effects			
		HMI	CMI	Host resistance models	Non-specific defences
Metals	Arsenic	+	+	+	ND
	Cadmium	+	+	+	+
	Lead acetate	+	+	+	+
	Lead nitrate	ND	+	+	ND
	Mercuric chloride	+	+	+ / –	ND
	Methylmercury	+	+ / –	+	ND
	Dioctyltin dichloride	+	+	+	+ / –
Polychlorinated phenols	Hexachlorobenzene	+	+ / –	+	+ / –
	Pentachlorophenol	+	+ / –	ND	+
Monocyclic and polycyclic aromatic hydrocarbons	Benzene	+	+	+	ND
	7,12-Dimethylbenz[a]anthracene	+	+	+	+
	Methylcholanthrene	+	+	ND	ND
	Benzo[a]pyrene	+	+ /-	ND	ND
Polyhalogenated biphenyls (PCB, PBB)	Aroclor 1248	+	+ / –	+	ND
	Aroclor 1254	+	+ / –	+	ND
	Firemaster FF-1	+	+	+ / –	ND
Isocyanates	Toluene di-isocyanate	+	+	ND	ND
Dibenzo-*p*-dioxins, dibenzofurans	2,3,7,8-Tetra-chlorodibenzo-*p*-dioxin	+	+	+	+
	1,2,3,4,6,7,8-Heptachloro-dibenzo-*p*-dioxin	+	+	ND	ND
	Tetrachlorodibenzofuran	+	+	ND	ND
Aliphatic hydrocarbons	Ethyl carbamate	+	+	+	+
	Methyl carbamate	+ / –	+ / –	+ / –	+ / –
	Dimethylnitrosamine	+	+	+	+
	Vinyl chloride	ND	+	ND	ND
	1,3-Butadiene	+	+	ND	ND
Gaseous air pollutants (inhalation exposures) mixtures	Ozone	+	+	+	+
	Nitrogen dioxide	+	+	+	ND
	SO_2, $(NH_4)_2SO_4$	+ / –	+	+	+
Miscellaneous chemicals	Trimellitic anhydride	ND	ND	ND	+
	Gallium arsenide	+	+	+	+
	4-Vinyl-1-cyclohexene diepoxide	+	+	+	+

+, Statistically significant effect; + / –, equivocal effect; ND, not determined.
Humoral-mediated immunity (HMI) includes T-dependent antibody response, B-cell proliferation, B-cell rosettes and immunoglobulin levels. Cell-mediated immunity (CMI) includes delayed-type hypersensitivity, T-cell mitogenesis and mixed lymphocyte culture. Non-specific defences include natural killer cell activity, macrophage phagocytosis and carbon clearance. Test species include mouse, rat, rabbit, cow, human and non-human primate. Host resistance models include pseudorabies, encephalomyocarditis, influenza, herpes viruses; *Salmonella* sp.; *Plasmodium berghei*; *Klebsiella pneumoniae*; *Streptococcus* sp.; *Listeria monocytogenes* bacteria; PYB6 sarcoma; B16F10 melanoma tumour cells, and bacterial endotoxin challenge.

[14], although reports of enhanced mitogen and antigen-induced lymphoproliferation following PCB exposure have also been reported [15,16]. PCB-mediated effects on immunoregulation may be responsible for some of the seemingly conflicting results. In this regard, significantly reduced CD4$^+$:CB8$^+$ lymphocyte ratios in monkeys fed a diet containing a PCB (Aroclor 1254) mixture for 23 months have been reported [12]. This change in CD4$^+$:CD8$^+$ ratios corresponded with suppression of antigen-specific serum antibodies following immunization of these animals with a T-dependent antigen. Decreased host resistance to viral and bacterial challenge has been a commonly reported finding in PCB-exposed animals [17,18]. However, both suppression and enhancement of tumour resistance in PCB-exposed rodents have been reported [18,19].

PBBs, which are commonly used in flame retardant formulations (e.g. Firemaster products), have been associated with altered immune function in both humans and animals. Perhaps the best example of environmental contamination resulting in substantial human exposure to PBBs occurred when these compounds were accidentally included in livestock feed in Michigan, thereby contaminating the food chain (see also Chapter 13). Human exposures were confirmed by the presence of high PBB levels in serum and adipose tissue. A number of immunological parameters were evaluated and found to be altered in PBB-exposed populations relative to controls. These parameters included altered lymphocyte numbers and subpopulations; altered mitogen-induced lymphoproliferative responses; increased serum immunoglobulin levels and skin-test responsiveness to recall antigens. Some changes were still apparent 15 years following the original incident [20]. It is unclear what influence, if any, these immunological alterations have had on susceptibility to infection in exposed populations.

Studies in laboratory animals with PBBs are limited; however, they indicate PBB exposure can suppress both humoral and cell-mediated immune responses in rodents. In contrast, PBBs appear to have little influence on host resistance to parasitic or bacterial challenges at levels in rodents where immune function changes have been observed [21–23].

Dibenzo-p-dioxins

Dibenzo-p-dioxins can occur naturally in the environment and also as contaminants from a number of industrial processes. The 2,3,7,8-tetrachlorodibenzo-p-dioxin (TCDD) isomer is the most potent from a toxicological (and immunotoxicological) standpoint and is often used in experimental studies as the prototype immunosuppressant for this class of compounds. Indeed, the effects of TCDD on both humans and laboratory animals as well as its mode of action is discussed further by several other authors in this book.

A 1976 industrial dioxin accident in Seveso, Italy, provided an opportunity to perform an immunological evaluation on 44 children living in the contaminated area [24]. Twenty of these children exhibited chlorance, indicating TCDD exposure. Serum immunoglobulin and complement levels, however, were within normal reference ranges, while mitogen-induced T- and B-cell blastogenesis was significantly elevated. A more recent incident involving accidental human exposure to TCDD occurred in a Missouri trailer park, where residents were exposed to dirt and dust contaminated with TCDD. The only significant immune abnormality reported was immunological anergy in response to skin testing with recall antigens [25]. In contrast, no immunological alterations were observed in US Air Force study of individuals involved in spraying Agent Orange (a herbicide containing up to 20 p.p.m. of TCDD as a contaminant) in Vietnam [26].

While the evidence of TCDD-related immune alterations in humans is limited, there is compelling evidence that TCDD and other related halogenated hydrocarbons are immunotoxic in rodents and other laboratory animal species. Since TCDD-mediated toxicity and immunotoxicity are believed to be genetically linked, and species sensitivity can differ by several orders of magnitude, it is possible that humans are less susceptible to the effects of TCDD than experimental animals. However, inadequate documentation of such parameters as exposure levels and routes of exposure in human studies, along with a consideration of the genetic variability within the human population, are factors making it difficult to determine the real risk associated with TCDD exposure in humans.

In laboratory animals, a sensitive end-point of TCDD-mediated toxicity is severe thymic atrophy. Suppression of antibody responses, delayed-type hypersensitivity and mitogen-induced lymphoproliferative responses are generally but not always observed at slightly higher dosages than those causing thymic atrophy [27]. Immune suppression can, however, also be demonstrated to occur in the absence of thymic atrophy [28].

Guinea pigs are extremely sensitive to toxicities associated with TCDD exposure. Cumulative doses of TCDD as low as $0.32\,\mu g\,kg^{-1}$ given over an 8-week period result in suppression of antibody and delayed-type hypersensitivity responses [29]. In studies by Clark *et al.* [30,31], however, cumulative doses of TCDD as low as $4\,ng\,kg^{-1}$ given to adult mice over a 4-week period resulted in multiple T-cell effects, including impaired generation of a cytotoxic T-lymphocyte response. Percentages of human $CD4^+$ and $CDW29^+$ (helper-inducer) T cells were suppressed *in vitro* at TCDD culture concentrations as low as $10^{-13}M$ [32].

The effects of TCDD on host resistance to bacterial and viral challenge are less clear-cut. Increased susceptibility to the facultative intracellular parasite *Salmonella typhimurium* but not to *Listeria monocytogenes*, pseudorabies virus or tumour cell challenge has been observed following TCDD exposure [33–35]. Studies by White *et al.* [36] support suppression of host resistance to non-facultative bacterial challenge in mice treated with TCDD and other immunotoxic dioxin isomers. Furthermore, House *et al.* [35] have recently demonstrated increased susceptibility of TCDD-exposed mice to challenge with influenza virus, an infectious agent requiring intact humoral immunity and interferon defence mechanisms [37,38] for its elimination.

TCDD-induced immunotoxicity is believed to be mediated through a stereospecific and irreversible binding to the cytosolic aromatic hydrocarbon (Ah) receptor. Targets for TCDD immunotoxicity may include the thymic epithelial cells, bone marrow cells and lymphocytes, all of which have been demonstrated to possess the appropriate receptor. Thymic effects mediated by TCDD may result in impaired T-cell maturation or differentiation, and possibly decreased production of thymic hormones produced by thymic epithelial cells.

It appears that other dibenzodioxins structurally similar to TCDD have similar mechanisms of toxicity. For example, certain of the dibenzofurans including 2,3,7,8-tetrachlorodibenzofuran (TCDF), not only bind with the Ah receptor, but also cause similar immunotoxic effects. Compared to TCDD, immunotoxicity studies with TCDF are limited; however, relatively higher doses of TCDF are usually required to produce immunotoxicity of similar magnitude to that produced by TCDD [39].

Polycyclic aromatic hydrocarbons

Polycyclic aromatic hydrocarbons (PAHs) consist of fused benzene rings containing carbon and hydrogen atoms. They are environmental contaminants found in coal tar and as byproducts of fossil fuel combustion. It is estimated that in the USA nearly 900 tons of one PAH alone, benzo[a]pyrene (BP), is emitted into the atmosphere yearly. The most widely studied PAHs include 3-methylcholanthrene (MCA), 7,12-dimethylbenz[a]anthracene (DMBA) and BP, all of which are both carcinogenic and immunosuppressive.

Exposure to each of these three compounds impairs antibody responses in rodents. Malmgren *et al.*[40] initially studied the effects of PAH exposure on the immune system. They reported significant depression of humoral T-cell-dependent serum antibody responses in mice exposed to MCA, 1,2-benzanthrene or 1,2,5,6-dibenzanthracene. MCA exposure in mice also alters cell-mediated immune responses including suppression of mitogen-induced T-cell proliferation and cytotoxic T-cell function [41] as well as prolongation of skin graft survival [42]. Additionally, depending upon the PAH, exposure in mice can result in prolonged immune suppression. Thus, Stjernsward [43] observed suppression of T-dependent antibody responses persisting for over 32 days in mice exposed to BP, while Ward *et al.* [44] described suppression of both humoral and cellular immune responses persisting for at least 90 days in mice exposed to DMBA.

Data from rodent studies indicate that there is some sensitivity of humoral relative to cell-mediated immune responses to BP-mediated immunosuppression [45,46]. Thus, BP exposure in mice suppresses primary antibody responses and mitogen-induced T- and B-cell lymphoproliferation, but does not alter delayed-type hypersensitivity responses, allograft rejection or allogeneic stimulation of lymphocytes in mixed leucocyte cultures. Challenge of these animals with infectious agents or tumour cells for which resistance is believed to be dependent upon cell-mediated immunity was unaltered in these studies—a result consistent with a somewhat selective effect of BP upon humoral immune responses.

DMBA is the most potent PAH in terms of both its carcinogenic and immunotoxic potentials. Suppression of both numbers of antibody-producing cells and cell-mediated responses including tumoricidal function of natural killer and cytotoxic T cells has been observed following DMBA exposure. Suppression of host immune tumoricidal mechanisms may play a role in the carcinogenicity of the PAHs. In this regard, there is a positive correlation between the carcinogenic and immunosuppressive potential of PAHs [47].

The mechanism of PAH-mediated immunosuppression is unclear; however, there appear to be multiple immune cell targets for these compounds. MCA, BP and DMBA all inhibit humoral immunity, affecting both B-cell proliferation and antibody production. DMBA exposure also significantly reduces splenic B-cell progenitors and/or their ability to proliferate. This suggests the immature B cell may represent at least one target of PAH immunosuppression. In addition to humoral immunosuppression, MCA and DMBA also inhibit cell-mediated immune responses. Recent studies suggest DMBA-associated alterations in T helper cell function may explain some of the suppressive effects of DMBA on cell-mediated immunity [48].

Solvents

Human data have linked occupational exposure to solvents with alterations in selected immune parameters. These changes have included decreased numbers of circulating T lymphocytes with a resultant decrease in the $CD4^+:CD8^+$ cell ratio [49], altered serum immunoglobulin and complement levels [50,51] and development of autoantibodies [51]. As with many human studies examining chemically induced immune changes, however, precise cause-and-effect relationships have often been difficult to demonstrate since, among other things, quantitative exposure data are often lacking and individuals are often simultaneously exposed to complex mixtures of solvents and other chemicals. Additionally, the clinical significance of the immunological changes observed in humans is usually unclear. One report [52], however, of immunological studies in families exposed to solvent-contaminated drinking water suggests an excess number of individuals with altered T-cell ratios, the presence of autoantibodies, infections and rashes. Among children of these families, an increased incidence of leukaemia was also reported.

The most thoroughly studied solvent from an immunotoxicological standpoint is benzene. Benzene has been used extensively as an industrial solvent, as an intermediate in pesticide and dye production and as a replacement for alkyl–lead compounds in unleaded gasoline. It has become a common environmental contaminant. Benzene is a mutagen and carcinogen, and exposure to benzene has been associated with a number of myelotoxicities and blood dyscrasias in animals and humans. These include leukopenia, pancytopenia, anaemia, aplastic/hypoplastic bone marrow, lymphocytopenia, granulocytopenia and thrombocytopenia [53].

Numerous studies also support a role for benzene metabolites in mediating at least some of the myelotoxic and immunotoxic effects associated with exposure [54]. Benzene and/or its metabolites have been demonstrated to alter lymphocyte subpopulations [55], inhibit mitogen-induced lymphoproliferation [56] and lymphokine production [57,58]. Furthermore, benzene affects differentiation and maturation of bone marrow lymphoid cell precursors [57,59]. In the latter regard, hydroquinone, an oxidative metabolite of benzene, has recently been shown to block the final stages of B-cell differentiation in bone marrow cell cultures [57] and can also inhibit production of interferon-γ [58]. Interferon-γ plays a regulatory role in B-cell maturation; thus, benzene may influence B-cell function, possibly through effects on lymphokine production.

Benzene exposure can suppress specific antibody responses in rabbits [53], and mice [60], and alter host resistance in mice to bacterial challenge [61]. Many of the immunotoxic and myelotoxic effects of benzene seen in laboratory animals are consistent with those observed in humans suffering from severe benzene toxicity. Often these individuals are subject to acute, overwhelming infections.

Metals

Several metals and metal salts have been demonstrated to modify the immune response. Metallic nickel, chromium and beryllium, as well as platinum, gold and mercury salts have been associated with adverse effects resulting from the interactions of these agents with the immune system. In both humans and laboratory animals, these compounds can result in one or more types of hypersensitivities. Immunotoxicity other than hypersensitivity responses (i.e. immunosuppression or immunopotentiation) induced by metals has been clearly demonstrated in laboratory animals, although the analogous human data are less compelling. Some metals, such as platinum complexes and gold salts, have been therapeutically used in humans for the treatment of certain diseases and these compounds may alter the immune response [62,63]. However, whether or not immunosuppression occurs in humans following occupational or environmental exposure to metals is unclear.

Lead is suspected of altering host resistance in children with elevated blood lead levels [64] and in smelter workers occupationally exposed to lead [65]. However, Kimber *et al.* [66] evaluated certain immune parameters (serum immunoglobulin levels, T-lymphocyte number, natural killer cell response) in occupationally exposed workers with elevated blood lead concentrations and observed no significant effect of lead on any of the parameters evaluated.

In laboratory animals, the most extensively studied metals in terms of their immunological effects are lead, mercury and cadmium. The most consistent immunological effects have been suppression of immune responses. However, metal-induced enhancement of immune function has also been reported [67,68]. Lead, cadmium and mercury have generally been shown to decrease host resistance to a

number of infectious agent or tumour challenges, although occasionally enhanced resistance to challenge with certain pathogens has been reported [69]. Lead exposure in rodents can decrease resistance to bacterial and viral challenges [70–72]. Similar results have been reported in rodents exposed to cadmium and challenged with bacteria or virus [67]. In addition, both inorganic and organic mercury exposure have been associated with decreased host resistance of rodents to viral challenge.

Suppression of antibody responses in rodents following lead and mercury exposure appears to be a more consistent observation than changes in cell-mediated immunity. For example, Luster *et al.* [73] demonstrated significant reductions in primary T-dependent antibody responses in rats perinatally exposed to lead. Similar results have been observed in mice following exposure to tetraethyl lead [74]. Likewise, cadmium and mercury have been demonstrated to depress antibody responses in laboratory animals. Chronic cadmium exposure has been reported to decrease both serum antibody titres and numbers of antibody-forming cells in rabbits [75] and mice [76], while several groups have demonstrated suppressive effects of mercury on primary antibody responses [77,78].

Metal-induced modulation of cell-mediated immune responses is less clearly defined. Faith and co-workers [79] reported that chronic lead exposure in rats depressed delayed-type hypersensitivity responses and mitogen-induced lymphoproliferation. These results were consistent with the decreased lymphoproliferative responses observed by Gaworski and Sharma [80] in mice subchronically exposed to lead, but inconsistent with the lack of lead-induced suppression of lymphoproliferation observed by other investigators [72,74,81].

A number of other metals, including nickel and tin, may reportedly act as immunotoxicants. Nickel exposure can alter host resistance to viral, bacterial and tumour cell challenges in laboratory animals [82–84]. Functional effects of nickel on macrophages and natural killer cells could represent at least part of the basis for the altered host resistance observed in nickel-treated animals,

The mechanism of metal-induced immunotoxicity appears to be complex and multi-faceted. However, studies with lead and tin suggest that these metals may bind sulphydryl groups associated with cell membrane or cytosolic components and disrupt cellular functions necessary for normal immune responses [69,85]. Experimental support for this possible mechanism of action comes in part from studies demonstrating that exogenous addition of sulphydryl reagents can reverse some of the *in vitro* functional alterations induced by lead [74]. The tin salts have been extensively studied in terms of their immunotoxic properties [86,87]. Because of this, and their wide range of industrial applications, they are discussed separately.

Organotins

Organotin compounds are used primarily as heat stabilizers in the production of polyvinyl chloride polymers, as industrial and agricultural biocides and as industrial catalysts for a variety of chemical reactions [86]. Studies in the 1960s provided the first indication of possible immunotoxicity associated with these compounds when Verscheuuren *et al.* [88] observed reduced numbers of circulating lymphocytes in guinea pigs and rats exposed to the hydroxide and acetate salts of triphenyltin. In guinea pigs, these compounds were also noted to cause thymic and splenic atrophy. More recent studies have demonstrated that certain of the diorganotin compounds can have similar effects [89]. Di-n-octyltin dichloride (DOTC) and di-n-butyltin dichloride (DBTC) have been observed to deplete thymic cellularity severely, reduce thymic weight and alter T-cell function in rats at dose levels not causing other toxicities. Thus, some of the organotins may exhibit sensitivity and specificity not only for the immune system, but apparently for specific components of the immune system (i.e. T cells) and immune response as well. Decreases in T-cell function associated with organotin exposure have been characterized as increased skin graft rejection times, reduced delayed-type hypersensitivity responses and decreased mitogen-induced T-cell proliferation [86,89]. Further evidence of specific T-cell dysfunction in DOTC- or DBTC-treated rats includes the observation of depressed antibody plaque responses to T-dependent, but not T-independent antigens in these animals. Suppression of T-cell responses correlates with depressed host resistance to *Listeria* challenge.

Immunotoxicity associated with organotin compounds tends to be species-specific. In this regard, neither extensive lymphoid tissue atrophy nor impairment of immune function was observed in mice or guinea pigs fed dialkyl tins [89]. However, thymic atrophy can be demonstrated in mice following parenteral exposure to either DOTC or DBTC; thus, interspecies variability in the immunotoxicity of these compounds may involve differences in their absorption, metabolism and elimination. This hypothesis is further supported by *in vitro* studies indicating that DOTC and DBTC added to cultures of immunoresponsive cells produce similar immunotoxic effects, regardless of species of cell origin.

Certain of the triorganotins, including tri-n-butyltin oxide (TBTO) and tri-n-butyltin chloride (TBTC) produce similar immunotoxicities as the active diorganotins. Vos and colleagues [90] noted that lymphocyte depletion and thymic effects as well as alterations in T-dependent immune function and host resistance in rats treated with TBTO and TBTC were similar to those observed following exposure to DOTC and DBTC. These similarities are not surprising since at least part of the thymic atrophy observed in rats following their exposure to tributyltin apparently results from a dibutyltin metabolite rather than the parent compound [91].

Current views as to the mechanism of organotin-mediated immunotoxicity centre on their direct effects on proliferating thymocytes which result in cellular depletion of the thymus and peripheral lymphoid tissues [85]. Anti-proliferative effects as well as some of the functional impairment observed in T cells following exposure to these compounds may involve interactions between dialkyl and sulphydryl groups of the target cell membrane and cytosol [85].

Adverse effects of pesticides on the immune system

Exposure to pesticides can provoke a variety of immune reactions. These reactions range from modulation of functional immune responses to development of hypersensitivity responses. The number of reviews on this subject attests to the interest in and concern for pesticide-induced immune alterations [31,52,92–96].

Table 4.5 Examples of pesticides reported to modulate immunity in experimental animals

Pesticide	Species	Summary of effects	References
Organophosphates			
Methylparathion	Rabbit	Thymus atrophy and reduced delayed-type hypersensitivity (DTH) response	[97]
	Mouse	Decreased host resistance to *Salmonella typhimurium* infection	[98]
Parathion	Mouse	Altered colony-forming activities of bone marrow haematopoietic stem cells	[99]
Malathion	Mouse	Suppression of cytotoxic T lymphocyte (CTL) response *in vitro*	[100]
Organochlorines			
2,2-*Bis*-(*p*-chlorophenyl)-1,1,1-trichloro ethane (DDT)	Rabbit	Thymus atrophy and reduced DTH response	[97]
Mirex	Chicken	Decreased IgG levels	[101]
Hexachlorobenzene	Mouse	Increased sensitivity to endotoxin and malaria challenge	[102]
	Rat	Increased humoral immune responses to tetanus toxoid and delayed-type hypersensitivity to ovalbumin	[103]
Dieldrin	Mouse	Decreased antibody-forming cell (AFC) response and increased susceptibility to viral infection	[104,105]
Chlordane	Mouse	Decreased contact hypersensitivity after *in utero* exposure	[106,107]
	Mouse	Suppression of AFC responses and T-cell activity in a mixed leucocyte culture (MLC) reaction following *in vitro* exposure	[108]
Pentachlorophenol	Mouse	Decreased host resistance to virus-induced tumour metastases	[109]
Chlorophenoxy compounds			
2,4-Dichlorophenoxyacetic acid (2,4-D)	Mouse	Enhanced T- and B-cell immune responses following dermal application	[110]
Carbamates			
Carbofuran	Rabbit	Reduced DTH response	[97]
	Mouse	Decreased host resistance to *S. typhimurium* infection	[98]
Aldicarb	Mouse	Decreased AFC response to sheep erythrocytes	[111]
	Human	Increased response to *Candida* antigen, increased number of lymphocytes expressing CD8 marker and decreased $CD4^+$:$CD8^+$ cell ratio	[112]
	Mouse	No alterations in splenic AFC response, B- or T-lymphocyte mitogenesis, mixed lymphocyte response, host resistance, or lymphocyte subsets	[113,114]
	Mouse	Inhibition of macrophage tumoricidal activity, IL-1 production	[115,116]
	Human	Persistent increase in $CD8^+$ lymphocytes	[117]
Organotin compounds			
Triphenyltin hydroxide (TPTH)	Rat	Reduced DTH response to tuberculin	[90]
Tributyltin oxide (TBTO)	Rat	Reduced T-cell-mediated, natural killer cell, and macrophage responses and decreased host resistance to *Trichinella spiralis* infection	[90]

Impairment of functional immunity

A number of different pesticide classes alter both antibody and cell-mediated immunity. Table 4.5 summarizes some human and experimental animal data for pesticide-induced impairment of immunity. These effects, in many cases, can be correlated with changes in host resistance to infection. Often these studies employed acute or relatively short-term exposures to the offending agent. Since many of these pesticides are stable, and are capable of persisting in the environment, they may represent a particularly important group of compounds from an immunotoxicological standpoint under chronic exposure conditions. In addition, pesticide impurities, although not discussed specifically in this section, may also result in immunotoxicity. O,O,S-trimethyl phosphorothiolate, a contaminant of malathion, and 2,3,7,8-tetrachlorodibenzo-*p*-dioxin, a contaminant of 2,4,5-trichlorophenoxyacetic acid, are two such compounds. The latter compound was discussed in detail in a previous section of this chapter.

Recent interest in the potential adverse effects of pesticides on the immune system has stemmed from studies in mice which were administered low levels of aldicarb, a carbamate pesticide, in drinking water—the route most common to human exposure. These studies reported that suppression of antibody responses occurred following exposure to levels of aldicarb as low as 1 p.p.b. for 34 days in drinking water [111]. Thomas *et al.* [113,114] in more comprehensive studies in mice, observed no aldicarb-related effects on the immune system. A recent report by Selvan and co-workers [115], however, showed that peritoneal macrophage tumour cell killing was impaired following exposure to low levels of aldicarb by the intraperitoneal route. Effects of anticholinesterase agents on mouse peritoneal macrophage metabolism, superoxide production and esterase activity may account for these results [118].

Epidemiological studies suggest that otherwise healthy women who have chronically ingested low levels of aldicarb-contaminated groundwater had altered numbers of T cells, including a decreased $CD4^+:CD8^+$ ratio [112]. No indication of altered disease status has been observed in these individuals. However, a follow-up study suggests that some of the immune changes have persisted [117]. These data are significant in the light of recent studies in California documenting food-poisoning outbreaks allegedly due to aldicarb sulphoxide at estimated dosage levels of 0.0011–0.06 mg kg^{-1} body weight [119].

Although there is sufficient evidence that pesticides affect certain functions of the immune and haematopoietic systems, it remains difficult to relate these changes to health risk. For example, even though morphological changes in blood were observed in humans exposed to pesticides under special occupational conditions (e.g. applications within greenhouses where high concentrations of pesticide are typically present), there was no indication of altered immune status [120]. However, in a study of pesticide workers exposed to combinations of four pesticides (malathion, parathion, dichlorodiphenyltrichloroethane and hexachlorocyclohexane), 73% showed signs of toxicity, including altered levels of serum immunoglobulin [121]. Increases in serum IgG but decreases in serum IgM and the C3 component of complement were reported in a study of 51 men exposed to chlorinated pesticides, as compared to a 28-man control group [122]. In each of these studies, however, a direct association with a change in health status is absent. In contrast, some studies do relate cause and effect with a possible mechanism of action. Marked impairment of neutrophil chemotaxis and an increased incidence of respiratory tract infection correlated with length of exposure in 85 workers exposed to organophosphate pesticides [123].

In summary, the data suggest that occupational exposure to pesticides can result in immune system disorders. There is insufficient information to support similar concerns regarding chronic, non-occupational exposure to pesticides.

Potential for inducing hypersensitivity

Contact sensitization. Over 40 pesticides of various chemical classes have been associated with contact dermatitis [6]. However, in spite of widespread occupational exposure, the incidence of documented allergic contact dermatitis cases for any particular pesticide is sporadic. The true incidence of pesticide-mediated contact dermatitis remains unclear. Occupational illness and injury reports suggest that the occurrence of allergic contact dermatitis in workers routinely exposed to pesticides is rare. One such report cites 342 cases of skin-related complaints reported in 1986 in California out of approximately 800 000 individuals commonly exposed to pesticides (agricultural workers and pesticide applicators) — i.e. 0.43 cases per 1000 workers. While contact dermatitis would account for only a fraction of the skin-related complaints, these figures do not reflect an additional 318 dermatitis cases reported in vineyard workers excluded from the incidence figures because of insufficient information to confirm a pesticide causal link. Additional studies have evaluated various environmental factors influencing the incidence of skin rashes in vineyard workers and found little correlation with pesticide exposure; most of the rashes were attributed to high temperatures during thinning and harvesting operations [124]. In contrast, 44% of 3717 Japanese reported experiencing specific allergic symptoms associated with agricultural pesticide use [125]. In a separate study of 200 people (50 of whom were agricultural workers) who were patch-tested for pesticide reactivity, 24 positive reactions were noted, primarily against the thiophthalimides, captan, folpet, and difolatan [126].

With respect to animal predictive testing, considerable guinea pig skin sensitization data exist for many pesticides, in part because governmental guidelines require this information for pesticide registration. Table 4.6 summarizes some of these data and data from human diagnostic patch-testing.

Dinitrochlorobenzene (DNCB), which is used as an algicide in cooling systems, is also frequently used experimentally as a prototype, strong contact sensitizer. Both Buehler-type (occluded patch) and guinea pig maximization tests (GPMT) identify DNCB as a potent sensitizer, although the incidence of sensitization at similar test concentrations is greater using the GPMT than the Buehler test [127,128]. Human studies support the potency of DNCB as a skin sensitizer. Following a single patch induction, Friedman *et al.* [129] demonstrated positive skin responses in humans tested at concentrations of DNCB below 0.2%. Diagnostic patch-testing of two workers with clinical dermatitis thought to be due to DNCB exposure gave moderately positive patch test reactions at concentrations as low as 1 p.p.m. [130].

GPMT data for benomyl, maneb, naled, malathion, captan and sodium chlorate classify all of these chemicals as strong to extreme sensitizers, at least at the highest concentrations tested. Sodium dichloropropionate was classified as a mild sensitizer (Table 4.6). Diagnostic patch-testing in isolated cases of presumed pesticide-related dermatitis has shown positive reactions to these chemicals at patch test concentrations as low as 1%. In the case of malathion, a survey of 200 workers with malathion exposure (at 1% diagnostic patch test level) showed a 3% incidence of positive responses [145]. However, this was not confirmed by an International Contact Dermatitis Research Group (ICDRG) survey of 455 individuals [6]. Reduction of a contaminant of technical-grade malathion, diethyl fumarate, has further reduced the potential for contact sensitization following exposure to this pesticide.

In summary, it is clear that many pesticides may act as contact sensitizers in both animals and humans. Predictive tests in guinea pigs may overestimate the human contact sensitization risk associated with pesticide exposure, since relatively few cases of human contact sensitization have been reported despite the widespread usage of pesticides. On the other hand, the true incidence of pesticide-induced contact sensitization is not known. This is due, in part, to difficulties in identifying, testing, tracking and documenting conditions and circumstances of exposure in occupationally exposed individuals.

Antibody-mediated allergic disease. Pesticides are generally low molecular weight compounds whose ability to act as sensitizers depends upon formation of stable immunogenic complexes with host proteins. There are few well controlled studies that investigate the ability of pesticides to induce and elicit immediate hypersensitivity (i.e. antibody-mediated) responses. Since symptoms of allergy to 2,4-dichlorophenoxyacetic acid (2,4-D) have been reported in humans, Cushman and Street [147] investigated the ability of this compound to induce allergic antibodies in mice. In these studies, female BALB/c mice were immunized with two intraperitoneal injections on day 1 and 28 with 2,4-D KLH

Table 4.6 Guinea pig skin sensitization predictive testing compared to human diagnostic patch-testing following exposure to selected pesticides

Material	Guinea pig skin sensitization				Human diagnostic patch test		
	Test	Positive* (%)	Grade*	Ref.	No. of subjects	Result[†] (challenge conc. %)	Ref.
Dinitrochlorobenzene	Buehler	100	NA	[127]	2	+ + → + + + (0.0001 → 0.1)	[130]
	GPMT	100	Extreme	[128]			
Barban	Buehler	100	NA	[131]	2	+ + → + + + (0,00001 → 0.1)	[94]
					1	+ + (10)	[138]
Benomyl	GPMT	100	Extreme	[132]	3	+ → + + + (1)	[139]
					1	Positive (1)	[140]
					4	+ + (10)	[141]
Maneb	GPMT	100	Extreme	[133]	3	+ + → + + + + (1-5)	[142]
					1	Positive (1)	[143]
Naled	GPMT	90	Extreme	[134]	3	Positive (60)	[144]
Malathion	GPMT	70	Strong	[134,135]	200	3% Positive (1)	[145]
Captan	GPMT	83	Extreme	[136]	509	3% Positive (1)	[6]
					200	4.0–5.5% Positive (0.5–1.0)	[126]
Sodium chlorate	GPMT	80	Strong	[137]	38	5.3–10.5% Positive (0.1–10.0)	[146]
Sodium dichloro-propionate	GPMT	10	Mild	[137]	38	10.5–13.2% Positive (0.1–10.0)	[146]

*Maximum incidence or grade observed in one or more tests using varying induction and challenge concentrations of the test material.
[†]Severity of diagnostic patch reaction: + → + + + + .
NA = not applicable; GPMT = guinea pig maximization test.

(keyhole limpet haemocyanin), or DNP (dinitrophenol)-KLH as a positive control. Presence of allergic antibodies specific for 2,4-D was demonstrated by passive cutaneous anaphylaxis (PCA) in rat skin. The highest antibody titres were detected 7 days after the secondary intraperitoneal immunization. In contrast, when sensitization was attempted with epicutaneous application of 2,4-D, mouse sera did not contain specific allergic antibodies.

Similar studies were conducted by Cushman and Street [148] with the pesticide malathion. Of the mice immunized intraperitoneally with malathion-KLH, 90% had detectable allergic antibody following the secondary intraperitoneal immunization as demonstrated by PCA and serological testing by a RAST (radioallergosorbent test). Like 2,4-D, malathion failed to induce allergic IgE antibody production when administered epicutaneously. Relatively high concentrations of the malathion conjugate were necessary for the development of an antigen-specific antibody response.

Evidence that insecticide or pesticide exposure in humans results in acute allergic reactions such as rhinitis, asthma, or anaphylaxis is difficult to confirm. Many atopic patients present with symptom exacerbation after exposure to pesticides, but most investigators consider such reactions to be irritative rather than allergic. Isolated case reports [149] however, provide some indication that allergic reactions to pesticides can occur, but the likelihood of this happening is rare.

At present, there is limited evidence that some patients may have asthmatic responses to pesticides. Although clinical characteristics of these responses suggest IgE sensitization, it is not established in humans that such sensitization occurs. Preliminary experiments in animals support the possibility of IgE sensitization to derivatives of pesticides and also indicate their potential role in allergic reactions. More studies are needed to estimate this involvement accurately and to determine the precise role of pesticides in allergic diseases and asthma.

Conclusions

Immunotoxicity assessment involves determination of a chemical's potential to act as a sensitizer or to alter the components of the immune system in an adverse manner. Many classes of chemicals to which humans are occupationally or environmentally exposed have been linked to hypersensitivity and/or immunomodulation.

Extensive human epidemiological and clinical data exist for a variety of chemicals and their capacity to produce immediate or delayed hypersensitivity responses. In terms of occupational or environmental exposure to chemical sensitizers, the skin and respiratory tract are frequent target organs. Contact sensitivity and asthma, rhinitis and urticaria are likely clinical manifestations of allergic immunotoxicity. Predictive methods for contact sensitizers have been developed in both laboratory animals and humans, while human diagnostic patch tests identify compounds to which an individual has been previously sensitized. Guinea pig skin sensitization data are commonly used in safety assessments for the identification and potency ranking of potential human contact sensitizers. In the USA, government regulatory guidelines exist calling for skin sensitization data for the registration of certain products, including pesticides. Thus, pesticides provide an example of a class of compounds for which there exist animal sensitization data as well as human predictive and diagnostic test information. It appears that guinea pig skin-testing methods are sensitive in predicting those pesticides likely to cause human contact sensitization. They may be overly sensitive, however, in that the high incidence of sensitization in guinea pigs to many of these chemicals might suggest higher incidences of human sensitization than the available human data would support. On the other hand, there are difficulties in determining the true incidence of sensitization to pesticides in those populations most likely to be exposed to pesticides, e.g. migrant farmworkers.

In contrast to hypersensitivity end-points of chemical immunotoxicity, limited human data exist concerning chemically induced modulation of immune function and other immune parameters. In those cases where alterations do exist following occupational or environmental exposure to immunotoxic chemicals their biological consequences are unclear (i.e. increased incidence of infections or neoplasias). It is not unreasonable, however, to consider those end-points as potential outcomes, particularly of chemical-induced immunosuppression. Human data from individuals with genetic or virally induced (e.g. human immunodeficiency virus-induced) immunodeficiencies as well as those being therapeutically immunosuppressed (e.g. organ transplant recipients) would support this concept. The substantial immunotoxicity database developed in experimental animals provides further evidence for the ability of several classes of chemicals to modulate the immune system and immune response, with consequential decreases in resistance to challenge with infectious agents or tumour cells.

Pesticides are a class of compounds for which there is limited human and substantial animal data, indicating the potential of some of these chemicals to alter the immune system. In laboratory animals, pesticide-induced changes in immune function clearly correlate with alterations in host resistance. In humans, the consequence of pesticide-mediated alterations in immune status is unclear; therefore, it is difficult to assess the immunotoxic risk associated with human exposure to pesticides. This problem carries over to other classes of immunotoxic chemicals as well. Areas of uncertainty associated with immunotoxicity risk assessment will need to be addressed in order that more knowledgeable decisions can be made as to chemical safety. As these uncertainties are reduced, risk assessments of immunotoxicity associated with chemical exposure will be more representative of real rather than perceived risks.

References

1 Kammuller ME, Bloksma N, Sienen W, eds. *Autoimmunity and Toxicology: Immune Disregulation Induced by Drugs and Chemicals.* Amsterdam: Elsevier, 1989.

2 Penn I. Tumors of the immunocompromised patient. *Ann R Med* 1985; 39:63–73.

3 Luster MI. Immunotoxicology and the immune system. *Health Environ Dig* 1989; 3:1–3.

4 Luster MI, Munson AE, Thomas PT *et al.* Development of a testing battery to assess chemical-induced immunotoxicity: national toxicology program's guidelines for immunotoxicity evaluation in mice. *Fund Appl Toxicol* 1988; 10:2–19.

5 Chan-Yeung M, Lam S. Occupational asthma. *Am Rev Resp Dis* 1986; 133(suppl): 686–703.

6 Cronin E. *Contact Dermatitis.* Edinburgh: Churchill Livingstone, 1980.

7 Kimbrough RD, ed. Halogenated biphenyls, terphenyls, naphthalenes, dibenzodioxins and related products. In: *Topics in Environmental Health.* vol. 4. New York: Elsevier/North-Holland Biomedical Press, 1980.

8 Chang KJ, Ching JS, Huang PC, Tung TC. Study of

patients with PCB poisoning. *J Formosan Med Assoc* 1980; 79:304–12.

9 Lee TP, Chang KJ. Health effects of polychlorinated biphenyls. In: Dean JH, Luster MI, Munson AE, Amos HE, eds. *Immunotoxicology and Immunopharmacology.* New York: Raven Press, 1985; 415–22.

10 Shigematsu N, Ishmaru S, Saito R, Ikeda T, Matsuba K, Sugiyama K, Masuda Y. Respiratory involvement in PCB poisoning. *Environ Res* 1978; 16:92–100.

11 Thomas PT, Hinsdill RD. Perinatal PCB exposure and its effects on the immune system of young rabbits. *Drug Chem Toxicol* 1980; 3:173–84.

12 Tryphonas H, Hayward S, O'Grady L, Loo JCK, Arnold DL, Bryce F, Zawidzha ZZ. Immunotoxicity studies of PCB (Aroclor 1254) in the adult rhesus (*Macaca mulatta*) monkey. Preliminary report. *Int J Immunopharmacol* 1989; 11:199–206.

13 Vos JG, Faith RE, Luster MI. *Immune Alterations.* New York: Elsevier/North-Holland Biomedical Press, 1980:241–66.

14 Talcott PA, Koller LD, Exon TH. The effect of lead and polychlorinated biphenyl exposure on rat natural killer cell cytotoxicity. *Int J Immunopharmacol* 1985; 7:255–61.

15 Silkworth JB, Loose LD. Cell-mediated immunity in mice fed either Aroclor 1016 or hexachlorobenzene. *Toxicol Appl Pharmacol* 1978; 45:326–7.

16 Silkworth JB, Loose LD. PCB and HCB induced alteration of lymphocyte blastogenesis. *Toxicol Appl Pharmacol* 1979; 49:86.

17 Dean JH, Luster MI, Boorman GA. Immunotoxicology. In: Sirois P, Rola-Pleszgyski M, eds. *Immunopharmacology* Amsterdam: Elsevier Biomedical Press, 1985; 349–97.

18 Lubet RA, Lemaire BN, Avery D, Kouri RE. Induction of immunotoxicity in mice by polyhalogenated biphenyls. *Arch Toxicol* 1986; 59:71–7.

19 Kerkvliet NI, Kimmeldorf DJ. Antitumor activity of a polychlorinated biphenyl mixture, Aroclor 1254, in rats inoculated with Walker 256 carcinosarcoma cells. *J Natl Cancer Inst* 1977; 59:951–5.

20 Bekesi JG, Roboz JP, Fischbeim A, Selikoff IJ. Clinical immunology studies in individuals exposed to environmental chemicals. In: Berlin A, Dean J, Draper MH, Smith EMB, Spreafico F, eds. *Immunotoxicology.* Dordrecht: Martinus Nijhoff Publishers, 1987; 347–61.

21 Luster MI, Boorman GA, Harris MW, Moore JA. Laboratory studies on polybrominated biphenyl-induced immune alterations following low-level chronic or pre/postnatal exposure. *Int J Immunopharmacol* 1980; 2:69–80.

22 Loose LD, Mudzinski SP, Silkworth JB. Influence of dietary polybrominated biphenyl on antibody and

host defense responses in mice. *Toxicol Appl Pharmacol* 1981; 59:25.

23 Fraker PJ. The antibody-mediated and delayed-type hypersensitivity response of mice exposed to polybrominated biphenyls. *Toxicol Appl Pharmacol* 1980; 53:1.

24 Reggiani G. Acute human exposure to TCDD in Seveso, Italy. *J Toxicol Environ Health* 1980; 6:27–43.

25 Hoffman RE, Stehr-Green PA, Webb KB *et al*. Health effects of long-term exposure to 2,3,7,8-tetrachlorodibenzo-p-dioxin. *JAMA* 1986; 255:2031–8.

26 Lathrop GD, Wolfe WH, Albanese RA, Moynahan PM. *Air Force health study (project ranch hand II). An epidemiologic investigation of health effects in air force personnel following exposure to herbicides, baseline morbidity study results.* vol. 16. Texas: USAF School of Aerospace Medicine, Brooks Air Force Base, 1984; 2-1-2-12.

27 Thomas PT, Faith RE. Adult and perinatal immunotoxicity induced by halogenated aromatic hydrocarbons. In: Dean JH, Luster MI, Munson AE, Amos HE, eds. *Immunotoxicology and Immunopharmacology.* New York: Raven Press, 1985; 305–13.

28 Silkworth JB, Vecchi A. Role of the Ah receptor in halogenated aromatic hydrocarbon immunotoxicity. In: Dean JH, Luster MI, Munson AE, Amos H, eds. *Immunotoxicology and Immunopharmacology.* New York: Raven Press, 1985; 263–75.

29 Vos JG, Moore JA, Zinkl JG. Effects of 2,3,7,8-tetrachlorodibenzo-p-dioxin on the immune system of laboratory animals. *Environ Hlth Perspect* 1973; 5:149–62.

30 Clark DA, Gauldie J, Szewczuk MR, Sweeney G. Enhanced suppressor cell activity as a mechanism of immunosuppression by 2,3,7,8- tetrachlorodibenzo-p-dioxin. *Proc Soc Exp Biol Med* 1981; 168:290–9.

31 Clark DA, Sweeney G, Safe S *et al*. Cellular and genetic basis for suppression of cytotoxic T-cell generation by haloaromatic hydrocarbons. *Immunopharmacology* 1983; 6:143–53.

32 Neubert R, Jacob-Müller U, Helge H, Stahlmann R, Neubert D. Polyhalogenated dibenzodioxins and dibenzofurans and the immune system. 2. *In vitro* effects of 2,3,7,8-tetrachlorodibenzo-p-dioxin (TCDD) on lymphocytes of venous blood from man and a non-human primate (*Callithrix jaccus*). *Arch Toxicol* 1991; 65:213–19.

33 Thigpen JE, Faith RE, McConnell EE, Moore JA. Increased susceptibility to bacterial infection as a sequela of exposure to 2,3,7,8-tetrachlorodibenzo-p-dioxin. *Infect Immun* 1975; 12:1319–24.

34 Dean JH, Lauer LD. Immunological effects following exposure to 2,3,7,8-tetrachlorodibenzo-p-dioxin: a re-

view. In: Lawrance WW, ed. *Public Health Risk of the Dioxins.* Los Altos, California: William Kaufmann, 1984:275–94.

35 House RV, Lauer DL, Murray MJ, Thomas PT, Ehrlich JP, Burleson GR, Dean JH. Examination of immune parameters and host resistance mechanisms in B6C3F1 mice following adult exposure to 2,3,7,8-tetrachlorodibenzo-p-dioxin. *Toxicol Environ Hlth* 1990; 31:203–15.

36 White KL, Lysy HH, McCay JA, Anderson AC. Modulation of serum complement levels following exposure to polychlorinated dibenzo-p-dioxins. *Toxicol Appl Pharmacol* 1986; 84:209–19.

37 Hoshino A, Takenaka H, Mizukoshi O, Imanishi J, Kishida T, Tovey M. Effect of anti-interferon serum on influenza virus infection in mice. *Antiviral Res* 1983; 3:59–68.

38 Vireligier J. Host defenses against influenza virus: the role of anti-hemagglutinin antibody. *J Immunol* 1975; 115:434–9.

39 Vecchi A. Some aspects of immune alternations induced by chlorodibenzo-p-dosing and chlorodibenzofurans. In: Berlin A, Dean J, Draper MH, Smith EMB, Spreafico F, eds. *Immunotoxicology.* Dordrecht: Martinus Nijhoff, 1987; 308–16.

40 Malmgren RA, Bennison BE, McKinley TW Jr. Reduced antibody titers in mice treated with carcinogenic and cancer chemotherapeutic agents. *Proc Soc Exp Biol Med* 1952; 70:484–8.

41 Wojdani A, Alfred LJ. *In vitro* effects of certain polycyclic hydrocarbons on mitogen activation of mouse T-lymphocytes: action of histamine. *Cell Immunol* 1983; 77:132–42.

42 DiMarco AT, Francheschi C, Xerri L, Prodi G. Depression of homograft rejection and graft-versus-host reactivity following 7,12-dimethyl-benz(a)anthracene exposure in the rat. *Cancer Res* 1971; 31:1446–50.

43 Stjernsward J. Effect of noncarcinogenic and carcinogenic hydrocarbons on antibody-forming cells measured at the cellular level *in vitro. J Natl Cancer Inst* 1966; 36:1189–95.

44 Ward EC, Murray MJ, Lauer LD, House RV, Dean JH. Persistent suppression of humoral and cell-mediated immunity in mice following exposure to the polycyclic aromatic hydrocarbon, 7,12-dimethyl-benz[a]anthracene. *Int J Immunopharmacol* 1986; 8:13–22.

45 Dean JH, Luster MI, Boorman GA, Lauer LD, Luebke RW, Lawson LD. Immune suppression following exposure of mice to the carcinogen benzo(a)pyrene but not the non-carcinogenic benzo(e)pyrene. *Clin Exp Immunol* 1983; 52:199–206.

46 Ball JK. Immunosuppression and carcinogenesis:

contrasting effects with 7,12-dimethylbenz(a)anthracene, benz[a]pyrene, and 3-methyl-cholanthrene. *J Natl Cancer Inst* 1970; 44:1.

47 Ward EC, Murray MJ, Dean JH. Immunotoxicity of nonhalogenated polycyclic aromatic hydrocarbons. In: Dean JH, Luster MI, Munson AE, Amos H, eds. *Immunotoxicology and Immunopharmacology.* New York: Raven Press, 1985; 291-304.

48 House RV, Pallardy MJ, Dean JH. Suppression of murine cytotoxic T-lymphocyte induction following exposure to 7,12-dimethylbenz[a]anthracene: dysfunction of antigen recognition. *Int J Immunopharmacol* 1989; 11:207-15.

49 Denkhaus W, Steldern DV, Botzenhardt U, Konietzko H. Lymphocyte subpopulation in solvent-exposed workers. *Int Arch Occup Environ Hlth* 1986; 57:109-15.

50 Lange A, Smolik R, Zatonski W, Szymanbska J. Serum immunoglobulin levels in workers exposed to benzene and xylene. *Int Arch Arbeitsmed* 1973; 31:37.

51 Cohen HS, Freeman ML, Goldstein BL. Invited review: the problem of benzene in our environment: clinical and molecular considerations. *Am J Med Sci* 1987; 275:124-36.

52 Byers VS, Levin AS, Ozonoff DM, Baldwin RW. *Cancer Immunol Immunother* 1988; 1:77-81.

53 International Agency for Research on Cancer. Evaluation of the carcinogenic risk of chemicals to humans: Some industrial chemicals and dyestuffs. *IARC Monogr* 1982; 29:93-148.

54 Luster MJ, Blank JA, Dean JH. Molecular and cellular basis of chemically induced immunotoxicity. *Annu Rev Pharmacol Toxicol* 1987; 27:23-49.

55 Irons RD, Moore BJ. Effect of short term benzene administration on circulating lymphocyte subpopulations in the rabbit: evidence of a selective B-lymphocyte sensitivity. *Res Commun Chem Pathol Pharmacol* 1980; 27:147-55..

56 Rozen MG, Snyder CA, Albert RE. Depressions in B- and T-lymphocyte mitogen induced blastogenesis in mice exposed to low concentrations of benzene. *Toxicol Lett* 1984; 20:343-9.

57 Tunek A, Olofess T, Berlin M. Toxic effects of benzene and benzene metabolites on granulopoietic stem cells and bone marrow cellularity in mice. *Toxicol Appl Pharmacol* 1981; 59:149-56.

58 Cheung SC, Nerland DE, Sonnenfeld G. Inhibition of interferon gamma production by benzene and benzene metabolites. *J Natl Cancer Inst* 1988; 80:1069-72.

59 King AG, Landreth KS, Wierda D. Hydroquinone inhibits bone marrow pre-B cell maturation *in vitro.* *Mol Pharmacol* 1987; 32:807-12.

60 Aoyama K. Effects of benzene inhalation on lymphocyte subpopulations and immune response in mice.

Toxicol Appl Pharmacol 1986; 85:92-101.

61 Rosenthal GJ, Synder CA. Modulation of the immune response to *Listeria monocytogenes* by benzene inhalation. *Toxicol Appl Pharmacol* 1985; 80:502-10.

62 Von Hoff DD, Slavik M, Muggia FM. Allergic reactions to cis platinum. *Lancet* 1976; i:90-3.

63 Harth M. Modulation of immune responses of gold salts. *Agents Actions* 1981; 8:464-76.

64 Sachs HK. Intercurrent infections in lead poisoning. *Am J Dis Child* 1978; 32:315-16.

65 Ewers U, Stiller-Winkler R, Idel J. Serum immunoglobulin, complement C3, and salivary IgA levels in lead workers. *Environ Res* 1982; 29:351-7.

66 Kimber I, Stonard MD, Gidlow DA, Niewola Z. Influence of chronic low-level exposure to lead on plasma immunoglobulin concentration and cellular immune function in man. *Int Arch Occup Environ Hlth* 1986; 57:117-25.

67 Koller LD. Immunotoxicology of heavy metals. *Int J Immunopharmacol* 1980; 2:269-79.

68 Lawrence DA. Immunotoxicity of heavy metals. In: Dean JH, Luster MI, Munson AE, Amos HE, eds. *Immunotoxicology and Immunopharmacology.* New York: Raven Press, 1985; 341-53.

69 Dean JH, Murray MJ. Toxic responses of the immune system. In: Klaassen CD, Amdur MO, Doull's J, eds. *Toxicology: The Basic Science of Poisons.* New York: Macmillan, 1991.

70 Hemphill RE, Kaeberle ML, Buck WB. Lead suppression of mouse resistance to *Salmonella typhimurium.* *Science* 1971; 172:1031-2.

71 Cook JA, DiLuzio NR, Hoffman EO. Factors modifying susceptibility to bacterial endotoxin: the effect of lead and cadmium. *CRC Crit Rev Toxicol* 1975; 3:201-29.

72 Lawrence DA. *In vivo* and *in vitro* effects of lead on humoral and cell mediated immunity. *Infect Immun* 1981; 31:136-43.

73 Luster MI, Faith RE, Kimmel CA. Depression of humoral immunity in rats following chronic developmental lead exposure. *J Environ Pathol Toxicol* 1978; 1:397.

74 Blakley BR, Archer DL. Mitogen stimulation of lymphocytes exposed to lead. *Toxicol Appl Pharmacol* 1982; 62:183-9.

75 Koller LD. Immunosuppression produced by lead, cadmium and mercury. *Am J Vet Res* 1973; 34:1457-8.

76 Koller LD, Exon JH, Roan JG. Antibody suppression by cadmium. *Arch Environ Hlth* 1975; 30:598-601.

77 Koller LD, Exon JH, Arbogast B. Methylmercury: effect on serum enzymes and humoral antibody. *J Toxicol Environ Hlth* 1977; 2:1115-23.

78 Blakley BR, Sicodia CS, Mukkur TK. The effect of

methylmercury, tetraethyl lead, and sodium arsenite on the humoral immune response in mice. *Toxicol Appl Pharmacol* 1980; 52:245–54.

79 Faith RE, Luster MI, Kimmel CA. Effect of chronic developmental lead exposure on cell mediated immune function. *Clin Exp Immunol* 1979; 35:413–24.

80 Gaworski CL, Sharma RR. The effects of heavy metals on ^{3}H-thymidine uptake in lymphocytes. *Toxicol Appl Pharmacol* 1978; 46:305–13.

81 Koller LD, Roan JG, Kerkvliet NI. Mitogen stimulation of lymphocytes in CBA mice exposed to lead and cadmium. *Environ Res* 1979; 19:177–88.

82 Adkins B, Richards JH, Gardner DE. Enhancement of experimental respiratory infections following nickel-inhalation. *Environ Res* 1979; 20:33–42.

83 Smialowicz RJ, Riddle MM, Rogers RR, Rowe DG, Luebke RW, Fogelson LD, Copeland CB. Immunologic effects of nickel: II. Suppression of natural killer cell activity. *Environ Res* 1985; 36:56.

84 Smialowicz RJ, Rogers RR, Rowe DG, Riddle MM, Luebke RW. The effects of nickel on immune function in the rat. *Toxicology* 1987; 44:271–81.

85 Penninks AH, Kuper F, Spit BJ, Seinen W. On the mechanism of dialkyltin-induced thymus involution. *Immunopharmacol* 1985; 10:1–10.

86 Snoeij NJ, Penninks AH, Seinen W. Biological activity of organotin compounds—an overview. *Environ Res* 1987; 44:335–53.

87 Boyer IJ. Toxicity of dibutyltin, tributyltin and other organotin compounds to humans and experimental animals. *Toxicology* 1989; 55:253–98.

88 Verschuuren HG, Kroes R, Vink HH, Van Esch GJ. Short-term toxicity studies with triphenyltin compounds in rats and guinea pigs. *Food Cosmet Toxicol* 1966; 4:35–45.

89 Seinen W, Penninks A. Immune suppression as a consequence of a selective cytotoxic activity of certain organometallic compounds on thymus and thymus-dependent lymphocytes. *Ann NY Acad Sci* 1979; 320:499–517.

90 Vos JG, Krajnc EI, Wester PW. Immunotoxicity of Bis(tri-n-butyltin) oxide. In: Dean J, Luster M, Munson A, Amos H, eds. *Immunotoxicology and Immunopharmacology*. New York: Raven Press, 1985; 327–40.

91 Snoeij NJ, Penninks AH, Seinen W. Dibutyltin and tributyltin compounds induce thymic atrophy in rats due to a selective action on thymic lymphoblasts. *Int J Immunopharmacol* 1988; 10:891–99.

92 Caspritz G, Hadden J. The immunopharmacology of immunotoxicology and immunorestoration. *Toxicol Pathol* 1987; 15:320–32.

93 Exon JH, Kerkvliet NI, Talcott PA. Immunotoxicity of carcinogenic pesticides and related chemicals. *En-viron Carcinogen Rev (J Environ Hlth)* 1987; C5:73–120.

94 Edmiston S, Maddy KT. Summary of illnesses and injuries reported in California by physicians in 1986 as potentially related to pesticides. *Vet Hum Toxicol* 1987; 29:391–7.

95 Koller LD. Effects of environmental contaminants on the immune system. *Adv Vet Sci Comp Med* 1979; 23:267–95.

96 Thomas PT, Busse WW, Kerkvliet NI *et al.* Immunologic effects of pesticides. In: Baker SR, Wilkinson CF, eds. *The Effects of Pesticides on Human health.* vol. XVIII. New York: Princeton Scientific Publishers, 1990; 261–95.

97 Street JC, Sharma RP. Alteration of induced cellular and humoral immune responses by pesticides and chemicals of environmental concern: quantitative studies of immunosuppression by DDT, Aroclor 1254, carbaryl, carbofuran, and methylparathion. *Toxicol Appl Pharmacol* 1975; 32:587–602.

98 Fan A, Street JC, Nelson RM. Immunosuppression in mice administered methyl parathion and carbofuran by diet. *Toxicol Appl Pharmacol* 1978; 45:235.

99 Gallicchio VS, Casale GP, Watts T. Inhibition of human bone marrow-derived stem cell colony formation (CFU-E, BFU-E, and CFU-GM) following *in vitro* exposure to organophosphates. *Exp Hematol* 1987; 15:1099–102.

100 Rodgers KE, Grayson MH, Imamura T, Devens BH. *In vitro* effects of malathion and O,O,S-trimethyl phosphorothioate on cytotoxic T-lymphocyte responses. *Pesticide Biochem Physiol* 1985; 24:260–6.

101 Rao DSVS, Glick B. Pesticide effects on the immune response and metabolic activity of chicken lymphocytes. *Proc Soc Exp Biol Med* 1977; 154:27–9.

102 Loose LD, Silkworth JB, Benitz KF, Mueller W. Impaired host resistance to endotoxin and malaria in polychlorinated biphenyl– and hexachlorobenzene-treated mice. *Infect Immun* 1978; 20:30–5.

103 Vos JG, Brouwer GMJ, Van Leewen FXR, Wagenaar SJ. Toxicity of hexachlorobenzene in the rat following combined pre– and postnatal exposure: comparison of effects on the immune system, liver and lung. In: Gibson G, Hubbard R, Park D, eds. *Immunotoxicology*. London: Academic Press, 1983; 219–30.

104 Bernier J, Hugo P, Krzystyniak K, Fournier M. Suppression of humoral immunity in inbred mice by dieldrin. *Toxicol Lett* 1987; 35:231–40.

105 Krzystniak K, Hugo P, Flippo D. Fournier M. Increased susceptibility to mouse hepatitis virus 3 of peritoneal macrophages exposed to Dieldrin. *Toxicol Appl Pharmacol* 1985; 80:397–408.

106 Spyker-Cranmer JM, Barnett JB, Avery DL, Cranmer MF. Immunoteratology of chlordane: cell-mediated

and humoral immune responses in adult mice exposed *in utero. Toxicol Appl Pharmacol* 1982; 62:402–8.

107 Barnett JB, Soderberg LSF, Menna JH. The effect of prenatal chlordane exposure on the delayed hypersensitivity response of BALB/c mice. *Toxicol Lett* 1985; 25:173–83.

108 Johnson KW, Kaminski NE, Munson AE. Direct suppression of cultured spleen cell responses by chlordane and immunocompetence. *J Toxicol Environ Hlth* 1987; 22:497–515.

109 Kerkvliet NI, Baecher-Steppan L, Schmitz JA. Immunotoxicity of pentachlorophenal (PCP). Increased susceptibility to tumor growth in adult mice fed technical PCP-contaminated diets. *Toxicol Appl Pharmacol* 1982; 62:55–64.

110 Blakely BR, Schiefer BH. The effect of topically applied n-butylester of 2,4-dichlorophenoxyacetic acid on the immune response in mice. *J Appl Toxicol* 1986; 6:291–5.

111 Olson LJ, Erickson BJ, Hinsdill RD, Wyman JA, Porter WP, Binning LK, Bidgood RC, Nordheim EV. Aldicarb immunomodulation in mice: an inverse dose-response to parts per billion levels in drinking water. *Arch Environ Contam Toxicol* 1987; 16:433–9.

112 Fiore MC, Anderson HA, Hong R, Golubjatnikov R, Seiser JE, Nordstrom D, Hanrahan L, Belluck D. Chronic exposure to aldicarb-contaminated groundwater and human immune function. *Environ Res* 1986; 41:633–45.

113 Thomas PT, Ratajczak HV, Eisenberg WC, Furedi-Machacek M, Ketels KV, Barbera PW. Evaluation of host resistance and immunity in mice exposed to the carbamate pesticide aldicarb. *Fund Appl Toxicol* 1987; 9:82–9.

114 Thomas PT, Ratajczak HV, Demetral D. Hagen K, Baron R. Aldicarb immunotoxicology: functional analysis of cell mediated immunity and quantitation of lymphocyte subpopulations. *Fund Appl Toxicol* 1990; 15:221–30.

115 Selvan RS, Dean TN, Misra HR, Nagarkatti PS, Nagarkatti M. Aldicarb suppression macrophages but not natural killer (NK) cell-mediated cytotoxicity of tumor cells. *Bull Environ Contam Toxicol* 1989; 43:676–82.

116 Dean T, Kakkanaiah V, Nagarkatti M, Nagarkatti P. Immunosuppression by aldicarb of T-cell response to antigen-specific and polyclonal stimuli results from defective IL-1 production by the macrophages. *Toxicol Appl Pharmacol* 1990; 106:408–17.

117 Mirkin IR, Anderson HA, Hanrahan L, Hong K, Golubjatnikov R, Belluck D. Changes in T-lymphocyte distribution associated with ingestion of aldicarb-contaminated drinking water—a follow-up study. *Environ Res* 1990; 51:35–50.

118 DeMaroussen P, Pipy B, Beraud M, Soqual MC, Forgue MF. The effects of carbaryl on the arachidonic acid metabolism and superoxide production by mouse resident peritoneal macrophages challenged by zymosan. *Int J Immunopharmacol* 1986; 8:155–66.

119 Goldman LR, Beller M, Jackson R. Aldicarb food poisonings in California, 1985–1988: toxicity estimates for humans. *Arch Environ Hlth* 1990; 45:141–7.

120 Kundiev YI, Krasnyuk EP, Viter V. Specific features of the changes in the health status of female workers exposed to pesticides in greenhouses. *Toxicol Lett* 1986; 33:85–9.

121 Kashyap SK. Health surveillance and biological monitoring of pesticide formulators in India. *Toxicol Lett* 1986; 33:107–14.

122 Wysocki J, Kalina Z, Owczarzy I. Serum levels of immunoglobulins and C-3 component of complement in persons occupationally exposed to chlorinated pesticides. *Med Pract* 1985; 36:111–17.

123 Hermanowicz A, Kossman S. Neutrophil function and infectious disease in workers occupationally exposed to phosphoorganic pesticides: role of mononuclear-derived chemotactic factor for neutrophils. *Clin Immunol Immunopathol* 1984; 33:13–22.

124 Winter CK, Kurtz PH. Factors influencing grape worker susceptibility to skin rashes. *Bull Environ Contam Toxicol* 1985; 35:418–26.

125 Ueda A, Ueda T, Matsushita T, Ueno T, Nomura S. Prevalence rates and risk factors for allergic symptoms among inhabitants in rural districts. *Sangyo Igaku* 1987; 29:3–16.

126 Lisi P, Caraffini S, Assalve D. A test series for pesticide dermatitis. *Contact Dermat* 1986; 15:266–9.

127 Buehler EV. A rationale of the selection of occlusion to induce and elicit delayed contact hypersensitivity in the guinea pig; a prospective test. In: Andersen KE, Maibach HI, eds. *Contact Allergy Predictive Tests in Guinea Pigs.* Basel: Karger, 1985; 39–58.

128 Wahlberg JE, Boman A. Guinea pig maximization test. In: Andersen KE, Maibach HI, eds. *Contact Allergy Predictive Tests in Guinea Pigs.* Basel: Karger, 1985; 59–106.

129 Friedman PS, Moss C, Shuster S, Simpson JM. Quantitative relationships between sensitizing dose of DNCB and reactivity in normal subjects. *Clin Exp Immunol* 1983; 53:709–15.

130 Adams RM, Zimmerman MC, Bartlett JB, Preston JF. 1-Chloro-2,4-dinitrobenzene as an algicide, report of four cases of contact dermatitis. *Arch Dermatol* 1971; 103:191–3.

131 Hogan DJ, Lane PR. Allergic contact dermatitis due to a herbicide (barban). *Can Med Assoc J* 1985; 132:387–9.

132 Matsushita T, Aoyama K. Cross-reactions between

some pesticides and the fungicide benomyl in contact allergy. *Ind Hlth* 1981; 19:77–83.

133 Matsushita T, Aoyama K. Dose–response relationship in delayed type contact sensitivity with maneb. An experimental model of "simple chemicals." *Ind Hlth* 1980; 18:31–9.

134 Matsushita T, Aoyama K, Yoshimi K, Fujita Y, Ueda A. Allergic contact dermatitis from organophosphorus insecticides. *Ind Hlth* 1985; 23:145–53.

135 Magnusson B, Kligman AM. The identification of contact allergens by animal assay. The guinea pig maximization test. *J Invest Dermatol* 1969; 52:268–76.

136 Marzulli FN, Maguire HC. Usefulness and limitations of various guinea pig test methods in detecting human skin sensitizers. Validation of guinea pig test for skin hypersensitivity. *Fund Chem Toxicol* 1982; 20:74–6.

137 Matsushita T, Arimatsu Y, Tomio T, Nomura S. Experimental study on contact dermatitis due to herbicides sodium chlorate and sodium 2,2-dichloropropionate. *Kumamoto Med J* 1975; 28:170–5.

138 Brancacia RB, Chamales MH. Contact dermatitis and depigmentation produced by the herbicide carbyne. *Contact Dermat* 1977; 3:108–9.

139 van Joost T, Haafs B, van Ketel WG. Sensitization to benomyl and related pesticides. *Contact Dermat* 1983; 9:153–64.

140 van Ketel WG. Sensitivity to the pesticide benomyl. *Contact Dermat* 1976; 5:290–1.

141 Savitt LE. Contact dermatitis due to benomyl insecticide. *Arch Dermatol* 1972; 105:926–7.

142 Nater JP, Terpstra H, Bleumink E. Allergic contact sensitization to the fungicide maneb. *Contact Dermat* 1979; 5:24–6.

143 Adams RM, Manchester RD. Allergic contact dermatitis to maneb in a housewife. *Contact Dermat* 1982; 8:271.

144 Edmundson WF, Davies JE. Occupational dermatitis from naled. *Arch Environ Hlth* 1967; 15:89–91.

145 Milby TH, Epstein W. Allergic contact sensitization to malathion. *Arch Environ Hlth* 1964; 9:434–7.

146 Matsushita T, Arimatsu Y, Misumi J, Tomio T, Nomura S. Skin disorders caused by herbicides sodium chlorate and sodium 2,2-dichloropropionate. *Kumamoto Med J* 1975; 28:164–9.

147 Cushman JR, Street JC. Allergic hypersensitivity to the herbicide 2,4-D in BALB/c mice. *J Toxicol Environ Hlth* 1982; 10:729–41.

148 Cushman JR, Street JC. Allergic hypersensitivity to the insecticide malathion in BALB/c mice. *Toxicol Appl Pharmacol* 1983; 70:29–42.

149 Newton JG, Breslin ABX. Asthmatic reactions to a commonly used aerosol insect killer. *Med J Anat* 1983; 1:378–80.

5

Adverse immunological effects of drugs and other chemicals and methods to detect them

HANS F. MERK, ERNST GLEICHMANN & HELGA GLEICHMANN

Introduction

Drug-induced toxicities can be divided into intrinsic and hypersensitivity reactions. Intrinsic reactions (type A) are related to the pharmacological properties of the drug and are based on studies with appropriate *in vitro* assays and animal experiments. Hypersensitivity (type B) is a major complication of drug therapy; this is related both to the drug and to individual host factors. In most cases such reactions cannot be predicted and at times may be fatal. This is especially true for immunologically mediated reactions, such as allergic reactions and autoimmune diseases induced by drugs. In clinical practice, it is usually difficult if not impossible to identify the agent eliciting the reaction because patients suffering from such drug-induced diseases are often receiving several drugs, each of which may have induced the reaction in question. In these cases it may be necessary to employ sophisticated assays or *in vivo* tests which are potentially harmful for the patient.

Both kinds of drug-induced diseases and the methods to detect them will be discussed in this chapter. The principal considerations of the immunological mechanisms involved are presented elsewhere in this book. In particular, we will emphasize examples of clinical diagnostic procedures in connection with allergic drug reactions and methods to investigate the mechanism of reaction as well as animal models which may be useful to predict such reactions in connection with autoimmune diseases.

Clinical signs and symptoms of drug-allergic reactions

About 30% of adverse reactions to drugs and chemicals have an immune or allergic pathogenesis [1–3]. In Table 5.1 adverse immune reactions are listed according to the time interval between the uptake of the compound and the onset of clinical signs and symptoms and involved effector mechanisms. This differentiation has been shown to be useful in clinical practice (see Chapter 2). Immediate-type reactions (type I) may start more or less simultaneously with drug administration. This is especially true in highly sensitized patients receiving β-lactam antibiotics intravenously or venom extracts during immunotherapy. The reaction is mediated by

Table 5.1 Classification of the effector mechanisms of adverse immune reactions

| Gell and Coombs 1963 | Immune effector mechanisms | | |
	Designation	Principal components	Harmful tissue reaction
Type I	Anaphylactic, reaginic, immediate-type hypersensitivity	IgE antibody, mediators released from mast cells	Asthma, urticaria, shock, hayfever
Type II	Cytotoxic	Antibody	Haemolysis, leukopenia, thrombocytopenia*
Type III	Immune complex	Antigen–antibody complexes	Vasculitis, glomerulonephritis, serum sickness, systemic lupus erythematosus
Type IV	Delayed hypersensitivity	T cells	Contact dermatitis

*There is evidence that in certain patients the immunologically mediated cytopenias are mediated by excessive activity of T suppressor cells rather than antibody.

immunoglobulin E (IgE) antibodies and some believe that IgG_4 antibodies may be involved [1,4]. IgE binds to a highly specific IgE receptor on mast cells and basophils. Antigen bridging between at least two IgE antibodies results in the activation of protein kinase C and the Ca^{2+}-dependent signal transduction system, which results in an explosive release of inflammatory mediators such as pre-formed histamine, platelet-activating factor (PAF), proteases such as tryptase and the synthesized metabolites of arachidonic acid generated after the cell-activating process [5]. Clinical signs and symptoms include urticaria, bronchoconstriction with wheezing, allergic conjunctivitis and rhinitis and finally anaphylactic shock. However, the identical clinical signs and symptoms may be evoked by release of these mediators following non-immunological stimuli such as morphine. The best known example is the intolerance reaction to non-steroidal anti-inflammatory drugs (NSAIDS). However, reactions especially to pyralozones and in some rare cases even to aspirin may be mediated by IgE antibodies [6]. Other examples are the intolerance to radiocontrast media, opiates which directly release histamine or dextran which binds non-specifically with IgG, thereby activating the complement cascade [7].

The late type of mainly humoral mediated reactions (types II and III) occurs 4–12 h after the administration of the antigen. One mechanism is mediated by IgG antibodies, in rare cases by IgA and IgM as well, and leads via immune complex formation (type III) or binding to target cells (type II) to complement activation, resulting in inflammation (vasculitis) or cytotoxicity (thrombocytopenia, etc.). This reaction cascade also plays a crucial role in autoimmune diseases such as systemic lupus erythematosus (SLE) as well. However, their pathogenesis is characterized by major disturbances of the T cells and will be discussed separately.

Another mechanism is the IgE late-phase reaction. Its signs and symptoms are similar to those of the immediate-type reaction; however, they are mediated by the release of inflammatory substances by basophils and not mast cells [8]. This is suggested by histamine release without an increase in prostaglandin D_2; the latter is only formed in mast cells and found in immediate types of allergic diseases. Histamine release without the appearance of prostaglandin D_2 is paralleled by an increase in infiltrating basophils in the skin [8].

The delayed type of immunological reactions (type IV) begins 24–96 h after drug administration and is mediated primarily by T lymphocytes. A typical clinical example is the allergic contact dermatitis which can be induced by topically applied drugs such as neomycin, diphenhydramine, chloramphenicol, benzocaine, sulphonamides, bufexamac (a topical NSAID) and even corticosteroids [9]. A special variant of these reactions is photosensitivity which may be photoallergic or phototoxic [10]. Elicitation of this reaction requires exposure to the drug plus solar radiation. Examples of topically or systemically applied drugs which may be involved in this reaction are, for example, chlorothiazides, NSAIDs such as peroxicam or nalidixic acid, sulphonamides and amiodarone [10].

Fixed drug eruption is linked to the cell-mediated delayed type of allergic drug reactions by most authors, although its pathogenesis is still unclear. It is characterized by a localized erythema, approximately 0.5–10 cm in diameter, that may lead to bulla formation. This typically recurs at the identical site after taking the responsible drug.

Cell-mediated hypersensitivity is also required for maculopapular eczematous eruptions and for Lyell's disease, which is characterized by epidermal necrolysis with bulla formation and desquamation and is associated with significant morbidity and mortality [11]. Ophthalmological involvement may be severe. Among the drugs associated with this syndrome are the antibiotics penicillin, pyrazolones, sulphonamides, and the anticonvulsant agents phenytoin, carbamazepin, and barbiturates.

Under clinical conditions several types of these immunological reactions are involved and sometimes it may be difficult to separate them exactly. For example, a patient who is allergic to penicillin will suffer from a contact dermatitis after topical application of the drug; he will also experience anaphylactic shock after intravenous application of the same drug. For all these types of drug allergies and others, including the IgE-dependent immediate type of hypersensitivity, it can hardly be overemphasized that in the vast majority of cases T lymphocytes play the key role in the control of whether or not antibodies are produced; if so, which class, and which amount.

Although every drug is theoretically capable of inducing an allergic reaction there are some which rarely if ever are the causative agent, e.g. androgens, oestrogens, progesterones, spironolactones, vitamins, antihistamines (an exception is contact dermatitis after topical application), atropine, digoxin, nystatin, tetracyclines, and dicoumarol. In contrast drugs which are often involved include β-lactam antibiotics, sulphonamides, pyrazolones, hydantoin, allopurinol, quinine and quinidine, D-penicillamine, hydralazine, and procainamide [9].

Autoimmunity versus allergy

Autoimmunity shares a number of features with allergic responses to drugs. First, in both allergy and autoimmunity the immune system is stimulated to specific responses that are harmful to the body. Second, there are very strong effects of genetic factors that predispose for both allergic and autoimmune reactions to chemicals. In genetically susceptible individuals, even trace amounts of a chemical can elicit an adverse immunological response, whereas genetically resistant individuals will tolerate much higher doses of the chemical without showing any adverse effects. Often these genetic effects are so strong that, when studying a mixed population consisting of susceptible and resistant individuals, the false impression may arise that there are no dose–effect relationships as far as allergic and autoimmune reactions to a chemical are concerned. Such relationships do become evident, however, when the susceptible population is studied alone.

Allergic and autoimmune reactions to chemicals can be distinguished as follows: in allergy, the adverse immune response is restricted to the offending exogenous agent present in the tissue. In chemically induced autoimmunity, by contrast, the adverse immune response is not restricted to the chemical compound inducing it, but involves responses to self-antigens as well. If the inducing agent is a non-specific immunostimulator, the adverse immune response may not be directed towards the inducing agent, but may be confined to anti-self responses.

Table 5.2 Examples of adverse immunological side-effects of drugs in humans*

Disease	Inducing drug
Drug-induced autoantibodies	
Autoimmune chronic active hepatitis, virus-negative	Halothane, tienilic acid
Autoimmune haemolytic anaemia of certain types	α-Methyldopa, L-dopa, captopril, cefalexin, mefenamic acid, penicillins
Goodpasture syndrome	D-penicillamine
Granulocytopenia of certain types	Aminopyrine, captopril, cefalexin, chloral hydrate, chlordiazepoxide, chlorpromazine, chlorpropamide, gold salts, mercurial diuretics, indomethacin, *p*-aminosalicylic acid, penicillins, sulphapyridine/sulphathiazol, thiouracils, tolazoline
Myasthenia gravis	D-penicillamine, possibly gold salts
Pemphigus vulgaris	D-penicillamine
Bullous pemphigoid	D-penicillamine
Systemic lupus erythematosus (SLE)	Gold salts, griseofulvin, hydralazine, phenytoin, practolol, D-penicillamine, procainamide, thiouracil, and others
Drug-induced immunological diseases with unknown pathogenesis	
Aplastic anaemia of certain types	D-penicillamine, phenytoin, quinacrine, phenylbutazone
Intrahepatic cholestasis/cholangitis	Chlorpromazine, chlorpropamide, erythromycin estolate, imipramine, nalidixic acid, nitrofurantoin
Hepatitis, non-viral	Aminosalicylic acid, amiodarone, captopril, isoniazid, phenytoin and other hydantoins, and others
Hypogammaglobulinaemia	Gold salts, phenytoin
Infectious mononucleosis-like syndrome	Aminosalicylic acid, dapsone, phenytoin
Interstitial nephritis	Azathioprine, cephalosporins, furosemide, penicillins (especially methicillin), phenindione, phenytoin, rifampicin, sulfinpyrazone, sulphonamides, thiazides, thiouracil
Lymphadenopathy/ (pseudo) lymphoma/Hodgkin's disease	Phenytoin and other hydantoins, possibly gold salts
Peripheral neuritis	Colchicine, gold salts, nitrofurantoin, sulphonamides
Serum sickness	Penicillins, cephalosporins, streptomycin, sulphonamides, and others
Skin: immunological drug reactions can mimic virtually all clinical and histological patterns of reaction	Antibiotics, barbiturates, diuretics, gold salts, anticonvulsants, tranquillizers, and many others

Continued

Table 5.2 *continued*

Disease	Inducing drug
Thrombocytopenia of certain types	Acetazolamide, acetylsalicylic acid, carbamazepine, cephalothin, chloramphenicol, digitoxin, gold salts, imipramine, levodopa, meprobamate, methyldopa, para-aminosalicylic acid, phenylbutazone, phenytoin, quinidine, quinine, rifampicin, spironolactone, stibophen, sulphonamides, sulphonylureas, thiazides
Vasculitis of different types	Allopurinol, busulphan, indomethacin, isoniazid, iodides, penicillin, phenothiazines, phenylbutazone, tetracyclines, thiazides, thiouracils
Examples of allergic reactions to chemicals (only reactions against non-self antigens are involved)	
Allergic asthma and related conditions	Different types of allergen inhaled at the workplace, such as the dust of manufactured antibiotics, ethylenediamine, formaldehyde, insecticides, isocyanates, salts of the heavy metals chromium, cobalt, mercury, nickel, platinum
Contact dermatitis	Very many topically applied drugs, such as antibiotics, antihistamines, local anaesthetics A great variety of other chemicals, including many different organic compounds and the salts of heavy metals, such as chromium, cobalt, gold, mercury, and nickel
Food allergy	Many different types of food additive, chemical contaminations of food

*Compounds are listed alphabetically and not according to the frequency of adverse immunological side-effects they induce.
Major sources of reference: [4,12,13].

Definition and classification of autoimmune diseases

A convenient, albeit somewhat arbitrary, classification of autoimmune diseases divides them into organ-specific and non-organ-specific or systemic ones. Organ-specific autoimmune diseases are limited to a single organ, e.g. the thyroid gland in autoimmune thyroiditis, and correspondingly, the autoantibodies in these conditions are directed towards tissue-specific antigens, such as thyroglobulin. Non-organ-specific autoimmune diseases, by contrast, involve autoantibodies to ubiquitous self-antigens and, in a varied pattern of expression, affect several organs. The autoantibodies most frequently looked for in the laboratory investigation of these patients are antinuclear antibodies and rheumatoid factors. An example of the non-organ-specific autoimmune diseases is systemic lupus erythematosus (SLE), in which high titres of IgG autoantibodies to a variety of nuclear antigens, in particular double-stranded DNA, are produced; this results in the formation of immune complexes which are deposited in the vessel walls and along basement membranes of different tissues and thus cause pathological alterations. Other examples of non-organ-specific autoimmune diseases are rheumatoid arthritis, Sjögren's syndrome, dermatomyositis, and scleroderma (progressive systemic sclerosis). Histologically, all these diseases are characterized by inflammatory lesions of the blood vessels and fibrinoid degeneration in the connective tissue; therefore, this family of diseases is also termed collagen-vascular diseases.

Chemicals as aetiological agents of human autoimmune diseases

In contrast to the pathogenesis of autoimmune

Table 5.3 Selected examples of human leucocyte antigen (HLA) phenotypes and other genetically determined traits that predispose to chemically induced autoimmune diseases in humans

Disease	Aetiological agent	Predisposing genetic factors		References
		HLA	Other	
Myasthenia gravis	D-penicillamine (anti-rheumatic drug)	DR1, Bw35	Slow sulphoxidizers	[16,17]
Glomerulonephritis due to granular IgG deposits at the basement membrane, proteinuria	D-penicillamine	DR3, DR4		[16,18]
Glomerulonephritis due to granular IgG deposits, proteinuria	Gold, sodium thiomalate (anti-rheumatic drug)	DR3, B8*		[18,19]
Autoimmune thrombocytopenia	Gold, sodium thiomalate	DR3		[20]
Drug-induced systemic lupus erythematosus	Hydralazine (anti-hypertensive drug)	DR4	Slow acetylators, female sex	[21]
Scleroderma-like lesions (sclerosis of the skin, Raynaud's phenomenon, arthralgia and arthritis, pulmonary and portal fibrosis, thrombocytopenia)	Vinyl chloride (industrial chemical)	DR5		[22]

*While HLA DR3 and DR8 are susceptibility factors, DR7 determines resistance.

diseases almost nothing is known about their aetiology. In those admittedly few cases, however, where an aetiological agent of human autoimmune disease can be identified, most often this agent is a chemical compound, and this, in turn, most often is a drug.

For three reasons it is not valid in the present state of ignorance to draw the reverse conclusion from these observations, namely that chemicals also are the main suspects for the many cases of autoimmune disease with unknown aetiology. First, there may be observer bias for drug-induced autoimmune diseases in that patients receiving drugs are under close medical supervision so that chances for such cases being noticed and reported are presumably greater than with other aetiological agents. Second, the natural history of autoimmune diseases induced by drugs is often different from that of the same disease developing spontaneously, because drug-induced autoimmune symptoms usually disappear after withdrawal of the drug, whereas idiopathic autoimmune diseases often progress or follow a course characterized by relapses and remissions. Third, it is conceivable that autoimmune diseases develop without an exogenous cause, due to spontaneously arising errors in the regulation of the immune system. This possibility is supported by the fact that there are inbred strains of animals that spontaneously develop autoimmune diseases.

In particular, drugs inducing SLE are well documented. As can be seen from Table 5.3, drugs can induce a great variety of organ-specific and non-organ-specific autoimmune diseases. Procainamide is the most common cause of drug-related lupus and associated with the formation of IgG-antibodies against the histone H2A–H2B complex [14]. Other drugs whose association with human SLE has been shown are hydralazine, isoniazid, methyldopa, chlorpromazine, and quinidine. A probable association exists for anti-convulsant agents, antithyroid drugs, penicillamine, sulphasalazine, β-blockers, lithium, para-aminosalicylic acid, oestrogens, gold salts, penicillin, griseofulvin, reserpine and tetracycline [15]. Several drugs can induce more than one kind of autoimmune disease (see, for instance, D-penicillamine and phenytoin), and certain drugs, such as penicillin or phenytoin, can induce both autoimmune disease and allergy (Table 5.4). With the exception of adverse immunological reactions to penicillin [23,24], very few drug reactions have been studied in a systematic fashion (see chapter 15). In particular, investigations of specific anti-drug reactions of T lymphocytes are scarce. Hence, in most instances of drug-induced autoimmunity it has not been proven if, indeed, T helper cells are involved in the pathogenesis, as one would postulate on theoretical grounds. (A reaction of T helper cells against the drug does not preclude, of course, that antibodies to that drug may be produced, too.) It is also unclear in the vast majority of cases if an adverse immunological reaction to a given drug is elicited by the compound or a metabolite.

Ptak *et al.* [25] showed that murine B cells were rendered foreign by trinitrobenzene sulphonic acid, a chemical that covalently binds to protein. Whether other chemicals, such as drugs, will spontaneously bind to the membrane of lymphoid cells *in vivo* and thus render them foreign is largely unknown. Some indirect evidence that this may, indeed, happen has been obtained from studies on sensitization to penicillin in humans [23] and D-penicillamine in mice [26]. In the latter case, it was shown that even after oral application of a high dose of D-penicillamine peritoneal macrophages of recipient mice were altered in such a way that they elicited reactions by specific T helper cells [27]. Whether this alteration is, indeed, responsible for the SLE-like autoimmune disease inducible by D-penicillamine in the rat [28] and for human autoimmune diseases induced by this drug (Table 5.3) is as yet unknown.

In contrast to the well documented potential of drugs to induce autoimmune side-effects, little is known about the autoimmune potential of occupational and environmental chemicals. Severe scleroderma-like lesions have been reported in workers exposed to vinyl chloride (Table 5.3) as well as workers exposed to quartz [29]. Moreover, scleroderma-like lesions, as well as SLE, have been reported in women carrying silicon-containing breast prostheses [30,31]. An SLE-like disease can also develop in humans exposed to a food additive, the azodye tartazine, or the industrial chemical hydrazin.

Mercurials as aetiological agents of autoimmunity and increased IgE production

A chemical studied in some depth is mercury, which has been shown to cause an SLE-like autoimmune syndrome as well as a marked increase in IgE formation in several rodent species. A prominent feature of the mercury-induced autoimmune syndrome in rodents is glomerulonephritis, and this disease has also been documented in humans exposed to mercurials (Table 5.5). The observations in humans were made in cases of mercury poisoning or exposure to mercury as a constituent of drugs or cosmetics. In all cases, people were exposed over a relatively short period of time to high concentrations of mercury. Whilst it is not known whether the

Table 5.4 Survey of human autoimmune diseases

Disease	Self-antigens*
Diseases in which pathogenic autoimmune reactions are certain or likely because the self-antigens involved have been relatively well defined	
Autoimmune chronic active hepatitis, virus-negative	Membrane and microsomes of liver cells, including P-450 cytochrome isoenzymes
Autoimmune haemolytic anaemia	Membrane components of erythrocytes
Bullous pemphigoid	Basement membrane of skin
Goodpasture's syndrome (glomerulonephritis and alveolitis with linear immunoglobulin deposits along the glomerular and alveolar basement membranes)	Components of the glomerular and alveolar basement membranes
Guillain–Barré syndrome	Myelin and other components of the sheets of peripheral nerves
Hashimoto's thyroiditis	Cytoplasmic or microsomal thyroid antigen, thyroglobulin
Idiopathic leukocytopenia	Membrane components of leucocytes
Idiopathic thrombocytopenia	Membrane components of platelets
Male infertility (certain cases)	Spermatozoa
Myasthenia gravis	Acetylcholine receptor at the neuromuscular synapsis
Pemphigus vulgaris	Desmosomes linking epithelial cells of the skin
Pernicious anaemia	Intrinsic factor (produced by parietal cells for absorption of vitamin B_{12})
Primary Addison's disease	Microsomal antigens in the adrenal cortex
Progressive systemic sclerosis (scleroderma)	Various antigens in cell nuclei, especially nucleoli
Systemic lupus erythematosus	Various nuclear antigens, especially double-stranded DNA; antigens on leucocytes and erythrocytes
Thyrotoxicosis	Thyroid-stimulating hormone receptors
Wegener's granulomatosis (inflammatory disease of veins and arteries, especially in the lung and kidneys)	Alkaline phosphatase-like material on endothelial cells and neutrophils
Diseases with immunological pathogenesis in which the relevant self-antigens are inadequately defined or unknown (in the latter case it cannot be excluded that the relevant antigens are foreign structures implanted into the tissue)	
Glomerulonephritis with granular deposits of immunoglobulin along the glomerular basement membrane	Antigens from the circulation, such as DNA, which have been implanted along the glomerular basement membrane Autochthonous membrane structures on the epithelial cells covering the glomerular basement membrane, e.g. glycoproteins belonging to the gp 330 family
Juvenile diabetes mellitus (type I diabetes)	Unknown antigens of the insulin-producing β cells in the pancreas

Continued

Table 5.4 *continued*

Disease	Self-antigens*
Rheumatoid arthritis	Antigens of articular cartilage, such as chondroitin sulphate and a care protein of proteoglycan; collagen; IgG
Morbus Sjögren (lymphocytic infiltration of salivary and lacrimary glands)	Unknown
Polymyositis (lymphocytic infiltration of striated muscles)	Unknown
Dermatomyositis	Unknown
Lichen ruber	Unknown
Uveitis, certain types	Unknown antigens of the ocular lens
Primary biliary cirrhosis	Inner mitochondrial membrane
Ulcerative colitis	Unknown
Multiple sclerosis	Unknown

*These are defined by the autoantibodies involved.

concentrations of mercury existing at the work place and in the environment constitute a risk with regard to immunopathology, it is noteworthy that the immunopathological signs inducible by mercury are not confined only to certain mercury compounds or to routes of administration of such compounds (Table 5.5). Moreover, the dosages of $HgCl_2$ that induce autoimmune disease and enhanced IgE formation in rodents are clearly below the dose range in which general toxicity is observed.

The pathogenesis of mercury-induced autoimmunity has been analysed in detail in the rat. In this species, there is stringent genetic control of $HgCl_2$-induced autoimmunity and increased IgE production which is determined by 3–4 independently segregating loci. One of these loci segregates with the major histocompatibility complex and exerts a strong effect; the others have not been identified. Out of 22 inbred strains of rat studied, the Brown Norway strain is the most susceptible, because it developed all the symptoms listed in Table 5.5; other strains were partially susceptible, and still others, such as Lewis, were resistant. In Lewis rats, even doses of $HgCl_2$ which induce acute tubular necrosis failed to induce autoimmune phenomena.

All autoimmune phenomena induced by $HgCl_2$ are T-cell-dependent because they fail to develop in $HgCl_2$-treated athymic rats. The pathological alterations of mercury-induced autoimmunity resemble those of chronic graft versus host disease [36,37]. Chronic graft versus host disease is caused by an excessive activation of T helper cells which secondarily activate other immune cells, in particular B cells; the latter then produce antibodies, especially SLE-like autoantibodies of the IgG isotype [45]. In mercury-induced autoimmunity there is also an excessive activation of T helper cells. This suggests that there is a common final pathway leading to SLE-like autoimmunity in chronic graft versus host disease and mercury-induced autoimmunity.

The popliteal lymph node assay

In the preclinical test phase there is a need for simple laboratory tests to predict the immunogenicity of chemicals for T cells. The popliteal lymph node (PLN) assay in laboratory rodents could suit this purpose [46]. A survey of results obtained by the PLN assay is described in several publications [46–48].

The assay monitors the ability of xenobiotics to induce immune activation by measuring increased

Table 5.5 Survey of autoimmune and other immunopathological symptoms induced by exposure to mercury compounds of humans and genetically susceptible strains of rat, respectively

Species studied	Mercury compounds studied	Route of application	Pathological symptom induced	Selected references
Humans*	Various Hg-containing drugs and ointments	Oral, percutaneous, and various routes of injection	Membranous glomerulonephritis with glomerular IgG deposits in the mesangium and at the glomerular basement membrane	[32,33]
			Contact dermatitis and other forms of dermatitis	[34]
			Enhanced IgE formation *in vitro*	[35]
Rat*†	$HgCl_2$, CH_3HgCl, Hg-containing drugs and ointments	Inhalation, intraperitoneal, oral, percutaneous, subcutaneous	Lymphadenopathy, splenomegaly	[36,37]
			Lymphocytic infiltration of salivary glands (similar to Sjögren's disease)	Aten & Weening (pers comm)
			Intravascular blood coagulation	[36]
			IgG autoantibodies against the glomerular basement membrane (similar to Goodpasture's syndrome)	[36,37]
			Membranous glomelonephritis with granular IgG deposits in the mesangium and at the glomerular basement membrane	[36–38]
			IgG deposits in the walls of blood vessels	[36,37]
			IgG autoantibodies to various nuclear antigens and other autoantibodies	[38]
			Polyclonal B cell stimulation	[36,37]
			Extreme increase in total serum IgE and, if antigen is administered simultaneously, formation of specific IgE antibodies	[36,37]

*Some of the abnormalities listed could also be induced in rabbits and guinea pigs exposed to $HgCl_2$ [39,40].
†Almost all the abnormalities induced in the rat can also be induced by $HgCl_2$ administration to susceptible strains of mouse [11,41–44].

PLN weight after a footpad injection; the popliteal node is the draining lymph site. During the primary PLN response to small chemicals or conventional antigens, the maximal response in the mouse hardly exceeds a PLN weight index of 10. In the rat, however, the values of PLN indices are usually higher than in the mouse. With most chemicals tested the primary PLN response, if inducible, peaked within the first 10 days after injection and returned back to normal at week 3–4; exceptions from this rule were seen with high dosages of heavy metals ($HgCl_2$, $CdCl_2$) and, in particular, quartz.

Quartz induced an ever progressing PLN enlargement so that after 6 months the weight increase of the draining PLN had reached values of up to 200 times that of the contralateral PLN [49]. Quartz also was exceptional in that the lymph node enlargement induced did not require the presence of T lymphocytes [50]; this fits the notion that quartz is not an antigen. Quartz is phagocytosed by macrophages and, since it is undigestible, it activates these cells to release factors which secondarily activate lymphocytes. Thus, in the case of quartz the PLN assay reflects non-specific immunostimulatory properties of the test compound.

By contrast, in all other instances where this was tested (phenytoin, D-penicillamine, streptozotocin, captopril, $AuCl_3$) the PLN response was not only T-cell-dependent, but also it was specific. Specificity was proven by the fact that primed mice showed an enhanced PLN response when given a second injection of the same, but not of another, compound [51,52].

Injection of chemicals into a hind footpad admittedly is an artificial manoeuvre. In real life, chemicals are taken up by different routes, such as the oral and the inhalation route, so that the mesenteric and mediastinal lymph nodes and the spleen, respectively, are the candidate lymphoid organs that may harbour sensitized T lymphocytes. It is of great practical importance, therefore, to have a simple test system in which mesenteric, mediastinal or splenic T lymphocytes from rodents, which received a chemical in the context of routine toxicity testing, can be assayed for possible sensitization to that chemical. Such a test system has recently been established in the form of the adoptive transfer PLN assay [46]. Potentially sensitized T cells were taken from donor mice that had received five intraperitoneal injections of streptozotocin and had then been rested for from 1 week up to 3 months. By histopathological criteria, the spleens of these mice were inconspicuous. Splenic T cells obtained from such donor animals were injected into the footpad of syngeneic rodents, together with a dose of streptozotocin which by itself is too low to induce a primary PLN response. At 2–5 days after the cell transfer, a specific PLN enlargement was seen in the recipient. In this experiment, the recipient is rather inert in that it serves to present the test compound to the donor's T cells and reflect (by PLN enlargement) their reaction. Thus, the adoptive transfer PLN assay showed that sensitized T cells present in the spleen of a donor mouse, which had been exposed to a drug by multiple intraperitoneal injections, can be demonstrated by specific restimulation in the PLN assay.

Methods to detect adverse immunological reactions to chemicals

Current tests to detect adverse immunological reactions to chemicals are usually performed a posteriori, i.e. after a presumed sensitization to a xenobiotic (Table 5.6).

In vivo tests

In tests with those drugs or chemicals which are suspected to have elicited the reaction in question the subject is challenged in order to reproduce the clinical signs and symptoms. If the response is similar to the observed one, e.g. the triple response of erythema, itch, and wheal in a skin test, it is concluded that an allergic reaction occurred. By immunological criteria this is of course far from proof and therefore it is difficult if not impossible to separate allergic from pseudoallergic reactions by these tests.

Table 5.6 Methods to detect adverse immunological reactions to drugs in humans

In vivo tests	*In vitro* tests
Prick test	Serological tests
Intradermal test	Radioallergosorbent test (IgE)
Patch test	Western blot
(photo patch test)	Cellular tests
Oral challenge test	Histamine release test
	Lymphocyte transformation test (LTT)
	LTT with drug-modified microsome
	Lymphocyte toxicity test

Skin-prick test. In order to perform this test the drug is dissolved in water or glycerol (1–10%) and one drop is placed on the skin surface. The tip of a stylet or small needle at a 15–20° angle is then introduced through the drop into the epidermis.

Intradermal test. This is performed by injecting 0.01–0.02 ml of a solubilized drug using a 27–30 gauge needle.

These tests preferentially detect the release of inflammatory mediators of cutaneous mast cells such as histamine, derivatives of arachidonic acid and enzymes such as tryptase or chymase as a result of binding of IgE antibodies formed against the drug to these mast cells. These skin tests are only helpful in penicillin allergy if polylysine adducts of the major and minor haptens are used and if an immediate type of allergic reaction had occurred [53]. With the intradermal test it is important to avoid non-specific irritant reactions.

Patch test. This approach is used not only to identify the cause of drug-induced contact dermatitis, but also in vasculitis, purpura, morbilliform drug eruptions and bullous drug eruptions such as Stevens–Johnson syndrome, Lyell's disease, and the fixed drug eruption. In the case of fixed drug eruption however one has to perform the patch test in the area where the eruption has occurred and the reactions must be checked 6, 24, 48, or 72 h thereafter. In the case of photosensitivity reactions the probable allergens are applied twice. 24 h after the application one part is irradiated with ultraviolet light [10].

If the need to know the cause of a drug reaction exceeds the risk of evoking a severe reaction, oral challenge testing is justified. Normally one starts with 1% or less of the therapeutic dose, followed by two- to 10-fold increments at 15–60 min intervals. This test should only be performed by experts with emergency equipment at hand [54]. Although this test is the 'gold standard', it does not permit differentiation between allergic and pseudoallergic reactions.

In vitro tests

Serological tests. For the determination of specific IgE antibodies, the radioallergosorbent test (RAST) is widely used to detect allergic reactions to the major hapten of penicillin, the penicilloyl derivative. This test is most useful in detecting IgE antibodies to ethylenoxide. Ethylenoxide is used to clean the equipment of dialysis machines and causes urticarial reactions and even anaphylactic shock in patients treated with haemodialysis. The RAST is much less specific in most other IgE-dependent drug reactions. Alternative tests have been recommended, such as a sepharose solid-phase system to detect IgE to trimethoprim or platinum salts; however it must be borne in mind that this test may lack specificity due to firm binding of IgE to sepharose. This may result in measurement of total rather than specific IgE [55].

Western blot techniques offer another approach to detection of IgE antibodies. These are limited to peptides or proteins. Examples are Orgotein, a superoxide dismutase which is used as an anti-inflammatory agent, or the protease trasylol [56]. Western blot techniques have also proven useful for detection of the involvement of drug metabolites in human hypersensitivity reactions and autoimmunity [54]. Thus, patients who developed a non-viral hepatitis after treatment with tienilic acid, a diuretic agent, had IgG autoantibodies directed against the cytochrome P-450 isoform P-450-8, also called P-450meph, obtained from human liver microsomes. These autoantibodies specifically inhibited the hydroxylation of tienilic acid by human liver microsomes, mediated by this enzyme. Such antibodies have been termed liver–kidney–microsome (LKM) antibodies [54].

Cellular tests. Beside the RAST, another way of detecting an allergen responsible for an immediate type of allergic reaction (type I) is to measure the release of inflammatory mediators, such as histamine, by mast cells or basophils after exposure to the antigens [57]. However there is only limited experience with this assay with respect to drug allergic reactions. Further progress may result by measuring mast cell-derived enzymes, such as tryptase or chymase, which are specific for human mast cell subtypes [58]. Radioimmunoassay for these substances and for histamine may become available soon [57].

In the vast majority of cases T-lymphocytes play the key role in the control of drug-allergic reactions because they are not only involved in the delayed type of allergic reactions but also in the immediate and late-type reactions (Table 5.1). In these reactions T lymphocytes control whether or not antibodies will be produced; if so, how much, and which class at which time. Therefore a test method demonstrating specific sensitization of human T helper cells to low molecular weight chemicals might be helpful. One approach is the lymphocyte transformation test (LTT). Sensitized lymphocytes undergo blastogenesis and generate lymphokines such as interleukin-2, which is followed by a proliferation response that can be measured by means of the incorporation of ^{14}C-thymidine during DNA synthesis [59,60]. In the LTT peripheral blood lymphocytes (essentially T cells) are obtained from a sensitized patient and cultured in the presence of the suspected drug. It has been shown that in penicillin-allergic patients primarily T helper cells are induced under the conditions of these tests [24]. This is of interest since it is likely that many chemicals known to cause autoimmune disease primarily trigger reactions by specific T helper cells which secondarily activate autoreactive B cells. Such a chemical or drug does not need to elicit contact dermatitis or the formation of antibodies specific for that chemical, let alone specific IgE antibodies. The LTT is the most frequently used *in vitro* diagnostic test in drug allergy beside the RAST.

However, a problem of the LTT in its present form is that it has produced many false-negative and also some false-positive results [1]. Nonetheless, the general opinion is that the accuracy of this test may be improved by further standardization [60] and, in particular, careful definition of the conditions required for presenting the test compound to the responder T cells.

Risk factors predisposing to human allergic and autoimmune diseases induced by drugs or occupational chemicals

It is clear from the few studies performed that genetic factors, both immunological (e.g. the major histocompatibility complex antigens) and pharmacological (e.g. enzyme polymorphism) can be involved in the development of drug-induced autoimmunity in humans. As to immunogenetic factor, the human leucocyte antigen (HLA) alleles of the respective patients have been determined, whilst the phar-

macogenetic traits studied have been those that are relevant for the metabolization of a particular drug.

One recognized risk factor is the association of autoimmune diseases with certain HLA alleles—the statistical chance of individuals possessing certain HLA alleles to develop a certain autoimmune disease is greater than that of individuals possessing different HLA alleles [17,19,20,61]. As opposed to such positive HLA associations, there are also negative HLA associations where possession of a certain HLA allele protects the carrier from developing a certain autoimmune disease [61]. This is also true for chemically induced autoimmune diseases (Table 5.3). The exact role of HLA structures in the pathogenesis of chemically induced autoimmune diseases is not known, however.

As with the HLA system (or the immunoglobulin gene superfamily), enzymes which are involved in the metabolism of xenobiotica such as drugs are characterized by an extensive polymorphism and at least 10 gene families with several subfamilies are found in mammalian species [62]. These enzymes are capable of activating drugs to highly reactive compounds.

Role of xenobiotica metabolism and their pharmacogenetic traits in adverse reactions

According to the hapten concept derived from the classical studies of Landsteiner, small molecules such as drugs require covalent binding to macromolecular proteins to become an immunogen [63]. Studies concerning the initiation of chemical carcinogenesis showed that a prerequisite for the binding of most xenobiotics to macromolecular substances compounds is their metabolism to highly reactive species [63]. Prior to the metabolic transformation, small molecular compounds are usually not very reactive and hence not immunogenic. Thus, in an immunological sense cytochrome P450–dependent enzymes may define the border between self and non-self. Therefore it seems reasonable to assume that similar mechanisms could play a role in some forms of drug hypersensitivity (prohapten concept) [2,64]. This concept is supported by experiments showing that known carcinogenic polycyclic hydrocarbons are able to induce contact dermatitis in guinea pigs and mice, in contrast to non-carcinogenic polycyclic hydrocarbons [65,66]. The metabolic pathway of xenobiotics such as drugs is dependent on the presence of cytochrome P450 isoenzymes, epoxide hydrases, and transferases, especially glutathione transferases, resulting in a delicate balance between detoxification of a substrate and its toxification [63]. It has also been shown that immunocompetent cells such as lymphocytes and especially monocytes possess cytochrome P450-dependent enzyme activities [67,68]. Not only do monocytes possess different cytochrome P450 isoenzymes compared to lymphocytes, placenta or liver tissue, as demonstrated by studies with monoclonal antibodies to specific P450 isoenzymes, but also a very strong inducibility compared with lymphocytes and even liver tissue [67].

It is of interest that some highly reactive metabolites, such as hydroxylamine derivatives of procainamide, may be generated alternatively by cytochrome P450 isoenzymes and activated oxygen species during the oxygen burst of neutrophils [69,70]. With certain drugs such as phenytoin, phenobarbital, pyralazones, and sulphonamides, evidence in favour of metabolites has been presented [53,71]. In retrospect, formation of autoantibodies such as the LKM antibodies (mentioned above) to cytochrome P450 is perhaps not totally surprising. Beaune and colleagues [72] have suggested that cytochrome P450, originally present in the endoplasmic reticulum of the hepatocyte, could be alkylated by a reactive metabolite and migrate on to the hepatocyte membrane surface. At this level, the modified protein could be recognized by specific T helper cells reacting to that part of the molecule derived from the reactive metabolite. These functionally active T helper cells, in turn, would allow formation of IgG autoantibodies that recognize the native protein. Beside the LKM2 which react with P450meph there are also LKM1 antibodies which are found in patients with severe hepatitis to halothane and the autoimmune chronic active hepatitis of children which is due to the cytochrome P450db (P450IID gene family) [73–76]. This is of special interest because cytochrome P450 isozymes are the main metabolizing enzymes and most often the first target for drugs and other xenobiotics.

Lymphocyte transformation test with drug-modified microsomes

In consideration of these aspects we have modified the LTT by preincubating human peripheral blood mononuclear cells with murine liver microsomes, which are the main subcellular structures that perform xenobiotic metabolism. The microsomes were prepared from NMRI mice which were pretreated intraperitoneally for a period of 3 days with 100 μl saline solution (control) or with 80 mg kg^{-1} 3-methylcholanthrene or with 50 mg kg^{-1} phenobarbital respectively in order to induce different hepatic cytochrome P450 isoenzymes. After this preincubation with microsomes, the cells were washed and utilized in a lymphocyte proliferation assay. The proliferative response to different antigens was measured by ^{3}H–thymidine incorporation in micro– or macrocultures, as previously described. Murine microsomes alone had no effect on the lymphocytes. In 25 out of 42 patients with an allergic reaction to drugs—proven by oral challenge or positive skin test result—we found an increased stimulation index in only 13 cases after the addition of microsomes and with NADPH as cofactor [77].

Perspectives

Hypersensitivity is a major problem in drug safety today. These reactions are unpredictable since individual patient factors play a major role. Further research and better understanding of these individual factors will improve drug safety, especially if we become able to predict an increased risk of hypersensitivity reaction by appropriate assay systems.

At the level of preclinical drug toxicity testing, a major progress might be to predict these reactions by appropriate animal tests such as the PLN assay. Therefore optimal conditions for the adoptive transfer PLN assay need to be worked out. It should be investigated, for instance, if the chemical will also be recognized by transferred memory T cells if it is administered to the prospective recipient not into the footpad along with the donor T cells, but via the route and at a dosage representing a more realistic exposure to that chemical. This would allow measurement of T cell reactions to immunologically relevant metabolites, provided these reach the circu lation. It is mandatory, however, that test systems, such as the PLN assay, be validated, before they can be used in routine toxicology to predict potential harmful hypersensitivity reactions of drugs in the preclinical phase of new drugs.

The findings with the microsomal drug-modified LTT mentioned above, as well as similar observations in practolol disease, halothane or tienilinic acid-induced hepatitis, suggest that the metabolism of drugs by different metabolizing enzymes, especially the multiple cytochrome P450 isoenzymes, plays an important role in drug-allergic reactions. They are subject to complex regulation, being dependent on both endogenous and exogenous factors [78]. Several human pharmacogenetic differences due to polymorphisms are now known [79]. The same is true for detoxifying enzymes such as the epoxide hydrases or transferases, e.g. the glutathione transferases.

The dependence of drug-allergic reactions on these metabolic pathways makes it possible that pharmacogenetic differences in xenobiotica metabolizing enzymes may influence the likelihood of allergic reactions in a patient [66,70]. Recently the use of recombinant DNA techniques such as the analysis of restriction fraction length polymorphism patterns of human P450 genes and genes regulating P450 levels were proposed to determine the xenobiotica metabolizing capacities of different individual patients [80]. If these and other methods become available for routine clinical investigations, it may become possible not only to diagnose sometimes harmful allergic reactions after their occurrence but also to predict the individual risk of a patient to whom we administer drugs before such reactions occur.

References

1 De Weck AL. Drug allergy. *Comp Immun* 1979; 355-79.

2 Park BK, Coleman JW, Kitteringham NR. Drug disposition and drug hypersensitivity. *Biochem Pharmacol* 1987; 36:581–90.

3 Pohl LR, Satoh H, Christ DD, Kenna JG. The immunologic and metabolic basis of drug hypersensitivities. *Annu Rev Pharmacol* 1988; 28:367–87.

4 Parker CW. Drug allergy. In: Parker CW, ed. *Clinical Immunology*. Philadelphia:WB Saunders, 1980:1219–60.

5 Ring J, Sedlmeier F, von der Helm D, Mayr T, Walz U, Ibel H, Riepel H, Przybilla B, Reimann H-J, Dorsch W. Histamine and allergic diseases. In: Ring J, Burg G, eds. *New Trends in Allergy.* Heidelberg: Springer, 1985:44–77.

6 Blanca M, Perez E, Garcia JJ, Miranda A, Terrados S, Vega JM, Suau R. Angioedema and IgE antibodies to aspirin: a case report. *Ann Allergy* 1989; 62:295–8.

7 Ring J. Mechanisms of pseudo-allergic reactions to drugs. In: Estabrook RW, Lindenlaub E, Oesch F, de Weck AL, eds. *Toxicological and Immunological Aspects of Drug Metabolism and Environmental Chemicals.* Stuttgart: Schattauer, 1988:569–95.

8 Charlesworth EN, Hood AF, Soter NA, Kagey-Sobotka A, Norman PS, Lichtenstein LM. Cutaneous late-phase response to allergen. *J Clin Invest* 1989; 83:1519–26.

9 Schulz KH. Allergische und pseudoallergische Reaktionen auf Arzneimittel. *Internist* 1986; 27:372–80.

10 Bickers DR. Photobiology 1937–1987. *J Invest Dermatol* 1989; 92:25S–31S.

11 Robinson GCJ, Balazs T, Egorov IK. Mercuric chloride-, gold sodium thiomalate-, and D-penicillamine-induced antinuclear antibodies in mice. *Toxicol Appl Pharmacol* 1986; 86:159–69.

12 Aaronson DW. Asthma: general concepts. In: Patterson RW, ed. *Allergic Diseases*. Philadelphia; JB Lippincott, 1980:231–78.

13 DeSwarte RD. Drug allergy. An overview. *Clin Rev Allergy* 1986; 4:143–69.

14 Totoritis MC, Tan EM, McNally EM, Rubin RL. Association of antibody to histone complex H2A–H2B with symptomatic procainamide-induced lupus. *N Engl J Med* 1988; 318:1431–6.

15 Hess E. Drug induced lupus. *N Engl J Med* 1988; 318:1460–2.

16 Dawkins RL, Christiansen FT, Zilko PJ, eds. In: *Immunogenetics in Rheumatology. Musculoskeletal Diseases and D-Penicillamine.* Amsterdam: Excerpta Medica, 1982:280–375.

17 Emery P, Panayi S, Huston G, Welsh KI, Mitchell SC, Shah RR, Idel JR, Smith RL, Waring RH. D-penicillamine induced toxicity in rheumatoid arthritis: the role of sulphoxidation status and HLA–DR3. *J Rheumatol* 1984; 11:626–32.

18 Wooley PH, Griffin J, Panayi GS, Batchelor JR, Welsh KI, Gibson TJ. HLA-DR antigens and toxic reaction to sodium aurothiomalate and D-penicillamine in patients with rheumatoid arthritis. *N Engl J Med* 1980; 303:300–2.

19 Hakala M, Van Assendelft AHW, Ilonen J, Javala S, Tiilikainen A. Association of different HLA antigens with various toxic effects of gold salts in rheumatoid arthritis. *Ann Rheum Dis* 1986; 45:177–82.

20 Adachi JD, Bensen WG, Singal DP, Powers PJ. Gold-

induced thrombocytopenia: platelet associated IgG and HLA typing in three patients. *J Rheumatol* 1984; 12:355–7.

21 Batchelor JR, Welsh KI, Mansilla Tinoco R, Dollery CT, Hughes GRV, Bernstein R, Ryan P, Naish PF, Aber GM, Bing RF, Russel GI. Hydralazine-induced systemic lupus erythematosus: influence of HLA-DR and sex on susceptibility. *Lancet* 1980; i:1107–9.

22 Black CM, Welsh KI, Walker AE, Bernstein RM, Catoggio LJ, McGregor AR, Lloyd Jones JK. Genetic susceptibility to scleroderma-like syndrome induced by vinyl chloride. *Lancet* 1983; i:53–5.

23 De Weck AL. Penicillins and cephalosporins. In: de Weck AL, Bundgaard JO, eds. *Handbook of Experimental Pharmacology.* vol. 63. *Allergic Reactions to Drugs.* Berlin:Springer, 1983:423–82.

24 Koponen M, Pichler WJ, de Weck AL. T cell reactivity to penicillin: phenotypic analysis of *in vitro* activated cell subsets. *J Allergy Clin Immunol* 1986; 78:645–52.

25 Ptak W, Rewicka M, Marcinkiewicz J. Induction of 'allogeneic effect'-like reaction by syngeneic TNP-modified lymphoid cells. *Immunobiol* 1984; 166:368–81.

26 Nagata N, Hurtenbach U, Gleichmann E. Specific sensitization of Lyt-1$^+$2$^-$ T cells to spleen cells modified by the drug D-penicillamine or a stereoisomer. *J Immunol* 1986; 136:136–42.

27 Vogeler S, Gleichmann E. Oral treatment of mice with the drug D-penicillamine (D-Pen) haptenates their peritoneal macrophages and primes their T cells. *Immunobiol* 1988.

28 Donker AJ, Venuto RC, Vladutiu AO, Brentjens JR, Andres GA. Effects of prolonged administration of D-penicillamine or captropril in various strains of rats. Brown Norway rats treated with D-penicillamine develop autoantibodies, circulating immune complexes, and disseminated intravascular coagulation. *Clin Immunol Immunopathol* 1984; 30:142.

29 Ziegler V, Haustein U-F, Mehlhorn J, Münzberger H, Rennau H. Ouarzinduzierte Sklerodermie. Sklerodermie-ähnliches Syndrom oder echte progressive Sklerodermie? *Dermatol Monatsschr* 1986; 172:86–90.

30 Guillaume JC, Roujeau JC, Touraine R. Lupus systemique apres protheses mammaires. *Ann Derm Vener* 1984; 111:703–4.

31 Kumagai Y, Shiokawa Y, Medsger TA Jr, Rodnan GP. Clinical spectrum of connective tissue disease after cosmetic surgery. Observations of 18 patients and a review of the Japanese literature. *Arth Rheum* 1984; 27:1–12.

32 Fillastre JP, Mery JP, Morel-Maroger L, Kanfer A, Godin M. Drug-induced glomerulonephritis. In: Solez K, Whelton A, eds. *Acute Renal Failure.* New York:

Marcel Dekker, 1985; 389–407.

33 Tubbs RR, Gephardt GN, Mc Mahon JT, Pohl MC, Vidt DG, Barenberg SA, Valenzuela R. Membranous glomerulonephritis associated with industrial mercury exposure. Study of pathogenetic mechanisms. *Am J Clin Pathol* 1982; 77:409–13.

34 Taugner M, Schütz R. Beitrag zun Quecksilber-Allergie. *Dermatologica* 1966; 133:245–61.

35 Kimata H, Shinomiy K, Mikawa H. Selective enhancement of human IgE production *in vitro* by synergy of pokeweed mitogen and mercuric chloride. *Clin Exp Immunol* 1983; 53:183–91.

36 Druet P, Sapin C, Druet E, Hirsch F. Genetic control of mercury-induced immune response in the rat. In: Porter GA, ed. *Nephrotoxic Mechanisms of Drugs and Environmental Toxins.* New York: Plenum, 1983; 425–35.

37 Druet P, Hirsch F, Pelletier L, Druet E, Baran D, Sapin C. Mechanisms of chemical-induced glomerulonephritis. In: Fowler BA, ed. *Mechanisms of Cell Injury: Implications for Human Health.* Chichester: John Wiley, 1987; 153–73.

38 Weening JJ, Hoedemaeker J, Bakker WW. Immunoregulation and antinuclear antibodies in mercury-induced glomerulopathy in the rat. *Clin Exp Immunol* 1981; 45:64–71.

39 Albini B. Ito S, Brentjens J. Andres G. Splenomegaly and immune complex splenitis in rabbits with experimentally induced chronic serum sickness. *J Reticuloendothel Soc* 1983; 34:485–500.

40 Polak L, Barnes JM, Turk JL. The genetic control of contact sensitization to inorganic metal compounds in guinea-pigs. *Immunology* 1986; 14: 707–11.

41 Fleuren GJ, DeHeer E, Burgers JV, Osnabrugge C, Hoedemaeker PJ. Mercuric-chloride-induced autoimmune glomerulopathy in BALB/c mice. *Kidney Int* 1985; 28:702.

42 Hultman P, Eneström S. The induction of immune complex deposits in mice by peroral and parenteral administration of mercuric chloride: strain dependent susceptibility. *Clin Exp Immunol* 1987; 67:283–92.

43 Mirtschewa J, Nürnberger W, Hallmann B, Stiller-Winkler R, Gleichmann E. Genetically determined susceptibility of mice to HgCl$_2$-induced antinuclear antibodies (ANA) and glomerulonephritis. *Immunobiol* 1987; 175:323–4.

44 Pietsch P, Allmeroth M, Gleichmann E, Vohr HW. Increased synthesis of IgE, but not IgM, in strains of mice susceptible to HgCl$_2$. *Immunobiol* 1987; 175:324.

45 Gleichmann E, Pals ST, Rolink AG, Radaszkiewicz T, Gleichmann H. Graft-versus-host reactions: clues to the etiopathology of a spectrum of immunological diseases. *Immunol Today* 1984; 5:324–32.

46 Gleichmann H, Klinkhammer C. Predictive tests in

immune reactions to drugs. In: Estabrook RW, Linden-laub E, Oesch F, de Weck AL, eds. *Toxicological and Immunological Aspects of Drug Metabolism and Environmental Chemicals.* Stuttgart: Schattauer, 1988:535–48.

47 Gleichmann E, Vohr H-W, Stringer C, Nuyens J, Gleichmann H. Testing the sensitization of T cells to chemicals. From murine graft-versus-host reactions (GVHRs) to chemical-induced GVH-like immunological diseases. In: Kammüller ME, Bloksma N, Seinen W, eds. *Autoimmunity and Toxicology. Immunedysregulation induced by Drugs and Chemicals.* Amsterdam: Elsevier, 1988.

48 Kammüller ME, Seinen W. Structural requirements for hydantoins and 2–thiohydantoins to induce lymphoproliferative popliteal lymph node reactions in the mouse. *Int J Immunopharmacol* 1988; 10:997–1010.

49 Stark M, Zaidi S, Hilscher B, Hilscher W, Gleichmann E. High– and low-responder mouse strains with respect to silica-induced fibrosis. *Immunobiol* 1988.

50 Zaidi SH, Hilscher B, Hilscher W, Brassel D, Grover R. Vergleichende morphometrische und autoradiographische Untersuchungen quarzinduzierter Läsionen bei nu/nu-Mäusen und Kontrollmäusen. In: *Ergebn Unters Geb Staub– und Silikosebekämpfung im Steinkohlenbergbau. Silikosebericht Nordrhein-Westfalen.* vol. 12. Essen: Verlag Glückauf, 1979; 187–92.

51 Hurtenbach U, Gleichmann H, Nagata N, Gleichmann E. Immunity to D-penicillamine: genetic, cellular, and chemical requirements for induction of popliteal lymph node enlargement in the mouse. *J Immunol* 1987; 139:411–16.

52 Klinkhammer C, Popowa P, Gleichmann H. Specific immunity to the diabetogen streptozotocin: cellular requirements for induction of lymphoproliferation. *Diabetes* 1988; 37:74–80.

53 Homburger HA. Diagnosis of allergy: *in vitro* testing. *CRC Crit Rev Clin Lab Sci* 1986; 23:279–314.

54 van Arsdel P. Allergy testing: position paper. American College of Physicians. *Ann Intern Med* 1989; 110:317–20.

55 Harle DG, Baldo BA, Smal MA, van Nunen SA. An immunoassay for the detection of IgE antibodies to trimethoprim in the sera of allergic patients. *Clin Allergy* 1987; 17:209–16.

56 Jugert F, Scholl P, Merk HF. Diagnose von Arzneimittel-Allergien mittels Western-Blot. *Allergologie* 1989; 12:85.

57 McBride P, Bradley D, Kaliner M. Evaluation of a radioimmunoassay for histamine measurement in biologic fluids. *J Allergy Clin Immunol* 1988; 82:638–46.

58 Schwartz LB, Metcalfe DD, Miller JS, Earl H, Sullivan T. Tryptase levels as an indicator of mast-cell activation in systemic anaphylaxis and mastocytosis. *N Engl J Med* 1987; 316:1622–6.

59 Crabtree GR. Contingent genetic regulatory events in T lymphocyte activation. *Science* 1989; 243:355–61.

60 Stejskal VDM, Olin R, Forsbeck M. The lymphocyte transformation test for diagnosis of drug-induced occupational allergy. *J Allergy Clin Immunol* 1986; 77:411–26.

61 Vesell ES. Pharmacogenetic perspectives: genes, drugs and disease. *Hepatology* 1984; 4:959–65.

62 Gonzalez FJ, Nebert DW. Evolution of the P-450 gene superfamily. *N Trends Genet* 1990; 6:182–6.

63 Guengerich FP, Liebler DC. Enzymatic activation of chemicals to toxic metabolites. *Crit Rev Toxicol* 1985; 14:259–307.

64 Remmer H, Schüppel R. The formation of antigenic determinants. In: Samter M, Parker CW, eds. *International Encyclopedia of Pharmacology and Therapeutics.* vol. 1. Oxford:Pergamon, 1972; 67–89.

65 Klemme J, Craig E, Mukhtar H. Induction of contact hypersensitivity to dimethylbenzanthracene and benz(a)pyrene in a tumor susceptible strain of mice. *Cancer Res* 1987; 47:6074–8.

66 Old LJ, Benacerraf B, Carswell E. Contact reactivity to carcinogenic polycyclic hydrocarbons. *Nature* 1963; 4886:1215–16.

67 Fujino T, Park SS, West D, Gelboin HV. Phenotyping of cytochrome P-450 in human tissues with monoclonal antibodies. *Proc Natl Acad Sci* 1982; 79:3682–6.

68 Song BJ, Gelboin HV, Park SS, Tsokos GC, Friedman FK. Monoclonal antibody-directed radioimmunoassay detects cytochrome P-450 in human placenta and lymphocytes. *Science* 1985; 228:490–2.

69 Rubin RL, Curnutte JT. Metabolism of procainamide to the cytotoxic hydroxylamine by neutrophils activated *in vitro. J Clin Invest* 1989; 83:1336–43.

70 Uetrecht JP, Sweetman RL, Woosley RL, Oates JA. Metabolism of procainamide to hydroxylamine by rat and human hepatic microsomes. *Drug Met Disp* 1984; 12:77–81.

71 Victorino RMM, Maria VA. Modifications of the lymphocyte transformation test in a case of drug-induced cholestatic hepatitis. *Diag Immunol* 1985; 3:177–81.

72 Beaune PH, Dansette PM, Mansuy D, Kiffel L, Finck M, Amar C, Leroux JP, Homberg JC. Human anti-endoplasmic reticulum autoantibodies appearing in a drug-induced hepatitis are directed against a human liver cytochrome P-450 that hydroxylates the drug. *Proc Natl Acad Sci* 1987; 84:551–5.

73 Gueguen M, Meunier-Rotival M, Bernard O, Alvarez F. Anti-liver kidney microsome antibody recognizes a cytochrome P450 from the IID subfamily. *J Exp Med* 1988; 168:801–6.

74 Gueguen M, Yamamoto AM, Bernard O, Alvarez F.

Anti-liver kidney microsome antibody type 1 recognizes human cytochrome P450 db1. *Biochem Biopys Res Commun* 1989; 159:542–7.

75 Homberg JC, Abuaf N, Bernard O, Islam S, Alvarez F, Khalil SH, Poupon R, Darnis F, Levy VG, Grippon P, Opolon P, Bernuau J, Benhamou JP, Alagille D. Chronic active hepatitis associated with antiliver/kidney microsome antibody type 1: a second type of 'autoimmune' hepatitis. *Hepatol* 1987; 7:1333–9.

76 Kiffel L, Loeper J, Homberg JC, Leroux JP. A human cytochrome P450 is recognized by anti-liver/kidney microsome antibodies in autoimmune chronic hepatitis. 1989; 159:283–9.

77 Merk HF, Schneider R, Scholl P. Lymphocyte stimulation by drug-modified microsomes. In: Estabrook RW, Lindenlaub E, Oesch F, de Weck AL, eds. *Toxicological and Immunological Aspects of Drug Metabolism and Environmental Chemicals.* Stuttgart:Schattauer, 1988.

78 Gonzalez FJ, Nebert DW. Evolution of the P-450 gene superfamily. *N Trends Genet* 1990; 6:182–6.

79 Gonzales FJ, Skoda RC, Kimura S, Umeno M, Zanger UM, Nebert DW, Gelboin HV, Hardwick JP, Meyer UA. Characterization of the common genetic defect in human deficient in debrisoquine metabolism. Nature 1988; 331:442–6.

80 Meyer UA. Molecular genetics and the future of pharmacogenetics. *Pharmacol Ther* 1990; 46:349–55.

6
Contact sensitivity

IAN KIMBER

Introduction

Contact sensitivity is probably the most frequently encountered toxicological consequence of the interaction of chemicals with the immune system, and certainly the most thoroughly investigated. The phenomenon of contact sensitivity can be viewed from a number of perspectives. To the immunologist it represents a convenient model for investigation of the initiation, expression and regulation of cellular immune responses. Indeed the study of contact sensitization has yielded information of fundamental importance to many areas of immunobiology. To the practising toxicologist, however, allergic contact dermatitis is a problem, a not infrequent reaction following dermal exposure to chemicals. Here the emphasis is on provision of accurate predictions of skin-sensitizing potential. Only recently has a new breed of applied immunologist, the immunotoxicologist, tackled the middle ground and examined the basic immunology of contact sensitivity not as a model system but as a means of addressing the toxicological (and clinical) challenges presented by allergic contact dermatitis. The purpose of this chapter is to provide a review of immunological mechanisms in contact sensitivity and to identify implications and applications for toxicological investigations.

Historical perspective

Ladislav Polak cites Jadassohn (1895) as being the first to describe the phenomenon of skin sensitization [1]. There have, in the intervening period, been a number of important milestones in our understanding of the biology of contact hypersensitivity. Progress has been facilitated by the availability of animal models of contact allergy and by an increasingly sophisticated appreciation of the molecular and cellular events which initiate and regulate immune responses in general, and delayed-type hypersensitivity in particular.

In 1935 Karl Landsteiner and John L. Jacobs reported the successful intradermal sensitization of guinea pigs to nitro- and chloro-substituted benzenes [2]. An observation fundamental to the understanding of contact sensitivity, and indeed to the understanding of cellular immune responses in general, came from the work of Landsteiner and Merrill Chase who successfully transferred cutaneous sensitization to naive guinea pigs with lymphoid cells from picryl chloride-sensitized donors [3]. Although much of the pioneering work on the immunobiology of contact allergy was accomplished with studies in the guinea pig, in recent years the focus of attention has moved largely to the mouse, in which species passive transfer of contact sensitization was first achieved by Crowle in 1959 [4]. The utility of the mouse as an experimental model for studies of contact sensitivity became firmly established in 1968 when Asherson and Ptak [5] developed a method whereby elicitation reactions can be measured quantitatively as a function of challenge-induced increases in ear thickness.

Contact allergy is a biphasic phenomenon comprising an induction or afferent phase during which sensitization is initiated, and an elicitation or efferent phase when, following subsequent exposure to the same chemical, the sensitized animal exhibits a cutaneous hypersensitivity reaction. Both the induction and elicitation phases are subject, or potentially subject, to a variety of immunoregulatory mechanisms which serve to modulate or contain the response. For the purposes of this review it is convenient to consider the subject under the headings induction, elicitation and immunoregulation.

The induction phase

There is now no doubt that contact sensitization is dependent upon the activation and clonal expansion of hapten-reactive T lymphocytes. The majority of evidence suggests that these events are initiated in the lymph nodes draining the site of sensitization. Frey and Wenk [6] demonstrated that destruction of the afferent lymphatics draining the exposed skin effectively prevented the appearance of contact sensitization in guinea pigs. Other circumstantial evidence lends weight to the argument that the critical interaction between antigen and lymphocytes takes place in the regional lymph nodes [7–9].

Turk and his colleagues demonstrated the appearance of large pyroninophilic blast cells in the paracortical areas of guinea pig lymph nodes draining the site of skin sensitization [10–12]. A similar development of T lymphoblasts in the draining nodes of mice sensitized to oxazolone (4-ethoxymethylene-2-phenyloxazol-5-one) was reported subsequently by Parrott and de Sousa [13]. Thymectomy was shown to prevent both the appearance of paracortical blasts [13–15] and the induction of contact sensitization [15]. Congenitally athymic (nude) mice are likewise unable to mount a lymphoproliferative response to oxazolone and fail to develop contact sensitization [16].

The afferent limb of contact allergy is complete when the animal is sensitized and able to mount an elicitation reaction upon challenge with the same chemical. The expanded population of reactive T lymphocytes which effect the elicitation phase are undoubtedly derived from the draining lymph nodes (splenectomy fails to influence the development of sensitization [17]) and rapidly become available systemically [18].

While it is surely the case that the extent of clonal expansion will directly influence the degree of sensitization achieved, such an association is, in practice, difficult to prove unequivocally. There are, however, several lines of circumstantial evidence that the vigour of proliferative responses following primary exposure correlate with the level of sensitization, and the severity of elicitation reactions. Recent studies in this laboratory have revealed that antigenic competition in experimental contact allergy is associated with, and probably a consequence of, a depressed primary proliferative response to the second chemical [19–21]. One inference that can be drawn is that modulation of the primary proliferative response may affect directly the outcome of sensitization.

Compatible with this is evidence which derives from studies of suppressor mechanisms which selectively inhibit the afferent limb of contact sensitization and result in impaired elicitation reactions. Such afferent-acting suppressor mechanisms, which may be induced by a variety of experimental manipulations, invariably inhibit lymphocyte proliferative responses [22–25]. The practical significance of these observations is that the quantitative assessment of T lymphocyte proliferation in draining lymph nodes may provide a realistic correlate of the potency of sensitization which a chemical at any given concentration is likely to cause.

An increased frequency of antigen-reactive T lymphocytes resulting from clonal expansion during the primary proliferative response can be demonstrated *in vitro*. Lymphocytes isolated from sensitized mice will mount a secondary proliferative response when cultured with the relevant hapten presented in an appropriate form [26–30]. Lymphocyte transformation tests (LTT) based on this phenomenon have been used by a number of laboratories for the investigation of human allergic contact dermatitis [31]. The clinical diagnosis of occupational and environmental contact allergy is conventionally performed using a patch test, frequently with a battery of allergens. Patch tests are not only sometimes difficult to interpret, but may also carry the risk of inadvertent sensitization of previously non-allergic individuals [32]. The potential value of the LTT is that it might provide a method for the diagnosis of allergic contact dermatitis, and identification of the causative allergen, without recourse to patch testing. The majority of studies have concentrated on nickel allergy where there has been some notable progress [33–38]. A limited number of other allergens have been examined using the LTT, including neomycin sulphate [38], chromium [39], 2,4-dinitrochlorobenzene (DNCB) [38,40–42] and urushiol [43]. The challenge for the future is for the development of robust methods to enable studies with lipophilic allergens which cannot be added directly to lymphocyte cultures.

Although the frequency of antigen-reactive T lymphocytes in naive mice will be considerably lower than in those which have been sensitized, there have been demonstrations of primary responses *in vitro*. Using the 'hanging-drop' culture technique, Knight and co-workers have shown that picryl chloride and fluorescein isothiocyanate (FITC) are capable of initiating primary proliferation *in vitro* [44,45]. The most convincing evidence for the ability of contact allergens to induce primary responses *in vitro* comes from the work of Hauser and Katz [46] who examined the capacity of cultured Langerhans cells to present antigen to naive lymphocytes. Autoreactive T cells stimulated by culture with unmodified Langerhans cells were eliminated by treatment with bromodeoxyuridine and light. The remaining T lymphocytes, while only minimally responsive to unmodified stimulator cells, were capable of mounting a significant proliferative response when cultured with hapten-modified Langerhans cells. That the hapten-induced proliferation observed was indeed attributable to the response of antigen-specific T lymphocytes is suggested by the fact that prior removal of trinitrophenol (TNP)-reactive T cells with bromodeoxyuridine and light prevented restimulation with this hapten, but not with FITC-derivatized Langerhans cells [46]. To date primary immune responses *in vitro* have been demonstrated only with potent skin allergens; it remains to be seen whether other skin-sensitizing chemicals will be able to provoke similar responses by naive lymphocytes. The *in vitro* assessment of the immunogenic potential of chemicals is therefore a possibility. If skin allergens are also capable of inducing primary proliferative responses by human lymphocytes then it may, in the future, be possible to perform prospective analyses of differential sensitivity to chemical sensitizers among human populations.

For the activation and expansion of reactive T lymphocytes antigen must reach the draining lymph nodes in an appropriate form. One can envisage that this could be achieved in one of several ways; in free form or bound to skin proteins or cells. In recent years most attention has focused on cellular transport and the role of Langerhans cells [47,48]. Epidermal Langerhans cells form part of a family of immunologically active dendritic cells (DC) found within both lymphoid and non-lymphoid tissues. Such cells are bone marrow-derived and express membrane class II histocompatibility (Ia) antigens [49–54]. Of particular interest is the fact that DC are potent, and in the case of primary T lymphocyte responses, possibly obligatory, antigen-presenting cells [53,55–57].

There is a body of evidence that Langerhans cells play an important role in the development of contact allergy. The efficiency of sensitization is impaired, or actively suppressed, when chemical is applied to areas of skin naturally poor in, or depleted of, Langerhans cells [58–62]. There is reason to believe, however, that the availability of Langerhans cells is not an absolute requirement for the initiation of contact hypersensitivity. Studies by Baker *et al.* in the guinea pig [63] and more recently by Streilein in the mouse [64] suggest that contact sensitization may proceed in the absence of epidermal Langerhans cells. One possibility is that there exists a second pathway of cutaneous antigen presentation. Compatible with this is the report by Tse and Cooper [65] of Ia$^+$ dendritic cells in the perivascular region of the mouse dermis which, when derivatized with hapten, can induce contact sensitivity in naive mice. The cautious conclusion which may be drawn is that Langerhans cells are sufficient, but not an absolute prerequisite, for the initiation of skin sensitization [64].

For some time it has been considered that the transport of antigen by Langerhans cells from the skin to the draining lymph nodes represents a major route of cutaneous sensitization [66]. In line with this is the observation that topical exposure of mice to 2,4-dinitrofluorobenzene (DNFB) caused a temporary, but marked, depletion of identifiable Langerhans cells from the epidermis [67]. In recent years it has become clear that within hours of contact sensitization there is an accumulation of DC in the lymph nodes draining the site of application [44,45,68–71]. Flow cytometric studies with skin-sensitizing fluorochromes such as FITC have provided evidence that a significant proportion of the DC which arrive in the draining nodes bear high levels of antigen [45,70,71].

For a number of reasons it seems likely that antigen-bearing DC play an important—even a decisive—role in the induction of contact sensitization. They are potent stimulators of both primary and secondary T lymphocyte proliferative responses *in vitro* [29,30,44,45,70] and small numbers will efficiently induce contact sensitization in naive animals [44,68,71,72]. Moreover, there exists a correlation between the number of DC which arrive in the draining lymph node within 24 h of skin sensitization and the vigour of the primary lymphocyte proliferative response [73]. The activation of T lymphocytes by DC occurs in two stages. Clonal selection of T lymphocytes is facilitated by a transient, antigen non-specific binding to DC [74–78]. This allows DC to sample and retain those T cells which possess receptors complementary for the antigen-Ia complex displayed by the antigen-presenting cell. A direct interaction between DC and T lymphocytes is a mandatory step in the activation process (soluble factors are apparently unable to substitute for cell contact [78]) and can be visualized as cluster formation. Recent studies in this laboratory [79] have shown that antigen-bearing DC isolated from the draining nodes of sensitized mice form clusters with T lymphocytes more effectively (or with greater stability) than do DC which lack demonstrable antigen.

The ultimate fate of antigen-bearing DC in lymph nodes is uncertain. The elevation in DC numbers is relatively transient. Following exposure to FITC levels return to control values within 6 days of sensitization [70]. It may be that either the appearance of hapten-specific antibodies [80] or the selective destruction of antigen-bearing DC by natural killer (NK) cells [81,82] compromises or eliminates antigen-presenting cell function.

No survey of cutaneous DC would be complete without examination of a second population of cells with a dendritic morphology which have been found to reside in murine epidermis. These cells are also bone marrow-derived but in contrast to Langerhans cells express the membrane glycoprotein Thy-1 and are Ia$^-$ [83–86]. The available data indicate that Thy-1$^+$ DC are primitive representatives of the T cell lineage. They are absent from SCID (severe combined immunodeficiency disease) mice [87], express the CD3-associated $\gamma\delta$-T-cell receptor (TCR) [88–90] and proliferate in response to concanavalin A and interleukin-2 (IL-2) [91]. No strictly analogous cells have been found in humans [92–94] although small numbers of $\gamma\delta$-TCR$^+$ lymphocytes reside in human epidermis [94]. It is relevant to examine the influence of Thy-1$^+$ DC on the induction of contact sensitization in mice as Bigby *et al.* [95] have suggested that the relative frequency of Langerhans cells and Thy-1$^+$ DC influences the intensity (but not the duration) of contact hypersensitivity. Moreover, adoptive transfer of hapten-derivatized Thy-1$^+$ DC [96] or Thy-1$^+$ DC lines [97] specifically down-regulates contact sensitization. In view of these data we were prompted to question whether any of the antigen-bearing DC which arrive in draining lymph nodes following skin sensitization express Thy-1. Conclusive evidence was obtained that, initially at least, all lymph node cells bearing high levels of the sensitizing antigen are dendritic, and all express membrane Ia. No antigen-bearing Thy-1$^+$ cells were observed [98]. These findings are of relevance with respect to a report by Okamoto and Kripke [99] in which it was found that suppression of contact sensitization with ultraviolet irradiation was associated with Thy-1$^+$, Ia$^-$ suppressor-inducer cells in the draining lymph node. A possible interpretation was that, as Thy-1$^+$ DC, in contrast to Langerhans cells, appear to be morphologically unaffected by local ultraviolet irradiation, the cells inducing suppression were migratory Thy-1$^+$ epidermal cells [99]. Our observations suggest that this explanation is unlikely [98]. While it is not possible to conclude that Thy-1$^+$ DC will not associate with antigen in the epidermis, it would appear that they fail to migrate and consequently will be unable to influence materially immune activation in draining nodes following skin sensitization.

Taken together, the most likely series of events which, under normal circumstances, occur following epicutaneous exposure to contact allergens is as follows. Langerhans cells form a reticuloepithelial trap for, and associate with, skin-sensitizing chemicals [100,101]. Interaction with chemical causes changes in Langerhans cells [102], which are stimulated to migrate, and carry antigen, via dermal lymphatics to the draining nodes [66].

Freshly isolated Langerhans cells are relatively poor stimulators of T-cell activation [103]. However, this property develops during culture and is associated with enhanced expression of membrane Ia antigen [103–107]. Interleukin-1 (IL-1) has been shown to enhance directly the activity of DC with respect to antigen presentation [108,109] and granulocyte–macrophage colony-stimulating factor (GM-CSF) to provide the stimulus necessary for the functional maturation of Langerhans cells *in vitro* [110–112]. As keratinocytes are able to produce both IL-1 [113,114] and GM-CSF [115,116], it is tempting to speculate that a functional maturation of Langerhans cells, analogous to that observed during culture, is initiated by the application of skin allergens and/or the migration of Langerhans cells to the local lymph nodes. Such functional maturation *in vivo* would account for the potent immunostimulatory properties exhibited by antigen-bearing lymph node DC [29,44,45,71,72].

As DC accumulation in lymph nodes represents an early event, possibly the earliest measurable cellular event, during the induction phase of contact sensitization, it is worthwhile considering whether this phenomenon has potential application as an alternative means of identifying contact allergens. In this laboratory we have recorded an increased frequency of lymph node DC following exposure of mice to a variety of skin allergens including FITC, rhodamine B isothiocyanate (RITC), oxazolone, DNCB, 2,4-dinitrothiocyanobenzene (DNTB) and cinnamic aldehyde [71,98]. Although substantial increases in the number of DC are observed after application of potent skin allergens, the response varies with the chemical used and weaker sensitizers

induce more modest responses [71]. In addition, the methodology required for accurate enumeration of lymph node DC is currently unsuitable for routine analyses, and it is not yet certain that only skin allergens are able to induce DC migration. Although the use of DC responses for predictive testing is some way off, there is no doubt that an appreciation of the role of DC during the induction phase of skin allergy will, in the future, pay dividends in elucidating the way in which chemicals interact with the immune system.

The elicitation phase

Elicitation reactions are induced following challenge of previously sensitized animals, with a peak response approximately 24 h following exposure. Reactions are characterized by an infiltration of mononuclear cells and in some instances basophils [117]. The sequence of events is thought to be as follows. In response to challenge, antigen associates with skin components (including Langerhans cells [118]), lymphocytes extravasate, migrate into the reaction site and, through lymphokine production, induce an amplified cellular infiltrate and local inflammation. Both CD4[+] and CD8[+] T lymphocytes are contained within the infiltrate, usually with the former predominating [119–121]. It is still not clear what role, if any, cytotoxic T cells play in the initiation of dermal reactions. The T lymphocyte infiltrate comprises both specific and non-specific elements. Studies by Scheper *et al.* [122], using expanded populations of dinitrophenol (DNP)-reactive T lymphocytes, showed that although there is a preferential accumulation of antigen-specific T lymphocytes at the challenge site there is also a significant infiltration by non-specific cells.

In recent years there has been considerable interest in the role of mast cells and vasoactive amines in the elicitation of contact allergy. The theory is that an early event following challenge is the degranulation of mast cells and the release of vasoactive amines such as histamine and serotonin. Vasodilation and the creation of gaps between adjacent endothelial cells then facilitates the entry of effector T lymphocytes which mediate the classical delayed hypersensitivity reaction [123]. Evidence supportive of this view comes from the observation by some investigators that challenge reactions in mice comprise both an early (1–2 h) and a late (24–48 h) phase of tissue swelling [124,125], and that the elicitation of contact sensitivity may be more effective in areas of skin rich in mast cells [126]. Moreover, reserpine, an agent that depletes mast cell serotonin, markedly impairs the elicitation of sensitization [127,128]. It has been proposed that the participation of mast cells in challenge reactions requires the sequential action of two independent T lymphocyte populations [123,129]. It is argued that the early component of the elicitation reaction is mediated by a T lymphocyte-derived antigen-binding factor that sensitizes tissue mast cells and possibly other vasoactive amine-containing cells [130–132]. Following challenge antigen is thought to bind to such sensitized cells, initiate degranulation and allow subsequent infiltration of the second population of T lymphocytes which cause the late-phase reaction [130,131]. For a number of reasons the role of vasoactive amines in delayed-type hypersensitivity remains controversial, however. It is clear, for instance, that mice genetically deficient in mast cells display 24-h challenge reactions comparable with normal animals [133–136]. Also, reserpine has been shown virtually to abolish the expression of contact reactions in mast cell-deficient mice [134,137], probably as the consequence of a direct effect of reserpine on T lymphocyte function [136,138].

The matter is therefore unresolved and currently the most realistic conclusion that one may draw is that while early-phase local inflammatory responses may contribute toward the expression of contact hypersensitivity, they do not appear to be essential. Whether or not mast cell degranulation represents a mandatory step in the process, there is no doubt that the inflammatory reaction induced following challenge will result in local vasoactive amine release. In the context of considering whether vasoactive amines provide a useful marker of the elicitation reaction in contact allergy it is unimportant whether mast cell degranulation is the cause or consequence of the hypersensitivity reaction. In agreement with a similar study by Kerdel *et al.* [139], we have found that there is a significant elevation in the serum concentration of histamine following challenge of sensitized mice [140]. Interestingly, in both studies,

the increase in histamine levels was biphasic with an early (1–2 h) and a late (24 h) response [139,140].

The availability of reliable serological markers of the elicitation reaction would be of some value in experimental studies of contact sensitivity. In guinea pigs challenge reactions are conventionally measured by visual assessment of erythema and/or induration, while in mice the preferred method is by measurement of challenge-induced increases in ear thickness [5]. Neither method is perfect; the evaluation of erythema is subjective and measurement of changes in ear thickness relatively difficult to perform. A serological method for the quantitative assessment of elicitation would facilitate batch analysis, interlaboratory comparisons and longitudinal studies. As one may operationally define cutaneous allergic reactions as those in which a sensitized animal can exhibit dermal inflammation following exposure to a chemical in the absence of primary irritancy, there are a number of ways in which challenge responses may be assessed by measurement of inflammatory mediators.

In addition to histamine, we have examined acute-phase protein responses during the elicitation of experimental contact hypersensitivity. Systemic injury, including acute inflammatory reactions, provokes rapid alterations in the hepatic synthesis and plasma concentration of a variety of proteins and glycoproteins known collectively as acute-phase proteins (APP) [141–144]. Studies in mice, using the potent skin allergens oxazolone and picryl chloride, revealed that increases in the serum concentration of two such APP, haptoglobin and serum amyloid A, correlated closely with challenge-induced increases in ear thickness [145]. No increases in APP concentration were found following challenge of naive mice, or in sensitized mice challenged with vehicle or a non-cross-reactive skin allergen [145].

The increased synthesis of APP during inflammatory reactions is mediated by cytokines. Although some studies have implicated IL-1 and tumour necrosis factor (TNF) as inducers of APP [146–148], more recent investigations indicate that interleukin–6 (IL-6) is of greater importance in this respect [149–151]. Not unexpectedly, therefore, it has been possible to demonstrate that contact hypersensitivity is also associated with a significant increase in the plasma concentration of IL-6 [152].

Although there is reason to speculate that serological evaluation of contact allergic responses will, in the future, be a practical proposition, there are two important considerations. Firstly, the use of changes in the concentration of mediators such as those described above requires that challenge is performed with non-inflammatory concentrations of the test chemical. This is not a major drawback as all other available methods for assessing elicitation reactions (based on challenge-induced erythema or oedema) are subject to the same constraint. Secondly, increases in the concentration of inflammatory mediators following challenge are likely to be obscured in experimental systems where Freund's complete adjuvant (FCA) is used to augment sensitization.

Immunoregulation

There is an enormous literature on the immunoregulation of contact sensitivity [153–155]. The difficulty, however, is that in many instances the immune system has been deliberately perturbed to provoke the appearance of immunoregulatory mechanisms. Thus, for example, suppression of contact sensitivity has been induced by the intravenous injection of soluble [22,24,25,156–158] or cell-associated [23,159–161] hapten, by the oral administration of allergen [162,163] and by the application of allergen following ultraviolet irradiation [59,164,165]. The results of such studies have revealed that active regulation of contact sensitivity can be achieved by suppressor cells which influence the induction stage of sensitization (afferent-acting suppressor cells) [22–25], by a complex network of interacting suppressor cells (and molecules) which inhibit the elicitation reaction (efferent-acting suppressor cells) [156,161,166], or by clonal inhibition [160]. In most but not all cases, suppressor cells active in contact sensitization have been characterized as T lymphocytes. In recent years the complexity of cellular interactions in induced immunoregulatory processes has been increased further by the description of contrasuppressor cells which modify suppression in an antigen-specific manner distinct from T-cell help [167,168]. Although there is no doubt that studies of this kind have done much to advance our understanding of the various cellular and molecular mechanisms which may serve to modulate the immune system, they provide little information about the regulatory events which actually influence the development and expression of contact allergy following conventional topical sensitization.

Inevitably the response to contact allergens, in common with other immune responses, is subject to a number of constraints, including the availability of the stimulating antigen and of growth factors necessary for the division and differentiation of T and B lymphocytes. The interesting question is whether there are, in addition, active homeostatic mechanisms which regulate responses. Indirect evidence for the appearance of regulatory mechanisms following epicutaneous exposure derives from experiments in which cyclophosphamide, given prior to sensitization, has been shown to augment contact allergic reactions, presumably through selective impairment or elimination of suppressor cells or their precursors [169–173]. Following conventional exposure to contact allergens there may therefore be both inducing or promoting signals and inhibitory (suppressive) effects with the balance between them influencing the severity and extinction of reactions and the longevity of sensitization. There is some evidence that exposure of animals to sub- (or supra-) optimal concentrations of skin-sensitizing chemicals may tip this balance and result in the appearance of cyclophosphamide-sensitive immunosuppression [174–177]. It has been suggested, but not proven, that some chemicals which in practice are relatively weak sensitizers are such, not due to any lack of inherent immunogenicity, but rather as a result of the induction of more active suppression [1]. If this were the case then a possible corollary might be that some chemicals fail to induce sensitization altogether and initiate only suppression (pure tolerogens). Some examples can be found in the literature. Studies in the mouse have shown that 5-methyl-3-pentadecylcatechol and other methylated analogues of 3-pentadecylcatechol (the active component of urushiol or poison ivy) have no, or only weak, skin-sensitizing activity, but act as epicutaneous tolerogens suppressing subsequent sensitization with 3-pentadecylcatechol [178,179]. Similar observations were made with the guinea pig [180]. Another example is the dinitrobenzene derivative DNTB. Studies in both the guinea pig [181] and mouse [182] had suggested that DNTB fails to cause sensitization, and instead results in specific hyporesponsiveness to the antigenically cross-reactive skin allergen DNFB. We subsequently re-examined this phenomenon and found that, in contrast to the previous reports, topical exposure to DNTB caused contact sensitization in the mouse, rat and humans [28]. Moreover, there was no evidence that DNTB caused tolerance in either the mouse or rat [28]. In the light of these results, and in the case of DNTB in particular, it may be imprudent to consider certain chemicals universal topical tolerogens; the balance between sensitization and regulation may in fact be very finely controlled and variable.

In the context of regulatory events which influence responsiveness following conventional sensitization there is evidence that topical exposure to some chemicals results in the appearance of mechanisms which affect lymphocyte proliferation [183–185]. We made a detailed study of this phenomenon in mice and found that epicutaneous exposure to potent skin allergens results in the appearance of two independent regulatory processes, both of which influence subsequent lymphoproliferative responses. There is a transient, antigen-non-specific mechanism together with a more persistent antigen-specific mechanism [20]. Their physiological role is, we speculate, to provide immune homeostasis and regulate, respectively, the primary and secondary proliferative responses to skin allergens [20]. A similar antigen-specific mechanism for regulation of proliferative responses to the inducing chemical has been found in guinea pigs; however, there was no evidence for the existence of antigen-non-specific effects in this species [186].

It should not be forgotten that while the development and expression of contact allergy is dependent upon the action of T lymphocytes, antibody responses may also be induced as the result of skin sensitization. Anti-hapten antibody of various classes has been found following topical exposure of mice and guinea pigs to strong skin allergens [187–190]. Antibodies directed against the inducing hapten may have the potential to influence contact allergy. It has been proposed that the inhibition of contact sensitization by polyclonal B cell mitogens [191,192] is due to the early appearance or vigorous production of anti-hapten antibodies, which in turn

activate suppressor T lymphocytes [193]. However, there is no compelling evidence that anti-hapten antibodies produced as a consequence of conventional sensitization affect contact hypersensitivity.

Of greater interest is the role of auto-anti-idiotypic antibody responses. Compared with guinea pigs, contact sensitivity in mice is relatively evanescent; sensitization is usually maximal 5 days following exposure, but has declined markedly by day 15. In an elegant series of experiments, Sy *et al.* [194] demonstrated that serum prepared from mice 9–15 days following sensitization to DNFB blocked the ability of DNFB-immune lymph node cells to transfer reactivity to naive recipients. The suppression was antigen-specific and attributable to immunoglobulin, but not to anti-hapten antibodies. The blocking effect could be absorbed by DNFB-immune lymphocytes, but not with normal lymph node cells and it was concluded that anti-receptor (anti-idiotype) antibodies were the cause of suppression and also responsible for the decline of contact sensitization in the intact mouse [194]. Auto-anti-idiotypic antibodies have also been shown to inhibit sensitization to picryl chloride in mice [195]. It appears possible that such antibodies do not interact with the effector T lymphocytes which mediate delayed hypersensitivity, but recognize idiotypes on other regulatory T cells induced following sensitization [196,197]. These findings provide an interesting example of idiotype–anti–idiotype interactions in immune regulation, as predicted by Jerne [198]. It may be that although anti-hapten antibodies do not influence responsiveness, anti-idiotypic antibody production directly affects the longevity (and possibly, magnitude) of skin sensitization.

Finally, it is instructive to consider briefly the inhibition of contact sensitization by ultraviolet B irradiation [199,200]. The biological mechanisms which impair the induction phase of skin allergy following exposure to ultraviolet do not necessarily reflect the nature of immunoregulatory processes which operate in the absence of such treatment. They do, however, provide some lessons and serve to illustrate the complexity of events which may influence cutaneous immunity and the difficulties involved in their accurate definition.

Toews *et al.* [59] reported that local exposure of mice to relatively low doses of ultraviolet B caused a depletion of identifiable Langerhans cells. Application of DNFB to the irradiated site did not cause contact sensitization. Furthermore, animals first exposed to the allergen via irradiated skin failed to exhibit contact allergy when sensitized with the same chemical on a distant, unirradiated site. The assumption was that not only are Langerhans cells necessary for effective skin sensitization, but also that their absence results in specific unresponsiveness [59]. Several other investigations confirmed that ultraviolet B compromised Langerhans cell function. It was found that exposure to ultraviolet B reduced Ia expression by epidermal Langerhans cells [201]. Stingl *et al.* [202] reported that ultraviolet B treatment of isolated Langerhans cells prevented their ability to act as antigen-presenting cells *in vitro*, and Sauder *et al.* [203] found that ultraviolet B inhibited the capacity of hapten-derivatized epidermal cells to induce contact sensitization *in vivo*.

Additional studies revealed that the systemic suppression of sensitization by ultraviolet B was associated with the appearance of afferent-acting suppressor T cells [164]. Such suppressor cells may arise in more than one way. It has been suggested that trans-urocanic acid acts as an epidermal photoreceptor and as the result of ultraviolet B irradiation undergoes an isomerization to the more soluble cis-form [204,205]. Cis-urocanic acid is immunosuppressive [204–206] and has been found to induce suppressor T cells that impair contact allergy and other forms of delayed hypersensitivity [207,208], possibly via production of soluble suppressor factors [208]. Alternatively, it could be argued that the ultraviolet B-resistant Thy-1[+] epidermal DC may initiate suppressor cells following exposure to antigen at irradiated sites [96]. However, the action of suppressor cells may not be the whole story. Different strains of mice exhibit variable susceptibility to the immunosuppressive effects of ultraviolet B [209,210]. Recently Glass *et al.* [211] have found that all strains of mice, irrespective of their susceptibility to ultraviolet B-mediated immunosuppression, induce antigen-specific, afferent-acting suppressor T cells following ultraviolet B treatment. Clearly, therefore, the appearance of such suppressor cells does not necessarily result in depression of contact sensitization. One possible explanation is that although suppressor cells are induced, effective contact

sensitization can still occur in some strains via a second, ultraviolet B-resistant (Langerhans cell-independent) pathway of cutaneous antigen presentation. As the dermis is considered to be relatively unaffected by low-dose ultraviolet B treatment, the Ia[+] dermal dendritic cells recently described by Tse and Cooper [65] may provide the mechanism. These observations are of some importance as they elegantly demonstrate that (in some strains at least) effective skin sensitization can proceed in the presence of functionally active suppressor cells. This lends weight to the argument that contact sensitization (and presumably all other immune responses) is subject to a variety of opposing influences with the balance between them determining the outcome of immunization. Changes in the nature or concentration of the chemical, the route of exposure, the availability and functional integrity of immunologically active cells, and no doubt other as yet undefined factors will alter this balance, and in some cases cause substantial depression, or even complete inhibition, of contact sensitization.

Predictive testing

The protocols used by Landsteiner and Jacobs for the intradermal sensitization of guinea pigs [2] were adapted by Draize *et al.* [212], who introduced a scoring system to evaluate erythematous reactions. The Draize test was the first assay developed specifically for the purpose of assessing skin-sensitizing potential and was used extensively for many years. Since then modifications to the original Draize test have been introduced [213,214], and a variety of new guinea pig predictive methods developed. Among these are the occluded patch test of Buehler [215–217], the ear-flank test [218], the guinea pig maximization test [219–221], the split adjuvant technique [222–224], the guinea pig optimization test [225–227], the TINA (*TI*erexperimenteller *NA*chweistest) test [228,229], the open epicutaneous test [230,231] and the FCA test [230,231].

All such tests are biphasic in nature, comprising both induction and elicitation phases. The procedures used for the induction of sensitization vary. While some tests rely on epicutaneous exposure (the occluded patch test of Buehler, the open epicutaneous test, the ear-flank test and the split adjuvant technique), others require intradermal injection (the Draize test, FCA test and the guinea pig optimization test) or a combination of both topical exposure and intradermal injection (the TINA test and the guinea pig maximization test). A number of the more sensitive methods employ FCA to augment sensitization. Following challenge, reactions are assessed visually and predictions of contact-sensitizing potential made from the frequency of test animals exhibiting a positive (erythematous) reaction.

The purpose of such tests is to identify and reduce the hazard of skin sensitization which might result from environmental or occupational exposure to chemicals. While there is no doubt that, within the context of toxicity testing, some guinea pig methods have provided, and will continue to provide, a valuable service, they are not without limitations [232–234]. There are a number of disadvantages, including the fact that the end-point is subjective and may be obscured when coloured materials are tested. Furthermore, it is necessary that challenge is performed with a non-irritant concentration (usually the maximum non-irritant concentration) of the test chemical. As a consequence direct comparisons between chemicals are frequently difficult, and it may only be possible to test highly irritant materials at low challenge concentrations. Finally, from a practical point of view, some tests, and particularly the more sensitive tests, are relatively costly and time-consuming to perform.

For these reasons, there has in recent years been a growing interest in the development of alternative predictive test methods which offer advantages compared with those currently available. The goal is a rapid, accurate and cost-effective assay which is sufficiently robust to be used in the prospective analysis of new chemicals. Initiatives in this area have been greatly facilitated by advances in our understanding of the cellular immune response to contact allergens and, perhaps for this reason, most attention has focused on the mouse, rather than the guinea pig, as an experimental model.

Elicitation reactions in mice can be assessed in a variety of ways. Assays based upon localization of ^{51}Cr-labelled lymphocytes [235], radioisotopic measurement of activated cells in challenged ears [236–240], the deposition of fibrin at the challenge site [135] and challenge-induced increases in ear weight

[241,242] have been described. It is, however, the measurement of changes in ear thickness following challenge which has been used most frequently to assess the contact-sensitizing potential of chemicals in the mouse [239,243–246], and recently several new predictive tests based on this method have been described. To date, the most thoroughly documented of these is the mouse ear-swelling test (MEST) described by Gad *et al.* [247]. Although the MEST employs a rigorous induction procedure (involving four consecutive daily applications to tape-stripped abdominal skin and the use of FCA) the incremental increase in ear thickness recorded with some skin allergens was relatively small [247]. While potent skin-sensitizing chemicals such as oxazolone and DNFB resulted in substantial ear swelling (challenge-induced increases of 34 and 68% respectively), weaker allergens provoked more modest responses (formalin 15%, cinnamic aldehyde 12% and phthalic anhydride 5%). Despite the fact that some other investigators have been unable, using MEST-type protocols, to obtain significant increases in ear thickness with chemicals such as eugenol and nickel sulphate which proved positive in MEST validation studies [240,248], this method clearly holds some promise for the future. Recently the use of a similar test, the mouse ear sensitization assay (MESA), has been discussed by Descotes [249]. It may prove possible to enhance the sensitivity of MEST and MESA protocols. Diets enriched for vitamin A acetate have been found to augment cell-mediated immune function [250,251] and to potentiate contact sensitization in mice [252]. Miller and her colleagues [253,254] have proposed that the use of mice maintained on a diet supplemented with vitamin A permits more sensitive identification of skin allergens in ear-swelling assays.

In this laboratory we have adopted another approach to the identification of contact allergens, the murine local lymph node assay which, in contrast to the methods described above, is based upon analysis of events which occur during the induction phase of sensitization [255–260]. The development of skin sensitization is critically dependent upon immune activation in lymph nodes draining the site of application [10–12,15], and in preliminary studies we found that mice previously exposed to skin allergens on the dorsum of the ear exhibited both an increased draining (auricular) lymph node weight and lymph node cell proliferation [255]. Exposure to non-sensitizing chemicals under the same conditions failed to result in similar changes [255]. Subsequently test conditions were optimized and comparisons made of various parameters of lymph node activation (increased lymph node weight, the frequency of pyroninophilic cells and the induction of lymphocyte proliferation). Studies performed with a battery of chemicals revealed that of the end-points examined, lymphocyte proliferative responses provided the most reliable and sensitive correlate of skin-sensitizing potential [256]. In these investigations proliferation was measured *in vitro* following culture of draining lymph node cells with ^{3}H-thymidine. The advantage afforded by this technique is that the proliferative activity of antigen-activated lymph node cell populations can be selectively enhanced by addition of an exogenous source of the T-cell growth factor IL-2. Unstimulated lymphocytes lack membrane receptors for this interleukin and addition of IL-2 causes little or no increase in the low levels of background ^{3}H-thymidine incorporation recorded in cultures of lymph node cells prepared from naive or vehicle-treated mice [256].

Recently, in an attempt to simplify the procedure and eliminate the requirement for cell culture, a modified local lymph node assay has been developed in which proliferative activity in the draining lymph nodes is measured *in situ* following intravenous injection of ^{3}H-thymidine [257,258]. In both cases the assay is performed using mice of CBA/Ca strain which, on the basis of comparative studies, were found to exhibit relatively vigorous T lymphocyte proliferative responses following sensitization [256].

Over 150 chemicals have now been tested and experience to date indicates that the local lymph node assay is able accurately to identify at least moderate and strong skin allergens, and shows a good, but not absolute, correlation with guinea pig tests [259]. The first phase of a national interlaboratory trial has recently been completed, the results of which demonstrate that the local lymph node assay is robust and 'travels well'. Using a panel of eight test chemicals the same predictions of skin-sensitizing potential were made by each of four collaborating laboratories [260].

The local lymph node assay offers a number of potential advantages. It is objective and quantitative. The frequently criticized visual assessment of erythema on which guinea pig tests rely is avoided. Compared with the majority of available guinea pig methods the assay is rapid and cost-effective. Exposure is via the relevant route, there is no requirement for adjuvant and comparatively small amounts of test material are needed. Importantly, the performance of the local lymph node assay is uninfluenced by the colour of the test chemical, and studies to date indicate that irritant, non-sensitizing agents fail to induce positive responses.

There is still much to be achieved. Currently a number of important issues (including the predictive value of the local lymph node assay with a wider range of test materials) are being addressed within the framework of more exhaustive interlaboratory trials. It is premature to suggest that the local lymph node assay will offer a realistic alternative to methods such as the guinea pig maximization test for all purposes and with all classes of chemicals. It is not unreasonable to conclude, however, that this assay can, in the context of industrial safety evaluation, provide an accurate and cost-effective method of identifying skin allergens, and may be of particular value in analysis of coloured and irritant materials.

Conclusions

Emerging opportunities to adopt more sophisticated approaches to the toxicological investigation of allergic contact dermatitis have paralleled an increased understanding of the cellular and molecular events which initiate and regulate contact sensitivity. The last two decades have witnessed remarkable advances in cellular immunology. The discovery of immunologically active DC (and renewed interest in epidermal Langerhans cells), an appreciation of the many and varied ways in which the immune system can be modified and is able to regulate itself, and a knowledge of the functional heterogeneity of T lymphocytes and their soluble products have all paid dividends in defining the immunological mechanisms of contact allergy. As described in this chapter there are already opportunities to develop new predictive test methods, to use immune and inflammatory mediators as serological markers of contact allergic reactions and to derive immunological correlates of skin-sensitizing potential. Other fascinating questions remain. What are the important events which occur immediately following interaction of sensitizing chemicals with the skin? How do the various skin cells capable of presenting antigen influence the development of contact sensitization? How can an increasingly precise understanding of immunological mechanisms in contact sensitivity be harnessed to allow more accurate risk assessment? Is it possible to distinguish between allergic and irritant dermatitic reactions? These, and many other challenges, make the phenomenon of contact sensitivity a fertile area of research for the immunotoxicologist.

References

1 Polak L. *Immunological Aspects of Contact Sensitivity. An Experimental Study. Monographs in Allergy.* vol. 15. Basel: Karger, 1980.

2 Landsteiner K, Jacobs JL. Studies on the sensitization of animals with chemical compounds. *J Exp Med* 1935; 61:643–6.

3 Landsteiner K, Chase MW. Experiments on transfer of cutaneous sensitivity to simple compounds. *Proc Soc Exp Biol Med* 1942; 49:688–90.

4 Crowle AJ. Delayed hypersensitivity in mice. Its detection by skin tests and its passive transfer. *Science NY* 1959; 130:159.

5 Asherson GL, Ptak W. Contact and delayed hypersensitivity in the mouse. 1. Active sensitization and passive transfer. *Immunol* 1968; 15:405–16.

6 Frey JR, Wenk P. Experimental studies on the pathogenesis of contact eczema in guinea pigs. *Int Arch Allergy Appl Immunol* 1957; 11:81–100.

7 Parker D, Turk JL. DNP conjugates in guinea pig lymph nodes during contact sensitization. *Immunol* 1970; 18:855–64.

8 Asherson GL, Mayhew B. Induction of cell-mediated immunity in the mouse: circumstantial evidence for highly immunogenic antigen in the regional lymph nodes following skin-painting with contact sensitizing agents. *Isr J Med Sci* 1976; 12:454–67.

9 McFarlin DE, Balfour B. Contact sensitivity in the pig. *Immunol* 1973; 25:995–1009.

10 Turk JL, Stone SH. Implications of the cellular changes in lymph nodes during the development and inhibition of delayed type hypersensitivity. In: Amos B, Koprowski H, eds. *Cell-Bound Antibodies*. Philadelphia: Wistar Institute Press, 1963: 51–60.

11 Oort J, Turk JL. A histological and autoradiographic study of lymph nodes during the development of

contact sensitivity in guinea pigs. *Br J Exp Pathol* 1965; 46:147–54.

12 Turk JL. Cytology of the induction of hypersensitivity. *Br Med Bull* 1967; 23:3–8.

13 Parrott DMV, de Sousa MAB. Changes in the thymus-dependent areas of lymph nodes after immunological stimulation. *Nature* 1966; 212:1316–17.

14 Davies AJS, Carter RL, Leuchars E, Wallis V. The morphology of immune reactions in normal, thymectomized and reconstituted mice. II. The response to oxazolone. *Immunol* 1969; 17:111–26.

15 de Sousa MAB, Parrott DMV. Induction and recall in contact sensitivity. Change in skin and draining lymph nodes of intact and thymectomized mice. *J Exp Med* 1969; 130:671–84.

16 Pritchard H, Micklem HS. Immune responses in congenitally thymus-less mice. I. Absence of response to oxazolone. *Clin Exp Immunol* 1972; 10:151–61.

17 Sy M-S, Miller SD, Kowach HB, Claman HN. A splenic requirement for the generation of suppressor T cells. *J Immunol* 1977; 119:2095–9.

18 Asherson GL, Zembala M. Anatomical location of cells which mediate contact sensitivity in the lymph nodes and bone marrow. *Nature* 1973; 244:176–7.

19 Kimber I, Pierce BB, Mitchell JA, Kinnaird A. Depression of lymph node cell proliferation induced by oxazolone. *Int Arch Allergy Appl Immunol* 1987; 84:256–62.

20 Kimber I, Shepherd CJ, Mitchell JA, Turk JL, Baker D. Regulation of lymphocyte proliferation in contact sensitivity: homeostatic mechanisms and a possible explanation of antigenic competition. *Immunol* 1989; 66:577–82.

21 Kimber I, Bentley AN, Ward RK, Baker D, Turk JL. Antigen-restricted antigenic competition induced by 2,4-dinitrochlorobenzene: association with depression of lymphocyte proliferation. *Int Arch Allergy Appl Immunol* 1990; 91:315–22.

22 Moorhead JW. Tolerance and contact sensitivity to DNFB in mice. IV. Inhibition of afferent sensitivity by suppressor T cells in adoptive transfer. *J Immunol* 1976; 117:802–6.

23 Miller SD, Sy M-S, Claman HN. Suppressor T cell mechanisms in contact sensitivity. II. Afferent blockade by alloinduced suppressor T cells. *J Immunol* 1978; 121:274–80.

24 Thomas WR, Watkins MC, Asherson GL. Suppressor cells for the afferent phase of contact sensitivity to picryl chloride: inhibition of DNA synthesis induced by T cells from mice injected with picryl sulphonic acid. *J Immunol* 1979; 122:2300–3.

25 Dieli F, Abrignani S, Salerno A. T suppressor afferent cells which regulate contact sensitivity to picryl chloride act across genetic barrier. *Immunol Lett* 1987;

14:49–52.

26 Phanuphak P, Moorhead JW, Claman HN. Tolerance and contact sensitivity to DNFB in mice. 1. *In vivo* detection by ear swelling and correlation with *in vitro* cell stimulation. *J Immunol* 1974; 112: 115–23.

27 Phanuphak P, Moorhead JW, Claman HN. Tolerance and contact sensitivity to DNFB in mice. II Specific *in vitro* stimulation with a hapten, 2,4-dinitrobenzene sulfonic acid (DNBSO₃Na). *J Immunol* 1974; 112:849–51.

28 Kimber I, Botham PA, Rattray NJ, Walsh ST. Contact sensitizing and tolerogenic properties of 2,4-dinitrothiocyanobenzene. *Int Arch Allergy Appl Immunol* 1986; 81:258–64.

29 Jones DA, Morris AG, Kimber I. Assessment of the functional activity of antigen-bearing dendritic cells isolated from the lymph nodes of contact-sensitized mice. *Int Arch Allergy Appl Immunol* 1989; 90:230–6.

30 Robinson MK. Optimization of an *in vitro* lymphocyte blastogenesis assay for predictive assessment of immunological responsiveness to contact sensitizers. *J Invest Dermatol* 1989; 92:860–7.

31 von Blomberg-van der Flier BME, Bruynzeel DP, Scheper RJ. Impact of 25 years of *in vitro* testing in allergic contact dermatitis. In: Frosch PJ, Dooms-Goossens A, Lachapelle J-M, Rycroft RJG, Scheper RJ, eds. *Current Topics in Dermatitis.* Heidelberg: Springer-Verlag, 1989: 569–77.

32 Agrup A. Sensitization induced by patch testing. *Br J Dermatol* 1968; 80:631–4.

33 Macleod TM, Hutchinson F, Raffle EJ. The uptake of labelled thymidine by leukocytes of nickel sensitive patients. *Br J Dermatol* 1970; 82:487–92.

34 Hutchinson F, Raffle EJ, Macleod TM. The specificity of lymphocyte transformation *in vitro* by nickel salts in nickel sensitive subjects. *J Invest Dermatol* 1972; 58:362–5.

35 Al-Tawil NG. Marcusson JA. Moller E. Lymphocyte transformation test in patients with nickel sensitivity: an aid to diagnosis. *Arch Dermatol Vener* 1981; 61:511–15.

36 von Blomberg-van der Flier M, van der Burg CKH, Pos O, van de Plassche-Boers EM, Bruynzeel DP, Garotta G, Scheper RJ. *In vitro* studies in nickel allergy: diagnostic value of dual parameter analysis. *J Invest Dermatol* 1987; 88:362–8.

37 Everness KM, Gawkrodger DJ, Botham PA, Hunter JAA. The discrimination between nickel-sensitive and non-nickel-sensitive subjects by an *in vitro* lymphocyte transformation test. *Br J Dermatol* 1990; 122:293–8.

38 Kimber I, Quirke S, Beck MH. Attempts to identify the causative allergen in cases of allergic contact dermatitis using an *in vitro* lymphocyte transformation test. *Toxic in Vitro* 1990; 4:302–6.

39 Yamada M, Niwa Y, Fujimoto F, Yoshinaga H. Lymphocyte transformation in allergic contact dermatitis. *Jpn J Dermatol* 1972; 82:94–7.

40 Miller AE, Levis WR. Studies on the contact sensitization of man with simple chemicals. I. Specific lymphocyte transformation in response to dinitrochlorobenzene sensitization. *J Invest Dermatol* 1973; 61:261–9.

41 Soeberg B, Anderson V. Hapten-specific lymphocyte transformation in humans sensitized with NDMA or DNCB. *Clin Exp Immunol* 1976; 25:490–2.

42 Levis WR, Whalen JJ, Powell JA. Specific blastogenesis and lymphokine production in DNCB-sensitive human leukocyte cultures stimulated with soluble and particulate DNP-containing antigens. *Clin Exp Immunol* 1976; 23:481–90.

43 Byers VS, Epstein WL, Castagnoli N, Baer H. *In vitro* studies of poison oak immunity. I. *In vitro* reaction of human lymphocytes to urushiol. *J Clin Invest* 1979; 64:1437–48.

44 Knight SC, Krejci J, Malkovsky M, Colizzi V, Gautam A, Asherson GL. The role of dendritic cells in the initiation of immune responses to contact sensitizers. I. *In vivo* exposure to antigen. *Cell Immunol* 1985; 94:427–34.

45 Macatonia SE, Edwards AJ, Knight SC. Dendritic cells and the initiation of contact sensitivity to fluorescein isothiocyanate. *Immunol* 1986; 59:509–14.

46 Hauser C, Katz SI. Activation and expansion of hapten- and protein-specific T helper cells from non-sensitized mice. *Proc Natl Acad Sci USA* 1988; 85:5625–8.

47 Friedman PS. The immunobiology of Langerhans cells. *Immunol Today* 1981; 2:124–8.

48 Wolff K, Stingl G. The Langerhans cell. *J Invest Dermatol* 1983; 80 (suppl): 17–21.

49 Steinman RM, Cohn ZA. Identification of a novel cell type in peripheral lymphoid organs of mice. I. Morphology, quantitation, tissue distribution. *J Exp Med* 1973; 137:1142–62.

50 Balfour BM, Drexhage HA, Kamperdijk EWA, Hoefsmit ECM. Antigen-presenting cells including Langerhans cells, veiled cells and interdigitating cells. In: Porter R, Whelan J, eds. *Microenvironments in Haemopoietic and Lymphoid Differentiation.* Ciba Foundation Symposium no. 84. London: Pitman Medical, 1981:281–301.

51 Steinman RM, Nussenzweig MC. Dendritic cells: functions and features. *Immunol Rev* 1981; 53:125–58.

52 Knight SC. Veiled cells—dendritic cells of the peripheral lymph. *Immunobiol* 1984; 168:349–61.

53 Austyn JM. Lymphoid dendritic cells. *Immunol* 1987; 62:161–70.

54 Steinman RM, Inaba K. Immunogenicity: role of dendritic cells. *BioEsssay* 1989; 10:145–52.

55 Inaba K, Steinman RM. Resting and sensitized T

lymphocytes exhibit distinct stimulatory (antigen-presenting cell) requirements for growth and lymphokine release. *J Exp Med* 1984; 160:1717–35.

56 Steinman RM, Inaba K, Schuler G, Witmer M. Stimulation of the immune response: contribution of dendritic cells. In: Steinman RM, North RJ, eds. *Mechanisms of Host Resistance to Infectious Agents, Tumors and Allografts*. New York: The Rockerfeller University Press, 1986:71–97.

57 Inaba K, Young JW, Steinman RM. Direct activation of CD8 $^+$ cytotoxic T lymphocytes by dendritic cells. *J Exp Med* 1987; 166:182–94.

58 Streilein JW, Toews GB, Bergstresser PR. Langerhans cells: functional aspects revealed by *in vivo* grafting studies. *J Invest Dermatol* 1980; 75:17–21.

59 Toews GB, Bergstresser PR, Streilein JW. Epidermal Langerhans cell density determines whether contact hypersensitivity or immunosuppression follows skin painting with DNFB. *J Immunol* 1980; 124:445–53.

60 Semma M, Sagami S. Induction of suppressor T cells to DNFB contact sensitivity by application of sensitizer through Langerhans cell-deficient skin. *Arch Dermatol Res* 1981; 271:361–4.

61 Rheins LA, Nordlund JJ. Modulation of the population density of identifiable epidermal Langerhans cells associated with enhancement or suppression of cutaneous immune reactivity. *J Immunol* 1986; 136:867–76.

62 Halliday GM, Muller HK. Sensitization through carcinogen-induced Langerhans cell-deficient skin activates specific long-lived suppressor cells for both cellular and humoral immunity. *Cell Immunol* 1987; 109:206–21.

63 Baker D, Parker D, Turk JL. Effect of depletion of epidermal dendritic cells on the induction of contact sensitivity in the guinea pig. *Br J Dermatol* 1985; 113:285–94.

64 Streilein JW. Antigen-presenting cells in the induction of contact hypersensitivity in mice: evidence that Langerhans cells are sufficient but not required. *J Invest Dermatol* 1989; 93:443–8.

65 Tse Y, Cooper KD. Cutaneous dermal Ia $^+$ cells are capable of initiating delayed type hypersensitivity responses. *J Invest Dermatol* 1990; 94:267–72.

66 Silberberg-Sinakin I, Thorbecke GJ, Baer RL, Rosenthal SA, Berezowsky V. Antigen-bearing Langerhans cells in skin, dermal lymphatics and in lymph nodes. *Cell Immunol* 1976; 25:137–51.

67 Bergstresser PR, Toews GB, Streilein JW. Natural and perturbed distributions of Langerhans cells: responses to ultraviolet light, heterotopic skin grafting and dinitrofluorobenzene sensitization. *J Invest Dermatol* 1980; 75:73–7.

68 Knight SC, Bedford P, Hunt R. The role of dendritic cells in the initiation of immune responses to contact sensitizers. II. Studies in nude mice. *Cell Immunol* 1985; 94:435–9.

69 Katz DR, Mukherjee S, Maisey J, Miller K. Vitamin A acetate as a regulator of accessory cell function in delayed-type hypersensitivity responses. *Int Arch Allergy Appl Immunol* 1987; 82:53–6.

70 Macatonia SE, Knight SC, Edwards AJ, Griffiths S, Fryer P. Localization of antigen on lymph node dendritic cells after exposure to the contact sensitizer fluorescein isothiocyanate. Functional and morphological studies. *J Exp Med* 1987; 166:1654–67.

71 Kinnaird A, Peters SW, Foster JR, Kimber I. Dendritic cell accumulation in draining lymph nodes during the induction phase of contact allergy in mice. *Int Arch Allergy Appl Immunol* 1989; 89:202–10.

72 Macatonia SE, Knight SC. Dendritic cells and T cells transfer sensitization for delayed-type hypersensitivity after skin painting with contact sensitizer. *Immunol* 1989; 66:96–9.

73 Kimber I, Kinnaird A, Peters SW, Mitchell JA. Correlation between lymphocyte proliferative responses and dendritic cell migration in regional lymph nodes following skin painting with contact sensitizing agents. *Int Arch Allergy Appl Immunol* 1990; 93:47–53.

74 Inaba K, Steinman RM. Accessory cell-T lymphocyte interactions: antigen-dependent and independent clustering. *J Exp Med* 1987; 163:247–61.

75 Inaba K, Steinman RM. Monoclonal antibodies to LFA-1 and to CD4 inhibit the mixed leukocyte reaction after the antigen-dependent clustering of dendritic cells and T lymphocytes. *J Exp Med* 1987; 165:1403–17.

76 Austyn JM, Morris PJ. T-cell activation by dendritic cells: CD18-dependent clustering is not sufficient for mitogenesis. *Immunol* 1988; 63:537–43.

77 Austyn JM, Weinstein DE, Steinman RM. Clustering with dendritic cells precedes and is essential for T-cell proliferation in a mitogenesis model. *Immunol* 1988; 63:691–6.

78 Inaba K, Romani N, Steinman RM. An antigen-independent contact mechanism as an early step in T cell-proliferative responses to dendritic cells. *J Exp Med* 1989; 170:527–42.

79 Cumberbatch M, Illingworth I, Kimber I. (manuscript in preparation).

80 Asherson GL, Colizzi V, Watkins MC. Immunogenic cells in the regional lymph nodes after painting with the contact sensitizers picryl chloride and oxazolone: evidence for the presence of IgM antibody on their surface. *Immunol* 1983; 48:561–9.

81 Shah PD, Gilbertson SM, Rowley DA. Dendritic cells that have interacted with antigen are targets for natural killer cells. *J Exp Med* 1985; 162:625–36.

82 Shah PD, Keij J, Gilbertson SM, Rowley DA. Thy-1 $^+$ and Thy-1 $^-$ natural killer cells. Only Thy-1 $^-$ natural

killer cells suppress dendritic cells. *J Exp Med* 1986; 163:1012–17.

83 Bergstresser PR, Tigelaar RE, Dees JH, Streilein JW. Thy-1 antigen-bearing dendritic cells populate murine epidermis. *J Invest Dermatol* 1983; 81:286–8.

84 Tschachler E, Schuler G, Hutterer J, Leibl H, Wolff K, Stingl G. Expression of Thy-1 antigen by murine epidermal cells. *J Invest Dermatol* 1983; 81:282–5.

85 Rowden G, Bishnupriya M, Mikol D, Higley H. An analysis of murine and human epidermal cell suspensions by means of immunoperoxidase staining of lymphocyte and Langerhans cell antigenic markers. *J Invest Dermatol* 1983; 80:343–4.

86 Chambers DA. The Thy-1 epidermal cell: perspective and prospective. *Br J Dermatol* 1985; 113 (suppl 28):24–33.

87 Nixon-Fulton JL, Witte PL, Tigelaar RE, Bergstresser PR, Kumar V. Lack of dendritic Thy-1$^+$ epidermal cells in mice with severe combined immunodeficiency disease. *J Immunol* 1987; 138:2902–5.

88 Kuziel WA, Takashima A, Bonyhadi M, Bergstresser PR, Allison JP, Tigelaar RE, Tucker PW. Regulation of T-cell receptor γ-chain RNA expression in murine Thy-1$^+$ dendritic epidermal cells. *Nature* 1987; 328:263–6.

89 Koning F, Stingl G, Yokoyama WM, Yamada H, Maloy WL, Tschachler E, Shevach EM, Coligan JE. Identification of T3-associated gamma-delta T cell receptor on Thy-1$^+$ dendritic epidermal cell lines. *Science* 1987; 236:834–7.

90 Steiner G, Koning F, Elbe A, Tschachler E, Yokoyama WM, Shevach EM, Stingl G, Coligan JE. Characterization of T cell receptors on resident murine dendritic epidermal T cells. *Eur J Immunol* 1988; 18:1323–8.

91 Nixon-Fulton JL, Bergstresser PR, Tigelaar RE. Thy-1$^+$ epidermal cells proliferate in response to concanavalin A and interleukin 2. *J Immunol* 1986; 136:2776–86.

92 Cooper KD, Breathnach SM, Caughman SW, Palini AG, Waxdal MJ, Katz SI. Fluorescence microscopic and flow cytometric analysis of bone marrow derived cells in human epidermis: a search for the human analogue of the murine dendritic Thy-1$^+$ epidermal cell. *J Invest Dermatol* 1985; 85:546–52.

93 Bos JD, Zonneveld I, Das PK, Krieg SR, Van der Loos ChM, Kapsenberg ML. The skin immune system (SIS): distribution and immunophenotype of lymphocyte subpopulations in normal human skin. *J Invest Dermatol* 1987; 88:569–73.

94 Bos JD, Tuenissen MBM, Cairo I, Krieg SR, Kapsenberg ML, Das PK, Borst J. T-cell receptor γδ bearing cells in normal human skin. *J Invest Dermatol* 1990; 94:37–42.

95 Bigby M, Kwan T, Sy M-S. Ratio of Langerhans cells to

Thy-1$^+$ dendritic epidermal cells influences the intensity of contact hypersensitivity. *J Invest Dermatol* 1987; 89:495–9.

96 Sullivan S, Bergstresser PR, Tigelaar RE, Streilein JW. Induction and regulation of contact hypersensitivity by resident bone marrow-derived dendritic epidermal cells: Langerhans cells and Thy-1$^+$ epidermal cells. *J Immunol* 1986; 137:2460–7.

97 Welsh EA, Kripke ML. Murine Thy-1$^+$ dendritic epidermal cells induce immunologic tolerance *in vivo*. *J Immunol* 1990; 144:883–91.

98 Cumberbatch M, Kimber I. Phenotypic characteristics of antigen-bearing cells in the draining lymph nodes of contact-sensitized mice. *Immunology* 1990; 71:404–10.

99 Okamoto H, Kripke ML. Effector and suppressor circuits of the immune response are activated *in vivo* by different mechanisms. *Proc Natl Acad Sci USA* 1987; 84:3841–5.

100 Shelley WB, Juhlin L. Langerhans cells form a reticuloepithelial trap for external contact allergens. *Nature* 1976; 261:46–7.

101 Shelley WB, Juhlin L. Selective uptake of contact allergens by the Langerhans cell. *Arch Dermatol* 1977; 113:187–92.

102 Hanau D, Fabre M, Schmitt DA, Lepoittevin J-P, Stampf J-L, Grosshans E, Benezra C, Cazenave J-P. ATPase and morphologic changes in Langerhans cells induced by epicutaneous application of a sensitizing dose of DNFB. *J Invest Dermatol* 1989; 92:689–94.

103 Schuler G, Steinman RM. Murine epidermal Langerhans cells mature into potent immunostimulatory dendritic cells *in vitro*. *J Exp Med* 1985; 161:526–46.

104 Inaba K, Schuler G, Witmer MD, Valinsky J, Atassi B, Steinman RM. Immunologic properties of purified epidermal Langerhans cells. Distinct requirements for stimulation of unprimed and sensitized T lymphocytes. *J Exp Med* 1986; 164:605–13.

105 Shimada S, Caughman SW, Sharrow SW, Stephany D, Katz SI. Enhanced antigen-presenting capacity of cultured Langerhans cells is associated with markedly increased expression of Ia antigen. *J Immunol* 1987; 139:2551–5.

106 Picut CA, Lee CS, Dougherty SP, Anderson KL, Lewis RM. Immunostimulatory capabilities of highly-enriched Langerhans cells *in vitro*. *J Invest Dermatol* 1988; 90:201–6.

107 Streilein JW, Grammer SF. *In vitro* evidence that Langerhans cells can adopt two functionally distinct forms capable of antigen presentation to T lymphocytes. *J Immunol* 1989; 143:3925–33.

108 Koide SL, Inaba K, Steinman RM. Interleukin 1 enhances T-dependent immune responses by amplifying the function of dendritic cells. *J Exp Med* 1987; 165:515–30.

109 Steinman RM. Cytokines amplify the function of accessory cells. *Immunol Lett* 1988; 17:197–202.

110 Witmer-Pack MD, Olivier W, Valinsky J, Schuler G, Steinman RM. Granulocyte/macrophage colony-stimulating factor is essential for the viability and function of cultured murine epidermal Langerhans cells. *J Exp Med* 1987; 166:1484–98.

111 Heufler C, Koch F, Schuler G. Granulocyte/macrophage colony-stimulating factor and interleukin 1 mediate the maturation of murine epidermal Langerhans cells into potent immunostimulatory dendritic cells. *J Exp Med* 1988; 167:700–5.

112 Koch F, Heufler C, Kampgen E, Schneeweiss D, Bock G, Schuler G. Tumour necrosis factor α maintains the viability of murine epidermal Langerhans cells, but in contrast to granulocyte/macrophage colony-stimulating factor, without inducing their functional maturation. *J Exp Med* 1990; 171:159–71.

113 Luger TA, Stadler BM, Luger BA, Mathieson BJ, Mage M, Schmidt JA, Oppenheim JJ. Murine epidermal cell-derived thymocyte-activating factor resembles murine interleukin 1. *J Immunol* 1982; 128:2147–52.

114 Kupper TS, Ballard DW, Chua AO, McGuire JS, Flood PM, Horowitz MC, Langdon R, Lightfoot L, Gubler U. Human keratinocytes contain mRNA indistinguishable from monocyte interleukin 1 α and β mRNA. Keratinocyte epidermal cell-derived thymocyte-activating factor is identical to interleukin 1. *J Exp Med* 1986; 164:2095–100.

115 Kupper TS, Coleman DL, McGuire J, Goldminz D, Horowitz MC. Keratinocyte-derived T cell growth factor. A T cell growth factor functionally distinct from interleukin 2. *Proc Natl Acad Sci USA* 1986; 83:4451–5.

116 Kupper TS, Lee F, Coleman D, Chodakewitz J, Flood P, Horowitz M. Keratinocyte derived T cell growth factor (KTGF) is identical to granulocyte macrophage colony stimulating factor (GM-CSF). *J Invest Dermatol* 1988; 91:185–8.

117 Dvorak HF, Mihm JC Jr. Basophilic leukocytes in allergic contact dermatitis. *J Exp Med* 1972; 135:235–54.

118 Silberberg I. Apposition of mononuclear cells to Langerhans cells in contact allergic reactions. An ultrastructural study. *Acta Dermatol Venereol* 1973; 53:1–12.

119 Ralfkiaer E, Wantzin GL. *In situ* immunological characterization of the infiltrating cells in positive patch tests. *Br J Dermatol* 1984; 111:13–22.

120 McMillan EM, Stoneking L, Burdick S, Cowan I, Husian-Hamzavi SL. Immunophenotype of lymphoid cells in positive patch tests of allergic contact dermatitis. *J Invest Dermatol* 1985; 84:229–33.

121 Wood GS, Volterra AS, Abel EA, Nickoloff BJ, Adams RM. Allergic contact dermatitis: novel immunohistologic features. *J Invest Dermatol* 1986; 87:688–93.

122 Scheper RJ, Van Dinther-Janssen ACHM, Polak L. Specific accumulation of hapten-reactive T cells in contact sensitivity reaction sites. *J Immunol* 1985; 134:1333–6.

123 Van Loveren H, Askenase PW. Delayed hypersensitivity is mediated by a sequence of two different T cell activities. *J Immunol* 1984; 133:2397–401.

124 Mackenzie AR, Pattison J, Hiller MA. Early and late reactions in contact sensitivity in the mouse. *Int Arch Allergy Appl Immunol* 1981; 65:187–97.

125 Van Loveren H, Meade R, Askenase PW. An early component of delayed-type hypersensitivity mediated by T-cells and mast cells. *J Exp Med* 1983; 157:1604–17.

126 Gershon RK, Askenase PW, Gershon MD. Requirement for vasoactive amines for production of delayed-type hypersensitivity skin reactions. *J Exp Med* 1975; 142:732–47.

127 Askenase PW, Bursztajn S, Gershon MD, Gershon RK. T cell-dependent mast cell degranulation and release of serotonin in murine delayed-type hypersensitivity. *J Exp Med* 1980; 152:1358–74.

128 Bäck O, Groth O. Reserpine and the suppression of both edema formation and cellular infiltrate of the contact sensitivity reaction in the mouse. *Arch Dermatol Res* 1983; 275:371–3.

129 Van Loveren H, Kato K, Meade R, Green DR, Horowitz M, Ptak W, Askenase PW. Characterization of two different Ly-1$^+$ T cell populations that mediate delayed-type hypersensitivity. *J Immunol* 1984; 133:2402–11.

130 Van Loveren H, Ratzlaff RE, Kato K, Meade R, Fergueson RT, Iverson GM, Janeway CA, Askenase PW. Immune serum from mice contact sensitized with picryl chloride contains an antigen-specific T cell factor that transfers immediate cutaneous sensitivity. *Eur J Immunol* 1986; 16:1203–8.

131 Meade R, Van Loveren H, Parmentier H, Iverson GM, Askenase PW. The antigen-binding T cell factor PCl-F sensitizes mast cells for *in vitro* release of serotonin. Comparison with monoclonal IgE antibody. *J Immunol* 1988; 141:2704–13.

132 Herzog WR, Meade R, Pettinicchi A, Ptak W, Askenase PW. Nude mice produce a T cell-derived antigen-binding factor that mediates the early component of delayed type hypersensitivity. *J Immunol* 1989; 142:1803–12.

133 Thomas WR, Schrader JW. Delayed hypersensitivity in mast cell-deficient mice. *J Immunol* 1983; 130:2565–7.

134 Galli SJ, Hammel I. Unequivocal delayed hypersensi-

tivity in mast cell-deficient and Beige mice. *Science* 1984; 226:710–13.

135 Mekori YA, Dvorak HF, Galli SJ. ^{125}I-fibrin deposition in contact sensitivity reactions in the mouse. Sensitivity of the assay for quantitating reactions after active or passive sensitization. *J Immunol* 1986; 136:2018–25.

136 Mekori YA, Chang JCC, Wershil BK, Galli SJ. Studies on the role of mast cells in contact sensitivity responses. Passive transfer of the reaction into mast cell-deficient mice locally reconstituted with cultured mast cells: effect of reserpine on transfer of the reaction with DNP-specific cloned T cells. *Cell Immunol* 1987; 109:39–52.

137 Askenase PW, Van Loveren H, Kraeuter-Kops S, Ron Y, Meade R, Theoharides TC, Nordlund JJ, Scovern H, Gershon MD, Ptak W. Defective elicitation of delayed-type hypersensitivity in W/W^v and S1/S1^d mast cell-deficient mice. *J Immunol* 1983; 131:2687–94.

138 Mekori YA, Weitzman GL, Galli SJ. Reevaluation of reserpine-induced suppression of contact sensitivity. Evidence that reserpine interferes with T-lymphocyte function independently of an effect on mast cells. *J Exp Med* 1985; 162:1935–53.

139 Kerdel FA, Belsito DV, Scotto-Chinnici BS, Soter NA. Mast cell participation during the elicitation phase of murine allergic contact hypersensitivity. *J Invest Dermatol* 1987; 88:686–90.

140 Kimber I, Cumberbatch M, Coleman JW. Serum histamine and the elicitation of murine contact sensitivity. *J Appl Toxicol* (in press).

141 Koj A. Acute phase reactants. Their synthesis, turnover and biological significance. In: Allison AC, ed. *Structure and Function of Plasma Proteins*. vol. 1. London: Plenum Press, 1974:74–131.

142 Kushner I. The phenomenon of the acute phase response. *Ann NY Acad Sci* 1982; 389:39–48.

143 Koj A. Metabolic studies of acute phase proteins. In: Mariani G, ed. *Pathophysiology of Plasma Protein Metabolism*. London: Macmillan, 1983:221–48.

144 Movat HZ. *The Inflammatory Reaction*. Amsterdam: Elsevier, 1985.

145 Kimber I, Ward RK, Shepherd CJ, Smith MN, McAdam KPWJ, Raynes JG. Acute-phase proteins and the serological evaluation of experimental contact sensitivity in the mouse. *Int Arch Allergy Appl Immunol* 1989; 89:149–55.

146 Dinarello CA. Interleukin 1 as mediator of the acute phase response. *Surv Immunol Res* 1984; 3:29–33.

147 Perlmutter DH, Dinarello CA, Punsal PI, Colten HR. Cachectin/tumor necrosis factor regulates hepatic acute-phase gene expression. *J Clin Invest* 1986; 78:1349–54.

148 Darlington GJ, Wilson DR, Lachman LB. Monocyte-conditioned medium, interleukin-1 and tumor necrosis factor stimulate the acute phase response in human hepatoma cells *in vitro*. *J Cell Biol* 1986; 103:787–93.

149 Morrone G, Gilberto G, Olivero S, Arcone R, Dente L, Content J, Cortese R. Recombinant interleukin 6 regulates the transcriptional activation of a set of human acute phase genes. *J Biol Chem* 1988; 263:12554–8.

150 Marinkovic S, Jahreis GP, Wong GG, Baumann H. IL–6 modulates the synthesis of a specific set of acute phase plasma proteins *in vivo*. *J Immunol* 1989; 142:808–12.

151 Castell JV, Gomez-Lechon MJ, David M, Andus T, Geiger T, Trullenque R, Fabra R, Heinrich PC. Interleukin 6 is the major regulator of acute phase protein synthesis in adult human hepatocytes. *FEBS Lett* 1989; 242:237–9.

152 Kimber I, Cumberbatch M, Humphreys M, Hopkins SJ. Contact hypersensitivity induces plasma interleukin 6 (IL–6). *Int Arch Allergy App Immunol*. 1990; 92:97–9.

153 Asherson GL, Zembala M, Thomas WR, Perera MACC. Suppressor cells and the handling of antigen. *Immunol Rev* 1980; 50:3–45.

154 Claman HN, Miller SD, Sy M-S, Moorhead JW. Suppressive mechanisms involving sensitization and tolerance in contact allergy. *Immunol Rev* 1980; 50:105–32.

155 Claman HN, Miller SD, Conlon PJ, Moorhead JW. Control of experimental contact sensitivity. *Adv Immunol* 1980; 30:121–57.

156 Asherson GL, Zembala M. Suppression of contact sensitivity by T cells in the mouse. I. Demonstration that suppressor cells act on the effector stage of contact sensitivity; and their induction following *in vitro* exposure to antigen. *Proc R Soc Lond B* 1974; 187:329–48.

157 Taborski U, Freitag W, Heremans H, Knop J. Inhibitory effects of interferon-γ on the suppressor T cell circuit in contact sensitivity. *Immunobiol* 1986; 171:329–38.

158 Marcinkiewicz J, Chain B. Antigen-specific inhibition of IL–2 and IL–3 production in contact sensitivity to TNP. *Immunol* 1989; 68:185–9.

159 Miller SD, Claman HN. The induction of hapten-specific T cell tolerance using hapten-modified lymphoid cells. I. Characteristics of tolerance induction. *J Immunol* 1976; 117:1519–26.

160 Miller SD, Sy M-S, Claman HN. The induction of hapten-specific T cell tolerance using hapten-modified lymphoid cells. II. Relative roles of suppressor T-cells and clone inhibition in the tolerant state. *Eur J Immunol* 1977; 7:165–70.

161 Miller SD, Sy M-S, Claman HN. Suppressor T cell mechanism in contact sensitivity. I. Efferent blockade by syn-induced suppressor T cells. *J Immunol* 1978; 121:265–73.

162 Chase MW. Inhibition of experimental drug allergy by prior feeding of the sensitizing agent. *Proc Soc Exp Biol Med* 1946; 61:257–9.

163 Asherson GL, Zembala M, Perera MACC, Mayhew B, Thomas WR. The production of immunity and unresponsiveness in the mouse by feeding contact sensitizing agents and the role of modulator cells in the Peyer's patches, mesenteric lymph nodes and other lymphoid tissues. *Cell Immunol* 1977; 33:145–55.

164 Elmets CA, Bergstresser PR, Tigelaar RE, Wood PJ, Streilein JW. Analysis of the mechanism of unresponsiveness produced by haptens painted on skin exposed to low dose ultraviolet radiation. *J Exp Med* 1983; 158:781–94.

165 Ullrich SE. Suppression of lymphoproliferation by hapten-specific suppressor T lymphocytes from mice exposed to ultraviolet radiation. *Immunol* 1985; 54:343–52.

166 Asherson GL, Dorf ME, Colizzi V, Zembala M, James BMB. Equivalence of conventional anti-picryl T suppressor factor in the contact sensitivity system and monoclonal anti–NP TsF$_3$: their final non-specific effect via the T acceptor cell. *Immunol* 1984; 53:491–7.

167 Ptak W, Bereta M, Marcinkiewicz J, Gershon RK, Green DR. Production of antigen-specific contrasuppressor cells and factor, and their use in augmentation of cell-mediated immunity. *J Immunol* 1984; 133:623–8.

168 Green DR, Ptak W. Contrasuppression in the mouse. *Immunol Today* 1986; 7:81–6.

169 Maguire HC, Ettore VL. Enhancement of dinitrochlorobenzene (DNCB) contact sensitization by cyclophosphamide in the guinea pig. *J Invest Dermatol* 1967; 48:39–43.

170 Turk JL, Parker D, Poulter LW. Functional aspects of the selective depletion of lymphoid tissue by cyclophosphamide. *Immunol* 1972; 23:493–501.

171 Turk JL, Polak L, Parker D. Control mechanisms in delayed-type hypersensitivity. *Br Med Bull* 1976; 32:165–170.

172 Polak L, Rinck C. Effect of elimination of suppressor cells in the development of DNCB contact sensitivity in guinea pigs. *Immunol* 1977; 33:305–11.

173 Parker D, Turk JL. Kinetics of the relation between suppressor and effector mechanisms in contact sensitivity in the guinea-pig. *Immunol* 1982; 47:61–6.

174 Lowney ED. Topical hyposensitization of allergic contact sensitivity in the guinea pig. *J Invest Dermatol* 1964; 43:487–90.

175 Lowney ED. Immunological unresponsiveness appearing after topical application of contact sensitizers to the guinea pig. *J Immunol* 1965; 95:397–403.

176 Sy M-S, Miller SD, Claman HN. Immune suppression with supraoptimal doses of antigen in contact sensitivity. I. Demonstration of suppressor cells and their sensitivity to cyclophosphamide. *J Immunol* 1977; 119:240–4.

177 Asherson GL, Perera MACC, Thomas WR. Contact sensitivity and the DNA response in mice to high and low doses of oxazolone: low dose unresponsiveness following painting and feeding and its prevention by pretreatment with cyclophosphamide. *Immunol* 1979; 36:449–59.

178 Dunn IS, Liberato DJ, Castagnoli N Jr, Byers VS. Contact sensitivity to urushiol: role of covalent bond formation. *Cell Immunol* 1982; 74:220–33.

179 Dunn IS, Liberato DJ, Castagnoli N Jr, Byers VS. Influence of chemical reactivity of urushiol-type haptens on sensitization and the induction of tolerance. *Cell Immunol* 1986; 97:189–96.

180 Stampf J-L, Benezra C, Byers V, Castagnoli N Jr. Induction of tolerance to poison ivy urushiol in the guinea pig by epicutaneous application of the structural analog 5-methyl-3-n-pentadecylcatechol. *J Invest Dermatol* 1986; 86:535-8.

181 Sommer G, Parker D, Turk JL. Epicutaneous induction of hyporeactivity in contact sensitization. Demonstration of suppressor cells induced by contact with 2,4-dinitrothiocyanatebenzene. *Immunol* 1975; 29:517–25.

182 Iijima M, Katz SI. Specific immunologic tolerance to dinitrofluorobenzene following topical application of dinitrothiocyanobenzene. Modulation by suppressor T cells. *J Invest Dermatol* 1983; 81:325–30.

183 Datta U, Barnet K, Asherson GL. DNA synthesis *in vitro* by cells from mice immunized with picryl chloride: effect of injection on immune cells. *Int Arch Allergy Appl Immunol* 1976; 50:574–82.

184 Wood P, Asherson GL, Mayhew B, Thomas WR, Zembala M. Control of the immune reaction: T cells in immunized mice which depress the *in vivo* DNA synthesis response in the lymph nodes to skin painting with the contact sensitizing agent picryl chloride. *Cell Immunol* 1977; 30:25–34.

185 Dunn IS, Liberato DJ, Castagnoli N, Byers VS. Induction of suppressor T cells for lymph node cell proliferation after contact sensitization of mice with a poison oak urushiol component. *Immunol* 1984; 51:773–81.

186 Baker D, Kimber I, Turk JL. Antigen-specific regulation of T lymphocyte proliferative responses to contact-sensitizing chemicals in the guinea pig. *Cell Immunol* 1989; 119:153–9.

187 Taylor RB, Iverson GM. Hapten competition and the nature of cell cooperation in the antibody response. *Proc R Soc Lond Biol* 1971; 176:393–418.

188 Thomas WR, Asherson GL, Watkins MC. Reaginic antibody produced in mice with contact sensitivity. *J Exp Med* 1976; 144:1386–90.

189 Takahashi C, Nishikawa S, Katsura Y, Izumi T. Anti-DNP antibody response after the topical application of DNFB in mice. *Immunol* 1977; 33:589–96.

190 Boerrigter GH, Bril H, Scheper RJ. Hapten-specific antibodies in allergic contact dermatitis in the guinea pig. *Int Arch Allergy Appl Immunol* 1988; 85:385–91.

191 Colizzi V, Bozzi L. A mechanism for the depression of contact sensitivity with B-cell mitogens. *Ann Immunol (Inst Pasteur)* 1979; 130C:659–73.

192 Benedettini G, De Libero G, Mori L, Campa M. *Staphylococcus aureus* inhibits contact sensitivity to oxazolone by activating suppressor B cells in mice. *Int Arch Allergy Appl Immunol* 1984; 73:269–73.

193 Campa M, De Libero G, Benedettini G, Mori L, Angioni MR, Marelli P, Falcone G. Polyclonal B cell activators inhibit contact sensitivity to oxazolone in mice by potentiating the production of anti-hapten antibodies that induce T suppressor lymphocytes acting through the release of soluble factors. *Int Arch Allergy Appl Immunol* 1985; 78:391–5.

194 Sy M-S, Moorhead JW, Claman HN. Regulation of cell-mediated immunity by antibodies: possible role of anti-receptor antibodies in the regulation of contact sensitivity to DNFB in mice. *J Immunol* 1979; 123:2593–8.

195 Shepherd GM, Gibbons JJ, Siskind GW, Thorbecke GJ, Goidl EA. Production of auto-anti-idiotypic antibody during the normal immune response. VIII. Effect of auto-anti-idiotypic antibody on contact sensitivity. *Cell Immunol* 1985; 94:512–20.

196 Moorhead JW. Antigen-receptors on murine T lymphocytes in contact sensitivity. III. Mechanisms of negative feedback regulation by autoanti-idiotypic antibody. *J Exp Med* 1982; 155:820–30.

197 Mustain EL, Claman HN, Moorhead JW. Antibody-mediated regulation of T cell responses. I. Characterization of a monoclonal antibody which specifically regulates contact hypersensitivity to DNFB in BALB/c mice. *J Immunol* 1986; 136:4372–8.

198 Jerne NK. Toward a network theory of the immune system. *Ann Immunol (Inst Pasteur)* 1974; 125C:373–89.

199 Haniszko J, Suskind RR. The effect of ultraviolet radiation on experimental cutaneous sensitization in guinea pigs. *J Invest Dermatol* 1963; 40:183–91.

200 Morison WL, Parrish JA, Woehler ME, Bloch KJ. The influence of ultraviolet radiation on allergic contact dermatitis in the guinea pig. I. UVB radiation. *Br J Dermatol* 1981; 104:161–4.

201 Aberer W, Schuler G, Stingl G, Honigsmann H, Wolff K. Ultraviolet light depletes surface markers of Langerhans cells. *J Invest Dermatol* 1981; 76:202–10.

202 Stingl G, Gazze-Stingl LA, Aberer W, Wolff K. Antigen presentation by murine epidermal Langerhans cells and its alteration by ultraviolet B light. *J Immunol* 1981; 127:1707–13.

203 Sauder DN, Tamaki K, Moshell AN, Fujiwara H, Katz SI. Induction of tolerance to topically-applied TNCB using TNP-conjugated ultraviolet light-irradiated epidermal cells. *J Immunol* 1981; 127:261–5.

204 De Fabo EC, Noonan FP. Mechanism of immune suppression by UV-irradiation in vivo. I. Evidence for the existence of a unique photoreceptor in skin and its role in photoimmunology. *J Exp Med* 1983; 157:84–98.

205 De Fabo E, Noonan F, Fisher M, Burns J, Kaiser H. Further evidence that the photoreceptor mediating UV-induced systemic immune suppression is urocanic acid. *J Invest Dermatol* 1983; 80:319.

206 Ross JA, Howie SEM, Norval M, Maingay J, Simpson T. UV-irradiated urocanic acid suppresses delayed-type hypersensitivity to herpes simplex virus in mice. *J Invest Dermatol* 1986; 87:630–3.

207 Ross JA, Howie SEM, Norval M, Maingay J. Two phenotypically distinct T cells are involved in ultraviolet-irradiated urocanic acid-induced suppression of the efferent delayed-type hypersensitivity response to herpes simplex virus, type 1 *in vivo*. *J Invest Dermatol* 1987; 89:230–3.

208 Harriott-Smith TG, Halliday WJ. Suppression of contact hypersensitivity by short-term ultraviolet irradiation:II. The role of urocanic acid. *Clin Exp Immunol* 1988; 72:174–7.

209 Bergstresser PR, Elmets CA, Streilein JW. Local effects of ultraviolet radiation on immune function in mice. In: Parrish JA, ed. *The Effect of Ultraviolet Radiation on the Immune System*. Skillman NJ: Johnson and Johnson, 1983; 73–86.

210 Streilein JW, Bergstresser PR, Genetic factors in ultraviolet-B-induced suppression of contact hypersensitivity in mice. *Immunogen* 1988; 27:252–8.

211 Glass MJ, Bergstresser PR, Tigelaar RE, Streilein JW. UVB radiation and DNFB skin painting induce suppressor cells universally in mice. *J Invest Dermatol* 1990; 94:273–8.

212 Draize JH, Woodward G, Calvery HO. Methods for the study of irritation and toxicity of substances applied topically to the skin and mucous membranes. *J Pharmacol Exp Ther* 1944; 82:377–90.

213 Sharp DW. The sensitization potential of some perfume ingredients tested using a modified Draize

procedure. *Toxicol* 1978; 9:261–71.

214 Johnson AW, Goodwin BFJ. The Draize test and modifications. In: Andersen KE, Maibach HI, eds. *Contact Allergy Predictive Tests in Guinea Pigs. Current Problems in Dermatology.* vol. 14. Basel: Karger, 1985; 31–8.

215 Buehler EV. Delayed contact hypersensitivity in the guinea pig. *Arch Dermatol* 1965; 91:171–7.

216 Ritz HL, Buehler EV. Planning, conduct and interpretation of guinea pig sensitization patch tests. In: Drill VA, Lazar P, eds. *Current Concepts in Cutaneous Toxicity.* New York: Academic Press, 1980; 25–40.

217 Buehler EV. A rationale for the selection of occlusion to induce and elicit delayed contact hypersensitivity in the guinea pig. A prospective test. In: Andersen KE, Maibach HI, eds. *Contact Allergy Predictive Tests in Guinea Pigs. Current Problems in Dermatology.* vol. 14. Basel: Karger, 1985; 39–58.

218 Stevens MA. Use of the albino guinea-pig to detect the skin-sensitizing ability of chemicals. *Br J Ind Med* 1967; 24:189–202.

219 Magnusson B, Kligman AM. The identification of contact allergens by animal assay, the guinea pig maximization test method. *J Invest Dermatol* 1969; 52:268–76.

220 Magnusson B, Kligman AM. *Allergic Contact Dermatitis in the Guinea Pig.* Springfield IL: Charles C. Thomas, 1970.

221 Wahlberg JE, Boman A. Guinea pig maximization test. In: Andersen KE, Maibach HI, eds. *Contact Allergy Predictive Tests in Guinea Pigs. Current Problems in Dermatology.* vol. 14. Basel: Karger, 1985: 59–106.

222 Maguire HC Jr. The bioassay of contact allergy in the guinea pig. *J Soc Cosmet Chem* 1973; 24:151–62.

223 Maguire HC Jr. Estimation of the allergenicity of prospective human sensitizers in the guinea pig. In: Maibach HI, ed. *Animal Models in Dermatology.* New York: Churchill-Livingstone, 1975: 67–75.

224 Maguire HC Jr, Cipriano D. Split adjuvant technique. In: Andersen KE, Maibach HI, eds. *Contact Allergy Predictive Tests in Guinea Pigs. Current Problems in Dermatology.* vol. 14. Basel: Karger, 1985; 107–13.

225 Maurer T, Thomann P, Weirich EG, Hess R. The optimization test in the guinea pig. A method for the predictive evaluation of the contact allergenicity of chemicals. *Agents Actions* 1975; 5:174–9.

226 Maurer T, Weirich EG, Hess R. The optimization test in the guinea pig in relation to other predictive sensitization methods. *Toxicol* 1980; 15:163–71.

227 Maurer T. The optimization test. In: Andersen KE, Maibach HI, eds. *Contact Allergy Predictive Tests in Guinea Pigs. Current Problems in Dermatology.* vol. 14. Basel: Karger, 1985: 114–51.

228 Ziegler V. Der tierexperimentelle nachweis allergener eigenschaften von industrieprodukten. *Derm Monatsch* 1977; 163:387–91.

229 Ziegler V, Suss E. The TINA test. In: Andersen KE, Maibach HI, eds. *Contact Allergy Predictive Tests in Guinea Pigs. Current Problems in Dermatology.* vol. 14. Basel: Karger, 1985: 172–92.

230 Klecak G, Geleick H, Frey JR. Screening of fragrance materials for allergenicity in the guinea pig. I. Comparison of four testing methods. *J Soc Cosmet Chem* 1977; 28:53–64.

231 Klecak G. The Freund's complete adjuvant test and the open epicutaneous test. In: Andersen KE, Maibach HI, eds. *Contact Allergy Predictive Tests in Guinea Pigs. Current Problems in Dermatology.* vol. 14. Basel: Karger, 1985: 152–71.

232 Andersen KE, Maibach HI. Guinea pig sensitization assays. An overview. In: Andersen KE, Maibach HI, eds. *Contact Allergy Predictive Tests in Guinea Pigs. Current Problems in Dermatology.* vol. 14. Basel: Karger, 1985: 263–90.

233 Oliver GJA, Botham PA, Kimber I. Models for contact sensitization—novel approaches and future developments. *Br J Dermatol* 1986; 115:53–62.

234 Kimber I. Aspects of the immune response to contact allergens; opportunities for the development and modification of predictive test methods. *Fd Chem Toxic* 1989; 27:755–62.

235 Sabbadini E, Neri A, Sehon AH. Localization of non-immune radioactively labelled cells in the lesions of contact sensitivity in mice. *J Immunol Meth* 1974; 5:9–19.

236 Eipert EF, Miller HC. Contact sensitivity in mice measured with thymidine labeled lymphocytes. *Immunol Comm* 1975; 4:361–72.

237 Vadas MA, Miller JFAP. Gamble J, Whitelaw A. A radioisotopic method to measure delayed type hypersensitivity in the mouse. I. Studies in sensitized and normal mice. *Int Arch Allergy Appl Immunol* 1975; 49:670–92.

238 Miller JFAP, Vadas MA, Whitelaw A, Gamble J. A radioisotopic method to measure delayed type hypersensitivity in the mouse. II. Cell transfer studies. *Int Arch Allergy Appl Immunol* 1975; 49:693–708.

239 Back O, Larsen A. Contact sensitivity in mice evaluated by means of ear swelling and a radiometric test. *J Invest Dermatol* 1982; 78:309–12.

240 Cornacoff JB, House RV, Dean JH. Comparison of a radioisotopic incorporation method and the mouse ear swelling test (MEST) for contact sensitivity to weak sensitizers. *Fund Appl Toxicol* 1988; 10:40–4.

241 Corsini AC, Belucci SB, Cost MG. A simple method of evaluating delayed type hypersensitivity. *J Immunol Meth* 1979; 30:195–200.

242 Chapman JR, Ruben Z, Butchko GM. Histology of quantitative assays for oxazolone-induced allergic contact dermatitis in mice. *Am J Dermatopathol* 1986; 8:130–8.

243 Moller H. Attempts to induce contact allergy to nickel in the mouse. *Contact Derm* 1984; 10:65–8.

244 Thorne PS, Hillebrand JA, Lewis GR, Karol MH. Contact sensitivity by diisocyanates: potencies and cross-reactivities. *Toxic Appl Pharmacol* 1987; 87: 155–65.

245 Tanaka K-I, Takeoka A, Nishimura F, Hanada S. Contact sensitivity induced in mice by methylene bisphenyl diisocyanate. *Contact Derm* 1987; 17:199–204.

246 Mor S, Ben-Efraim S, Leibovici J, Ben-David A. Successful contact sensitization to chromate in mice. *Int Arch Allergy Appl Immunol* 1988; 85:452–7.

247 Gad SC, Dunn BJ, Dobbs DW, Reilly C, Walsh RD. Development and validation of an alternative dermal sensitization test: the mouse ear swelling test (MEST). *Toxic Appl Pharmacol* 1986; 84:93–114.

248 Stephens TJ, Drake K, Renskers KJ, Teal J, Penney D, Kaminsky M, Grey T, Northroot H. Preliminary evaluation of the mouse ear swelling test (MEST). *The Toxicologist* 1987; 7:83.

249 Descotes J. Identification of contact allergens: the mouse ear sensitization assay. *J Toxicol—Cut Ocul Toxicol* 1988; 7:263–72.

250 Malkovsky M, Dore C, Hunt R, Palmer L, Chandler P, Medawar PB. Enhancement of specific antitumor immunity in mice fed a diet enriched in vitamin A acetate. *Proc Natl Acad Sci USA* 1983; 80:6322–6.

251 Malkovsky M, Edwards AJ, Hunt R, Palmer L, Medawar PB. T-cell-mediated enhancement of host-versus-graft reactivity in mice fed a diet enriched in vitamin A acetate. *Nature* 1983; 302:338–40.

252 Miller K, Maisey J, Malkovsky M. Enhancement of contact sensitization in mice fed a diet enriched in vitamin A acetate. *Int Arch Allergy Appl Immunol* 1984; 75:120–5.

253 Maisey J, Miller K. Assessment of the ability of mice fed on vitamin A supplemented diet to respond to a variety of potential contact sensitizers. *Contact Derm* 1986; 15:17–23.

254 Maisey J, Purchase R, Robbins MC, Miller K. Evaluation of the sensitizing potential of 4 polyamines present in technical triethylenetetramine using 2 animal species. *Contact Derm* 1988; 18:133–7.

255 Kimber I, Mitchell JA, Griffin AC. Development of a murine local lymph node assay for determination of sensitizing potential. *Fd Chem Toxicol* 1986; 24:585–6.

256 Kimber I, Weisenberger C. A murine local lymph node assay for identification of contact allergens. Assay development and results of an initial validation study. *Arch Toxicol* 1989; 63:274–82.

257 Kimber I, Hilton J, Weisenberger C. The murine local lymph node assay for identification of contact allergens. A preliminary evaluation of *in situ* measurement of lymphocyte proliferation. *Contact Derm* 1989; 21:215–20.

258 Kimber I, Weisenberger C. A modified local lymph node assay for identification of contact allergens. In: Frosch PJ, Dooms-Goossens A, Lachapelle J-M, Rycroft RJG, Scheper RJ, eds. *Current Topics in Contact Dermatitis.* Heidelberg: Springer-Verlag. 1989: 592–5.

259 Kimber I, Hilton J, Botham PA. Identification of contact allergens using the murine local lymph node assay: comparisons with the Buehler occluded patch test in guinea pigs. *J Appl Toxicol* 1990; 10: 173–80.

260 Kimber I, Hilton J, Botham PA, Basketter DA, Scholes EW, Miller K, Robbins MC, Harrison PTC, Gray TJB, Waite SJ. The murine local lymph node assay. Results of an inter-laboratory trial. *Tox Letters* 1990; 55:203–13.

7

The lung as a target organ

DAVID E. BICE

Introduction

The goal of this chapter is to help the reader understand how inhaled pollutants might alter pulmonary immune responses, leading to either suppression of pulmonary defences, or the induction of pulmonary hpersensitivity. To achieve this goal, it is necessary to understand the mechanisms responsible for the induction of pulmonary immunity. Therefore, a description of the cells and tissues responsible for pulmonary immune responses and their functions is presented. Examples of the suppression of pulmonary immune responses by inhaled toxicants, as well as examples of pulmonary disease induced by inhaled chemicals are presented.

The goal of toxicology studies is to obtain a better understanding of biological processes in humans and how these processes provide protection or lead to disease. Therefore, animal models selected to study the effects of inhaled toxicants must have the same cellular and molecular responses in the induction and regulation of pulmonary immunity as humans. Otherwise, data from the animal model cannot be used to estimate possible effects on human pulmonary immunity. Because of the need to accurately predict the possible effects of inhaled toxicants on the lungs of humans, differences in pulmonary immunity among laboratory animal models and humans are also discussed.

Mechanisms of pulmonary immune responses

An understanding of the mechanisms responsible for the induction of pulmonary immunity is necessary to determine how inhaled pollutants may either suppress immune defences in the lung or stimulate levels of pulmonary immunity that would result in disease. A review of data from studies designed to define the mechanisms responsible for the induction of immunity after exposure of the lungs to antigen is presented below.

Primary antibody responses after pulmonary immunization

Studies completed during the last several years have evaluated immunity produced in response to the localized deposition of antigen in the lungs of a variety of species. The results of these studies have provided information concerning the lymphoid tissues in which primary immune responses are produced after pulmonary immunization, the mechanisms responsible for the translocation of antigen from the lung to these tissues, the accumulation of antigen-specific antibody and immune cells in the lung, and the roles of immune cells that accumulate in the immunized lung in providing immune defence.

In pulmonary immunity studies that have used small laboratory species, antigen is usually instilled directly into the trachea, exposing the entire lung [1–3]. In larger animals (e.g. dogs and non-human primates) antigen can be instilled into selected airways of a single lung lobe by using a fibreoptic bronchoscope. Saline or other control materials can be instilled into different lung lobes of the same animal [4–7]. A variety of antigens have been used, although particulate antigens, such as sheep red blood cells (SRBC) or rabbit red blood cells (RRBC), are frequently used. Highly antigenic-soluble antigens (e.g. keyhole limpet haemocyanin) have also been used [8].

Lung-associated lymph nodes. The instillation of antigen into the lungs of rodents, as well as into selected lung lobes of dogs, results in the production of antigen-specific, antibody-forming cells (AFC) and antibody in the lung-associated lymph nodes [2,3,9–11]. The lung-associated lymph nodes function as effective filters to remove particulate materials that clear from the lower respiratory tract via the lymphatics [12,13]. The lung-associated lymph

nodes are responsible for the induction of primary immune responses after instillation of antigen into the lung [14]. Lymphoid tissues that do not drain the lung are not normally involved in producing immunity after lung immunization. Therefore, only background numbers of antigen-specific AFC are present in spleen or lymph nodes that do not receive lymphatic drainage from the lung.

Although it is clear that the lung-associated lymph nodes are responsible for the induction of immunity after a primary immunization with particulate antigen, how antigen leaves the lung and reaches these tissues is not completely understood. It is likely that most of the instilled particulate antigen deposited in the terminal airways and alveoli is cleared by phagocytosis by pulmonary alveolar macrophages and polymorphonuclear (PMN) leucocytes that then transport the foreign material up the mucociliary escalator and out of the lung [12,15,16]. However, some antigen is transported to the lung-associated lymph nodes where immunity is produced.

Cell populations in the lung change in response to pulmonary immunization, and these changes may be important in the translocation of antigen to the lung-associated lymph nodes. Inflammation is produced in the lung in response to particulate antigen instilled into the lung in primary immunizations [4–6,9,17–22]. PMN that enter the lung during an inflammatory response can phagocytos particles in the lung and carry them to the lymph nodes that receive lymphatic drainage from the lung [20]. Therefore, the production of lung inflammation and the accumulation of PMN in the lung may enhance the transport of materials from the lung to the lung-associated lymph nodes. In addition, alveolar macrophages also phagocytos particles in the alveoli and carry phagocytosed particles to the lung-associated lymph nodes [18,19]. It seems likely that it is the transport of antigen from the lung in PMN and/or alveolar macrophages that allows antigen to be presented to antigen-sensitive lymphocytes in the lung-associated lymph nodes. The cells that carry antigen from the lung to the lung-associated lymph nodes (e.g. alveolar macrophages or PMN) may also function as antigen-presenting cells in these tissues. However, it is also possible that dendritic cells and/or lymph node macrophages are the cells responsible for antigen presentation in the lung-associated lymph nodes, and that alveolar macrophages and PMN from the lung serve only to transport antigen to these tissues.

Antibody immunity in blood after lung immunization. Antibody produced in the lung-associated lymph nodes is released into the blood, providing systemic immune protection. In addition to increased levels of antigen-specific antibody in the blood, large numbers of specific immunoglobulin M (IgM) and IgG AFC are found in the blood of dogs, cynomolgus monkeys, and chimpanzees after localized pulmonary immunization [4–7,9,17] (Table 7.1). Published data indicate that the most likely source of antigen-specific immune cells in the blood is by immune stimulation of the lung-associated lymph nodes with a release of AFC into the efferent lymphatics [4,10,11,22,23]. Distant lymphoid tissues contain few or no AFC after pulmonary immunization, and no observable histological changes occur in airway or alveolar lymphoid nodules or aggregates in dog lungs after primary immunization that would suggest that these tissues are the source of blood AFC after a primary exposure to antigen [23,24]. Immune cells released from the lung-associated lymph nodes would be distributed to all tissues of the body, including lung. Memory lymphocytes are probably also released into blood and would provide immune memory to lymphoid tissues distant from the lung.

Changes in lung cell populations after pulmonary immunization. The instillation of particulate antigen into the lungs of dogs and non-human primates changes both the number of cells present in lung lavage fluid, as well as the distribution of the cell types present (e.g. PMN, lymphocytes, and macrophages). These cellular changes follow specific patterns and persist from a few hours to 2 or more weeks after a single antigen exposure.

An increase in the number of PMN in the lavage fluid from immunized lung lobes is the first cellular change observed after exposure of the lung to particulate antigen [4–7,9,17,25]. The increased number of inflammatory cells is accompanied by increased levels of serum proteins that enter the lung from the vascular bed [6,7,9,26,27]. Neutrophils enter the lungs of dogs and non-human primates in the first few hours after exposure to antigen, with an initial peak of number of PMN in lavage fluid from immunized lung lobes of dogs at 1 day after immunization [25]. However, few lymphocytes enter the lung at this time. A second PMN response is observed around 7 days after immunization, and lymphocytes and AFC begin to enter the lung at this time [7,25].

The numbers of alveolar macrophages and lymphocytes also increase in the immunized lung lobes of dogs and non-human primates after a localized pulmonary immunization [4–7,9,17]. The peak responses of these cell types, with a mean of 64%

Table 7.1 Antibody-forming cells/10^6 lymphoid cells* in lung-associated lymph nodes, blood and distant lymphoid tissues after primary lung immunization

Species	Antigen	LALN	Blood	Distant lymph node or spleen
Mouse	SRBC	>500	<20	
Rat	SRBC	>600	<50	<10
Chinese hamster	SRBC	>300	<10	
Syrian hamster	SRBC	>300	<20->700	
Guinea pig	SRBC	>500	<10	<20
Rabbit	SRBC	>600	<20	<10
Sheep	HRBC		<10	
Dog	SRBC	>200	>500	<20
Cynomolgus monkey	SRBC		>500	
Chimpanzee	SRBC		>400	
Human	Various		>500	

*Antibody-forming cells were immunoglobulin M (IgM), IgG, and/or IgA, depending on the study. LALN, lung-associated lymph nodes; SRBC, sheep red blood cells; HRBC, horse red blood cells.

pulmonary alveolar macrophages and a mean of 25% lymphoid cells, occurs between 7 and 14 days after immunization [4–7,9,17]. The number of lymphocytes present in lavage fluid from the immunized lung lobes of some animals may be as high as 50% of the cells lavaged from the lung.

Antibody responses in the lung after instillation of antigen. As indicated above, large numbers of lymphocytes are found in the lungs of dogs and non-human primates after a primary immunization by instillation of particulate antigen (Table 7.2). Many of the lymphoid cells are actively producing specific antibody. Published data indicate that blood is the source of AFC present in the lung after a primary immunization [4,22,23]. The number of AFC in the blood of dogs and non-human primates peaks consistently earlier than in the lung, suggesting that in primary immune responses the blood is likely the source of immune cells in the alveoli [4–7,9,17].

Historically, it was believed that immune responses could be produced in the lung in the absence of any regional or systemic immunity. However, the results of a study that used two distinct antigens for simultaneous immunization of two lung lobes indicate that AFC enter the lung from the blood in primary immune responses, rather than being produced locally in lymphoid tissues in the lung (e.g. bronchus-associated lymphoid tissues) [4]. The results of other studies also support this concept [21,22]. In addition, the results of detailed studies of the histological changes in the lung and lung-associated lymph nodes after primary lung immunization showed no changes in lymphoid aggregates or nodules that would suggest a local production of AFC in primary immune responses in the lung [23,28].

The mechanisms responsible for the accumulation of antibody and immune cells into immunized lung lobes from the blood of dogs and non-human primates are not completely understood. The results of one study suggest that the recruitment of T lymphocytes into the lung is antigen-specific [29]. However, the recruitment of AFC into the lung is not antigen-specific [4]. In addition, the AFC produced in lymphoid tissues that do not drain the lung enter an immunized lung lobe at the same rate as AFC produced in the lung-associated lymph nodes [21]. Apparently, after a primary immunization, AFC enter the lung due to non-specific changes resulting from the release of mediators and/or the induction of inflammation by exposure of the lung to particulate antigen. The exact changes and cellular events that allow AFC and immune cells to enter an area of the lung exposed to antigen are not known.

Large numbers of AFC (1000 IgM, and 10 000 IgG AFC/10^6 lymphoid cells) are found in lavage fluid from immunized lung lobes of dogs. Similar responses are observed in the lungs of non-human primates after localized pulmonary immunization (Table 7.2). Although significantly lower numbers of AFC are found in the saline-exposed control lung lobes, immune cells are present in lung lobes that were exposed only to saline [4–7,9,17].

Species	Antigen	Primary response		Secondary response	
		Lavage	Tissue	Lavage	Tissue
Mouse	SRBC		<100	>800	>400
Rat	SRBC	<10	<10	<10	<10
Guinea pig	SRBC	<10	<100		
Rabbit	SRBC	<10	<10		
Sheep	HRBC			<100	
Dog	SRBC	>1000		>5000	
Cynomolgus monkey	SRBC	>1000		>10 000	
Chimpanzee	SRBC	>1000			
Human	None	>1000			

Table 7.2 Antibody-forming cells/10^6 lymphoid cells* in lung lavage and lung tissue after primary lung immunization and antigen challenge

*Antibody-forming cells were immunoglobulin M (IgM), IgG, and/or IgA, depending on the study. SRBC, sheep red blood cells; HRBC, horse red blood cells.

Some immune cells that enter immunized lung lobes after a primary exposure to antigen mature to plasma cells [30] and produce antibody locally. This local production of antibody significantly increases the specific antibody in the alveoli [26]. The results of a study that evaluated the effects of this locally produced antibody on the phagocytic function of alveolar macrophages indicated that cytophilic and opsonizing antibody were significantly higher in immunized dog lung lobes than in control lung lobes [27]. In addition, significantly more SRBC instilled into an immunized lung lobe were phagocytased than SRBC instilled into control lung lobes [27]. These data all indicate that antibody produced by the immune cells in the immunized lung is important in pulmonary immune defence.

Secondary antibody responses after pulmonary immunization

Immune memory in previously immunized lung lobes. Memory lymphocytes are recruited into the immunized lung lobes of dogs and non-human primates during the development of a primary immune response [6,7,31]. Although a large number of immune cells enter the lung from the blood, there appears to be no production of immune cells in the lung after a primary exposure to antigen. However, immune memory cells recruited into the lung during a primary immune response respond locally to subsequent antigen challenges. The function of these pulmonary immune memory cells can be demonstrated by the measurement of secondary immunity after challenge of a previously immunized lung lobe with a dose of antigen too low to induce a primary immune response. Instillation of the same low dose of antigen into a control lung lobe does not result in a measurable response [31]. Although the lung-associated lymph nodes are the immune tissues that respond after a primary lung immunization [4,7,11,22,23], preliminary data suggest that the local response by memory cells to antigens in the lung may eliminate the need for immune responses in the lung-associated lymph nodes after an antigen challenge.

Antigen presentation in secondary immune responses in the lung. After primary lung immunization, AFC

are prosduced in the lung-associated lymph nodes. It could be assumed that antigen presentation in the lung-associated lymph nodes is by either macrophages or dendritic cells, as in all other lymph nodes. However, the response of memory cells in the lung to antigen challenge indicates that cells in the lung assume the role of antigen presentation. The alveolar macrophage might seem the most likely cell responsible for antigen presentation in these secondary immune responses, and numerous publications report the results of studies that used *in vitro* testing to evaluate the function of pulmonary alveolar macrophages as an antigen-presenting cell. Although the results of some studies suggest that the pulmonary alveolar macrophage will support antigen-stimulation of lymphocytes *in vitro* [32–34], other studies indicate that the pulmonary alveolar macrophage may actually suppress cellular [35–37] and antibody immunity [38,39]. The implication of the latter studies is that one possible function of the pulmonary alveolar macrophage is to control the development of excessive immune reactions that might develop in the alveoli and damage the lung. However, there are other cells and mediators that may also play a role in regulating immune responses in the alveoli [40].

Although antigen presentation in the alveoli could be by alveolar macrophages, the results of recent studies suggest that dendritic cells in the interstitial tissues of the alveoli might be responsible for antigen presentation in the lung [41]. In addition, cells responding to antigen challenge are in the interstitial tissues, rather than the alveoli, supporting the possibility that dendritic cells and/or tissue macrophages are the antigen-presenting cells [7]. If these observations are correct, the primary role of the alveolar macrophage is in the phagocytosis and clearance of materials from the lung, and possibly in immunoregulation, with little or no role in antigen presentation.

Long-term antibody production in the lung. The results of recent studies suggest that antibody production can continue in the lung for years after exposure to antigen [42]. It became apparent from the results of studies of immune memory in the lung that the levels of specific antibody in immunized and challenged lung lobes did not return to background levels 180 days after the last exposure to antigen. Therefore, we evaluated the levels of antibody in lavage fluid from the immunized and control lung lobes of ogs that were last exposed to antigen 3 or 5 years previously. We also determined the amounts of antibody being produced by cells lavaged from these lung lobes. Significantly more antibody was observed in the lavage fluid from immunized lung lobes, although antibody was also present in serum and lavage fluid from control lung lobes. However, cells producing antibody were found only in the immunized lung lobes. Studies are underway to determine if retention of antigen in the lung is responsible for maintenance of antibody production.

Induction of lung disease by inhaled materials

Immunosuppressive effects

Air contains a large variety of pollutants that are inhaled. In addition, specific toxicants are also inhaled by workers in various occupations. Immunotoxicology experiments have examined the possibility that environmental or occupational inhalation exposures could damage pulmonary defences, leading to increased pulmonary infections and/or lung tumours. Results from these studies indicate that toxic materials deposited in the lung can suppress immune responses in lymph nodes that drain the lung. Studies have evaluated the effects of particulate materials, including pulmonary exposures to carbon [43,44], silica [45,46], fly ash [45], benzo-a-pyrene [2], diesel exhaust [47], cigarette smoke [48–50], and radioactive particles [51,52] on the development of immunity. These studies measured effects on immune responses in the lung-associated lymph nodes, as well as on immunity in distant lymphoid tissues. After either acute or chronic exposures, the immune functions of lung-associated lymph nodes can be suppressed. In some studies, the damaged immune functions of these lymph nodes was permanent [45]. Damage of lung tissues by inhaled toxic gases can also suppress the induction of immunity after lung immunization [53,54].

In contrast to animal studies that frequently use high exposure doses, there are limited data suggesting that the inhalation of environmental pollutants suppresses pulmonary immune defences. The role of environmental exposures in the aetiology of human infectious diseases and cancer is not understood. In addition to an increased incidence of lung cancer, individuals who smoke have an increased number of pulmonary infections [55,56], and there appears to be a higher rate of pulmonary infections in residents of highly polluted cities [57–60]. However, additional data are needed to determine if inhalation of environmental pollutants can significantly suppress pulmonary immunity.

Induction of pulmonary hypersensitivity after inhalation exposure

Although the data supporting the suppression of pulmonary immunity by inhaled environmental or occupational pollutants are limited, the incidence of hypersensitivity lung diseases is relatively common. Hypersensitivity to inhaled materials is by far the most problematic manifestation of inhaled toxicants. In some individuals, these lung immune responses can lead to serious lung disease. Despite the relatively high morbidity and long history of these disorders, much of the pathophysiology remains to be elucidated. Although animal models have been devised to study pulmonary hypersensitivity, there are species differences that have made the extrapolation of data from these studies to human disease difficult. Some of the problems with using animal models to study pulmonary immune responses are discussed below.

Lung diseases induced by inhaled antigens or chemicals can be divided into three general categories. Examples of these diseases include IgE-mediated asthma or rhinitis, hypersensitivity pneumonitis, where cellular immunity, or a combination of cellular and humoral immunity induce disease, and chronic beryllium lung disease induced by cell-mediated immune responses. An important consideration that will be discussed is that in most situations, only a small percentage of the exposed individuals develop responses to these antigens or chemicals that result in disease. General considerations of these hypersensitivity diseases are discussed below.

Occupational asthma, rhinitis. Rhinitis and asthmatic reactions to inhaled environmental allergens are common. In addition to the organic allergens in the environment that lead to atopy in sensitive individuals, inhaled chemicals can also cause asthma (see Chapter 12). Asthma induced by inhaled chemicals is defined as variable airway obstruction causally related to exposure to sensitizing (i.e. not irritating) concentrations of substances present in the environment [61,62]. Sensitizing chemicals are found more frequently in industrial work situations than in the environment. It is estimated that between 50 000 and 100 000 workers in the USA are regularly exposed to diisocyanates at any given time [63]. Chemicals leading to sensitivity are also found as indoor and outdoor pollutants, but not as frequently and usually in lower concentrations than in industry.

Clinically relevant pulmonary responses to inhaled chemicals can be produced by several different mechanisms. The chemical may act as a non-specific irritant, as an allergen causing immediate hypersensitivity, or it may stimulate a non-specific release of pharmacological mediators. In many examples of occupational asthma, the actual mechanisms that cause disease remain to be elucidated.

Many agents leading to occupational asthma are low molecular weight chemicals such as nickel, platinum, palladium, toluene diisocyanate, or trimellitic anhydride [64–66]. However, complex organic molecules including bacterial enzymes used in detergents can also induce occupational asthma [67].

Hypersensitivity pneumonitis. Hypersensitivity pneumonitis is characterized by a spectrum of lymphocytic and granulomatous, interstitial and alveolar-filling pulmonary disorders associated with intense and often prolonged exposure to a wide range of inhaled antigens, and possibly some haptens, that are found in a variety of industries. The number of organic materials that can induce hypersensitivity pneumonitis continues to grow, with disease classification based on the material inhaled. It appears that chronic inhalation of high levels of nearly any organic dust can lead to hypersensitivity pneumonitis [68].

Data indicating that hypersensitivity pneumonitis can be induced by inhaled chemicals are limited. However, it appears that immune responses to proteins altered by chemical binding or immune responses to hapten–protein conjugates may induce hypersensitivity pneumonitis. Toluene diisocyanate, trimellitic anhydride, diphenylmethane diisocyanate and heated epoxy resin are examples of chemicals that may induce hypersensitivity pneumonitis [63,68]. Pulmonary opacities resulting from diisocyanate exposure have been reported [69], and diisocyanate exposure was suspected to be the cause of several cases of hypersensitivity pneumonitis [70]. Additional reports implicate methylene diphenyl diisocyanate and hexamethylene diisocyanate as the cause of reactions similar to hypersensitivity pneumonitis [66,71–75]. One report described the presence of isocyanate-specific IgG antibody in an individual with pulmonary disease similar to hypersensitivity pneumonitis [76].

Histological features in the lungs of individuals with hypersensitivity pneumonitis are compatible with cell-mediated immune reactions. The pathology of the disease is a granulomatous pneumonitis, consisting of patchy infiltration of the bronchiolar and alveolar walls with epithelioid, lymphoid, and giant cells, the latter with characteristic cytoplasmic clefts [77]. Granuloma formation is a feature of cellular immunity, but can also be produced by insoluble antigen-antibody complexes [78] and by particulate antigens [79]. High levels of antigen-specific antibody are usually present and may also be involved in the induction of hypersensitivity pneumonitis. However, the roles of cellular and antibody-mediated immune responses in hypersensitivity pneumonitis is not completely clear [68]. Some data are available indicating that lymphocytes from immune animals can passively transfer sensitivity that results in lung lesions after pulmonary challenge [80–82]. The results of these studies show that immune cells can transfer cellular immunity to the lung. However, the responses produced are transient and may not be representative of immune reactions in the lungs of the few individuals who develop hypersensitivity pneumonitis with lung damage.

Chronic beryllium lung disease. Although asthma and hypersensitivity pneumonitis were recognized centuries ago, the recognition of lung disease caused by inhaled beryllium is more recent. Beryllium disease is a product of the 20th-century arrival of the high technologies of nuclear power, aerospace, and electronics. Beryllium was not produced commercially in the USA until the 1930s [83]; however, numerous cases of disability and death from beryllium poisoning occurred among workers in the fluorescent lamp industry after the introduction of beryllium as a component of phosphors [84]. Because of the difficulties of associating beryllium with lung disease, it was not until 1949 that air standards were set for beryllium; these are essentially unchanged today [85]. For workplace air, an 8-h time-weighted, average maximum permissible level of $2.0\,\mu g/m^3$ was established, along with a peak 30-min level of $25\,\mu g/m^3$. The adoption of adequate standards and hygienic practices to control human exposure to beryllium was delayed by disagreement about the cause of the disease observed in and around the beryllium plants in the 1940s. Although the incidence of exposure has been greatly reduced by these standards, the amount of beryllium produced and used has greatly increased, and new cases of chronic beryllium lung disease continue to be diagnosed.

Two different diseases are produced by inhaled beryllium. Acute beryllium lung disease, a severe chemical pneumonitis, is due directly to the toxicity from the inhalation of relatively high levels of beryllium. In contrast, chronic beryllium lung disease is caused by the induction of immunity to low levels of inhaled beryllium. Only chronic beryllium lung disease and immune responses produced to this chemical will be discussed.

Pollutants and increased incidence of pulmonary hypersensitivity

The possibilities that inhaled pollutants could damage the immune system, or that inhaled antigenic materials could lead to hypersensitivity lung disease, are frequent considerations in pulmonary immunotoxicology studies. However, epidemiological data suggest that the incidence of allergic lung disease (e.g. asthma or rhinitis induced by pollen inhalation) is increasing, as is the number of deaths due to asthmatic responses [86–88]. The factors responsible for this increasing incidence are unknown.

Even though experimental data show that inhaled toxicants can suppress immunity after lung immunization, elevated immune responses are most frequently observed in the lung-associated lymph nodes after immunization of the lungs of animals exposed to a variety of pollutants [2,45,47,53,54]. Whether immune responses to antigens deposited in the lungs of animals exposed to pollutants will be suppressed or elevated appears to be determined by several factors. For example, the dose and toxicity of the material inhaled are important factors. Frequently, suppression is observed only at high doses of highly toxic materials [46,47]. Exposures to lower doses or less toxic pollutants frequently elevate immunity to antigens in the lung [45,47]. In addition, the time of exposure in relation to when antigen is deposited in the lung also seems important. A single acute exposure can either suppress or elevate immunity to antigen deposited in the lung depending on when the animals are immunized in relation to the exposure [2,52,54].

Based on these data and on the results of other studies that have evaluated the effects of environmental pollutants on the induction of hypersensitivity [89,90], it seems possible that inhaled pollutants might be responsible for the observed increased incidence of allergic lung disease to commonly inhaled allergens. Data suggest that children raised in the homes of smokers have a higher incidence of asthma [91]. Additional studies are needed to determine if the inhalation of environmental pollutants elevates the levels of immunity to common allergens, leading to an increased incidence of pulmonary hypersensitivity.

Possible mechanisms—suppression of pulmonary immunity or induction of hypersensitivity

Possible suppression or stimulation of primary immunity by inhaled toxicants

Based on the concepts of pulmonary immunity described above, there are a variety of cells and tissues associated with the lung that could be damaged, or their immune functions altered, by inhaled toxic materials. Listed below are changes induced by inhaled pollutants that could lead to immune suppression or hypersensitivity.

Changes in antigen clearance. Changes in the clearance of antigen from the lung could suppress pulmonary immunity. Damage to the pulmonary epithelial cells (e.g. type I and/or type II) and/or changes in numbers of epithelial cells (e.g. type II cell hyperplasia) could alter the lymphatic clearance of antigens from the lung to the lung-associated lymph nodes [53]. Changes in the numbers and functions of alveolar macrophages and neutrophils that enter the lung could also alter clearance of antigen from the lung [19, 20].

Data are also available to support the possibility that exposure of the lung to toxicants can cause elevated immune responses to antigens deposited in the lung. Experimental inhalation exposure to environmental pollutants increases the level of immune responses in lung-associated lymph nodes after pulmonary immunization, suggesting that exposure increased the clearance of antigen from the lung to these tissues [2,45,47,54]. However, no data are available to determine if exposure to pollutants in the environment increases the clearance of allergens to the lung-associated lymph nodes. An increased clearance of antigen from the lung could explain the observed increase in the rate of allergic lung disease in individuals living in high polluted areas [89,90].

Changes in function of lung-associated lymph nodes. Some inhaled toxic particulates are cleared from the lung to the lung-associated lymph nodes. The accumulation of toxic particles in the lung-associated lymph nodes may alter not only the number and subpopulations of lymphocytes in these tissues but also the functions of these cells [45]. In addition, the numbers and functions of antigen-handling cells in the lung-associated lymph nodes could also be changed. Published data show that inhaled insoluble particles that translocate to the lung-associated lymph nodes remain in these tissues with a long half-life [13]. The retention of toxic particles in the lung-associated lymph nodes may permanently alter the immune functions of these tissues [45].

As discussed above, elevated immune responses could be produced if exposure increases the clearance of antigen from the lung to the lung-associated lymph nodes. However, it is also possible that altered functions of the cells in the lung-associated lymph nodes by inhaled particulates that translocate to these tissues may also cause an increased level of

immunity after pulmonary immunization. The cellularity of the lung-associated lymph nodes is generally increased after exposures to particulate materials, and if antigen is deposited in the lungs of these animals, an elevated immune response is observed [2]. Therefore, inhaled toxicants could cause an increased rate of immunity to commonly inhaled antigens (e.g. allergens) by two mechanisms. The first would be an increased clearance of antigen to the lung-associated lymph nodes, and second would be cellular changes in these tissues that would elevate immune responses to antigens that clear from the lung. However, it must be noted that the concentrations of pollutants used in experimental studies that have provided these data are high in comparison to environmental exposures. Low doses might have no effect on antigen clearance or function of the lung-associated lymph nodes, and it is not known if environmental exposures increase the levels of immune responses in these lymph nodes.

Changes in recruitment of immune cells into the lungs. The mechanisms responsible for recruiting immune cells into the lung are not completely understood. However, our data suggest that changes in vascular permeability are important in the recruitment of lymphoid cells and AFC into the lung [4]. Therefore, the induction of inflammation and/or damage to lung tissues could alter the recruitment of immune cells and antibody from the blood into the lung. There are no data available to determine whether inhalation of environmental pollutants increases the recruitment of immune cells into the human lung.

Changes in antibody production by cells in the lung. Large numbers of AFC are present in lavage fluid from immunized lung lobes [4,17]. Because plasma cells are found in the alveoli and interstitial tissues of the lung [20], these cells are at risk to inhaled pollutants. Damage of these cells could reduce the levels of local antibody production important in pulmonary defences against pathogens.

Although the number of AFC is highest after primary immunization or antigen challenge, we have identified cells producing antibody in immunized lung lobes 3–5 years after the last antigen exposure [42]. The long-term maintenance of AFC in the lung would provide high levels of antibody in the fluids lining the lung. This antibody could be essential to eliminate inhaled pathogens before clinical infection is produced. The location of these cells in the alveoli and interstitial tissues of the lung suggests that inhaled pollutants could disrupt long-term antibody production. There are no experimental or human data that can be used to determine if exposures to environmental pollutants damage immune cells responsible for local production of antibody in the lung.

Possible alteration of secondary antibody responses by inhaled toxicants

Changes in function of immune memory cells in the lung. The long-term production of antibody in the lung should be important in providing immune memory pulmonary defence. In addition cells responsible for long-term antibody production, immune memory cells, are also recruited and/or produced locally after pulmonary immunization [6,7,31]. Our data suggest that these immune memory cells could provide pulmonary immune defence by responding to inhaled or aspirated pathogens. These immune memory cells are found in the interstitial tissues of the lung [7] and the damage of these cells, or pulmonary cells responsible for antigen presentation, could result in a loss of pulmonary immune memory. It seems possible that a loss of immune memory in the lung would increase the incidence of recurrent pulmonary infections.

Induction of pulmonary immunity and hypersensitivity

In the early studies of hypersensitivity, it was assumed that hypersensitivity lung disease would result whenever a pulmonary immune response was induced to antigens that cause hypersensitivity. However, more recent data suggest that exposure to these antigens almost always results in immunity and that these immune responses can be maintained for long times without the development of clinical disease. Only a small percentage of exposed individuals that become immune develop lung disease. The following is a discussion of the induction of pulmo-

nary immunity to antigens that can cause pulmonary disease and, based on the limited data available, of how disease may be produced.

Induction of pulmonary immunity to hypersensitivity antigens or haptens

To induce pulmonary immune responses, the chemicals or organic materials inhaled must be of a respirable size and deposit in the lower respiratory tract [68]. Particles greater than 10 µm generally do not induce pulmonary immunity or hypersensitivity lung disease. Low molecular weight chemicals apparently act as haptens, binding host proteins to form complete antigens that can induce hapten- or carrier-specific antibodies. Some highly reactive chemicals (e.g. isocyanates or anhydrides) may induce the formation of neoantigens that stimulate antibody production [75,92]. Therefore, immune responses to inhaled chemicals may be directed against a broad range of antigen specificities, from haptens to altered host protein neoantigens.

Atopy is a predisposing factor for the development of occupational asthma induced by high molecular weight sensitizers (e.g. enzymes, flour, animal products) [67]. However, no relationship exists between atopy and the induction of lung disease by low molecular weight sensitizers such as toluene diisocyanate, plicatic acid, and trimellitic anhydrides. Other factors that may be important in the initiation of disease include the presence of pre-existing bronchial hyper-reactivity [93–96], altered adrenergic tone [97], recent or concurrent respiratory viral infections [98], or alterations in the integrity of tight junctions of basal membranes [99]. There are no data that can be used to determine if environmental pollutants increase sensitivity to these inhaled antigens. However, smoking does not appear to be a predisposing factor [61,62]. Many of the antigens that cause hypersensitivity pneumonitis have adjuvant properties that may be important in the induction of disease [100], and frequently, chemicals or organic materials also induce inflammation that could increase the chance that an immune response will be produced.

The details of the induction of immunity to these chemicals or antigens are not completely understood. However, it seems likely that a portion of the antigens deposited in the airways or lower respiratory tract are cleared to lung-associated lymph nodes or lymph nodes draining exposed mucosal surfaces. Immune cells produced in these tissues are released into the circulatory system and recruited from blood into the lung or mucosal tissues [14]. It is likely that immune memory cells would also be recruited as observed in experimental studies of pulmonary immunity, and that long-term antibody production would be established. Thus, locally produced antibody and immune cells would be available to respond to future antigen exposures.

Importance of local pulmonary responses in hypersensitivity

The local response (e.g. local production of IgE or recognition of antigen by T lymphocytes) is probably much more important in the induction of pulmonary hypersensitivity disease than is systemic immunity. The local amplification of beryllium-sensitized lymphocytes in the lung, and the activation of these cells by beryllium, leads to a local secretion of lymphokines that could be responsible for the induction of lung granulomas. Although interstitial granulomas are typically found only in the lungs, non-caseating granulomas may also occur in the skin, liver, spleen, lymph nodes, myocardium, skeletal muscles, kidney, bone, and salivary glands [101].

Pulmonary immunity versus hypersensitivity

A complicating fact in understanding the role of immunity in hypersensitivity lung disease is that antibody produced to inhaled antigens can be identified in the blood of most individuals exposed to antigens that can cause hypersensitivity pneumonitis, even though only a small percentage of those exposed develop hypersensitivity pneumonitis. Therefore, the levels of antibody in blood do not correlate with disease [77] and the induction of immunity to inhaled antigens may only indicate that an individual has been exposed. Not only do many individuals exposed to antigens that can cause hypersensitivity pneumonitis have elevated antibody levels with no symptoms, but clinically normal individuals can have significantly elevated numbers

of lymphocytes in their lungs for extended periods of time [102,103]. Although pulmonary hypersensitivity could not be induced in the absence of an immune response, other factors may determine whether or not disease is produced. The observations that there is no correlation between disease and the presence of antibody, the level of cellular immunity, or elevated numbers of lymphocytes in the lung suggest that disorders in the regulation of immunity, rather than the induction of immunity, are responsible for the induction of hypersensitivity pneumonitis. It is also possible that the levels of locally produced antibody in the lung may be more important in the production of disease than levels measured in blood.

Because beryllium ions are too small to be antigenic *per se*, it has been assumed that they must bind to a protein to form a hapten–carrier complex. As indicated above for hypersensitivity pneumonitis and other antigens deposited in the lung, it is likely that the initial immune response to inhaled beryllium occurs in the lung-associated lymph nodes [10,104]. Immune cells produced and released into the blood would likely be recruited into the exposed lung. The local response of these immune cells would amplify the immune response to beryllium retained in the lung [31,105]. This local immune response to beryllium retained in the lung, and the relatively long retention of beryllium, may be important in the development of granulomatous lung disease.

Only a small percentage—approximately 3–4%—of individuals who are exposed to antigens or chemicals that function as haptens that can cause pulmonary hypersensitivity actually become clinically ill. As described above, most individuals exposed to organic antigens become immune. With chemicals such as beryllium, it is possible that this 3–4% represents only those individuals who are genetically capable of recognizing beryllium immunologically. However, it is also possible that greater numbers of individuals exposed to inhaled beryllium develop immunity, but that the immune responses are not measured, because they never become clinically ill. Too little data are available from the examination of individuals exposed to beryllium, but who have no clinical disease, to determine if this possibility is real. The possibility that a larger percentage of exposed individuals may become immune is supported by recent results from animal studies, showing that a larger percentage of animals that inhaled BeO developed immunity to beryllium [104]. Lung lavage fluids from exposed dogs contained 40–70% lymphocytes, and cultures of these cells responded to beryllium in lymphocyte stimulation assays. Histopathology showed that dogs exposed to beryllium had tissue changes characteristic of chronic beryllium lung disease. Although these dogs were immune to beryllium and had histopathology characteristic of chronic beryllium lung disease, they were not clinically ill, and after 12 months the pulmonary lesions had nearly resolved [104]. Therefore, as with hypersensitivity pneumonitis, induction of immunity to beryllium may be less important in the production of permanent pulmonary disease than is regulation of the immune response induced to beryllium.

Species comparisons–pulmonary immunity

Immunity in lung-associated lymph nodes

The concepts of pulmonary immunity presented above are based predominantly on the immune responses observed after lung immunization of dogs and non-human primates. Although there are species differences in the immune responses produced in the lungs of laboratory animals, probably all laboratory animals produce a primary immune response in the lung-associated lymph nodes after pulmonary immunization (Table 7.1). Therefore, it is likely that any animal could be used to evaluate the effects of inhaled toxicants on immune responses in the lung-associated lymph nodes. A number of studies (discussed above) have shown that exposure of the lungs to a variety of pollutants can either suppress or elevate immune responses in the lung-associated lymph nodes. Although it is clear that immune responses in the lung-associated lymph nodes can be altered, the mechanisms responsible for the observed changes are poorly understood.

Lymphocytes and antibody-forming cells in lungs after immunization

The production of immunity in the lung-associated lymph nodes is only the first step leading to immune responses in the lung. In dogs and non-human primates, AFC are released from the lung-associated lymph nodes, and large numbers are found in the blood [4,17,22]. These AFC and other lymphocytes are recruited from the blood mainly into the immunized lung lobe [4,17,22]. Although all species develop immune responses in the lung-associated lymph nodes, resulting in systemic humoral immunity after lung immunization, there are major species differences in the numbers of AFC in blood, and in the numbers of AFC and lymphocytes that enter the lungs after pulmonary immunization (Tables 7.1 and 7.2).

After lung immunization of dogs and non-human primates, a high percentage of the cells in lavage fluid from the lung are lymphocytes (30–50% at 7–12 days after immunization). In addition, large numbers of these cells are actively producing antigen-specific antibody. Although studies involving pulmonary immunization have not been carried out in humans, humans do have large numbers of lymphocytes and AFC in lung lavage fluids [106,107].

In contrast, rodents generally have no increase in the percentage of lymphocytes in lavage fluid after lung immunization, and there is no increase in the number of AFC in the lung (Table 7.2). The reasons for the small number of AFC in the lungs of rodents is apparently because these species have few AFC in the blood, and because inflammation produced in the lung after instillation of antigen does not generally result in the entry of large numbers of lymphocytes into the lung [14]. Of the rodents evaluated, only mice had increased AFC in their lungs after antigen challenge. The numbers were small compared to dogs and non-human primates, and were found only after high doses of antigen, or after antigen challenge of immune mice [108, 109].

Selection of species to study immunotoxicology of inhaled pollutants

As indicated above, the lung-associated lymph nodes are the tissues responsible for the induction of immunity after primary lung immunization of any species. Therefore, any animal species could probably be used to evaluate the effects of inhaled toxicants on the induction of immunity in the lung-associated lymph nodes. However, in the measurement of the effects of inhaled toxicants on the recruitment of immune cells into the lung or on the functions of these cells in the lung, the selection of the animal model becomes more important. Because large numbers of immune cells accumulate in the lungs of non-human primates and dogs, these animals should be used. The immune responses that develop in these animals appear to be most like the responses observed in humans after pulmonary exposure to antigenic materials.

Animal models used to evaluate occupational asthma

The guinea pig has frequently been used to evaluate asthmatic responses to chemicals [110,111] (Chapter 12). Genetically hyper-responsive rats and dogs, ozone-exposed, hyper-responsive dogs and sheep, mice, and rabbit models of late allergic reactions have also been used to study bronchial hyper-responsiveness [112,113]. However, few animals spontaneously develop a response to inhaled antigens that is the same as asthma in humans. Primates may be a good model, because they do develop pulmonary hypersensitivity diseases. Dogs develop IgE-mediated skin disease to allergens [114], and recent publications suggest that injections of ragweed antigen with aluminium hydroxide as an adjuvant, starting within 24 h of birth, may offer a valid model of asthma [115,116]. Therefore, the dog may also provide a good model to study the induction of occupational asthma.

Frequently, the doses of chemicals used in animal studies of occupational asthma are high. The use of high doses that would cause a non-specific release of mediators could result in non-specific asthmatic-like responses, rather than in the induction of asthma by the production of IgE to the chemical being studied. It is usually difficult to measure specific IgE in these animal models [113].

Animal models used to evaluate hypersensitivity pneumonitis

Several animal species have been used to evaluate pulmonary responses to antigens that can cause hypersensitivity pneumonitis [117–121]. Studies carried out with these animal models have provided data concerning the induction of inflammation and immunity by either inhalation or instillation of antigens that can cause hypersensitivity pneumonitis. These data provide useful information concerning the cellular responses to antigen deposited in the lung and the development of pulmonary immunity. However, there is no ideal model of hypersensitivity pneumonitis. Whether animals are immunized systemically by the injection of antigen in adjuvants, and then challenged by lung exposure, or if all exposures are delivered to the lung as aerosols, none of the experimental animals develop hypersensitivity pneumonitis with permanent lung damage, as seen in humans. Rather, the animals appear to develop immune responses that are like those observed in exposed humans who do not develop disease. In other words, when animals are exposed to these antigens, the response produced is the same as observed in approximately 97% of exposed humans. However, there is no animal model that will develop fibrotic lung disease after single or multiple exposures to antigens that can cause hypersensitivity pneumonitis in humans. In fact, after multiple exposures, the accumulation of cells in the lung in response to antigen exposure can disappear [122]. Therefore, it appears that the animal models used to date provide information about the events that occur in normal humans after exposure to these antigens.

Animal models used to evaluate sensitivity to beryllium

Rats and guinea pigs have been used to evaluate the induction of immunity to instilled or inhaled beryllium, as well as the production of pulmonary lesions [123–126]. Different strains of guinea pigs that are either sensitive or non-sensitive for the induction of granulomas after instillation of beryllium have also been used. Some species require the instillation of relatively large doses of beryllium to induce immunity and/or lung lesions [123–125], and in some animals, the histopathology of the lesions produced is not similar to the lesions observed in humans [126].

A recent animal model of beryllium lung disease

in dogs showed that this species develops pulmonary immunity to beryllium and lung lesions that mimic the responses observed in the human lung [104]. As described above, there are significant differences in cellular responses in the lungs of various animals after lung immunization [14]. Because immune responses in the lungs of dogs appear to be the same as those observed in non-human primates, dogs may prove especially useful as a model for evaluating the effects of lung immunity on the development of pulmonary disease. However, a criticism of this model may be the same as that for other animal models used to study the induction of hypersensitivity pneumonitis—that the responses observed may represent the responses of normal individuals who do not develop chronic beryllium lung disease, rather than the responses of an individual who does develop chronic beryllium lung disease.

Acknowledgements

The authors thank the personnel at the Inhalation Toxicology Research Institute for their suggestions and assistance in the preparation of this manuscript. This review is based in part on research performed under Department of Energy Contract No. DE-AC04-76EV01013 and was conducted in facilities fully accredited by the American Association for Accreditation of Laboratory Animal Care.

References

1 Bice DE, Schnizlein CT. Cellular immunity induced by lung immunization of Fischer 344 rats. *Int Arch Allergy Appl Immunol* 1980; 63:438–45.

2 Schnizlein CT, Bice DE, Mitchell CE, Hahn FF. Effects on rat lung immunity by acute lung exposure to benzo(a)pyrene. *Arch Environ Health* 1982; 37:201–6.

3 Stein-Streilein J, Gross GN, Hart DA. Comparison of intratracheal and intravenous inoculation of sheep erythrocytes in the induction of local and systemic immune responses. *Infec Immun* 1979; 24:145–50.

4 Bice DE, Degen MA, Harris DL, Muggenburg BA. Recruitment of antibody-forming cells in the lung after local immunization is nonspecific. *Am Rev Respir Dis* 1982; 126:635–9.

5 Bice DE, Harris DL, Muggenburg BA, Bowen JA. The evaluation of lung immunity in chimpanzees. *Am Rev Respir Dis* 1982; 126:358–9.

6 Mason MJ, Bice DE, Muggenburg BA. Local pulmo-nary immune responsiveness after multiple antigenic exposures in the Cynomolgus monkey. *Am Rev Respir Dis* 1985; 132:657–60.

7 Mason MJ, Gillett NA, Bice DE. Comparison of sytemic and local immune responses after multiple pulmonary antigen exposures. *Regional Immunol* 1989; 2:149–57.

8 Weissman DN, Bice DE, Siegel DW, Schuyler MR. Murine lung immunity to a soluble antigen. *Respir Cell Molec Biol* 1990; 2:327–33.

9 Bice DE, Muggenburg BA. Effect of age on antibody responses after lung immunization. *Am Rev Respir Dis* 1985; 132:661–5.

10 Bice DE, Harris DL, Muggenburg BA. Regional immunologic responses following localized deposition of antigen in the lung. *Exp Lung Res* 1980; 1:33–41.

11 Turner FN, Kaltreider HB. Immunology of the lower respiratory tract. III. Concentrations of antigen and of antibody-forming cells in pulmonary and systemic lymphoid tissues of dogs after intrapulmonary or intravenous administration of sheep erythrocytes. *Clin Exp Immunol* 1978; 33:128–35.

12 Morrow PE. Lymphatic drainage of the lung in dust clearance. *Ann NY Acad Sci* 1972; 200:46–65.

13 Snipes MB, Boecker BB, McClellan RO. Retention of monodisperse or polydisperse aluminosilicate particles inhaled by dogs, rats and mice. *Tox Appl Pharmacol* 1983; 69:345–62.

14 Bice DE, Shopp GM. Antibody responses after lung immunization. *Exp Lung Res* 1988; 14:133–55.

15 Brain JD, Golde DW, Green GM, Massaro DJ, Valberg PA, Ward PA, Werb Z. Biologic potential of pulmonary macrophages. *Am Rev Respir Dis* 1978; 118:435–43.

16 Green GM, Jakab GJ, Low RB, Davis GS. Defense mechanisms of the respiratory membrane. *Am Rev Respir Dis* 1977; 115:479–514.

17 Bice DE, Harris DL, Hill JO, Muggenburg BA, Wolff RK. Immune responses after localized lung immunization in the dog. *Am Rev Respir Dis* 1980; 122:755–60.

18 Cory D, Kulkarni P, Lipscomb M. The migration of bronchoalveolar macrophages into hilar lymph nodes. *Am J Pathol* 1984; 115:321–8.

19 Harmsen AG, Muggenburg BA, Snipes MB, Bice DE. The role of macrophages in particle translocation from lungs to lymph nodes. *Science* 1985; 230:1277–80.

20 Harmsen AG, Mason MJ, Muggenburg BA, Gillett NA, Jarpe MA, Bice DE. Migration of neutrophils from lung to tracheobronchial lymph nodes. *J Leuk Biol* 1987; 41:95–103.

21 Hillam RP, Bice DE, Muggenburg BA. Lung localization of antibody-forming cells stimulated in distant

peripheral lymph nodes. *Immunol* 1985; 55:257–61.

22 Kaltreider HB, Barth E, Pellegrini C. The effect of splenectomy on the appearance of specific antibody-forming cells in lungs of dogs after intravenous immunization with sheep erythrocytes. *Exp Lung Res* 1981; 2:231–8.

23 Brownstein DG, Rebar AH, Bice DE, Muggenburg BA, Hill JO. Immunology in the respiratory tract. Serial morphologic changes in the lungs and tracheo-bronchial lymph nodes of dogs after intrapulmonary immunization with sheep erythrocytes. *Am J Pathol* 1980; 98:499–514.

24 Kaltreider HB, Caldwell JL, Adam E. The fate and consequence of an organic particulate antigen instilled into bronchoalveolar spaces of normal canine lungs. *Am Rev Respir Dis* 1977; 116:267–80.

25 Bice DE, King-Herbert AP, Morris MJ, Hanna N, Haley PJ. Inflammation and recruitment of immune cells into the lung. *Reg Immunol* 1990; 2:376–84.

26 Hill JO, Bice DE, Harris DL, Muggenburg BA. Evaluation of the pulmonary immune response by analysis of bronchoalveolar fluids obtained by serial lung lavage. *Int Arch Allergy Appl Immunol* 1983; 71:173–7.

27 Harmsen AG, Bice DE, Muggenburg BA. The effect of local antibody responses on *in vivo* and *in vitro* phagocytosis by pulmonary alveolar macrophages. *J Leuk Biol* 1985; 37:483–92.

28 Van Der Brugge-Gamelkoorn GJ, Claassen E, Sminia T. Anti-TNP-forming cells in bronchus-associated lymphoid tissue (BALT) and paratracheal lymph node (PTLN) of the rat after intratracheal priming and boosting with TNP-KLH. *Immunol* 1986; 57:405–9.

29 Lipscomb MF, Lyons CR, O'Hara RM, Stein-Streilein J. The antigen-induced selective recruitment of specific T lymphocytes to the lung. *J Immunol* 1982; 128:111–15.

30 Bice DE, Gray RH, Evans MJ, Muggenburg BA. Identification of plasma cells in lung alveoli and interstitial tissues after localized lung immunization. *J Leuk Biol* 1987; 41:1–7.

31 Bice DE, Muggenburg BA. Localized immune memory in the lung. *Am Rev Respir Dis* 1988; 138:565–71.

32 Lipscomb MF, Toews GB, Lyons CR, Uhr JW. Antigen presentation by guinea pig alveolar macrophages. *J Immunol* 1981; 126:286–91.

33 Schuyler MR, Todd LS. Accessory cell function of rabbit alveolar macrophages. *Am Rev Respir Dis* 1981; 123:53–7.

34 Weinberg DS, Unanue ER. Antigen-presenting function of alveolar macrophages: uptake and presentation of *Listeria monocytogenes*. *J Immunol* 1981; 126:794–9.

35 Ansfield MJ, Benson BJ, Kaltreider HB. Immunosup-pression by surface-active material: lack of species specificity. *Am Rev Respir Dis* 1979; 120:949–52.

36 Holt PG. Inhibitory activity of unstimulated alveolar macrophages on T-lymphocyte blastogenic response. *Am Rev Respir Dis* 1978; 118:791–3.

37 Demenkoff JH, Ansfield MJ, Kaltreider HB, Adam E. Alveolar macrophage suppression of canine broncho-alveolar lymphocytes: the role of prostaglandin E_2 in the inhibition of mitogen-responses. *J Immunol* 1980; 124:1365–70.

38 Lawrence EC, Theodore BJ, Martin RR. Modulation of pokeweed-mitogen-induced immunoglobulin secretion by human bronchoalveolar cells. *Am Rev Respir Dis* 1982; 126:248–52.

39 Pennline KJ, Herscowitz HB. Dual role for alveolar macrophages in humoral and cell-mediated immune responses: evidence for suppressor and enhancing functions. *J Reticuloendothel Soc* 1981; 30:205–17.

40 Sitrin RG, Ansfield MJ, Kaltreider HB. The effect of pulmonary surface-active material on the generation and expression of murine B- and T-lymphocyte effector functions *in vitro*. *Exp Lung Res* 1985; 9:85–97.

41 Nicod LP, Lipscomb MF, Weissler JC, Lyons CR, Albertson J, Toews GB. Characterization of a potent accessory cell not obtained by bronchoalveolar lavage. *Am Rev Respir Dis* 1987; 136:818–23.

42 Bice DE, Muggenburg BA. Long-term maintenance of localized antibody immunity in the lung. *Am Rev Respir Dis* 1989; 139:A455.

43 Miller SD, Zarkower A. Effects of carbon dust inhalation on the cell-mediated immune response in mice. *Infect Immun* 1974; 9:534–9.

44 Zarkower A. Alterations in antibody response induced by chronic inhalation of SO_2 and carbon. *Arch Environ Hlth* 1972; 25:45–50.

45 Bice DE, Hahn FF, Benson J, Carpenter RL, Hobbs CH. Comparative lung immunotoxicity of inhaled quartz and coal combustion fly ash. *Environ Res* 1987; 43:374–89.

46 Miller SD, Zarkower A. Silica-induced alterations of murine lymphocyte immunocompetence and suppression of B lymphocyte immunocompetence: a possible mechanism. *J Reticuloendothel Soc* 1976; 19:47–61.

47 Bice DE, Mauderly JL, Jones RK, McClellan RO. Effects of inhaled diesel exhaust on immune responses after lung immunization. *Fund Appl Toxicol* 1985; 5:1075–86.

48 Sopori ML, Cherian S, Chilukuri R, Shopp GM. Cigarette smoke causes inhibition of the immune response to intratracheally administered antigens. *Toxicol Appl Pharmacol* 1989; 97:489–99.

49 Thomas WR, Holt PG, Keast D. Recovery of immune system after cigarette smoking. *Nature* 1974; 248:358–9.

50 Thomas WR, Holt PG, Keast D. Development of alterations in the primary immune response of mice by exposure to fresh cigarette smoke. *Int Arch Allergy* 1974; 46:481–6.

51 Bice DE, Harris DL, Schnizlein CT, Mauderly JL. Methods to evaluate the effects of toxic materials deposited in the lung on immunity in lung-associated lymph nodes. *Drug Chem Toxicol* 1979; 2:35–47.

52 Galvin JB, Bice DE, Guilmette RA, Muggenburg BA, Haley PJ. Pulmonary immune response of dogs after exposure to ^{239}PuO$_2$. *Int J Rad Biol* 1989; 55:285–96.

53 Hillam RP, Bice DE, Hahn FF, Schnizlein CT. Effects of acute nitrogen dioxide exposure on cellular immunity after lung immunization. *Environ Res* 1983; 31:201–11.

54 Schnizlein CT, Bice DE, Rebar AH, Wolff RK, Beethe RL. Effect of lung damage by acute exposure to nitrogen dioxide on lung immunity in the rat. *Environ Res* 1980; 23; 362–70.

55 Finklea JF, Hasselbald V, Riggan WB, Nelson WC, Hammer EI, Newill VA. Cigarette smoking and hemagglutination inhibition response to influenza after natural disease and immunization. *Am Rev Respir Dis* 1971; 104:368–76.

56 Finklea JF, Sandifer SH, Peck FB, Manos JP. A clinical and serologic comparison of standard and purified bivalent inactivated influenza vaccines. *J Inf Dis* 1969; 120:708–19.

57 Bouhuys A, Beck GJ, Schoenberg JB. Do present levels of air pollution outdoors affect respiratory health? *Nature* 1978; 276:466–71.

58 Green GM. Air pollution, host immune defenses, and asthma; a review. In: Findel AJ, Duel WC, eds. *Clinical Implications of Air Pollution Research.* Acton, MA: Publishing Sciences, 1974:147–63.

59 Levy D, Gent M, Newhouse MT. Relationship between acute respiratory illness and air pollution levels in an industrial city. *Am Rev Respir Dis* 1977; 116:167–73.

60 Lloyd OL. Respiratory-cancer clustering associated with localized industrial air pollution. *Lancet* 1978; i:318–20.

61 Chan-Yeung M, Lam S. Occupational asthma. *Am Rev Respir Dis* 1986; 133:686–703.

62 Cotes JE, Steel J. Occupational asthma. In: *Work-Related Lung Disorders.* Oxford: Blackwell Scientific Publications, 1987:345–72.

63 Musk AW, Peters JM, Wegman DH. Isocyanates and respiratory disease: current status. *Am J Indust Med* 1988; 13:331–49.

64 McConnell LH, Fink JN, Schlueter DP, Schmidt MG. Asthma caused by nickel sensitivity. *Ann Intern Med* 1973; 78:888–90.

65 Pepys J, Pickering CA, Hughes EG. Asthma due to inhaled chemical agents—complex salts of platinum. *Clin Allergy* 1972; 2:391–6.

66 Zeiss CR, Patterson R, Pruzansky JJ, Miller MM, Rosenberg M, Levitz D. Trimellitic anhydride-induced airway syndromes: clinical and immunologic studies. *J Allergy Clin Immunol* 1977; 60:96–103.

67 Newhouse ML. Tagg B, Pockock SJ, McEwan AC. An epidemiological study of workers producing enzyme washing powders. Lancet 1970; i:689–93.

68 Salvaggio JE. Hypersensitivity pneumonitis. *J Allergy Clin Immunol* 1987; 79:558–71.

69 Blake BL, Mackay JB, Rainey HB, Weston WJ. Pulmonary opacities resulting from diisocyanate exposure. *J Coll Rad Aust* 1965; 9:45–8.

70 Charles J, Berstein A, Jones B, Jones DJ, Edwards JH, Seal RME, Seaton A. Hypersensitivity pneumonitis after exposure to isocyanates. *Thorax* 1976; 31:127–36.

71 Baur X, Dewair M, Rommelt H. Acute airway obstruction followed by hypersensitivity pneumonitis in an isocyanate (MDI) worker. *J Occup Med* 1984; 26:285–7.

72 Fink JN, Schlueter DP. Bathtub refinisher's lung: an unusual response to toluene diisocyanate. *Am Rev Respir Dis* 1978; 118:955–9.

73 Malo JL, Ouimet G, Cartier A, Levitz D, Zeiss CR. Combined alveolitis and asthma due to hexamethylene diisocyanate (HDI), with demonstration of crossed respiratory and immunologic reactivities to diphenylmethane diisocyanate (MDI). *J Allergy Clin Immunol* 1983; 72:413–19.

74 Malo JL, Zeiss CR. Occupational hypersensitivity pneumonitis after exposure to diphenylmethane diisocyanate. *Am Rev Respir Dis* 1982; 125:113–16.

75 Zeiss CR, Kanellakes TM, Bellone JD, Levitz D, Pruzansky JJ, Patterson R. Immunoglobulin E-mediated asthma and hypersensitivity pneumonitis with precipitating anti-hapten antibodies due to diphenylmethane diisocyanate (MDI) exposure. *J Allergy Clin Immunol* 1980; 65:346–52.

76 Le Quesne PM, Axford AT, McKerrow CB, Jones AP. Neurological complications after a single severe exposure to toluene di-isocyanate. *Br J Ind Med* 1976; 33:72–8.

77 Pepys J. Occupational allergic lung disease caused by organic agents. *J Allergy Clin Immunol* 1986; 78:1058–62.

78 Spector WG, Heesom N. The production of granulomata by antigen-antibody complexes. *J Pathol* 1969; 98:31–9.

79 Boros DL, Warren KS. The bentonite granuloma. Characterization of a model system for infection and foreign body granulomatous infiltration using soluble mycobacterial, histoplasma and schistosoma antigens.

Immunol 1973; 24:511–29.

80 Bice DE, Salvaggio JE, Hoffman E. Passive transfer of experimental hypersensitivity pneumonitis with lymphoid cells in the rabbit. *J Allergy Clin Immunol* 1976; 58:250–62.

81 Schuyler M, Cook D, Listrom M, Fengolio-Preiser C. Blast cells transfer experimental hypersensitivity pneumonitis in guinea pigs. *Am Rev Respir Dis* 1988; 137:1449–55.

82 Schuyler M, Subramanyan S, Hassan M. Experimental hypersensitivity pneumonitis: transfer with cultured cells. *J Lab Clin Med* 1987; 109:623–30.

83 Drury JS, Shriner CR, Lewis EB, Towill LE, Hammons AS. *Reviews of the Environmental Effects of Pollutants: VI. Beryllium.* Cincinnatti: USEPA, Health Effects Research Laboratory (NTIS no. EPA-600/1-78-028), 1978.

84 Hardy H. Beryllium disease: a clinical perspective. *Environ Res* 1980; 21:1–9.

85 Eisenbud M. Origins of the standards for control of beryllium disease (1947–1949). *Environ Res* 1982; 27:79–88.

86 EPA. *Air Quality Criteria for Ozone and Other Photochemical Oxidants.* vol. V. EPA-600/8-84-020A. Research Triangle Park, NC 27711: Environmental Criteria and Assessment Office, 1984.

87 Menzel DB. Ozone: an overview of its toxicity in man and animals. *J Tox Environ Hlth* 1984; 13:183–204.

88 National Center for Health Statistics. *Current Estimates from the National Health Interview Survey.* United States, series 10, no. 173. 1989. Rockville: DHEW Publications.

89 Osebold JE, Gershwin IF, Lee YC. Studies on the enhancement of allergic lung sensitization by inhalation of ozone and sulfuric acid aerosol. *J Environ Pathol Toxicol* 1980; 3:221–34.

90 Riedel F, Kramer M, Scheibenbogen C. Effects of SO_2 exposure on allergic sensitization in the guinea pig. *J Allergy Clin Immunol* 1988; 82:527–34.

91 Tager IB. Health effects of "passive smoking" in children. *Chest* 1989; 96:1161–4.

92 Butcher BT, Mapp C, Reed MA, O'Neill CE, Salvaggio JE. Evidence for carrier specificity of IgE antibodies detected by isocyanate-protein conjugates in sera of isocyanate sensitive individuals. *J Allergy Clin Immunol* 1982; 69 (suppl):123.

93 Butcher BT, O'Neil CE, Reed MA, Salvaggio JE, Weill H. Development and loss of toluene diisocyanate reactivity: immunologic, pharmacologic, and provocative challenge studies. *Allergy Clin Immunol* 1982; 70:231–5.

94 Lam S, Wong R, Yeung M. Nonspecific bronchial reactivity in occupational asthma. *J Allergy Clin Immunol* 1979; 63:28–34.

95 O'Brien IM, Newman-Taylor AJ, Burge PS, Harries JG, Fawcett IW, Pepys J. Toluene di-isocyanate-induced asthma II. Inhalation challenge tests and bronchial reactivity studies. *Clin Allergy* 1979; 9:7–15.

96 Van Ert M, Battigelli MC. Mechanism of respiratory injury by TDI (toluene diisocyanate). *Ann Allergy* 1975; 35:142–7.

97 Szentivanyi A. The beta adrenergic theory of the atopic abnormality in bronchial asthma. *J Allergy Clin Immunol* 1968; 42:203–32.

98 Empey DW, Laitinen LA, Jacobs L, Gold WM, Nadel JA. Mechanisms of bronchial hyperreactivity in normal subjects after respiratory tract infection. *Am Rev Respir Dis* 1976; 113:131–9.

99 McFadden ER. Pathogenesis of asthma. *J Allergy Clin Immunol* 1984; 73:413–24.

100 Bice DE, McKarron K, Hoffman EO, Salvaggio JE. Adjuvant properties of *Micropolyspora faeni. Int Arch Allergy Appl Immunol* 1977; 55:267–74.

101 Freiman DG, Hardy HL. Beryllium disease: the relation of pulmonary pathology to clinical course and prognosis based on a study of 130 cases from the US beryllium case registry. *Hum Pathol* 1970; 1:25–44.

102 Cormier Y, Belanger J, Beaudoin J, Laviolette M, Beaudoin R, Hebert J. Abnormal bronchoalveolar lavage in asymptomatic dairy farmers. *Am Rev Respir Dis* 1984; 130:1046–9.

103 Cormier Y, Belanger J, Laviolette M. Persistent bronchoalveolar lymphocytosis in asymptomatic farmers. *Am Rev Respir Dis* 1986; 133:843–7.

104 Haley PJ, Finch GL, Mewhinney JA, Harmsen AG, Hahn FF, Hoover MD, Bice DE. A canine model of beryllium-induced granulomatous lung disease. *Lab Invest* 1989; 61:219–27.

105 Rossman MD, Kern JA, Elias JA, Cullen MR, Epstein PE, Preuss OP, Markham TN, Daniele RP. Proliferative response of bronchoalveolar lymphocytes to beryllium. A test for chronic beryllium disease. *Ann Intern Med* 1988; 108:687–93.

106 Rankin JA, Naegel GP, Schrader CE, Matthay RA, Reynolds HY. Air-space immunoglobulin production and levels in bronchoalveolar lavage fluid of normal subjects and patients with sarcoidosis. *Am Rev Respir Dis* 1983; 127:442–8.

107 Rankin JA, Walzer PD, Dwyer JM, Schrader CE, Enriquez RE, Matthay RA. Immunologic alterations in bronchoalveolar lavage fluid in the acquired immunodeficiency syndrome (AIDS). *Am Rev Respir Dis* 1983; 128:189–94.

108 Kaltreider HB, Byrd PK, Daugherty TW, Shalaby MR. The mechanism of appearance of specific antibody-forming cells in lungs of inbred mice after intratracheal immunization with sheep erythrocytes. *Am Rev*

Respir Dis 1983; 127:316–21.

109 McLeod E, Caldwell JL, Kaltreider HB. Pulmonary immune responses of inbred mice. Appearance of antibody-forming cells in C57BL/6 mice after intrapulmonary or systemic immunization with sheep erythrocytes. *Am Rev Respir Dis* 1987; 118:561–71.

110 Karol MH, Hauth BA, Riley EJ, Magreni CM. Dermal contact with toluene diisocyanate (TDI) produces respiratory tract hypersensitivity in guinea pigs. *Tox Appl Pharmacol* 1981; 58:221–30.

111 Karol MH. Concentration-dependent immunologic response to toluene diisocyanate (TDI) following inhalation exposure. *Tox Appl Pharmacol* 1983; 68:229–41.

112 Tse CST, Chen SE, Bernstein IL. Induction of murine reaginic antibodies by toluene diisocyanate. An animal model of immediate hypersensitivity reactions to isocyanates. *Am Rev Respir Dis* 1979; 120:829–35.

113 Woolcock AJ. Asthma—what are the important experiments? *Am Rev Respir Dis* 1988; 138:730–44.

114 Kleinbeck ML, Hites MJ, Loker JL, Halliwell RE, Lee KW. Enzyme-linked immunosorbent assay for measurement of allergen-specific IgE antibodies in canine serum. *Am J Vet Res* 1989; 50:1831–9.

115 Kepron W, James JM, Kirk B, Sehon AH, Tse KS. A canine model for reaginic hypersensitivity and allergic bronchoconstriction. *J Allergy Clin Immunol* 1977; 59:64–9.

116 Becker AB, Hershkovich J, Simons FER, Simons KJ, Lilley MK, Kepron MW. Development of chronic airway hyperresponsiveness in ragweed-sensitized dogs. *J Appl Physiol* 1989; 66:2691–7.

117 Kawai T, Salvaggio J, Lake W, Harris JO. Experimental production of hypersensitivity pneumonitis with bagasse and thermophilic actinomycete antigen. *J Allergy Clin Immunol* 1972; 50:276–88.

118 Keller RH, Calvanico NJ, Stevens JO. Hypersensitivity pneumonitis in nonhuman primates. I. Studies on the relationship of immunoregulation and disease activity. *J Immunol* 1982; 128:116–22.

119 LeFever AV, Abramoff P. Pulmonary immune effector cells: II. Antigen-specific blastogenic responsiveness of lymphocyte populations during pulmonary immune complex disease. *Exp Lung Res* 1984; 7:23–39.

120 Peterson LB, Braley JF, Calvanico NJ, Moore VL. An animal model of hypersensitivity pneumonitis in rabbits. Development of chronic pulmonary inflammation and cell-mediated hypersensitivity after repeated aerosol challenge. *Am Rev Respir Dis* 1979; 119:991–9.

121 Richerson HB, Seidenfeld JJ, Ratajczak HV, Richards DW. Chronic experimental interstitial pneumonitis in the rabbit. *Am Rev Respir Dis* 1978; 117:5–13.

122 Butler JE, Swanson PA, Richerson HB, Ratajczak HV, Richards DW, Suelzer MT. The local and systemic IgA and IgG antibody responses of rabbits to soluble inhaled antigen. *Am Rev Respir Dis* 1982; 126:80–5.

123 Barna BP, Chiang T, Pillarisetti SG, Deodhar SD. Immunologic studies of experimental beryllium lung disease in the guinea pig. *Clin Immunol Immunopathol* 1981; 20:402–11.

124 Barna BP, Deodhar SD, Chiang T, Gautam S, Edinger M. Experimental beryllium-induced lung disease. I. Differences in immunologic response to beryllium compounds in strains 2 and 13 guinea pigs. *Int Arch Allergy Appl Immunol* 1984; 73:42–8.

125 Barna BP, Deodhar SD, Gautam S, Edinger M, Chiang T, McMahon JT. Experimental beryllium-induced lung disease. II. Analysis of bronchial lavage cells in strains 2 and 13 guinea pigs. *Int Arch Allergy Appl Immunol* 1984; 73:49–55.

126 Schepers GWH, Durkan TM, Delahant AB, Creedon FT. The biological action of inhaled beryllium sulfate. A preliminary chronic toxicity study on rats. *Arch Ind Hlth* 1957; 15:32–58.

8
Intolerance and allergic reactions to food components and additives

STEPHEN NICKLIN

Introduction

An expanding literature catalogues our increasing awareness of food intolerance. Early sceptics now accept food allergy and intolerance as a real phenomenon and what appeared to clinicians 50 years ago to be the work of the devil has gained scientific credibility. Over the last decade in particular the diverse spectrum of food-associated disorders has been more precisely characterized, problems of terminology have been resolved and the importance of pseudoallergic reactions is increasingly appreciated.

Historical perspective

Intolerance to foods and dietary constituents is a well established and long recognized phenomenon. Reactions clearly associated with food intake were known to the Greeks and Hippocrates [1] was one of the first to recognize that cow's milk could cause gastric upset and urticaria in susceptible individuals. Later Galen [2] described a child who developed similar allergic symptoms following the ingestion of goat's milk. However, despite this early appreciation of food intolerance the first reports of systematic studies into food intolerance did not appear in the literature until the early part of the 20th century when the more severe symptoms of anaphylactic allergy were linked with the ingestion of particular foods. In 1912 Schloss [3] reported that a child who presented adverse reactions following the ingestion of certain foods gave a positive skin reaction when aqueous extracts from these foods were applied to traumatized skin. At about the same time Talbot [4] in the USA reported that certain children with asthma produced by so-called egg poisoning also gave positive skin reactions following dermal challenge with egg extract. Park in 1920 [5] went on to demonstrate that an elimination diet which precluded cow's milk effectively controlled shock reactions in a milk-sensitive child. Since similar reactions could be induced and elicited in experimentally sensitized animals it was postulated that food intolerance was probably an immunologically specific disorder [4,5]. Further supportive evidence for an immune aetiology for food intolerance was provided by the pioneering studies of Prausnitz and Kustner [6] who demonstrated that the factor responsible for sensitivity to fish, now known to be antigen-specific immunoglobulin E (IgE), was present in the serum of the fish-sensitive individual.

Following these early studies the reports of intolerance to various foods and dietary components increased, as did the range of symptoms attributed to food intolerance. Today symptoms characteristic of food intolerance have been claimed to occur in susceptible individuals following the ingestion of not only novel foods but also various food additives used to colour, flavour or preserve our foods. The reported reactions mirror symptoms caused by classical food allergy and include intestinal discomfort, vomiting, diarrhoea or both and are often associated with non-alimentary responses including urticaria, angioedema, erythema and respiratory problems. Other symptoms so vague as to be almost impossible to define include nausea, lassitude, anxiety, migraine headaches and hyperactivity and irritability in children (Table 8.1). This broadening spectrum of diverse clinical symptoms, the lack of clear cause and effect, and a defined dose–response relationship have gradually led to the realization that food intolerance is a multifaceted syndrome caused by a number of different agencies acting via various reaction pathways. Unfortunately, although the symptoms of food intolerance are fairly well recognized the mechanisms which elicit these reactions remain elusive.

Table 8.1 Symptoms believed to be associated with food intolerance

Gastrointestinal	Respiratory
Pain	Laryngeal oedema
Colic	Rhinitis
Distension	Asthma
Nausea	Otitis media
Vomiting	Apnoea
Diarrhoea	Rhinorrhoea
Steatorrhoea	
Cutaneous	Other symptoms
Erythema	Anaphylaxis
Pruritis	Hypertension
Eczema	Migraine headache
Atopic dermatitis	Hyperactivity
Urticaria	Joint pains
Angioedema	Malaise

Terminology

In popular language any adverse or untoward reaction to a particular substance is commonly referred to as an allergy. Unfortunately this general usage is scientifically incorrect and, as will be seen below, the majority of food reactions have no true allergic basis. Much of this confusion arises from inappropriate or inaccurate nomenclature. Over the years both clinical descriptions and lay terms used for the classification of intolerance reactions have varied widely and the precise terminology as currently used by allergologists and immunologists is often not synonymous with that used by clinicians and general public. In an attempt to avoid this confusion, food intolerance is taken in this chapter to mean all non-psychologically based adverse or unpleasant reactions initiated following the ingestion of a specific food or food component. The reactions are reproducible and may be elicited following blind challenge. The term encompasses both immune and non-immune (pseudoallergic) reactions. Immunological reactions require by definition that the sensitive individual has been previously exposed to a particular food antigen and that this encounter has resulted in antigen-specific recognition. Pseudoallergic reactions on the other hand require no previous encounter and are the result of natural or added chemicals that produce an effect akin to that of a drug or biologically active agent.

This chapter sets out to highlight the existing but often separate areas of knowledge pertaining to food intolerance. It does not attempt to create a single model of food intolerance *per se* but rather sets out to explore the underlying nature of the problem so that limitations as well as the utility of our present knowledge may be better appreciated and communicated to the non-allergologist. The chapter essentially divides into two sections. The first deals with immune recognition of dietary constituents; the second is concerned with pseudoallergic processes. Food intolerance encompasses both processes.

Immunological processing of dietary antigen

Virtually all food constituents including additives, drugs and environmental contaminants can, under appropriate conditions, act as antigens. The host response to ingested components is, therefore, central to our understanding of the mechanisms governing the induction and regulation of the food-allergic condition. It is clearly not feasible within the confines of this text to give a full account of all the processes associated with normal gastrointestinal immune reactivity. The following sections are therefore designed to present a general overview of the relevant features of the gastrointestinal immune system, focusing in particular on antigen uptake, processing and immunoregulation. The reader is, however, directed to more specialized sources of information as and where appropriate.

Intestinal barrier

The epithelial lining of the gastrointestinal tract provides in extensive surface area for the absorption of digested food components necessary for the nutritional well-being of the organism, yet it simultaneously presents a barrier to a vast number of itinerant micro-organisms, exogenous antigens and toxins that continuously pass through the gastrointestinal tract as part of the daily dietary intake. Food undoubtedly represents the largest antigenic load confronting the immune system. Indeed, it has been estimated that approximately 100 tons of food passes through the human gastrointestinal tract during an average lifespan [7]. Whilst the bulk of undigested material is quantitatively excluded, small but immunologically significant quantities of dietary antigen (including food additives) continuously enter the body tissues. Accordingly, the gut has evolved a gut-associated lymphoid tissue (GALT) both to generate immune effector functions and to monitor and regulate antigen uptake [8].

Antigen uptake

The free or uncontrolled entry of intestinal antigen into the GALT is of course a rare event. Nevertheless, controlled antigen sampling of lumenal contents is a well documented occurrence (see [9] for further information). Qualitatively, the most important route of entry for intestinal antigen appears to be via the specialized epithelium cells overlying the Peyer's patches. These structures are macroscopic aggrega-

tions of lymphoid tissue located immediately beneath the epithelium of the small intestine. Ultrastructurally Peyer's patches present a villus-free single layered epithelium, overlying a dense lymphoid core. The unique feature of the epithelium is the presence of specialized columnar epithelial cells [9]. These cells have the capacity to sample small quantities of material from the gut lumen and direct this material to the cells of the lymphoid core below. The mesenteric lymph nodes receive and filter the cells and lymph collected in the wall of the intestine and conveyed to them by the afferent lymphatics. As these nodes lie downstream of both the lamina propria and the Peyer's patches, small lymphocytes, immunoblasts and macrophages are conveyed in significant numbers to this extra-intestinal site [10].

Only in the case of injury or pathological changes could macromolecules enter the tissues directly although, of course, small molecules such as haptens and metabolites may be absorbed directly into the portal circulation. Non-specific uptake does nevertheless occur and is facilitated by a damaged or inflamed gut [11], alcohol [12], various drugs, including cytostatics [13], as well as a range of naturally occurring plant-derived toxins (see the section on pseudoallergic reactions, below). The clinical significance of these processes as they relate to intestinal immunity and disease is of course difficult to evaluate because, associated with local damage, the intercurrent protective capacity of both the local and systemic immune system must also be considered.

Immunoregulation

As outlined above, antigen sampling of a variety of soluble and particulate antigens is a well recognized phenomenon. The process occurs continuously and appears to be a prerequisite for the initiation of both intestinal antibody production [14] and, perhaps more importantly, the induction of systemic antigen-specific immune tolerance [15]. This state of tolerance involves a number of mechanisms, the most important of which stem from the generation of antigen-specific suppressor/contrasuppressor cells. These lymphocytes block the initiation/elicitation of hypersensitivity reactions and help maintain a status quo within the intestinal environment. The fact that oral immunization may lead to the simultaneous induction of a local secretory antibody response on the one hand and systemic tolerance on the other suggests that the primary function of the regulatory mechanisms is to facilitate protective immunity at the level of the gastrointestinal tract, yet block or at least precisely control the initiation of potentially damaging systemic reactions against intestinal antigen that may gain access to body tissues either via an inappropriate route or in a form likely to initiate an adverse reaction [15]. Although oral tolerance induction appears to be a most efficient mechanism—an ability endorsed by the comparative rarity of food allergy in the population as a whole—such regulatory mechanisms can none the less be circumvented and, as indicated, the gut is often the initiation point for a spectrum of hypersensitivity reactions.

Immunologically mediated reactions to foods and food constituents

Allergic reactions are designated types I–IV, on the basis of the underlying immunological mechanism (discussed in Chapters 7 and 12). Although such a classification remains universally accepted it is important to note that the reactions seldom occur in isolation from each other and in many instances responses are mixed. The essential basis of these reactions and their role in food allergic reactions are considered below.

Hypersensitivity reactions

Type I hypersensitivity reaction. When immune recognition of antigen results in the formation of antigen-specific cytophilic IgE antibodies, these bind to and specifically sensitize mast cells and circulating basophils [16]. Whereas traditionally the mast cells have been considered as a single entity, it is now apparent that the mast cell population is in fact quite heterogeneous and composed of a number of distinct subtypes (reviewed in [17]). To date the best characterized of these subsets are the rat and mouse mucosal mast cells (MMC) found within the intestinal lamina propria and the connective tissue mast cells (CTMC) distributed within the skin, lung, peritoneal cavity and other tissue sites. In addition

to their location and distinct staining profiles, the MMC and CTMC also differ with respect to function, morphology and biochemistry (Table 8.2). Immunologically however one of the most striking differences in these cell types is the fact that the MMC expand during T-cell-dependent responses to parasite infection and allergens. This is in marked contrast to CTMC which exhibit no T-cell dependence, being found in equal numbers in both athymic and normal animals. In addition to their considerable role in IgE-mediated hypersensitivity, mast cells are also now known to be involved in the late-phase components of both type 3 and 4 reactions (see below) and in the leukotriene regulation of immunity in general [16]. The pluripotent capacity of mast cells stems from their ability to discharge a wide range of highly potent mediators in response to both specific (IgE) and/or non-specific stimuli (see the section on pseudoallergic reactions, below).

As described in Chapter 5, mast cells, depending on type, contain a wide variety of pharmacologically and biologically active mediators including histamine, serotonin, proteoglycans, various proteins and hydrolases as well as neutrophil and eosinophil chemotactic factors [17]. Histamine and the associated vasoactive amines act on local blood vessels to increase their permeability and other preformed mediators such as proteases destabilize the intracellular junctions between gut enterocytes, allowing further ingress of antigen [18–20]. Mast cell activation also releases arachidonic acid from membrane-

Table 8.2 Mast cell characteristics

Marker	Mucosal mast cell	Connective tissue mast cell
Alcian blue	+ ve	+ ve
Saffron	–ve	+ ve
Berberine sulphate	–ve	+ ve
Granule structure	Variable density	Uniformly dense
Major proteoglycan	Chondroitin	Heparin
Histamine content	+	+ + +
Serotonin content	+	±
PGD2/LTC4 ratio	1:25	40:1
T-cell dependent	Yes	No
High affinity IgE(rec)	Yes	Yes
Sensitivity of SCG	No	Yes

SCG, sodium cromoglycate.

bound phospholipids. As a consequence prostaglandins are synthesized via the cyclo-oxygenase pathway and leukotrienes via the 5-lipoxygenase pathway. These highly potent mediators possess varied regulatory and pro-inflammatory activities which modulate vascular permeability, cause smooth muscle contraction and attract and activate neutrophils and phagocytes [21] (Fig. 8.1). Local effects may in addition induce a general 'leakiness' in the gut, favouring the absorption of bystander antigens [22,23]. In this way, hypersensitivity to a particular component may lead to the ingress of unrelated antigens and immune recognition of a progressively expanding repertoire of ingested antigenic materials.

Type II hypersensitivity. Although type II reactions do not appear to play a major role in food allergy, antibodies against various food protein antigens are associated with a range of inflammatory diseases. However, as similar antibodies are also seen in a proportion of normal controls, their pathogenic significance in the aetiology of the disease process remains open to speculation [24]. Nevertheless, the existence of dietary-specific antibodies, regardless of their specificity, isotype or amount must be considered as significant and indicative of immune recognition. The presence of such antibodies within the circulation clearly raises questions concerning the possible role of type III immune complex-mediated reactions both in inflammatory bowel disease and in food allergy in general.

Type III hypersensitivity. The manifestations of classical type III hypersensitivity, also referred to as immune complex-mediated hypersensitivity, stems from the combination of free antigen with circulating antibody and the subsequent deposition of immune complexes (microprecipitates) in and around small blood vessels. This deposition initiates platelet agglutination, activates the complement cascade and triggers tissue-damaging inflammatory processes. As described above, C3a and C5a, byproducts of complement activation, have anaphylactoid properties and facilitate mast cell activation.

Normal individuals form immune complexes containing food antigen and antigen-specific IgA or IgG which appear easily and effectively removed from the circulation. In contrast, it has been demonstrated that food-allergic individuals not only have higher circulating levels of anti-food antibodies but the immune complexes that are formed are both qualitatively and quantitatively different from non-allergic counterparts [25]. Circulating immune complexes containing specific food antigens have been demonstrated in patients with IgA deficiency [26] and in patients with cow's milk allergy [25]. Tissue deposits of milk-specific antigens, complement and both IgG and IgM antibodies have also been demonstrated in a variety of milk-intolerant individuals [27].

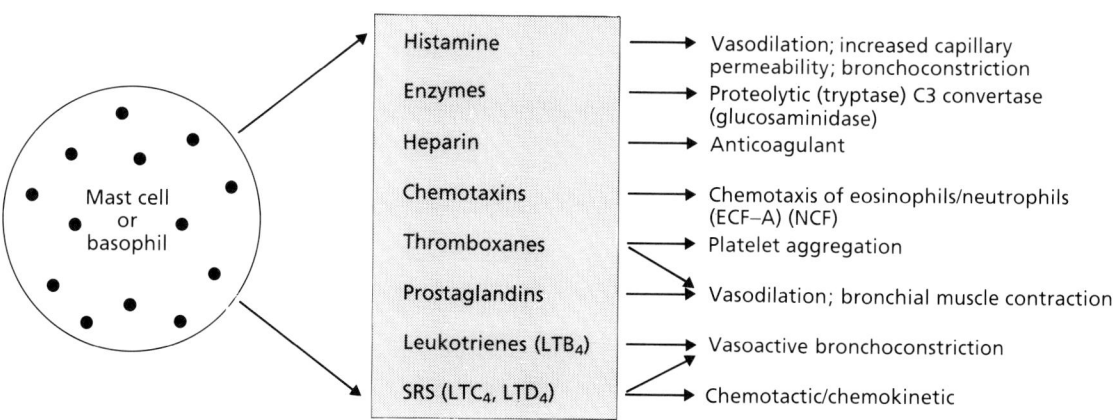

Fig. 8.1 Products and consequences of mast cell or basophil activation.

Whereas it is most likely that type III reactions clearly have some role to play in food-allergic reaction, precise mechanisms need to be determined. Diagnosis of type III reactivity is difficult. The demonstration of circulating anti-food antibodies is only of value if they are significantly elevated; unfortunately, as such antibodies are present in normal individuals there is no consensus of opinion as to what should be considered normal.

Type IV hypersensitivity. It is now apparent that type IV reactions play a role in a number of disease processes, including food allergy. Increased numbers of intra-epithelial lymphocytes have thus been reported in the intestine of individuals suffering cow's milk intolerance [28,29] and peripheral blood lymphocytes from such individuals also respond to milk proteins *in vitro* [30,31]. Contact reactions to food and food components provide even more compelling evidence for the involvement of T cells in food allergy. Whilst there are numerous examples of naturally occurring sensitizing agents (poison ivy, poison oak, primula, etc.) it is also apparent that sensitized individuals also react following dermal contact with various food products. Thus various plant-derived flavouring and fragrance agents such as vanillin, geranium oil, Peru balsam, cinnamon oils and orange and lemon oils have all been shown to possess sensitizing properties [32]—even the lowly cabbage and potato have been reported to cause occupational allergy in housewives [33,34].

True occupational responses are also not uncommonly reported amongst herdsmen and veterinary surgeons following contact with milk proteins; bakers and confectioners following exposure to flour, nuts and egg white and chefs after preparing dishes containing fish or crustacea [35].

Prevalence

Estimates as to the overall prevalence of allergy are highly variable. This is due to the fact that diagnostic methods and screening procedures vary and diagnosis often depends on subjective methods and cognizance of the patients' views as well as their previous history. The pattern of allergies also differs from patient to patient; some become latent, lulling a patient into a false sense of security only to reappear later in life, others resolve completely, whereas others spread a phenomenon in which certain food-allergic patients become increasingly intolerant to a range of foods, having been previously sensitive to only one or two. Retrospective analysis of children with confirmed IgE-mediated food allergies indicates that many infants become tolerant to the offending antigens and gradually outgrow their allergy. At the same time, however, it is clear that allergies to certain foods resolve more easily than others: milk and egg allergies, for example, are more often outgrown than allergies to fish or nuts [36]. Such processes are impossible to predict and are often further influenced by age and the natural evolution of fashionable, educated or ethnic eating habits. Conservative estimates put the incidence of food allergy in the overall population to be in the region of 1–10% but, as indicated above, accurate estimates of prevalence are difficult and any views or the extrapolation of selected figures should be tempered accordingly.

Reactions against defined protein antigens

Defined food allergies, such as cow's milk intolerance, in young children are somewhat more easily quantified and have been variously estimated from 0.2–7.5% [37]. It is now well established that infants and children are more likely to suffer from food allergies than adults. Bock and Martin [27] reported that out of a group of 500 randomly selected infants, 4% developed varying degrees of cow's milk allergy, as judged by both double-blind trial and specific immunological tests within the first 3 years of life. The majority of these cases were transitory and in many instances sensitivity was lost within a few weeks of onset [36]. Children born to allergic parents are of course statistically more likely to develop food allergies than counterparts born to normal parents and, as one might predict, the overall incidence of food allergy is significantly higher in atopic children (often approaching 25% of those with diagnosed infantile eczema) [38]. Focusing on adult atopics, 24% of affected individuals report symptoms after eating or handling foods to which they believe themselves to be sensitive. However, in both adults and children double-blind challenges with suspected foods have revealed that only approximately one-third of patients react [39]. Although there are a number of explanations of the 'no-show' effect the fact remains that up to 10% of atopic adults may reproducibly react to food or dietary components.

Some of the most commonly cited foods associated with adverse reactions are presented in Table 8.3. Cow's milk tops the league of allergens, and for obvious reasons is the most common allergenic food amongst bottle-fed infants. From the data currently available it appears that casein and β-lactoglobulin represent the major allergens to be found in cow's milk, whereas ovalbumin appears to be the major allergen in eggs. Lesser proteins cannot of course be necessarily ruled out, and milk, for example, is known to contain at least 20 separate antigenic proteins [40]. In Scandinavian countries fish, particularly cod, is commonly implicated in food hypersensitivity reactions [40]. Indeed asthma, angioedema and even anaphylaxis have been reported to occur even following inhalation of the steam aerosol from cooking fish. The active allergen involved has been isolated and identified as allergen M, a 12 000 Da, water-soluble, paravalbumin protein unique to fish and amphibian muscle [41]. Soya products used as possible cow's milk substitute have also been examined in some detail. Of the four globulin subfractions, designated 15, 11, 25, and 28 fractions, which comprise the bulk of the soya bean protein, the 25 subfraction has been proven to be the most allergenic [42]. The whey fraction of soya bean protein also contains several biologically active substances including a haemagglutinin, a urease, and a soya bean trypsin inhibitor (see below).

Effects of food processing

Food-processing techniques and the cooking process itself can also modify the antigenic character of food components. Heating food is known to denature

Table 8.3 Foods associated with adverse reactions

Milk products	Citrus fruits
Egg products	Mangos/bananas
Fish/crustacea/molluscs	Chocolate
Meat/derived products	Beverages
Nuts/grains/seeds	Additives

labile proteins; for example bovine serum albumin, bovine γ-globulin and α-lactalbumin are all rendered less antigenic following heating. Alpha casein and β-lactoglobulin on the other hand are more heat-stable and less affected by processing. Furthermore some methods of food processing actually enhance allergenicity. Gentle heating of milk in the presence of lactose, the so-called Browning reaction, links carbohydrate moieties to the β-lactoglobulin backbone and thereby enhances allergenicity. Tomatoes also become increasingly allergenic on ripening but their capacity to elicit reactions in sensitive individuals is neutralized by cooking [40].

Enzymic digestion of foods has also been demonstrated to alter allergenicity. Novel antigenic determinants in milk proteins are uncovered following *in vitro* treatment with proteolytic enzymes [43]. This phenomenon has led to the suggestion that such allergens may be in part responsible for so-called delayed-onset reactions. Support for this premise is indeed available and IgE antibodies have been demonstrated in delayed-onset responders with specificity to pepsin/trypsin-digested β-lactoglobulin but not to undigested β-lactoglobulin [44].

The plethora of potential allergens superimposed upon an individual's unique and particular degree of immune responsiveness currently clouds diagnostic processes. Nevertheless it is anticipated that the increasing availability of purified allergens will allow many of the unanswered questions concerning food allergy to be addressed. This includes the sequence of events that occurs following the ingestion of allergen, the site and mechanism of absorption, conditions regulating recognition and finally the site of allergen–mast cell/basophil interaction. It is further envisaged that diagnostic tests utilizing a panel of purified antigens will yield better and more meaningful correlations with clinical symptomatology than do tests currently applied using crude food extracts.

Reactions to food additives

Clinical responses suggestive of food allergy have been reported following dietary exposure to a range of chemicals used to colour, flavour or preserve foods [45]. In recent years the synthetic food colours have received increasing attention and tartrazine

(FD & C yellow no. 5) in particular remains the azo-pyrazole-based dye most frequently implicated in food intolerance studies. Intolerance to tartrazine was first reported by Lockey in 1959 [46]; this was subsequently confirmed by numerous other studies [45]. Reactions to tartrazine usually take the form of asthma or urticaria, and less commonly rhinitis, angioedema, headache, gastrointestinal colic or shock. Intolerance to tartrazine often accompanies chronic asthma or chronic urticaria and may occur in parallel with intolerance to other food additives.

Whilst reports of intolerance to food colours have steadily increased over the last decade, to date there is little hard evidence of a direct association between clinically identified intolerance to tartrazine and the presence of a circulating tartrazine-specific IgE antibody [47]. Tartrazine (as discussed later) can however function as a hapten when conjugated to protein, and induce the formation of specific IgG and IgE antibodies in rabbits [48], and rats respectively [49]. Delayed hypersensitivity (type IV) responses to tartrazine have also been reported in both humans [50] and experimental animals [51], and others using lymphocyte transformation tests have demonstrated significant transformation of lymphocytes from patients with chronic urticaria to tartrazine and foodstuffs [52].

Whereas tartrazine remains the most commonly implicated food colour in patients with adverse reactions to additives, some allowance must be made for the selective usage of the colour in clinical testing regimens; in fact various other dyes, including amaranth, sunset yellow, indigo carmine and ponceau 4R have all been linked with adverse reactions in patients with chronic urticaria [45]. Cross-reactions with drugs such as aspirin and other dietary components, including benzoic acid, food flavourings, anti-oxidants and stabilizers have also been commonly reported.

The presence of multiple reactivity among food-intolerant individuals clearly raises some important questions—either reactions are occurring via parallel but separate pathways or there is some form of true cross-reactivity between the molecules. As the offending compounds are often structurally distinct (Fig. 8.2), reactivity must stem either from active/antigenic sites or shared epitopes within these molecules, possibly mediated by the sulphanilic or

naphthionic acid residues in the azo dyes, or the reactivity is directed against shared subsidiary reaction products, contaminants or impurities present in some food additives. This is particularly important with respect to food colours where in some instances the dyes need only contain 65% of the parent colour. Although guidelines are set for the levels of permitted subsidiary reaction products/unreacted reagents, the final colour contains a complex mixture of components, the number and relative proportions of which may vary from batch to batch and between manufacturers. Furthermore, adverse reactions may involve responses against metabolites rather than the parent compound *per se*. Indeed in the majority of cases it is only metabolites generated by caecal bacteria or at best trace amounts of the parent compound that actually gain entrance to the body tissues [53].

In recent years the safety of food anti-oxidants and preservatives has also been reviewed in terms of their apparent ability to provoke adverse reactions in sensitive individuals [54]. The use of gallate esters for example has given cause for concern and controversy with regard to their potential allergenicity and continued use as food anti-oxidants. Lauryl gallate in particular was implicated in topically elicited dermatitis in workers exposed to materials containing this product [54,55]. Dodecyl gallate, a currently permitted food additive, has also been reported to be a potent skin sensitizer [56]. Nevertheless it is important to note that strong reactions were only seen to occur in previously contact-sensitized individuals working or repeatedly exposed to the food product or additive. It is also important to note that in normal animals the repeated ingestion of even potent contact-sensitizing agents most often results in lifelong tolerance to the agent [15]. In this condition the animal is effectively protected from initiating allergic reactions, even following parenteral challenge. Indeed there is evidence to suggest that this also applies to the gallate esters [45].

Pseudoallergic reactions

As indicated above, allergic reactions require that the affected individual has been previously exposed to a particular food antigen and that this encounter has resulted in sensitization. Pseudoallergic reac-

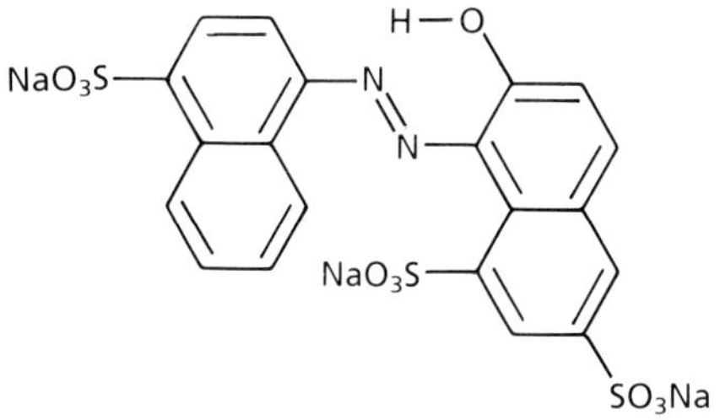

Ponceau 4R

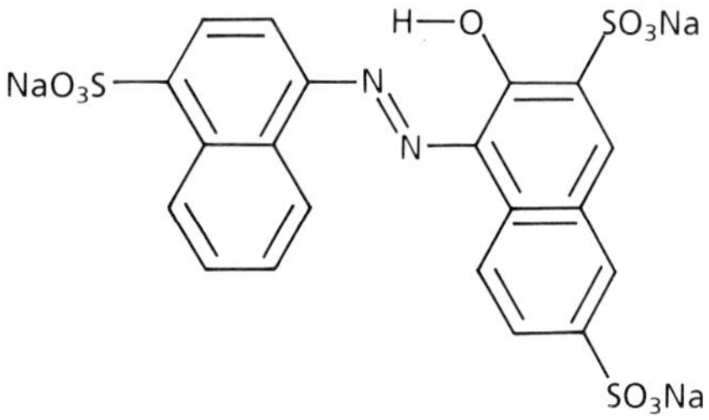

Amaranth

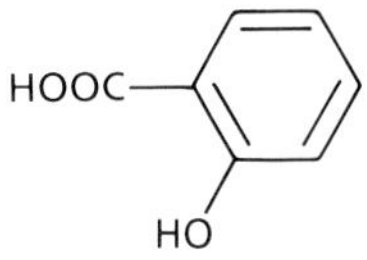

Salicylic acid

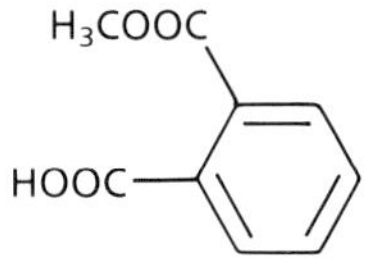

Acetylsalicylic acid

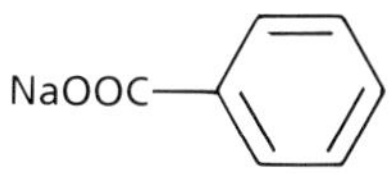

Sodium benzoate

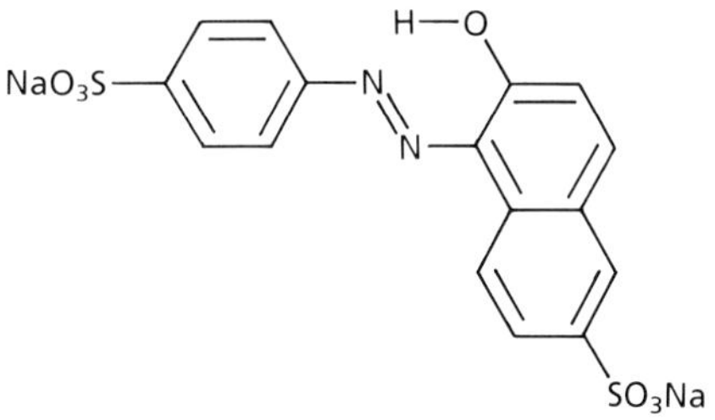

Sunset yellow

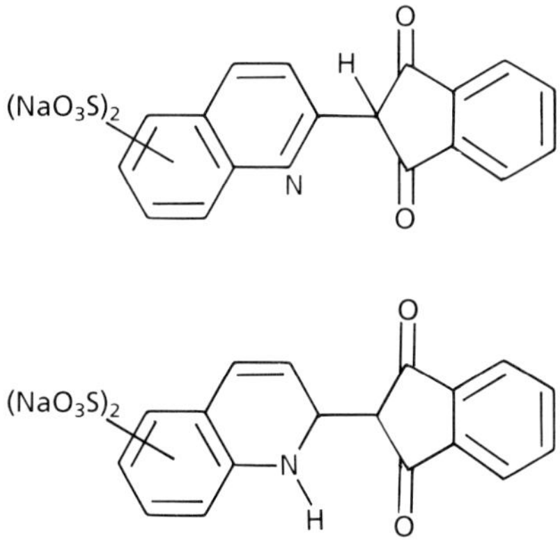

Quinoline yellow

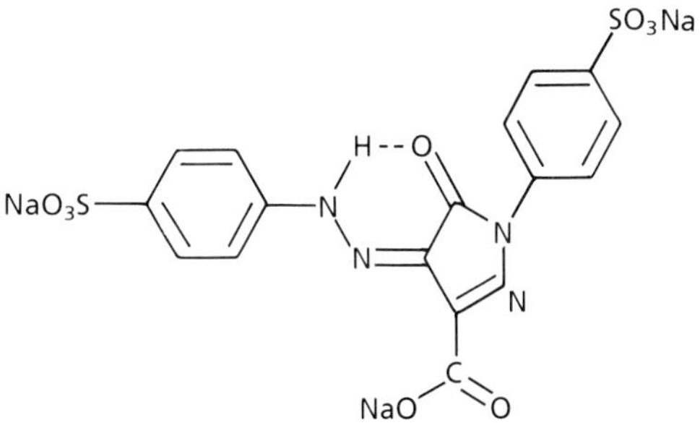

Tartrazine

Fig. 8.2 Structural comparison of cross-reactive agents associated with adverse reactions.

tions are non-immune responses and require no previous encounter. It has been suggested that the food-allergic reactions may, in the first instance, need to be triggered by a non-specific process which may involve, for example, direct mast cell damage, localized gut lesions, altered surface charge and/or enhanced membrane permeability. It is then envisaged that these effects either alone or in combination cause enhanced uptake of protein antigens facilitating immune recognition/hypersensitivity reactions. Some of the processes currently thought to underlie pseudoallergic reaction pathways are discussed below.

Pharmacological effects of food and food additives

Pharmacological reactions are by definition responses produced by natural or added chemicals that mediate effects akin to those of a drug or pharmacologically active agent. In contrast to true allergic reactions, pharmacological reactions are dose-dependent and usually only occur when relatively large amounts of a problem food are ingested. A surprising variety of foods contains vasoactive amines and other pharmacologically active agents capable of eliciting a wide range of symptoms that, in particular, affect the gastrointestinal tract and central nervous system. Symptoms may include skin rashes, recurrent vasomotor headache or migraine, facial flushing, abdominal pain and recurrent diarrhoea.

Vasoactive/biogenic amines. Low levels of vasoactive agents (see Table 8.4 for details) are naturally present within many foods. Significantly higher levels of amines can also be produced by bacteria that can decarboxylate amino acids; these may be part of the food itself, as in many cheeses, or present as a contaminant, scombroid fish-poisoning being the classic example of the latter phenomenon. As the name implies, this syndrome is mainly associated with scombroid fish, e.g. mackerel, tuna, bonito; however, other species including sardines, mahi-mahi and blue fish have also been implicated. The muscle tissues of these fish contain naturally high levels of histidine which can be rapidly metabolized to histamine by contaminating bacteria if the fish are not properly refrigerated [57]. Symptoms resulting from this form of poisoning include headache, flushing, urticaria, abdominal pain and vomiting. However, in order to circumvent the problem of histamine in the diet humans evolved a protective mechanism in the form of histamine-*N*-methyltransferase (HMT) and diamine oxidase (DOA) enzyme systems. In most individuals the combined activity of these enzymes is sufficient to neutralize the levels of histamine normally present in the diet. In histamine intoxication, however, these enzymic defences are overwhelmed or in some instances inhibited by secondary protein decomposition products, e.g. putrescine and cadaverine, both of which are known to potentiate histamine toxicity [58].

Tyramine also possesses a wide range of biological activities and like histamine may either be present in food or produced from tyrosine by micro-organisms. In addition to being a potent vasoconstrictor, tyramine also releases histamine and prostaglandin

Histamine	Fermented products, especially cheeses; wines; vegetables etc.; tinned/smoked fish products; tomatoes; spinach; yeast extract
Histidine	Pork sausage meat; roast venison; Camembert; parmesan cheese; fish products; peanuts; avocado
Tyramine	Cheddar cheese; Brie; Gruyère; Camembert; yeast; herring; pickles
Phenylethylamine	Chocolate; Cheddar cheese
Dopamine	Chocolate
Dihydroxyphenylalanine	Broad beans
Glutamate	Monosodium glutamate; soy sauce; oriental cuisine; snacks/processed foods

Table 8.4 Dietary sources/precursors of vasoactive amines

mediators from mast cells and noradrenaline from adrenergic neurons [59].

Non-specific mast cell activation. In addition to the antigen-specific activation discussed above, mast cells can be activated by a diverse range of other stimuli such as the C5a and C3a anaphylotoxins generated as part of type III hypersensitivity reaction or following the direct interaction between food components and complement itself. Recent studies suggest that adverse reactions to certain food colours including tartrazine may occur via such a mechanism [60]. Colours have also been shown to facilitate non-specific histamine release from both human basophils [61] and human intestinal MMC [62]. Other non-physiological secretagogues such as compound 48/80, mellitin, calcium ionophore A2317 and a range of drugs, modified proteins and synthetic peptides, also have the capacity to activate mast cells directly [63,64] (Fig. 8.3). As described previously, ethanol also causes non-specific release of histamine from the gut and intestinal mast cells, thereby promoting intestinal 'leakiness', an effect often further compounded by the presence of natural histamine in certain wines [11].

Additional research has also established that a range of neuroendocrine peptides/hormones and interleukins has the capacity to induce mast cell mediator release, thereby linking various aspects of the nervous/immune/inflammatory and endocrine systems. Peptides with secretagogue activity include somatostatin, substance P, vasoactive intestinal pep-tide, neurotensin, bradykinin, adrenocorticotrophic hormone and parahormone [63,65–67]. The opiate peptides, dynorphin, α-neoendorphin and β-endorphin have also been reported to induce histamine release from rat peritoneal mast cells but all fail to activate isolated mucosal mast cells [65,68]. The significance of this differential responsiveness amongst the mast cell subgroups remains open to speculation, as do the reports of direct innervation of mast cells [69,70]. Morphologically however it is apparent that intestinal mast cells are intimately associated with amyelinic fibres which following axon-triggering liberate substance P and somatosta-tin into the mast cell environment [67]. The above data, when considered together with evidence dem-onstrating that both histamine and serotonin can act as neurotransmitters [71] and data that suggests that histamine release can be conditioned [72], provide strong support for the link between the nervous system and non-specific mast cell activation.

Natural toxicants and anti-nutritional dietary factors

Contrary to popular belief, risks to health posed by naturally occurring plant/microbial toxins far out-weigh those associated with pesticide residues or synthetic food additives. The seriousness of the risks they pose ranges from trivial gastrointestinal dis-comfort and flatulence, such as caused by legume oligosaccharides, to life-threatening acute/chronic illness as produced by cyanogenic and ptaquiloside glycosides. In the UK and Europe as a whole the risk

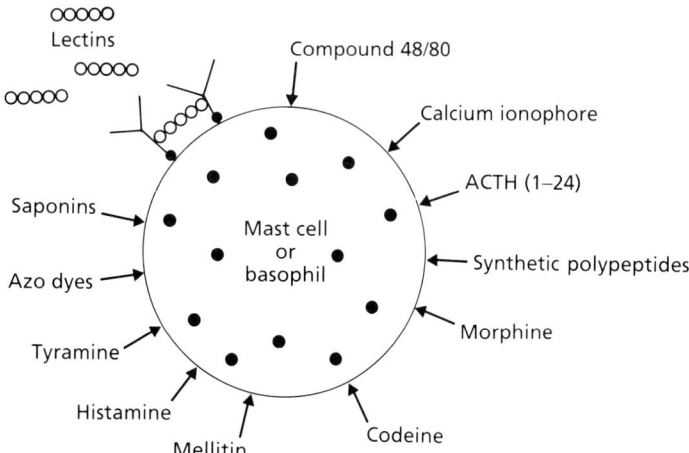

Fig. 8.3 Non-immunologically mediated mast cell activation.

of poisoning from natural food constituents is rare. Nevertheless changes in culinary fashions clearly may pose new risks. It is envisaged that increased public perception of healthy eating and dietary issues will lead to an increased intake of fresh and uncooked vegetables and diverse cereal types. In parallel, advances in food-processing technology will lead to increased availability and palatability of novel food forms.

An in-depth analysis of plant toxins is outside the scope of the present review; the following discussion is therefore restricted to those agents capable of inducing adverse rather than overtly toxic reactions.

Membranolytic food components. A significant proportion of conventional European diets, as well as foods consumed by ethnic minorities, vegetarians and health-conscious consumers contain bioactive or membranolytic components. The most active of these include glycoalkaloid toxins from potatoes and saponins and lectins from legumes. These if eaten in quantity or in a raw state may result in intestinal irritation or local damage and may well aggravate existing gastrointestinal diseases such as inflammatory bowel disease, gastritis, ulcerative colitis, or Crohn's disease. The possibility that glycoalkaloids, present in potatoes, may modify the absorption of other food constituents and xenobiotics from the gut was first suggested by McMillan and Thompson in 1979 [73]. This postulate is now fully supported by recent studies which indicate that the potato-derived glycoalkaloids, α-chaconine and α-solanine are highly potent membranolytic agents [74]. These two compounds, which exhibit synergy in their biological activity, are present in potatoes at 2.5–15 mg 100 g^{-1} fresh weight. Whilst peeling reduces the risk of intake the ingestion of modern snack products containing potato skins or purposely eating skin in the mistaken belief that it is a rich source of fibre and vitamins significantly increases the intake of these agents.

Appreciation of the well known surface active properties of the saponins present in legumes and other plant-derived food products stimulated more recent research which has demonstrated that various of these glycosides have the capacity both to increase intestinal permeability *in viro* [75] and to modify mucosal cell proliferation *in vivo* [74]. Further work on the ability of glycoalkaloids to facilitate the uptake of intestinal antigen seems particularly warranted.

Lectins. Lectins represent a heterogeneous group of naturally occurring plant-derived proteins and glycoproteins (Table 8.5). Legumes are a particularly rich source of lectins. Indeed the anti-nutritive effects of uncooked legumes, referred to as scours in cattle, has been known to livestock farmers since antiquity. The realization that a similar syndrome could occur in humans [76], apparently as a side-effect of healthy eating, prompted a detailed programme of lectin analysis in a range of footstuffs. Whereas the vast majority of the lectins identified (over 100 to date) were heat-labile, several isolated from common foods, including avocado, maize, wheat, bran, carrot, apple, pumpkin seeds, banana, nuts and various breakfast cereals were autoclave-resistant [77]. Whilst all such food products have been fully and appropriately tested, several workers have commented on year-to-year and batch-to-batch variations in the overall lectin content of the various foods; thus it is possible that untoward reactions could still occur with certain batches of foods normally considered to be safe.

Table 8.5 Source and specificity of selected dietary lectins

Source	Lectin	Sugar specificity
Wheat	Wheat germ agglutinin	*N*-Acetylglucosamine
Jackbeans	Concanavalin A	α-Mannose, α-glucose
Lentils	*Lens culinaris* agglutinin	α-Mannose, α-glucose
Green pea	*Pisum sativum* agglutinin	α-Mannose, α-glucose
Soybean	Soya bean agglutinin	*N*-Acetylgalactosamine
Peanut	Peanut agglutinin	Galactose
Kidney beans	Phytohaemagglutinin	No simple sugar inhibitor
Edible snail	*Helix pomatia* agglutinin	*N*-Acetylgalactosamine

The bioactivity of lectins stems from their ability to bind or interact with, and/or activate glycoprotein/oligosaccharide receptors expressed on the surface membranes of the gastrointestinal tract as well as a wide range of other cell types including lymphocytes. Certain lectins agglutinate cells; many act as lymphocyte mitogens causing non-specific polyclonal transformation; others are lytic or toxic and produce cell membrane damage. In addition to their ability to cause gut damage several lectins are capable of initiating mast cell and basophil activation either by acting as antigens themselves in type I reaction, by cross-linking cell-bound IgE or by cross-linking the membrane-associated IgE Fc receptor [78].

Mitogenic lectins also have the capacity to stimulate B cells to initiate IgE production and this facilitates type I sensitization [79]. Indeed lectins as a group have been proven to possess a range of immunomodulatory properties and, depending on dose, timing and route of administration, have been demonstrated either to enhance [80] or suppress humoral and cellular responses [80,81]. A number of lectins have the capacity to direct non-specific cytotoxicity in T cells in a manner akin to the normal antibody-dependent driven mechanism [82] and some non-specifically endow macrophages with cytotoxic potential [83]. Perhaps more importantly however natural killer cell activity has been shown to be able to be inhibited by simple sugars [84], suggesting that recognition events in the natural killer process may involve a sugar-specific recognition mechanism. Clearly the possibility that dietary lectins may interfere with components of natural immunity is a matter of some concern. Indeed it has been suggested that their capacity both to produce intestinal lesions and to interfere with normal immunoregulatory processes may under defined conditions abrogate local tolerogenesis mechanisms and thereby facilitate systemic sensitization [85].

Carrageenans. Another class of naturally occurring food additives that has attracted attention in recent years is the carrageenans. The carrageenans are high molecular weight sulphated polygalactans isolated from various species of red seaweed. They are used extensively in the food industry as thickening, gelling and protein-suspending agents [86]. Initially, all grades of carrageenan were considered safe by the US Food and Drug Administration and were permitted for use as regulated food additives. However, subsequent reports implicated degraded forms of carrageenan (30 000 mol wt) in the induction of ulcers and metaplastic changes in the intestinal tract of a number of animal species [87,88]. In guinea pigs it was shown that the ulcerogenic capacity of the carrageenan was related to the ability of intestinal macrophages to endocytose the material [89]. It was suggested that following uptake, carrageenan caused lysosomal enzyme release with resultant local tissue damage and ulceration.

Although the food-grade carrageenans have not been associated with the induction of ulcers, they have been shown to cross the intestinal epithelial barrier. Using a carrageenan-specific Alcian blue staining technique, we have demonstrated that small quantities of food-grade carrageenan given at 0.5% in drinking water could penetrate the intestinal epithelium of adult inbred rats [90]. Subsequent studies also demonstrated the absorption of ^{3}H-labelled carrageenan across the lamina propria, its transport through the Peyer's patches and its subsequent arrival in the mesenteric lymph node [91].

Since the uptake of carrageenan occurred in the absence of inflammatory or pathological changes, it seems probable that the Peyer's patch cells were fulfilling a normal role in sampling antigenic components from the intestinal lumen and transporting the material to the GALT. Whilst there is no evidence to suggest that the persorption of small quantities of carrageenan across the epithelial barrier poses an acute toxic hazard, carrageenans are biologically active molecules and several authors have reported that parenterally administered carrageenans can markedly affect a number of normal immune responses. These studies include the suppressive effect of carrageenans on macrophage function [92], antibody production [93] and cell-mediated immune responses [94,95]. The oral administration of carrageenan to rats has also been demonstrated to result in a dose-dependent suppression of lymphocyte responsiveness *in vitro* [96] and an impaired humoral immunity against sheep red blood cells *in vivo* [91].

Although the above effects were initially attributed to the selective toxic effect of carrageenans on antigen-processing macrophages, more recent data have demonstrated that by the correct adjustment of dosage, route and time of administration, carrageenans also have the capacity to enhance both cell-mediated and humorally mediated immune responses [97,98].

The fact that carrageenan can enhance some responses but suppresses others implies that macrophages exposed to carrageenan may modify immune responses by the timed release of specific immunoregulatory products. Evidence in support of this possibility came from studies which demonstrated that carrageenan-treated macrophages could, depending on conditions and time of administration, lead to the release of either stimulatory and/or inhibitory factors. The former was shown to be the immunostimulatory agent interleukin; the latter was shown to be a prostaglandin [99,100].

At present it is impossible to relate these studies directly to the human situation. While it is likely that uptake of high molecular weight material also occurs across the human gut there is no evidence to suggest that the limited uptake of carrageenan that may occur in humans in any way interferes with normal immune competence. Nevertheless, increased exposure may of course occur during allergic reactions and following episodes of gastrointestinal disease. It is also relevant that experimental studies to date have all been performed in animals with an intact gastrointestinal tract and it might be expected that non-specific damage associated with infection, allergy or mast cell degranulation or gastrointestinal lesions may be associated with an increased uptake of carrageenan. Further studies under such conditions are clearly necessary in order better to predict possible immunological consequences associated with enhanced uptake.

Interactions between food additives and neuroendocrine receptors

It has been variously estimated that 0.1–0.23% [101] of the population react to additives. The reactions produced are diverse and variable but may include urticaria, rhinitis, angioedema, headache and gastrointestinal disturbances. It has also been suggested that the ingestion of excessive amounts of additives is associated with hyperactivity in children [102]

and although this view still remains controversial it does seem to have gained some credence in certain situations [103,104].

Whereas a number of food chemical additives have been shown to be immunogenic in their own right it would appear that most reactions are pharmacological rather than immunological in nature. Whereas it has been known for some time that parenterally administered tartrazine can initiate bronchospasm [105] and increase both the firing rate of carotid sinus nerves [106] and arterial blood pressure in guinea pigs [107], more recent studies also suggest that orally administered tartrazine may interact directly with acetylcholine receptors present within the intestinal mucosa [108]. Similarly xanthine and erythrosine have also been demonstrated to possess neuromodulatory functions by facilitating the release of both cholinergic and dopaminergic transmitters at neuromuscular junctions [109,110]. Continuing on this theme, monosodium glutamate, a widely used culinary prerequisite in various Chinese cuisines, has been linked with the aptly termed Chinese restaurant syndrome [111]. In sensitive individuals monosodium glutamate produces flushing, sweating, confusion, and in some instances, collapse—all symptoms consistent with acetylcholine intoxication. Since glutamic acid and sodium are precursors in the acetylcholine pathway it has been suggested that the rapid rise in plasma sodium/glutamate level is reflected by a surge in acetylcholine production [112]. Furthermore, additional data link glutamate and aspartate with 'excitoneurotoxicity' in newborn rats [113]. In *in utero* mice studies butylated-hydroxytoluene and -hydroxyanisole have been demonstrated to reduce cerebral serotonin and noradrenaline and initiate behavioural difficulties in later life [114].

Conclusions

Adverse reactions to food and food constituents remain an important general health issue that affects allergic and non-allergic individuals of all ages but especially young children. Responses are triggered by a variety of routes and stimuli but are all broadly divisible into hypersensitivity (immunologically mediated reactions) and intolerance (pseudoallergic non-immunological reactions).

The diverse range of possible reactions superimposed on an individual's idiosyncratic constitution often renders diagnosis and interpretation of individual responses impossible. At present the diagnosis of food intolerance is dependent upon the amelioration of symptoms following the elimination of the suspect food or food constituent from the diet and the elicitation of a positive reaction following subsequent oral challenge.

Despite a plethora of information concerning antigen uptake across the gut, immunoregulation, tolerance induction and the genesis of the secretory response, our understanding of the complex way in which the gastrointestinal tract processes food allergens remains incomplete. The fact that adverse reactions may also be initiated by pseudoallergic processes at first sight may be considered only to compound our difficulties. However the growing realization that adverse reactions may in addition be mediated by a variety of non-immunological processes offers a much needed fillip to our appreciation of the complexities of food intolerance, since it helps resolve the enigma of food allergy without antibody.

It is hoped that this chapter has shown that there is some order in the problem of food sensitivity. As always, the way forward lies in continued research and a better understanding of the underlying mechanisms.

References

1 Hippocrates. *The Hippocratic Collection, Encyclopedia Britannica.* Alley AK, Hanson DG eds, vol. 8. Chicago: Encyclopedia Britannica, 1983:942–3.

2 Galen JD. *De Sanitate Tuenda (Hygiene).* Translated by Green RM, Springfield IL: Charles C. Thomas, 1951:210–12.

3 Schloss OM. A case of allergy to common foods. *Am J Dis Child* 1912; 3:341–6.

4 Talbot FB. Idiosyncrasy to cow's milk: its relationship to anaphylaxis. *Boston Med Surg J* 1916; 175:409–12.

5 Park EA. A case of hypersensitiveness to cow's milk. *Am J Dis Child* 1920; 19:46–9.

6 Prausnitz C, Kustner H. Studien uber die Ueberemfindlichkeit. *Zentralbl Bakteriol Orig* 1921; 86:160–9.

7 Johannson SGO, Dannaeus A, Lilja G. The relevance of anti-food antibodies for the diagnosis of food allergy. *Ann Allergy* 1984; 53:665–70.

8 Parrott DMW. The structure and organisation of lymphoid tissue in the gut. In: Brostoff J, Challacombe SJ, eds. *Food Allergy and Intolerance.* London: Bailliere Tindall, 1987:3–26.

9 Nicklin S. Intestinal uptake of antigen: immunological consequences. In: Miller K, Nicklin S, eds. *Immunology of the Gastrointestinal Tract.* Florida: CRC Press, 1987:129–45.

10 Hall JG. The gut associated lymphoid tissue as a model of a specialized immune subsystem. In: Berlin A, Dean J, Draper MH, Smith EMB, Spreafico F, eds. *Immunotoxicology.* Amsterdam: Martinus Nijhoff; 1987:171–91.

11 Nicklin S, Miller K. Local and systemic immune response to intestinally presented antigen. *Int Arch Allergy Appl Immunol* 1983; 77:87–91.

12 Draper LR, Gyure LA, Hall JG, Robertson D. Effects of alcohol on the integrity of the intestinal epithelium. *Gut* 1983; 24:399–402.

13 Rainsford KD. Side-effects of anti-inflammatory analgeric drugs. In: Rainsford KD, Velo GP, eds. *Side Effects of Anti-Inflammatory Drugs.* Lancaster: MTP Press, 1987:3–33.

14 Challacombe SJ. The induction of secretory IgA responses. In: Brostoff J, Challacombe SJ, eds. *Food Allergy and Intolerance.* London: Bailliere Tindall, 1987:269–85.

15 Challacombe SJ, Tomassi TB. Oral tolerance. In: Brostoff J, Challacombe SJ, eds. *Food Allergy and Intolerance.* London: Bailliere Tindall, 1987:255–68.

16 Ishizaka K. Basic mechanisms of IgE-mediated hypersensitivity. *Curr Op Immunol* 1989; 1:625–9.

17 Galli S. Biology of disease: new insights into "the riddle of the mast cells": microenvironmental regulation of mast cell development and phenotype heterogeneity. *Lab Invest* 1990; 62:5–33.

18 King SJ, Miller HRP. Anaphylactic release of mucosal mast cell protease and its relationship to gut permeability in *Nippostrongylus*-primed rats. *Immunol* 1984; 51:653–60.

19 Marquardt DL. Histamine. *Clin Rev Allergy* 1983; 1:343–51.

20 Beaven MA. Histamine: its role in physiological and pathological processes. *Monogr Allergy* 1978; 13:1–113.

21 Schwartz LB, Austen KF. Structure and function of the chemical mediators of mast cells. *Progr Allergy* 1984; 34:271–321.

22 Kilshaw PJ, Slade H. Passage of ingested protein into the blood during gastrointestinal hypersensitivity reactions: experiments in the preruminant calf. *Clin Exp Immunol* 1980; 41:575–82.

23 Scadding G, Bjarnason I, Brostoff J, Levi JA, Peters TJ. Intestinal permeability to ^{51}Cr-labelled EDTA in food-intolerant subjects. *Digestion* 1989; 42:104–9.

24 Targan SR, Kagnoff MF, Brogan MD, Shanahan F.

Immunologic mechanisms in intestinal disease. *Ann Intern Med* 1987; 106:853–70.

25 Pagnelli R, Levinsky RJ, Brostoff J, Wraith DG. Immune complexes containing food proteins in normal and atopic subjects after oral challenge and the effect of sodium cromoglycate on antigen absorption. *Lancet* 1979; i:1270–727.

26 Cunningham-Rundles C, Brandeis WE, Good RH. Bovine antigens and the formation of circulating immune complexes in selective immunoglobulin A deficiency. *J Clin Invest* 1979; 64:272–9.

27 Bock SA, Martin M. The incidence of adverse reactions to foods—a continuing study. *J Allergy Clin Immunol* 1983; 71:98.

28 Phillips AD, Rice SJ, France NE, Walker-Smith JA. Small intestinal intraepithelial lymphocyte levels in cow's milk protein intolerance. *Gut* 1979; 20:509–12.

29 Stern M, Dietrich M, Muller J. Small intestinal mucosa in coeliac disease and cow's milk protein intolerance. Morphometric and immunofluorescent studies. *Eur J Pediatr* 1982; 139:101–5.

30 Ashkenazi A, Levin S, Idar D, Or A, Rosenberg I, Handzel ZT. *In vitro* cell mediated immunologic assay for cow's milk allergy. *Pediatr* 1980; 65:399–402.

31 Minor JD, Tolber SG, Frick OL. Leukocyte inhibition factor in delayed-onset food allergy. *J Allergy Clin Immunol* 1980; 66:314–21.

32 Miller K, Nicklin S. Adverse reactions to food additives and colours. In: Watford J, ed. *Developments in Food Colours 2.* London: Elsevier Applied Science, 1984:207–32.

33 Pearson RSB. Potato sensitivity: an occupational allergen in housewives. *Acta Allergol* 1966; 21:507–9.

34 Blaiss MS, McCant ML, Lehrer SB. Anaphylaxis to cabbage: detection of allergen. *Ann Allergy* 1987; 58:248–51.

35 Hjorth N. Wilkinson DS. Type I and type IV allergy in contact dermatitis. *Br J Dermatol* 1973; 88:103–9.

36 Bock SA. Adverse reactions to foods during the first three years of life. *J Allergy Clin Immunol* 1985; 75:178.

37 Bahna SI, Gandhi MD. Milk hypersensitivity. II. Practical aspects of diagnosis, treatment and prevention. *Ann Allergy* 1983; 50:295–301.

38 Heiner DC. Allergy to cow's milk. *N Engl Soc Allergy Proc* 1981; 2:192.

39 Bock SA, Buckley J, Holst A, May CD. Proper use of skin tests with food extracts in diagnosis of hypersensitivity to food in children. *Clin Allergy* 1978; 7:189.

40 Andersson JA, Soyn D, eds. American Academy of Allergy and Immunology Committee on adverse reactions to foods. US DHSS NIH Publication no. 84–2442. 1984:115–17.

41 Elsayed S, Bennich H. The primary structure of allergen M from cod. *Scand J Immunol* 1975; 4:203–8.

42 Shibasaki M, Suzuki S, Tajima S, Nemoto H, Kuroume T. Allergenicity of major component proteins of soybean. *Int Arch Allergy Appl Immunol* 1980; 61:441–8.

43 Spies JR, Stevan MA, Swtein WJ, Coulson EJ. The chemistry of allergens. XX. New antigens generated by pepsin hydrolysis of bovine milk proteins. *J Allergy* 1970; 45:208–19.

44 Haddad ZH, Kalra V, Verma S. IgE antibodies to peptic and peptic-tryptic digests of betalactoglobulin. Significance in food hypersensitivity. *Ann Allergy* 1979; 42:368–71.

45 Miller M. Intolerance to food colours and other additives. In: Miller K, Nicklin S, eds. *Immunology of the Gastrointestinal Tract.* Florida: CRC Press, 1987: 85–94.

46 Lockey SD. Allergic reaction due to FD & C yellow no. 5 tartrazine, an aniline dye used as a colouring and identifying agent in various steroids. *Ann Allergy* 1959; 17:719.

47 Weliky N, Heiner DC. Hypersensitivity to chemicals. Correlation of tartrazine hypersensitivity with characteristics serum IgD and IgE response patterns. *Clin Allergy* 1980; 10:375–89.

48 Johnson HM, Smith BG. Haptenic relationships of p-azobenzene-sulphonate and some structurally-related food dyes. *Immunochem* 1972; 9:253–61.

49 Nicklin S, Miller K. Induction of a transient reaginic antibody response to tartrazine in the rat. *Int Arch Allergy Appl Immunol* 1985; 76:185–7.

50 Warrington RJ, Sauder PJ, McPhillips S. Cell-mediated immune response to artificial food additives in chronic urticaria. *Clin Allergy* 1986; 16:527–33.

51 Safford RJ, Goodwin A. Immunogenicity of tartrazine and its metabolites. *Int Arch Allergy Appl Immunol* 1985; 77:331–7.

52 Valverde E, Vich JM, Garcia-Calderon JV, Garcia-Calderon PA. *In vitro* stimulation of lymphocytes in patients with chronic urticaria induced by additives and food. *Clin Allergy* 1980; 10:691–9.

53 Walker R. The metabolism of Azo compounds: a review of the literature. *Fd Cosmet Toxicol* 1980; 8:659–76.

54 Food additives and contaminants committee. Report on the antioxidants in Food Regulations 1966 and 1974. London: Ministry of Agriculture, Fisheries and Food, 1982.

55 World Health Organisation. *Tech Rep Ser Wld Hlth Org* 539, Geneva: WHO, 1974; 417–21.

56 VanDer Meeren HLM. Dodecyl gallate, permitted in food, is a strong sensitizer. *Contact Derm* 1987;

16:266–72.

57 Taylor SL. Food allergies. *Food Technol* 1985; 39:98–105.

58 Hui JY, Taylor SL. Inhibition of *in vivo* histamine metabolism in rats by foodborne and pharmacologic inhibitors of diamine oxidase, histamine N-methyltransferase and monoamine oxidase. *Toxicol Appl Pharmacol* 1985; 81:241–9.

59 Hanington E. Migraine. In: Lessof MH, ed. *Clinical Reactions to Food.* Chichester, John Wiley: 1983:155–80.

60 Nicklin S, Hutchinson AP, Miller K. Interactions between food colours and the complement system. *Toxicol* 1989; 9:820–1.

61 Murdoch RD, Lessof MH, Pollock I, Young E. Effects of food additives on leukocyte histamine release in normal and urticaria subjects. *J R Coll Phys* 1987; 21:251–6.

62 Schaubschulager WW, Zabel P, Schlaark M. Tartrazine-induced histamine release from gastric mucosa. *Lancet* 1987; ii:800–1.

63 Foreman JC, Piotrowski W. Peptides and histamine release. *J Allergy Clin Immunol* 1984; 74:127–31.

64 Stanworth DR. Mechanisms of hypersensitivity. In: Gibson GG, Hubbard R, Parke DV, eds. *Immunotoxicology.* London: Academic Press, 1983:71–86.

65 Shanahan F, Lee TDG, Bienenstock J, Befus AD. The influence of endorphins on peritoneal and mucosal mast cell secretion. *J Allergy Clin Immunol* 1984; 74:499–504.

66 Casale TB, Bowman S, Kaliner M. Induction of human cutaneous mast cell degranulation by opiates and endogenous opioid peptides: evidence for opiate and non-opiate receptor participation. *J Allergy Clin Immunol* 1984; 73:775–90.

67 Payan DG, Levine JD, Goetzl EJ. Modulation of immunity and hypersensitivity by sensory neuropeptides. *J Immunol* 1984; 132:1324–601.

68 Sugiyama K, Furuta H. Histamine release induced by dynorphin(1–13) from rat mast cells. *Jpn J Pharmacol* 1984; 35:247–52.

69 Newson B, Dahlstrom A, Enerback L, Ahlman H. Suggestive evidence for a direct innervation of mucosal mast cells. *Neurosci* 1983; 10:565–70.

70 Wiesner-Menzel L, Schulz B, Vakilzadeh F, Czarnetzki BM. Electron microscopical evidence for a direct contact between nerve fibres and mast cells. *Acta Derm Venereol* 1981; 61:465–9.

71 Weiner RI, Ganong WF. Role of brain monoamines and histamine in regulation of anterior pituitary secretion. *Physiol Rev* 1978; 58:905–76.

72 Russell M, Dark KA, Cummins RW, Jones R. Learned histamine release. *Science* 1984; 225:733–4.

73 McMillan M, Thompson JC. An outbreak of suspected solanine poisoning in schoolboys. *Q J Med* 1979; 48:227–43.

74 Gee JM, Johnson IT. Effects of some purified saponins on transmural potential difference in mammalian small intestine. *Toxicol In Vitro* 1989; 3:85–90.

75 Johnson IT, Gee JM. Interactions between haemolytic saponins, bile salts and small intestinal mucosa in the rat. *J Nutr* 1988; 116:2270–7.

76 Noah ND, Bender AE, Reaidi GB, Gilbert RJ. Food poisoning from raw red kidney beans. *Br Med J* 1980; ii:236–7.

77 Nachbar MS, Oppenheim JD. Lectins in the US diet: a survey of lectins in commonly consumed foods and a review of the literature. *Am J Clin Nutr* 1980; 33:2338–45.

78 Helin RM, Froese A. Binding of the receptors for IgE by various lectins. *Int Arch Allergy Appl Immunol* 1981; 65:81–4

79 Astorquiza MI, Sayago S. Modulation of IgE response by phytohemagglutinin. *Int Arch Allergy Appl Immunol* 1984; 73:367–9.

80 Romball CG, Weigle WO. The enhancing effect of mitogens in the *in vivo* immune response in rabbits. *J Immunol* 1975; 115:556–60.

81 Nirmul G, Severin C, Taub RN. *In vivo* effects of con A. I. Immunosuppressive effects. *Transplant* 1972; 14:91–5.

82 Yue CL, Tanimoto K, Horinchi Y. Characterization and possible mechanisms of mitogen-induced cell-mediated cytotoxicity. *Scand J Immunol* 1981; 14:397–408.

83 Rothlein R, Yoon Berm Kim. Porcine alveolar macrophages discriminate between self and non-self in lectin-mediated cellular cytotoxicity. *Cell Immunol* 1982; 68:368–76.

84 MacDermott RP, Kienker LJ, Bertovich MJ, Muchmore AV. Inhibition of spontaneous but not antibody dependent cell-mediated cytotoxicity by simple sugars. *Immunol* 1981; 44:143–52.

85 Pusztai A, Clarke EMW, Grant G, King TP. The toxicity of *Phaseolus vulgaris* lectins. Nitrogen balance and immunochemical studies. *J Sci Food Agric* 1981; 32:1037–46.

86 Towle GA. Carrageenan. In: Whistler RL, Bemiller JN, eds. *Industrial Gums.* New York: Academic Press, 1973:105–19.

87 Sharratt M, Grasso P, Carpanini F, Gangolli SD. Carrageenan ulceration and ulcerative colitis. *Gastroenterol* 1971; 61:410–17.

88 Watt J, Marcus R. Hyperplastic mucosal changes in the rabbit colon produced by degraded carrageenan. *Gastroenterol* 1970; 59:760–71.

89 Abraham R, Fabian RJ, Goldberg L, Coulston F. Role of lysosomes in carrageenan-induced caecal ulcer-

ation. *Gastroenterol* 1974; 67:1169–74.

90 Nicklin S, Miller K. Effect of orally administered food-grade carrageenans on antibody-mediated and cell-mediated immunity in the inbred rat. *Fd Chem Toxicol* 1984; 22:615–21.

91 Nicklin S, Baker KC, Miller K. Intestinal uptake of carrageenan: distribution and effects on humoral immune competence. *Adv Exp Med Biol* 1988; 237:813–19.

92 Di Rosa M. Biological properties of carrageenan. *J Pharmacol* 1972; 24:89–102.

93 Thomson AW, Fowler EF. Carrageenan: a review of its effect on the immune system. *Agents Actions* 1981; 1:265–73.

94 Sakemi T, Kuroiwa A, Nomoto K. Effect of carrageenan on the induction of cell-mediated cytotoxic responses *in vivo*. *Immunol* 1980; 41:297–305.

95 Rumjanek VM, Brent L. Immunosuppressive activity of carrageenan for cell-mediated responses in the mouse. *Transplant* 1978; 26:113.

96 Bash JA, Vago JR. Carrageenan-induced suppression of T lymphocyte proliferation in the rat: *in vivo* suppression induced by oral administration. *J Reticuloendothel Soc* 1980; 28:213–25.

97 Niclin S, Atkinson HAC, Miller K. Iota-carrageenan induced reaginic antibody production in the rat. I. Characterisation and kinetics of the response. *Int J Immunopharmacol* 1985; 7:677.

98 Richou R, Lallouette P, Legger H. La carrageenan substance adjuvante et stimulante de l'immunitite. *CR Hebd Acad Sci* 1968; 267:257–64.

99 Nicklin S, Baker K, Miller K. Carrageenan induced changes in the immunomodulatory capacity of macrophages an *in vitro* study. *Adv Exp Med Biol* 1988; 237:821–32.

100 Bash JA, Cochran FR. Carrageenan-induced suppression of T lymphocyte proliferation in the rat: *in vitro* production of a suppressor factor by peritoneal macrophages. *J Reticuloendothel Soc* 1980; 28:203–15.

101 Commission of the European Communities. *Report of a Working Group of Adverse Reactions to Ingested Additivies, 111, 556-81-EN*. Brussels: Commission of the European Communities, 1981:14–27.

102 Feingold B. *Why your Child is Hyperactive*. New York; Random House, 1978:101–14.

103 Egger J, Carter CM, Graham PJ, Barnett D. Controlled trial of oligoantigenic treatment in the hyperkinetic syndrome. *Lancet* 1985; i:540–5.

104 Swansea JM, Kinsbourne M. Food dyes impair performance of hyper-reactive children on a laboratory learning test. *Science* 1980; 207:1485–6.

105 Biggs DF, Peterson MA, Aaron TH. Tartrazine induced airway constriction in anesthetised paralysed guinea pigs. *Proc West Pharmacol Soc* 1981; 24:363–5.

106 D'Souza SJA, Biggs DF. Tartrazine and indomethacin increase firing rates in the carotid sinus nerves of guinea-pigs. *Proc West Pharmacol* 1985; 28:133–7.

107 D'Souza SJA, Biggs DF. Aspirin indomethacin and tartrazine increase carotid-sinus nerve activity and arterial blood pressure in guinea-pigs. *Pharmacol* 1987; 34:96–103.

108 Hutchinson AP, Carrick B, Miller K, Nicklin S. Interaction between synthetic food colours and neurochemical receptors in the guinea pig ileum. *The Toxicologist* 1991 (in press).

109 Augustine JG, Levitan H. Neuro-transmitter release from a vertebrate neuro-muscular synapse affected by a food dye. *Science* 1980; 207:1489–90.

110 Lafferman JA, Silbergerd EK. Erythrosin B inhibits dopamine transport in rat caudate synaptosomes. *Science* 1968; 205:410–12.

111 Kwok RHM. Chinese restaurant syndrome. *N Engl J Med* 1968; 278:796.

112 Ghadimi H, Kumar S, Konturek SJ, Kusche J. Studies on monosodium glutamate ingestion: biochemical explanations of Chinese restaurant syndrome. *Biochem Med* 1971; 5:447–56.

113 Olney JW, Labruyer J. Brain damage in mice from voluntary ingestion of glutamate and aspartate. *Neurobehav Toxicol* 1980; 2:125–9.

114 Stokes JD, Scudder CL. The effect of butylated hydroxyanisole and butylated hydroxytoluene on behaviour development of mice. *Dev Psychobiol* 1974; 7:343–50.

9
The effect of nutrition on the immune system

JACOB SHOHAM

Introduction

The impact of nutrition on host defence mechanisms, particularly those related to the immune response, was recognized long ago, in connection with conditions of severe malnutrition. Lower resistance to infection and severe thymic atrophy were observed early in this century in children suffering from protein-calorie malnutrition (PCM) [1]. The research conducted since then focused on PCM conditions. However, it was soon realized that naturally occurring states of malnutrition are difficult to interpret, because deficiencies usually involve multiple dietary factors and because infection, anorexia and debilitation further complicate this condition [2].

Humans require six basic categories of dietary components [3]. Three of them are regarded as macronutrients (proteins, carbohydrates and fats), supplying the main building blocks (amino acids and some fats) for the body, as well as energy for growth and metabolism. Two others are micronutrients (vitamins and minerals) which are needed in small quantities, but are nevertheless essential for well-being. In recent years, additional essential micronutrients, needed in ultratrace amounts, were recognized [4]. The sixth component is water, with its obvious vital role in life. A suitable amount and combination of these food constituents is needed for the maintenance of normal body activities, including those of the immune system.

The realization that marked reduction in food intake, characteristic of PCM, is commonly associated with vitamin and mineral deficiencies led many investigators to analyse the effect of single nutrient deficiencies on the immune system [5–12]. This can be properly done only in defined, controlled animal experiments. The selection of assay system to assess immune dysfunctions is also of obvious importance. Since many nutritional deficiencies may be complicated by infections [13], which, in turn affect immune functions [14], this perturbing influence should be eliminated. Finally, in deriving conclusions from animal experiments to clinical situations, one should bear in mind that a given combination of nutrients or their combined deficiencies may have an effect which is different from that observed with each one of them alone. Isolated deficiencies of certain micronutrients can occur also in clinical medicine (e.g. iron, vitamin A etc.). The study of lymphocyte growth requirements *in vitro* [15] may provide clues for possible dietary needs of the immune system.

In recent years it became clear that not only deficiencies but also excesses of macro- and micronutrients can profoundly affect the immune response [5,16,17].

This chapter summarizes the main current trends in the research on nutrition and the immune system. It starts with the main clinical prototype of this research—that on PCM, a multinutrient deficiency state. The rest of the chapter deals with the effects of deficiency or excess of specific nutrients on the immune system. When enough data are available on a given nutrient, direct information on the immune system [lymphoid tissue cellularity and composition of immune cells, humoral immunity, cell-mediated immunity (CMI) and phagocytic cell function] is produced first, followed by data on immune-related disease conditions (infection, cancer and autoimmunity). Data on animal experiments and clinical studies are compiled together.

Protein-calorie malnutrition

PCM is not a discrete, all-or-none phenomenon, but rather it spans an entire spectrum, ranging from subclinical malnutrition compatible with adequate life, to extreme lethal stages of nutritional deficiency [18]. In dealing with PCM one should differentiate between primary and secondary ones. Primary PCM is a situation where energy and protein intake are apparently the most limiting factors in malnutrition, although vitamin and mineral deficiencies are also present to a varying degree. Secondary PCM is the consequence of a primary disease that leads either to

inadequate food intake or utilization, or to increased nutritional requirements. Examples of secondary PCM are diseases inducing cachexia of metabolic, infectious or neoplastic origin, gastrointestinal problems including malabsorption, and endocrine or psychological disorders. Severe PCM may be manifested as an oedematous (kwashiorkor) or nonoedematous (marasmus) variety; in the former there is more protein deficiency and hypoalbuminaemia, while in the latter there is more calorie deficiency, with clinical manifestations of extreme weight reduction and muscle wasting. In these cases, as well as in chronic mild-to-moderate PCM, the condition is characteristically a multinutrient deficiency, including micronutrients whose individual effects will be discussed below. In addition, the concentration of certain hormones such as adrenaline, corticosteroids, insulin and thyroxine is altered during PCM and its accompanying stress. Primary PCM will be in the focus of the present discussion.

Each of the deficiencies which compose PCM, and their interacting effects, may have important consequences on the immune response. Moreover, a major proportion of people suffering from PCM suffer also heavy burdens of infection and both interfere with normal immune responses. Infections, particularly chronic ones, deplete the host's metabolic energy and contribute a parameter of secondary PCM to the picture. Most of the studies have been on clinical PCM in human subjects [19–39]. However, several studies were performed on experimental animals [40–48]. A particularly interesting model is the dormant fasted black bear (*Ursus americanus*) who survives up to 5 months without food and water, showing no signs of nutritional deficiencies or increased incidence of infection. These bears exhibit diminished lymphocyte proliferation but normal phagocytic function during dormancy [49].

Lymphoid tissue cellularity is profoundly affected in PCM. The thymus is the most vulnerable organ in this situation and the degree of its atrophy serves as a barometer of the severity of malnutrition. The effect can be so severe that the term nutritional thymectomy can be justified [50]. Histologically the clear distinction between the densely packed thymic cortex and the sparse medulla is ill defined. Hassall's corpuscles appear degenerated but the epithelial stromal component is relatively preserved, in contrast to its appearance in the primary immunodeficiency syndrome named after Di George. The histological changes in the thymus are most marked in patients who show lymphopenia before death.

All other lymphoid organs become involuted, although not to the same degree as the thymus. In the spleen the periarteriolar cuff of lymphocytes is less prominent. In lymph nodes, thymus-dependent areas are depleted [51] while plasma cells and germinal centres remain relatively intact.

The absolute number of lymphocytes is moderately reduced but the number of T lymphocytes is markedly reduced (15–25% of lymphoid cells forming E rosettes, with sheep red blood cells (RBC), as compared to 60–75% in normal subjects [52]. Within the population of T cells there is a reduction in the proportion of CD4 and an increase in CD8 cells, the helper and cytotoxic/ suppressor cell populations, respectively [24,53]. These changes are reflected also in the functional activity of T cells (see below). Since the number of B cells is normal [54] and that of T cells is markedly reduced the proportion of null cells which lack markers of both cell types is markedly increased. Many of these null cells may represent T-cell progenitors, for two reasons. Firstly, the enzyme terminal deoxynucleotidyl transferase is elevated in peripheral blood mononuclear cells of PCM subjects [54]. This enzyme is a marker of T cells at early maturational stages and in PCM its level was found to correlate directly with the proportion of null cells. Secondly, serum thymic hormone activity is decreased is PCM [23], probably because of the extreme thymic involution. The *in vitro* addition of a thymic hormonal preparation to PCM lymphocytes resulted in increased percentage of E rosette-forming cells [55–57]. These changes can be probably attributed to the severe restriction of active cell division which is characteristic of lymphoid tissue. In addition, lymphoid cell death may also be accelerated, particularly in the thymus, because of changes in hormonal milieu. For example, plasma cortisol levels are often raised and adrenalectomized animals have been found to survive prolonged protein deficiency without profound involution of lymphoid tissue. Part of the cortisol effect may be related to the hypoalbuminaemia of PCM, since a large proportion of the hormone is unbound and physiologically active. Finally, infections which are most common in PCM contribute to the changes in lymphoid tissues.

Humoral immunity appears to be only minimally affected by PCM [58]. The number of B cells is normal and the cells are able to mount a relatively adequate antibody response after immunization. However, responses to antigens requiring the help of T lymphocytes, macrophages or both are affected. Apparently, some mechanisms exist that enable cells selectively to utilize amino acids to favour host survival. Whereas serum albumin is markedly reduced during PCM, children with infection are able to divert sufficient amino acids from other potential uses to manufacture immunoglobulins and acute-phase proteins. Accordingly, serum immunoglobulin levels are usually normal. Moreover, in many cases of PCM hypergammaglobulinaemia [often predominantly of immunoglobulin M (IgM) type] is present, accompanied by detectable IgE levels, which are normally absent in individuals with adequate dietary intake. These abnormalities may reflect decreased T-cell functions, chronic or recurrent infections or parasitic infestation and increased gastrointestinal permeability to food antigens. On the other hand, secretory IgA level is low in PCM [20,59]. This may be correlated with the increased incidence of Gram-negative septicaemia in such patients. The secretory IgA level is probably related to reduced synthesis of the secretory component by gut epithelial cells, since serum IgA levels are normal. In severe cases of PCM, a reduction in all antibody-producing cells occurs. This is particularly true for children suffering from nutritional marasmus, whereas patients with kwashiorkor have high immunoglobulin values. The antibodies produced in PCM are of low affinity [25], resulting in the frequent occurrence of immune complexes in the serum. These complexes may inhibit other immune functions and cause immune complex disease.

Production of complement components is also reduced in PCM [60,61]. However, the main reason for the observed decreased complement levels is most probably increased consumption.

CMI is profoundly impaired [37]. This is evident from the typical changes in lymphoid tissue cellularity; the composition of lymphoid cell subpopulations (see above); the pattern of micro-organisms recovered from these patients, and the tests for T-cell function. These tests include:

1 Delayed-type hypersensitivity (DTH) skin reactions both to recall antigens and to primary sensitization. The recall antigens, such as mumps, tetanus, trichophyton or tuberculin evaluate the memory T cells and inflammatory (phagocytic) cells, both depressed in PCM. The primary sensitization is performed with dinitrochlorobenzene (DNCB) or keyhole limpet haemocyanin and tests the afferent limb of CMI which is also defective in PCM. These skin tests are sensitive measures of CMI depression in PCM, even in its milder forms [30,38,62,63].

2 Lymphocyte proliferative response (PR) to mitogens is frequently reduced [29,37]. More consistent reduction is seen when autologous sera are used for culture, suggesting that PCM serum contains inhibitory factors and/or lacks supporting factors for cell proliferation [19,64,65].

3 Lymphokine production is also frequently impaired. Synthesis of interleukin-2 and of interferon is reduced [66], whereas production of leucocyte or macrophage migration inhibition factors is normal or only slightly reduced [31].

The substantial reduction in CMI, which is much more profound than in humoral immunity, is related not only to the aforementioned decrease in T cells but also to the appearance of inhibitors of immune response such as endotoxins, antigen-antibody complexes and C-reactive protein. In addition, a reduction in the production of thymic hormones and regulatory lymphokines contributes to impaired T-cell function.

Phagocytic cell functions were also impaired in PCM [26,32,67]. Cell number and phagocytosis are usually normal. However, the oxidative and glycolytic activities of these cells are reduced and this is accompanied by impaired bactericidal activity by neutrophils and macrophages [68]. The enzymes myeloperoxidase, lysozyme and NADPH oxidase are reduced in PCM, probably in connection with the respective deficiency of iron or vitamin A (see below) or the increased levels of plasma cortisol. Myeloperoxidase is an iron-dependent enzyme;

NADPH oxidase level is modified by cortisol. In addition, the macrophages in PCM are not able to process antigen properly—a defect which may contribute to the appearance of immune complexes. This defect, together with the reduced production of lymphokines and chemotactic factors, contributes to the decreased DTH mentioned before.

Susceptibility to infections is substantially increased in PCM [14], and represents a major hallmark of this condition. PCM is accompanied by a high incidence of infections, particularly with mycobacteria, viruses and fungi, in which CMI is more important than humoral response. The reduction of natural defence mechanisms at surface areas of lungs and intestines (e.g. secretory IgA, lysozyme), the impairment in phagocytic inflammatory cell function and the decreased complement activity further contribute to the frequency and severity of infections in PCM, and the infections, in turn, aggravate PCM and immune dysfunction, creating a vicious cycle [69].

PCM during pregnancy may have deleterious effects on the development of lymphoid organs, particularly the thymus, in the foetus, with marked suppression of both cellular and humoral immunity and increased vulnerability to infection during the neonatal period [70–73].

Extreme variations in the expression of immune dysfunctions in PCM may exist, including in the degree and the relative emphasis on impairment of humoral or cellular immunity [32,38]. This may be related to the time and extent of protein or calorie deprivation, to the type and extent of concomitant nutrient deficiencies (e.g. vitamins, minerals), and to accompanying conditions, particularly infections.

Renourishment of severely malnourished human subjects or animals results in a rapid restoration of immune functions [33]. Moreover, malnourished animals provided with low amounts of protein may preferentially utilize the nitrogen supply to restore immune functions at the expense of restoration of body stores [74]. Immune response to a mucosally encountered antigen recovers very quickly with renourishment, even to the extent of allowing an enhanced rebound of the PFC response [75]. Malnourished children who underwent nutritional therapy preserved all corrected immune functions even at 10 years after therapy [76].

Protein and amino acid deficiencies (experimental)

The creation of protein or individual amino acid deficiencies is highly artificial and can be generated experimentally in animals as a tool for the better understanding of clinical malnutrition, in particular of the various forms of PCM.

Protein deficiency

Protein deficiency in animals chronically fed a low-protein diet caused immune dysfunction which was different in young and adult animals [77–80]. Such a diet at *young age* caused mainly T-cell dysfunction, including involution of the thymus and other lymphoid organs, DTH response to primary sensitization and recall antigens, skin allograft rejection, *in vitro* response to allogeneic cells and mitogens and cytotoxic T-cell activity. Antibody response to T-cell-dependent antigens (e.g. sheep RBC) was decreased and could be restored by injection of normal syngeneic thymocytes, suggesting defective helper T-cell function. On the other hand, immunoglobulin levels and induction of antibody response to B-cell-dependent antigens were normal. However, when extremely low amounts of proteins were used in animal feeding, both humoral and cellular immunity were decreased.

When *adult* animals were chronically fed with a low-protein diet, a different profile of immune dysfunction emerged. Humoral immunity was profoundly reduced, with lower levels of immunoglobulins and increased susceptibility to bacterial infections. A low-protein diet (10% ovalbumin) increased the susceptibility of guinea pigs to infection with *Mycobacterium bovis* [81–83]. On the other hand, efficacy of vaccination against *Listeria monocytogenes* was not impaired under such conditions [84]. The main defect was in the number of antibody-forming cells, since immunoglobulin production per antibody-forming cell was unchanged. Secretory IgA response was found to be reduced in Balb/c mice fed isocaloric diets containing 2–4% protein [85]. This can be attributed in part to stimulation of suppressor T cells in such animals [86]. In contrast, CMI was enhanced, including increased number and competence of T cells, with enhanced capacity for allograft rejection, graft versus host reaction, and *in vitro* PR to T-cell mitogens. A similar situation, different from classical PCM, was described in children with chronic protein deprivation, who had increased T-cell-mediated immune responses and reduced B-cell functions. These observations, which contradict those in PCM, may be related to the chronicity and extent of the deficiency and differences in accompanying deficiencies, which allows a different pattern of adaptation.

Moderate protein deprivation (4% casein) resulted in delay in tumour development and increased generation of tumour cytolytic T cells [87].

The effect of protein deprivation on the development of autoimmune disorders was studied in NZB mice which were prone to develop a systemic lupus erythematosus (SLE)-like syndrome. Chronic, partial protein restriction (6% casein) on an isocaloric diet postponed the onset of SLE symptoms but did not prolong life [88]. The diet prevented thymic involution, splenomegaly and aberrations in immune response observed in the control, normally fed (22% casein) NZB mice. Protein restriction was less effective than calorie deprivation in prolonging the survival of NZB/W mice [89] (NZB/W develop autoimmune manifestations earlier than NZB).

Amino acids

The role of individual amino acids in the maintenance of a competent immune system was studied in experimental animals by feeding diets with isolated deficits or excesses of a single essential amino acid or an imbalance among essential amino acids. Most amino acid deficiencies are associated with a reduction in humoral immunity, particularly the antibody response to new antigens and not with CMI impairment. Amino acid imbalances may have a similar effect. With long-lasting amino acid deficits the entire immune system is affected. Continued deficiencies of branched chain or sulphur-containing amino acids lead to a depletion of cells from lymphoid tissues [90]. Isolated tryptophan [91,92] or phenylalanine [92] deficiencies resulted in depressed antibody response to sheep RBC; a combined deficiency of both led also to partial atrophy of the spleen and thymus [93]. On the other hand, a diet supplemented with tryptophan caused a significant decrease in chick mortality to *Escherichia coli* [94]. The combined restriction of tyrosine and phenylalanine in the diet of human healthy volunteers resulted in an increase in the number and activity of natural killer cells and in an increased proportion of T cells of both CD4 and CD8 phenotype [95]. An isolated deficiency of valine, threonine or isoleucine or a combined deficiency of methionine and cysteine or phenylalanine and tyrosine also caused profound suppression of antibody response, whereas isolated deficiency of arginine, histidine or lysine caused only moderate impairment of antibody response [91]. On the other hand, in a study on mice, diet supplemented with arginine enhanced PR to *Listeria monocytogenes*, and to phytohaemagglutinin (PHA) but not to concanavalin A (Con A), and enhanced production of interferon-γ [96]. However, the *in vivo* immuno-enhancing effects of arginine do not reflect the direct effects of arginine *in vitro* [97].

Leucine deficiency had no effect on antibody response, but, in contrast to all other amino acid deficiencies or imbalances, increased the activity of cytotoxic T lymphocytes (CTL) directed against inoculated tumour cell antigens [98]. On the other hand, diet rich in leucine given to rats fed a protein-poor diet did reduce antibody response, serum IgG levels and lymphopoiesis. The combined effects of a leucine overload with a protein-poor diet were comparable to that produced by complete elimination of protein from the diet [99,100]. The effect of leucine excess may be related to activation of enzymes involved in the catabolism of valine and isoleucine. Indeed, the addition of small amounts of these two amino acids to the leucine-rich, protein-poor diet prevented the immune system effects of the latter [100].

An interesting connection was found between amino acids in diet and autoimmunity. Partial deprivation of selected amino acids, e.g. phenylalanine and tyrosine, prolonged survival and inhibited autoimmune pathology in lupus-prone NZB/W mice [101,102]. Moreover, a fully synthetic amino acid diet had a profound effect in decreasing SLE pathology in NZB/W female mice [103] or autoimmune diabetes in Wistar BB rats [104]. It may be that antigens associated with dietary proteins may be involved in the development of autoimmune disorders. Such antigens are capable of inducing cross-reactive

autoimmunity in a way similar to that of infectious agents or pharmacological substances [105–114].

In summary, the most prominent change observed in animals fed single amino acid-deficient diets is some reduction in *de novo* production of antibody to a new antigen. This relatively minor immune impairment may be attributed to a disturbed amino acid distribution required for protein synthesis by a new clone of antibody-producing cells. This is only the final step in a complex immunogenic sequence which starts with antigen recognition and processing, and continues with clonal expansion. Only the final stage of immunoglobulin synthesis is deficient in animals subjected to brief periods of amino acid imbalance. More profound amino acid deficit combined with other nutrient deficiencies will ultimately bring us closer to the situation of chronic clinical malnutrition.

Lipids

In the immune system lipids serve two major functions: as the main structural building blocks of the cell membranes, like other cells of the body, and as intercellular mediators [115]. The lipid fraction of the lymphocyte (and phagocytic cell) surface membrane is composed of phospholipids, cholesterol and small amounts of glycolipids. The exact composition of the lipid bilayer of the membrane can affect lymphocyte function in two major ways: by modifying cell membrane fluidity which influences ligand (e.g. antigen, mitogen, lymphokine, hormone) and membrane receptor interaction, as well as cell-to-cell interactions, permeability and enzyme activity, and by changing the availability of eicosanoid precursors for prostaglandins, leukotrienes and thromboxane-strong modulators of immune responsiveness [116,117].

Cell membrane fluidity is dependent on two determinants—the molar ratio of cholesterol to phospholipids and the degree of saturation of fatty acids in the phospholipid fraction. The more cholesterol or saturated fatty acids in the surface membrane structure, the more rigid it becomes, with a profound effect on the functional status of the cell. Since fatty acid carbon chains have an angular bend at the site of each unsaturated double bond, they require more space in the lipid bilayer than straight chain saturated fatty acids, with resultant increased fluidity [118]. Cell membrane fluidity is also affected by the translocation of phospholipids from the inside to the outside of the cell membrane, which is caused by phospholipid methylation, stimulating lectins, immunoglobulins and chemotactic proteins [119]. Two phosphoglycerides (phosphatidylcholine and phosphatidylethanolamine) are the major phospholipids in lymphocyte surface membrane. Phosphatidylinositol is a minor component, but of much importance for lymphocyte activation [120]. The lymphocyte surface membrane is also rich in sphingomyelin. The glycolipids serve functions similar to those of surface proteins and glycoproteins, i.e. as cell-surface antigens and receptors. As such they are involved in the mediation of cellular recognition and interactions [121,122].

The main trigger for lymphocyte activation is the binding of a ligand (antigen, mitogen) to its receptor on the cell surface, followed by aggregation or capping of the receptors. These events cause profound changes in membrane composition with a high turnover of fatty acyl moieties, changes in phosphatidylinositol metabolism, initiation of eicosanoid biosynthesis pathways, changes in ion permeability including calcium, with subsequent induction of RNA, protein and finally DNA synthesis and cell proliferation. The changes in fatty acyl moieties introduce more polyunsaturated fatty acids (PUFA) into the membrane structure with resultant increased fluidity and availability of eicosanoid precursors. The composition of the lipids in the diet may accordingly have a major direct impact on key processes during the development of the immune response. Various lipid constituents may have this impact by actual incorporation into the lipid bilayer of the membrane, by enzyme induction or even by a detergent effect. The following discussion will concentrate first on total lipids and then on the major constituents: PUFA (compared with saturated fatty acids) and cholesterol and their effect on the immune system. The effect of dietary phospholipids was not systematically studied.

Total lipids, specific fatty acids and obesity

Both total lipid intake and the presence of specific fatty acids in a given concentration may influence discrete immune functions. The presence of unsaturated bonds changes entirely the function of the fatty acid molecule with a progressively greater impact on the immune system as the number of bonds increases from one (oleic acid) to two (linoleic acid), three (linolenic acid) or four (arachidonic acid) double bonds. Generally, diets high in PUFA are more immunosuppressive than diets high in saturated fats. Obesity is also being dealt with in this connection. Although obesity may not be caused by fat intake only, excessive dietary lipids and obesity are nevertheless related and should be discussed together.

Lymphoid tissue cellularity is reduced in genetically obese mice—C57B1/6j (*ob/ob*). The thymic and splenic tissues are small in size and contain fewer than normal mononuclear cells and the proportion of immunocompetent cells is changed [123]. PUFA, particularly arachidonic acid and its precursors, cause a decrease in splenic and thymic weights [124,125]. The arachidonic acid effect is prevented by inhibitors of prostaglandin synthesis and not by adrenalectomy.

Humoral immunity is also changed in the obese mice with slight-to-moderate reduction in the number of splenic IgG-producing cells [123]. Antigen challenge of mice infused with methyl palmitate was not followed by antibody production [126]. On the other hand, PUFA deficiency inhibited IgM and IgG response to primary and secondary immunization against sheep RBC in mice [127], to be corrected by inclusion of PUFA in the diet. Moreover, a diet rich in PUFA increased IgG (but not IgA or IgM) response as compared to normally fed controls.

CMI is impaired in obese individuals, as measured *in vivo* and *in vitro*. Obese mice immunized *in vivo* with lymphoma cells show a diminished capacity to generate cytotoxic T cells, although their natural killer cell activity is increased [123]. High levels of PUFA suppressed CMI, including prolongation of skin allografts in mice or rats [128–133], decreased DTH reaction to B_{16} melanoma in mice [134], suppressed graft versus host response, decreased susceptibility to induction of experimental allergic encephalomyelitis in rats by injection of brain homogenate in adjuvant [135,136] and decreased PR to PHA, Con A or PPD and cytotoxic activity in mouse spleen cells [129,131,137–139].

The dose, composition and route of administration of PUFA are critical determinants of experimental outcome. For example, feeding mice a diet rich in α-linolenic acid enhances cell-mediated cytotoxic response to a viral challenge. Excess dietary PUFA improved kidney transplant survival in humans [140,141]. PUFA-deficient diets caused effects which were opposite to those described above [128–132,135,136,142,143], an effect which was not found to be correlated with decreased prostaglandin synthesis [144].

Phagocytic cell function may be decreased as a result of lipid overload. Intravenous infusion of methyl palmitate [126] or ethyl stearate [145] inhibited phagocytic function and clearance of colloidal carbon. Chemotactic, phagocytic and bactericidal activities of human neutrophils were inhibited by infusion of soybean oil emulsion to healthy subjects or by adding this emulsion [146] or free fatty acids bound to albumin [147] to neutrophil suspensions *in vitro*. Saturated or unsaturated fatty acids added *in vitro* inhibited to a varying degree macrophage colony formation from murine bone marrow cells stimulated by colony-stimulating factor-1 (CSF-1) [148]. Macrophage mobility stimulated by PPD [130,149] was diminished in the presence of PUFA *in vitro*. However, this may be a toxic rather than physiological effect [150], since PUFA was dissolved into the medium in alcohol in these studies, instead of using it as albumin-bound molecules [151]. The proportions of α-linolenic to linoleic acids in diet affected prostaglandin metabolism in peritoneal macrophages which in turn modulate ariginase activity in these cells [152], important for ornithine and consequently DNA synthesis [153]. On the other hand, conflicting results exist as to the correlation between prostaglandin levels and phagocytosis in such macrophages [152,154]. Changes in PUFA proportions also modify the types of leukotrienes produced by macrophages [155,156]. Similar studies were performed in humans [157].

Susceptibility to infection was assessed in several studies with conflicting results. Susceptibility was increased in obese dogs who developed paralytic encephalitis when inoculated with distemper virus [158]. Dogs on a high-fat diet developed more severe experimental viral hepatitis than their normally fed litter-mates [159]. On the other hand, the use of saturated vegetable oil as the sole source of dietary fat increased the resistance of mice to experimental tuberculosis [160]. The use of fat as an isocaloric substitute for carbohydrates in rats increased their resistance to infection by several bacteria and parasites.

Autoimmune disorders were significantly improved by using low-fat diets. In NZB/W mice, a high-fat diet (regardless of the type of fatty acid) enhanced the appearance of immune complex nephritis and promoted early death, whereas a low-fat diet had the opposite effect [161–165]. The low-fat diet also decreased manifestations of Sjögren's syndrome in these mice. The degree of fat saturation influenced the type of autoantibodies produced [161], the type and location of glomerular deposition [163], helper T-cell function and prostaglandin levels in lymphoid tissues [166]. The usual forms of prostaglandins and leukotrienes derived from arachidonic acid are potent inflammatory mediators. On the other hand, eicosapentaenoic acid (EPA), a minor precursor of arachidonic acid, is the source of anti-inflammatory forms of prostaglandins and leukotrienes (PGE_3 and LTD5). Indeed, safflower oil, rich in arachidonic acid precursors (e.g. linoleic acid), enhanced autoimmune symptomatology in NZB/W or MRL/1rp mice, whereas the absence of arachidonic acid precursors in the diet as well as supplementation with EPA (fish oil) resulted in depression of autoimmune manifestations and increased survival [161,167–171]. The results of initial clinical studies, testing the use of EPA in rheumatoid arthritis, are compatible with the animal studies [172–174].

In summary, the consistent beneficial effect of a low-fat diet on autoimmune disorders can be explained by the connection between fatty acids and prostaglandin and leukotriene production, by the regulatory effects of lipoproteins on lymphocytes [175] and by the direct action of lipids on the composition and fluidity of lymphocyte surface membranes [6].

Tumour development is enhanced by high-fat diets rich in PUFA [176–179]. In chemically induced breast tumours in rats, each doubling of dietary fat concentration approximately doubled the chance of tumour development [178]. In another study, the rate of growth of a transplantable mammary tumour was greater with higher (10–20%) dietary fat content as compared to low (2–5%) ones. The tumour-promoting effects of the high-fat diets were completely abrogated by indomethacin treatment [180]. In addition, natural killer cell activity was diminished in tumour-bearing rats fed a high-fat diet [181]. On the other hand, EPA-rich fish oil reduced the incidence and volume of tumour development [182–184]. These results are compatible with epidemiological data on the correlation between dietary fat and breast cancer.

There is evidence that some of the tumour-promoting effects of dietary lipids are immune-mediated. Two pathways for these effects may be conceived: modification of lipid composition of the target tumour cell membranes, which influences their response to cytolytic attack by either various cytotoxic cells or by complement-mediated lysis [179,185,186], and regulatory and cell membrane effects on lymphocytes, which affect recruitment of cytotoxic T cells and their frequency [187,188] or of natural killer cells [189]. The regulatory effects are prostaglandin-mediated and therefore indomethacin-inhibited [190,191].

Cholesterol

The cholesterol content of the cell membrane determines membrane fluidity—the higher its concentration in the membrane, the less fluid it is. Decreased membrane fluidity interferes with receptor movement.

Effects of cholesterol on the immune system were studied only in its excess, by introducing it in the diet or by parenteral administration.

Humoral immunity is modified by cholesterol excess. However, conflicting results exist as to the direction of change. In some studies hypercholesterolaemia in mice or rabbits caused a decrease in antibody response [192,193], whereas in others antibody titres were increased [194,195].

DTH skin test reaction is increased in hypercholesterolaemic monkeys or rabbits [192,194]. The PR to PHA and the cytotoxic activity induced by allogeneic cells are dependent on cholesterol from either endogenous synthesis or uptake from plasma or medium when bound to lipoprotein [196,197].

Conflicting results also exist in respect to phago-cytic cell functions. Phagocytosis was found to be reduced in one study [198], increased in another [192] and unchanged in still another [199]. Obviously, the exact conditions of the experiments influence their outcome. However, it seems plausible to conclude that the influence of cholesterol availability and/or metabolism on the phagocytic capabilities of cells may be related to the requirement for a net synthesis of cell membrane cholesterol and phospholipid after phagocytic activity [200].

The existence of conflicting data may be explained by the fact that a balance is needed between plasma, membrane and intracellular cholesterol content (and synthesis) in order to achieve optimal lymphocyte response and phagocytic functions. On the one hand, cholesterol synthesis plays an important role in lymphocyte proliferation and accordingly, an excess of exogenous cholesterol turns off endogenous cholesterol synthesis needed for lymphocyte response to antigen. On the other hand, the cholesterol-induced decrease in membrane fluidity is associated with enhanced T-cell activity.

Lipoproteins

Plasma lipoproteins were shown to have a regulatory effect on the immune response [201]. The effects are mediated via direct contact with immune cell membranes or by regulating the supply of lipids such as cholesterol. The various lipoproteins have different but overlapping effects on the immune system.

High density lipoproteins (HDL) combine with lymphocytes and facilitate cholesterol removal. Membrane fluidity and endogenous cholesterol synthesis are modified as a result. It was shown by us to be a vital culture medium constituent for the growth of several human or mouse thymic stromal cell subpopulations grown in serum-free defined medium on extracellular matrix [202,203].

Intermediate density lipoproteins (IDL) have a strong effect on the PR of human lymphocytes ([204] and see below).

Low density lipoproteins (LDL) transport cholesterol and regulate its biosynthesis in human lymphocytes. The PR is suppressed by LDL, an activity which can be attributed to the apoprotein ([205,206] and see below).

Very low density lipoproteins (VLDL) inhibit the

initiation of protein synthesis and subsequent DNA synthesis in lymphocytes. It inhibits the primary haemagglutinin response of mice to sheep RBC [207].

Other effects which were ascribed to lipoproteins include:

1 Suppression of the PR of T cells. All classes of lipoproteins can suppress the PR of human [204] or mouse [208] lymphocytes to allogeneic cells or to the lectins PHA and Con A. The order of inhibitory potency was: IDL > VLDL > LDL > HDL. The inhibitions took place with low physiological levels of the lipoproteins, suggesting an important modulatory effect on circulating lymphocytes *in vivo*. The lipid part, probably cholesterol, appeared to be the active inhibitory part of the lipoprotein molecule, since delipidation of the lipoproteins eliminated their activity [208]. A subclass of LDL was found to be particularly inhibitory to PR, either because of the presence in it of oxygenated cholesterol or the activity of the apoprotein [205]. LDL was shown to interact with the lymphocyte surface membrane, most probably via specific receptors and prevent calcium accumulation in the stimulated lymphocytes and thus inhibit their subsequent activation. Cord blood LDL or HDL of neonates had a two- to fourfold lower inhibitory effect on adult lymphocyte PR [209].

2 Suppression of tumoricidal activity of macrophages by a high level of lipoproteins.

3 Reduction in T-cell rosetting.

4 Inhibition of attachment of certain complement components to cell surfaces.

Taking all the data on lipids and the immune system together it is clear that the relative availability of the various lipids to the body can profoundly influence immune functions because they are vital components of cell membrane, or interact with the cell surface and because some of them serve as precursors of the prostaglandin or leukotriene and thromboxane series of molecules which are potent regulators of immunological and inflammatory processes. We are just beginning to appreciate the dynamic role lipids can play in regulating immune responses.

Water-soluble vitamins

The water-soluble vitamins consist of members of the vitamin B complex and vitamin C (ascorbic acid). The vitamin B complex comprises a large number of compounds that differ extensively in chemical structure and biological action. The reason for grouping them in a single class was their original isolation from the same sources, notably liver and yeast. Because of their somewhat similar distribution in foods there is a tendency for dietary deficiency to involve several members of the vitamin B complex in the same patient. These vitamins function in intermediary metabolism in many essential reactions.

The interaction between B complex vitamins and the immune system was noticed in the 1920s [210] with the appearance of lymphopenia and lymphoid tissue atrophy in deficient mice. However, only recent work has identified specific isolated vitamin B effects on the immune system. In practice the incidence of isolated vitamin B deficiency state is extremely low today. However, combined multinutrient deficiencies always include some B-group vitamins. Accordingly, the mechanism of specific vitamin B effects on immune functions should be studied in experimental animals and on cultured cells. The discussion of each vitamin will be preceded by a short description of its biochemistry, physiology and clinical pathology. More details can be found in [3].

Thiamine (vitamin B₁)

Thiamine, a molecule containing a pyrimidine and a thiazole nucleus, functions in the body in carbohydrate metabolism in the form of the coenzyme thiamine pyrophosphate. Its deficiency may cause beri-beri with polyneuritis and cardiac failure. Milder deficiency conditions may be manifested by anorexia and constipation. In alcoholics, thiamine deficiency causes Wernicke–Korsakoff encephalopathy.

Thiamine has a moderate effect on the immune system in animals [211–213]. Inhibition of splenic plaque-forming cell formation was observed in thiamine-deficient rats after immunization with sheep RBC. An overt excess of thiamine [up to 100-fold more than the recommended daily allowance (RDA)] can stimulate neutrophil chemotaxis and motility *in vivo* or *in vitro* [214–217]. Other host defence functions (e.g. antibody response, PR to PHA, DTH, neutrophil counts) do not seem to be altered by a high intake of thiamine, as judged from an epidemiological study on elderly patients who took high levels of multivitamin preparations [218].

Riboflavin (vitamin B₂)

Riboflavin (vitamin B₂)

Riboflavin is a yellow pigmented compound of the flavin group which carries out its functions in the body in one of two coenzyme forms: flavin mononucleotide (FMN) and flavin adenine dinucleotide (FAD). These coenzymes are part of a wide variety of respiratory flavoproteins. Its deficiency causes angular stomatitis, seborrhoeic dermatitis and other epidermal mucosal derangements.

The main effect of riboflavin deficiency on the immune system is diminished antibody response to test antigens, e.g. depressed haemagglutinating antibody responses to human RBC, diphtheria toxin or staphylococcal antigen [211]. The diminished response could be corrected by additional boost immunizations [219]. Thymic weight may be decreased in such animals. Overt excess (5–100-fold over RDA) of riboflavin did not enhance immune parameters in elderly subjects [218].

Niacin (nicotinic acid; vitamin B₃)

Niacin (nicotinic acid; vitamin B₃)

Nicotinic acid functions in the body after conversion to nicotinamide adenine dinucleotide (NAD), to serve as a coenzyme for a wide variety of proteins that catalyse oxidation–reduction reactions essential for tissue respiration. Its deficiency leads to the clinical condition known as pellagra, which is characterized by dermatitis, diarrhoea and dementia.

The effects of niacin on the immune system were studied both *in vivo* and *in vitro*. Reduced levels of niacin in chicken's diet did not affect the immune response in several tests [220]. On the other hand it did serve as an adjuvant to antibody production against bacterial α-amylase in guinea pigs, when given in moderate excess [221]. It did not have an effect on DTH. However, it was shown to have a mitogenic, or a co-mitogenic (with PHA) effect on lymphocyte PR [221,222].

Pyridoxine (vitamin B₆)

Pyridoxine (vitamin B₆)

Pyridoxine, a molecule based on the pyridine ring, exists in three molecular forms: pyridoxine (free alcohol), pyridoxal (aldehyde) and pyridoxamine (contains the aminomethyl group). The last two forms are the physiologically active ones when phosphorylated. Pyridoxine serves as a coenzyme for a wide variety of metabolic transformations of amino acids and nucleic acids and is essential for cell multiplication. The main deficiency symptoms are hypochromic anaemia and central nervous system lesions. It may also cause cheilosis, glossitis and dermatitis, a potential source of infections. The antagonist deoxypyridoxine can be used rapidly to induce experimental deficiency. The other alternative, which can be used also in combination with the antagonist, is a pyridoxine-deficient diet.

Because of the central role of pyridoxine in amino acid and nucleic acid metabolism, pyridoxine deficiency causes more profound effects on the immune system than deficiencies of any other B-group vitamin [223,224]. The effects include lymphoid tissue depletion and suppression of both humoral and CMI.

Lymphoid tissue depletion was observed as a decrease in thymic weight of deficient rats [225], as splenic hypoplasia in foetuses of deficient pregnant rats [226] and as lymphopenia measured in many species [90].

A diminished antibody response to primary or even secondary immunization with several antigens or to influenza virus infection was observed in pyridoxine-deficient rats or guinea pigs [211,227]. The antibodies produced by such animals had a diminished binding affinity [224]. It should be emphasized that even when the primary response was normal before induction of pyridoxine deficiency, the secondary response was abrogated. On the other hand, if the vitamin is absent during a primary immunization, anamnestic responses will not occur even when the nutritional deficiency is restored. Repeated immunization did not help to improve the response. Even a diet with a reduced pyridoxine amount (0.1–0.3 of regular dose) showed some impairment of antibody response [228]. A diminished response was also observed in pyridoxine-deficient human volunteers immunized with tetanus toxoid or typhoid vaccine [229]. A combination of pyridoxine and pantothenic acid deficiency caused complete inhibition of antibody response [230]. On the other hand, pyridoxine deficiency did not alter anaphylactic reactions of guinea pigs immunized and challenged with bovine serum albumin [231].

Pyridoxine-deficient guinea pigs showed a diminished DTH response to PPD despite previous exposure to the antigen [224,232]. However, in contrast to the humoral response, the sensitization mechanism was not inhibited in the deficient animals; if sensitized during the period of pyridoxine deficiency, guinea pigs regained their normal responsiveness after correction of the deficiency [233]. Pyridoxine-deficient mice inoculated with P815 tumour cells showed a significantly reduced CTL response to the tumour cells [234]. Natural killer cell activity was not impaired. Serum thymic factor level was decreased in pyridoxine-deficient animals [235]. Reduced immunocompetence, as evidenced by decreased T-cell rosette formation and by reduced PR to PHA, in haemodialysis patients, could be corrected by excess pyridoxine in diet [236].

Allograft survival is prolonged in pyridoxine-deficient animals. Returning the recipient animals to a normal diet 3–4 weeks after transplantation did not increase the incidence of rejection [237]. The ability of thoracic duct lymphocytes to respond *in vitro* to allogeneic cells was diminished in deficient rats [238,239]. However, no impairment in the response to lipopolysaccharide was observed [240].

Phagocytic cell functions were improved by pyridoxine therapy, including oxidative burst activity and chemotaxis [236]. On the other hand, pyridoxine deficiency was shown to reduce phagocytosis by alveolar macrophages and production of macrophage-activating factor (MAF) in rats [241].

Immunity against tumours was impaired in pyridoxine-deficient mice challenged with Molony sarcoma virus or inoculated with P815 tumour cells, as judged by increased tumour incidence and size and by reduced CTL to the tumour cells [234,242].

Susceptibility to infections was increased in pyridoxine-deficient rats [243].

Pyridoxine excess has not been shown to improve (or decrease) the immune response in animals or in humans [218,234].

In summary, pyridoxine deficiency affects primarily T and B cell functions with a smaller effect on phagocytic and natural killer cell functions. Pyridoxine excess is of no value for the immune system.

Pantothenic acid

Pantothenic acid, an organic acid, functions in the body following its incorporation into coenzyme A which serves as a cofactor for a variety of enzyme-catalysed reactions involving transfer of acetyl (two carbon) groups. The main deficiency symptoms include fatigue, headache, nausea, paraesthesias and incoordination.

The effect of deficiency on the immune system is related primarily to humoral response, not to CMI. In rats the impairment could not be corrected by increasing the immunizing antigen dose but was prevented by correcting the vitamin deficit. Several antigens were used, including *Salmonella pullorum* [244], influenza virus and human or sheep RBC [245]. Studies in pantothenic acid-deficient human volunteers [229,230,246] revealed only a slight reduction in antibody response to vaccination with influenza virus or tetanus toxoid and no effect on allograft rejection. However, combined pyridoxine and pantothenic acid deficiency caused a profound reduction in antibody response.

Biotin

Biotin, an organic acid, serves as a coenzyme for several enzyme-catalysed carboxylation reactions and plays an important role in both carbohydrate and fat metabolism. The main symptoms of deficiency include nausea, depression, muscle pain, anaemia, dermatitis, atrophic glossitis and hyper-aesthesia.

In experimental biotin deficiency in rats the main immune disorder was found to be impairment in antibody response [211,247]. However, other studies also showed an impaired CMI. Biotin-deficient guinea pigs had a reduction of B and T lymphocytes to about half of the normal numbers, whereas the number of neutrophils was doubled [248]. Biotin-deficient rats showed a marked reduction in thymus size and cellularity, but not in that of the spleen [249]. These rats failed to develop experimental allergic encephalomyelitis, a typical CMI response.

An extensive combination of immunodeficiencies was found in siblings with an inherited disorder of biotin-dependent carboxylase enzymes which catabolize branched chain amino acids [250,251]. These children had a low serum IgA concentration, a lack of T-cell-independent antibody response (e.g. pneumococcal polysaccharide vaccine), a diminished T-cell proliferation response *in vitro* to *Candida* antigen and an absence of DTH reaction. The children also suffered from central nervous system dysfunction, alopecia and conjunctivitis. The discrepancy between the derangements in experimental biotin deficiency and the inherited disorder suggests additional metabolic defects in the latter.

An increase in high-affinity rosette formation by T lymphocytes of healthy human subjects was noticed after *in vitro* incubation of peripheral blood mononuclear cells (PBMC) with Con A and biotin [252].

Folic acid (pteroilglutamic acid)

The chemical structure of folic acid is based on the pteridine ring linked by a methylene bridge to a para-amino benzoic acid which is joined by an amide linkage to glutamic acid. The active metabolic form is tetrahydrofolic acid which acts as an acceptor of a one carbon unit. It is a key coenzyme in several important reactions in amino acid and nucleic acid metabolism. The main manifestation of deficiency is megaloblastic anaemia.

Folic acid deficiency results in a widespread impairment of the immune system including both humoral and CMI as well as diminished resistance to infection.

The antibody response to *Rickettsia typhi* was diminished in vitamin-deficient rats, but corrected by increased antigen dose or by boosting with the antigen [219]. A similar reduction was observed in the number of splenic plaque-forming cells in folate-deficient rats immunized with sheep RBC [90,247].

A decrease in thymus size and a reduction in the number of T cells in the spleen and peripheral blood was observed in folate-deficient rats [90,253]. The response to PHA was reduced both *in vivo* (skin test) and *in vitro* (proliferation of spleen cells) [90]. Methotrexate, a folic acid antagonist, can block the development of contact sensitivity development in mice [254].

Folic acid deficiency-induced megaloblastic anaemia in humans is accompanied by immune dysfunctions, including an impaired proliferative response to PHA *in vitro* and a DTH response to dinitrochlorobenzene *in vivo* [255]. Phagocytic and bactericidal activities in such patients were normal [256]. However, in a more recent study [257,258] neutrophil phagocytosis and bactericidal activity were impaired in PCM patients. Folic acid therapy resulted in correction of phagocytosis but not bactericidal activity, with good temporal correlation between folic acid levels and the degree of correction of phagocytosis. However, another report suggests that impaired phagocytosis is related to vitamin B_{12}, not folic acid, deficiency [259].

Susceptibility to infections was profoundly increased in folate-deficient guinea pigs. Inoculation of 10^9 *Shigella flexneri* bacteria caused an 89% mortality in these animals (there were no deaths in the control group) [260]. Similarly, folic acid-deficient mice were more susceptible to murine rotavirus infection [261].

Vitamin B_{12} (cyanocobalamin)

Vitamin B_{12} has a complex structural formula; the core portion is a porphyrin-like ring-structure with four reduced pyrrole rings linked to a central cobalt atom and extensively substituted with methyl, acetamide and propiononamide residues. The active coenzymes, methylcobalamin and 5-deoxyadenoylcobalamin, are essential for cell growth and replication and the maintenance of normal myelin throughout the nervous system. When concentrations of vitamin B_{12} are inadequate, folate becomes trapped as methyltetrahydrofolate to cause functional deficiency of other intracellular forms of folic acid. In addition, the coenzyme forms of vitamin B_{12} are essential for the formation of methionine and in lipid and carbohydrate metabolism. The main deficiency phenomena include megaloblastic anaemia and an irreversible damage to the nervous system, which results from progressive demyelination of neurons in the spinal column and cerebral cortex. This may be caused either by nutritional deficiency or by lack of intrinsic factor needed for intestinal absorption of the vitamin (pernicious anaemia).

Vitamin B_{12} deficiency cannot be induced in animals and the evaluation of its effect on the immune function relies primarily on studies on patients with untreated pernicious anaemia. Because of the rarity of this condition today few studies have been carried out. Some reduction in proliferative response to PHA [262] but not to gastric mucosal homogenates [263] was observed. The T lymphocyte number in peripheral blood was normal. In another study [264] lymphocytes from pernicious anaemia patients did not exhibit the normal suppression of PR to PHA in the presence of deoxyuridine, a defect which could be corrected by *in vitro* addition of the vitamin to the lymphocyte cultures. *In vivo* treatment by vitamin B_{12} corrected this defect only after 3 months. More recent *in vitro* studies were done on lymphocytes obtained from healthy subjects. Methyl-B_{12} ($0.1–10\,\mu g\,ml^{-1}$ in culture medium) enhanced the T-cell PR to suboptimal concentrations of Con A as well as pokeweed mitogen (PWM)-induced antibody production by B lymphocytes [265]. Similar results were observed with mouse spleen cells [266]. Similar *in vitro* treatment reversed nitrous oxide-induced cellular depletion of the B_{12}-dependent enzyme thymidilate synthetase [267]. Other studies also suggest the need for vitamin B_{12} in the DNA synthetic phase of lymphocyte proliferation.

Phagocytic cell number and function were found to be impaired in patients with megaloblastic anaemia and low serum B_{12}, including neutropenia, ultrastructural changes and reduced bactericidal activity [259,268]. However, more recent studies [269] could not detect differences in neutrophil function between normal subjects and pernicious anaemia patients. An increased susceptibility to *Trypanosoma lewisi* infection was observed in rats fed a vitamin B_{12}-deficient diet [270].

Vitamin C

Vitamin C, L-ascorbic acid, a hexuronic acid, has several known physiological functions, including those related to the synthesis of collagen, catecholamines and steroids. It functions as a growth factor in wounds and neonatal tissues, as a modulator of the hexose monophosphate shunt and as a general reducing agent [271].

Humans, other primates and guinea pigs cannot synthesize vitamin C from glucose and require the vitamin exogenously. The RDA of vitamin C is $60\,mg\,day^{-1}$ for adults. However, much larger doses (even $5–10\,g\,day^{-1}$) are well tolerated. The main deficiency symptoms are related to scurvy with petechial haemorrhages, bleeding gums, poor wound healing and anaemia. Vitamin C is passively absorbed from the gastrointestinal tract and is distributed in all body tissues. Leucocytes are considered as a labile storage pool which contains $60–70\,\mu g\,10^{-8}$ cells [272].

Vitamin C had generated a great deal of interest with regard to its effect on immune functions and host defence against infections. Pauling's claims regarding vitamin C effects in the common cold [273] further stimulated the interest in the relationship between this compound and the immune system.

Vitamin C has no effect on lymphoid tissue structure or on lymphocyte counts in peripheral blood [274]. The effect on the antibody response in either animals or humans is inconsistent. Different studies demonstrated some increase, no effect or even an inhibition of antibody production [275–279]. At any rate, no evidence for a clinically important improvement in humoral immune responsiveness could be demonstrated in subjects taking large doses of vitamin C. Inconsistent results exist also in connection with the vitamin C effect on complement levels [280–282]. On the other hand, a large body of data suggests an important effect of vitamin C on CMI and phagocytic functions, and probably also on some other immune functions.

In scorbutic guinea pigs vitamin C was shown to decrease the ability to induce experimental allergic encephalomyelitis, a typical CMI disease [283], to reduce or eliminate DTH response to mycobacteria [284] and to prolong allograft survival [285]. It was, however, interesting to find out that the failure to develop skin reactivity to tuberculin could be corrected by vitamin C supplementation, without the need to repeat primary sensitization [283]. Moreover, lymphocytes taken from such anergic animals were able to respond to tuberculin *in vitro* with typical mitosis and to transfer PPD hypersensitivity to healthy control animals. Conversely, sensitized lymphocytes from healthy controls did not induce

DTH if transferred to scorbutic guinea pigs [286,287]. These data suggest defects in inflammatory response, rather than in genuine T-cell functions. Indeed, defective or decreased inflammatory response was generated in scorbutic guinea pigs using non-specific irritants [286,287] or histamine and in Arthus-type dermal hypersensitivity [275]. Impaired inflammatory responses in such animals can be attributed to deficiencies in the mobilization and function of phagocytic cells (see below) and/or vascular endothelial changes, known to be associated with vitamin C deficiency. However, some studies indicated depressive effects of vitamin C deficiency on T-cell functions measured *in vitro*, including responsiveness to T-cell mitogens [288] and cell-mediated cytotoxicity [289]. Moreover, an excess of vitamin C given to guinea pigs or to Balb/c mice [290,291] resulted in an increase in T-cell number and in response to Con A or PHA.

Studies in humans demonstrated similar effects. Most of the studies indicate that vitamin C at physiological concentrations enhanced the *in vitro* response of human mononuclear cells to stimulation by specific antigens, T-cell mitogens and allogeneic cells. The enhanced responses included T-cell proliferation and cytotoxicity, as well as suppressor cell and natural killer cell activities [292,293]. In another study, vitamin C was shown to counteract influenza virus-induced depression of lymphoid cell responses to PHA, probably a macrophage-mediated effect [294]. These effects may be related to vitamin C modulation of cyclic guanosine monophosphate levels in mononuclear cells [295], an effect which was also documented in other blood-formed elements [296,297]. *In vivo* experiments in humans with either deprivation or supplementation of vitamin C lend further support to the documented effect of this vitamin on CMI responses [279,298].

Some of the studies described in the previous section (e.g. [294]) indicate an effect of vitamin C on monocyte/macrophage functions. The interaction between vitamin C and phagocytic cells is evident in many other studies. The very fact that such cells normally contain high concentrations of vitamin C [272], that under *in vitro* conditions they can take it up and that its level falls during phagocytosis [299,300] suggest significant relationships. It was recognized a long time ago [301] that the appropri-

ate phagocytic activity in guinea pigs depends on an adequate level of ascorbic acid. In more recent studies it was shown that the addition of ascorbate to cultures of normal macrophages increased the cellular concentrations of cyclic guanosine monophosphate and of hexosemonophosphate shunt activity [302,303], as well as phagocytic and chemotactic activities and motility [280,281,303,304]. Similar observations were done also on human neutrophils and eosinophils [281,305,306]. Vitamin C can decrease auto-oxidation by oxidative burst products in phagocytic cells without decreasing the intracellular concentration of reactive bactericidal molecules [307].

Vitamin C has been used to treat some clinical phagocytic cell dysfunctions. In Chediak-Higashi syndrome, which is characterized in part by defective neutrophil functions, vitamin C treatment resulted in improved neutrophil chemotaxis, improved bactericidal activity, reduction of cyclic adenosine monophosphate levels and reduction of days of clinical illness [308,309]. However, in other cases these effects could not be achieved [310]. Vitamin C was found to be beneficial also in chronic granulomatous disease [306] in hyper-IgE syndrome [311] and in recurrent pyogenic infections [312].

Immediate hypersensitivity (type I) reactions seem to be affected by vitamin C; the effect may be either weak or inconsistent. In animals, the release of histamine and slow-reacting substances of anaphylaxis from sensitized lung fragments of vitamin C-deficient guinea pig are reduced; it is restored to normal by vitamin C supplementation [313]. Other studies [314] were not able to reproduce such an effect in experimental reactions. In clinical studies vitamin C intake reduced histamine [315] or metacholine-induced bronchospasm [316], but was ineffective in clinical allergic reactions such as ragweed antigen-induced bronchospasm in known asthmatics [317], or cutaneous and nasal reactivities to allergens in symptomatic patients [318]. It can be concluded that vitamin C may have some effects on immediate hypersensitivity by affecting various relevant cellular mechanisms (e.g. calcium chelation, cyclic nucleotides, phosphodiesterase or prostaglandins) but most probably it does not have a significant clinical effect in such conditions.

Interferon production by induced mouse [319] or human [320] fibroblast cultures was increased by the addition of vitamin C into the medium. A similar *in vivo* effect on interferon production in mice was also observed [321]. The clinical significance of these observations is unknown.

Thymic reticular cell activity and the production of thymic hormones are probably dependent on appropriate vitamin C supplementation [322].

Many studies were conducted to evaluate the value of vitamin C in various doses (including megadoses) in the treatment and prophylaxis of common upper respiratory illnesses [280,323–325]. The studies showed only minor and insignificant effects on disease prevention. However, the duration and severity of symptoms were reduced.

Although vitamin C is an essential micronutrient, it has only minimal interaction with lymphoid cell functions. It has, however, an important role in phagocytic cell function, mostly cell mobility, probably related to the synthesis and assembly of microlobular structures of these cells. This effect may be the basis of the other effects of vitamin C on T-cell function and on resistance to infection.

Fat-soluble vitamins

Of the four fat-soluble vitamins (A,D,E and K), only two (A and E) are of established importance for proper immune function; one (vitamin D) has some relevance in this connection, whereas vitamin K does not appear to play any role in the immune system. Since fat-soluble vitamins cannot be excreted by the kidneys, as can the water-soluble ones, situations of hypervitaminosis can develop much more easily with toxic consequences on different body organs, including the immune system. More details of the biochemistry, physiology and clinical pathology of these vitamins can be found in [3].

Vitamin A

Vitamin A exists in a variety of forms. Retinol (vitamin A_1), a primary alcohol, is present in esterified form in the liver of fishes and animals; 3-dehydroretinol (vitamin A_2) occurs mixed with retinol. Retinoic acid (vitamin A acid), in which the alcohol group has been oxidized, shares some but not all of the actions of retinol. The plant pigment carotenes are vitamin A precursors (provitamin A, e.g. β-carotene; see below).

Vitamin A has a number of important functions in the body. It plays an essential role in the function of the retina, in the growth and differentiation of epithelial tissues, in bone growth, in reproduction and in embryonic development. It also has a stabilizing effect on various membranes and acts to regulate membrane permeability. It has important effects on RNA, glycoprotein and glycolipid synthesis.

Vitamin A deficiency and protein malnutrition are the two most serious nutritional deficiency diseases in the world today. The main deficiency symptoms include night blindness and lesions in epithelial surfaces (skin, lung, genitourinary and gastrointestinal).

The toxic manifestations of hypervitaminosis A include irritability, fatigue, typical skin and bone changes, and hepatosplenomegaly with ultimate cirrhosis.

Both vitamin A deficiency and excess have major influences on the immune system and on host resistance to infection.

The cellularity of lymphoid organs was affected by vitamin A. Vitamin A deficiency in rats resulted in atrophy of spleen and thymus [326]. In the thymus the cortical areas were particularly affected with almost complete depletion of thymocytes. In the spleen, the germinal centres were the most affected areas. In contrast, mice receiving daily vitamin A supplementation for 21 days had a significant increase in the weight of lymph nodes and thymus but not the spleen. Histologically, the lymph nodes exhibited hypertrophy with relative enlargement of the paracortical areas.

Humoral immunity was impaired in vitamin A-deficient rats immunized with diphtheria toxoid, sheep RBC [211,326] or pneumococcal polysaccharide [327]. Such impairment was also observed in vitamin A-deficient lambs injected with human γ-globulins, and it could not be corrected by 2-week repletion with vitamin A [328]. The impairment was monitored by lower levels of specific serum antibodies and splenic plaque-forming cells. These parameters were increased in normal animals given large acute doses of vitamin A, during or before primary or secondary immunizations [329,330]. In one such study [329], mice were injected with vitamin A 4 days before immunization with sheep RBC. At 4 days after immunization, plaque-forming assay was performed on spleen cells. Vitamin A caused a fivefold increase in plaque-forming cells at 3000 iu day^{-1} but not with the 9000 iu day^{-1} dose, which was apparently toxic. Furthermore, vitamin A (3000 iu) given concomitantly with low (but not high) doses of hydrocortisone prevented hydrocortisone-induced immunosuppression [329]. The time relationship between vitamin A administration and immunization is critical. Vitamin A given daily for 5 days before or after immunization has an enhancing effect on antibody response. The effect disappeared if vitamin A was given from day 6 on, after immunization [330].

In a study performed on undernourished non-vaccinated children in Bangladesh [331], the children were immunized with tetanus toxoid with or without a single dose of vitamin A (200 000 iu). No subsequent differences were observed in the antibody response between the two groups. It should be mentioned, however, that none of these children were overtly vitamin A-deficient. Vitamin A may have an adjuvant effect when administered with antigen [326,329,332]; the mechanism of this action may be related to increased lymphocyte proliferation or improved antigen presentation.

CMI is also affected by vitamin A. *In vivo* tests included DTH and allograft rejection [330,333]. This effect was abrogated by treating the mice with antithymocyte antiserum, suggesting that vitamin A exerts its effect on T lymphocytes.

In vivo tests were done on lymphocytes taken from vitamin A-deficient rats and assayed for PR to PHA and Con A. A significant reduction in PR was observed in the spleen cells (but not thymocytes) of deficient animals, to be corrected within 3 days of vitamin supplementation [334]. PR was also enhanced by *in vitro* addition of vitamin A into the stimulated cultures of normal human lymphocytes [335]. In another study on surgical patients [336], a 7-day course of vitamin A therapy avoided postoperative depression of lymphocyte counts or PR to allogeneic stimulation which was seen in the untreated control patients.

Few but conflicting data [326,337] exist as to the effect of vitamin A on macrophage–monocyte func-

tion, and at any rate these do not seem to be a major target of this vitamin.

Autoimmune manifestations in NZB mice are exacerbated by vitamin A deficiency [338].

Tumour development in mice could be prevented by treatment with vitamin A prior to tumour cell inoculation. The effect, which could be seen in some tumours [339], but not in other ones [340], could be abrogated by antilymphocyte antiserum, indicating a role for CMI in the antitumour effect of vitamin A. Moreover, vitamin A treatment before tumour cell inoculation resulted in enhancement of tumour-specific cytotoxic activity. A bell-shaped dose–response curve was observed for the vitamin A effect on cytotoxicity, with peak enhancement at 25–100 μg day^{-1} and suppression at doses higher than 300 μg day^{-1} [341]. In another study [340] it was found that chemically induced skin papillomas regressed by 61% in mice treated by 100 mg kg^{-1} week^{-1} vitamin A, or by 86% using 400 mg kg^{-1} week^{-1}. On the other hand, the incidence of colon and liver cancer was increased in vitamin A-deficient rats exposed to dimethylhydrazine or to aflatoxin B [342].

Resistance to infection is also dependent on vitamin A [343,344]. This is related in part to the role of vitamin A in maintaining the functional integrity of epithelial and mucosal surfaces and the production of mucus secretion. Production of lysozyme is vitamin A-dependent [345]. Obviously, the impairment of immune response in vitamin A deficiency has a major impact on host susceptibility to infection. Indeed, vitamin A-deficient rats were much more susceptible to intestinal infection with *Angiostrongylus cantonesis* with more severe illness and lower acquisition of immunity against subsequent reinfection [344]. Vitamin A-deficient rats were also most susceptible to malaria parasites (*Plasmodium berghei*), with rapid development of parasitaemia and death. Oral vitamin A treatment allowed complete recovery. Similarly, vitamin A-deficient chickens were more susceptible to Newcastle disease virus [346]. In contrast, vitamin A supplementation of normal mice (3000 iu day^{-1} for 4 days before infection) resulted in increased resistance to infection with *Pseudomonas aeruginosa*, with clearance of administered bacteria from the blood within 5 h. In 24 h all control animals were dead, whereas the vitamin A-treated group was sterile and alive [337]. Similar results were observed in mice infected with *Candida albicans* or *Listeria monocytogenes*.

Carotenoids, like β-carotene, were referred to only in connection of their being precursors to vitamin A. However, recent studies have shown that carotenoids—even those which lack provitamin A activity—can function as antioxidants, inactivate highly reactive molecules (e.g. singlet oxygen and free radicals), an activity not shared by vitamin A. In doing so, the carotenoids can protect cells from oxidation damage, including auto-oxidation in phagocytic cells, without affecting their bactericidal capability [347]. Beta-carotene was shown to prevent stress- and radiation-induced thymic involution and lymphopenia [347] and to increase helper T-cell (OKT4 +) number in human PBMC [348], and graft versus host response in animals [349]. Cantaxanthin and β-carotene enhanced T- and B-cell proliferation [350]. However, the most consistent and significant effect of carotenoids is related to their ability to augment several aspects of antitumour immunity, including enhanced regression of virally induced tumours and increased cytotoxic activity of macrophages, natural killer cells and T cells against tumours [347,351,352]. Moreover, different carotenoids were recently shown to prevent or inhibit the gross development of squamous cell carcinoma induced in the hamster buccal pouch by 7,12-dimethyl benz(a)anthracene. Histologically, there were areas of tumour lysis and inflammatory infiltrate consisting of cytotoxic lymphocytes and macrophages [353–356].

Vitamin D

Vitamin D is a product of ultraviolet cleavage (in the skin) of the provitamin dehydrocholesterol and is further activated by sequential hydroxylation in the liver and kidney. Its main physiological role is as a positive regulator of calcium metabolism. Vitamin D deficiency causes rickets in children and osteomalacia in adults. Hypervitaminosis is toxic mainly because of the resultant hypercalcaemia.

Vitamin D has only a small effect on the immune system. Vitamin-deficient rats had some impairment of antibody production to diphtheria toxoid but not

to human RBC [211,357,358]. Rachitic baby pigs had a lower antibody response to *Salmonella pullorum* antigen [103].

Vitamin E (tocopherols)

Eight naturally occurring tocopherols with vitamin E activity are known, the most abundant and active one being α-tocopherol. The exact mechanism of action of vitamin E is still unknown. A most important feature of tocopherols is their anti-oxidant activity, and this seems to be its major nutritive and therapeutic value. In acting as an anti-oxidant vitamin E presumably prevents oxidation of essential cellular constituents, prevents the formation of toxic oxidation products, such as those formed from unsaturated fatty acids and destroys free radicals generated during cellular metabolism or biotransformation of xenobiotics. In this way vitamin E protects the structural integrity of cells and prevents damage to membranes and enzymes [359]. The anti-oxidant activity is shared by selenium and sulphur-containing amino acids as well as by ascorbic acid (vitamin C) and by β-carotene (provitamin A). Moreover, vitamin E, as the major vitamin anti-oxidant in plasma and tissues, protects other micronutrients, including those with immuno-enhancing properties, from oxidative damage [360]. In addition, although there are several anti-oxidants, as mentioned before, some of the symptoms of vitamin E deficiency are not alleviated by the other anti-oxidants; presumably, vitamin E has more specific actions as well, and may be as a repressor that regulates the synthesis of specific enzymes or other proteins required for the differentiation or adaptation of tissues.

Symptoms of deficiency in experimental animals include structural and functional abnormalities in many organs and organ systems, including the reproductive, muscular, cardiovascular and haematopoietic. The consequences of deficiency and the results of vitamin E treatment in humans are much less clear.

The effects of vitamin E on the immune system were studied primarily in animals with only very few studies performed in humans. Most of the studies are concerned with vitamin E added to food rather than its deficiency.

Antibody response and the number of plaque-forming cells to sheep RBC were significantly enhanced in animals receiving a diet rich in vitamin E [361]. The effect was observed in both young and adult chicks and was more pronounced in hypoxic ones. Hypoxia is a known immunopoietic stimulation and it acted synergistically with vitamin E probably in its role as an anti-oxidant. A study on guinea pigs [362] immunized with attenuated Venezuelan equine encephalomyelitis virus vaccine also indicated the enhancement of antibody production by vitamin E administration. Studies on mice immunized with foreign RBC or with tetanus toxoid [361] showed vitamin E-dependent enhancement of antibody production, stronger on primary than on secondary immunization and on IgE synthesis than on IgM. IgG response was almost completely suppressed in vitamin E-deficient mice. The anti-oxidant diphenyl-*p*-phenylene diamine could not substitute for vitamin E. In all these studies the highest doses of vitamin E used gave the best results. Vitamin E also had an *in vitro* enhancing effect on plaque-forming cells taken from sheep RBC-immunized mice; the addition of vitamin E allowed antibody production to occur in the absence of adherent cells [361].

CMI was modified by vitamin E. A positive correlation was found between splenic vitamin E level and the mitogenic activity of splenocytes in mice [363]. In studies on vitamin E-deficient animals, the response to mitogen stimulation [364] or mixed lymphocyte responses [365] were severely depressed. The presence of the antioxidant 2-mercaptoethanol in the lymphocyte cultures did not correct depressed PR of the deficient animals, suggesting an additional role of vitamin E, beside its anti-oxidant activity. In contrast, lymphocyte PR to PHA or Con A (less so to lipopolysaccharide) was enhanced by vitamin E supplemented either *in vitro* or *in vivo* [366]. The effect was more pronounced at suboptimal concentrations of the stimulating agent, with high doses of vitamin E and when PUFA in the diet was low. Vitamin E enhancement of PR is thymus-dependent. When lymphocytes from congenitally athymic mice were cultured with lipopolysaccharide (a B-cell mitogen) and vitamin E, the responses were less than those from mice with normal thymuses [366]. This may be related to the need for thymic factors or thymus-derived helper T cells. A double-blind placebo-controlled clinical study on 32 elderly healthy subjects, whose food was supplemented with 800 iu day^{-1} α-tocopherol for 30 days, indicates a significant improvement in DTH and in PR response to Con A, accompanied by increased interleukin-2 production, and a decrease in prostaglandin E$_2$ production [367]. In contrast to most of the studies showing a beneficial effect of vitamin E even when given in megadoses, a study of Prasad [368] who gave megadoses of the vitamin (300 mg day^{-1} for 4 days) to young volunteers showed suppression of PR to PHA, although the DTH response to PHA was not changed.

Macrophage number and function were also modulated by vitamin E. In vitamin E-deficient rabbits, a 10-fold reduction in the number of peritoneal cells accumulating 48 h after intraperitoneal injection of mineral oil was observed [369]. Chemotactic activity was not changed. In another study. vitamin E-deficient rats had a lower bactericidal activity of pulmonary macrophages [370]. Macrophage membrane receptors were altered in such animals [371]. Chemotaxis, ingestion of complement-coated beads and protection from autoxidative damage were reduced in vitamin E-deficient rats [372]. On the other hand, vitamin E-supplemented diets in mice caused an increase in phagocytic activity against *Diplococcus pneumoniae* in immunized mice [373]. RES clearance of carbon particles from blood was also enhanced [373], indicating non-immunogenic enhancement in phagocytic activity. In humans, the ingestion of 1600 iu vitamin E for 7 days resulted in increased phagocytic activity of neutrophils, but decreased bactericidal capacity. This may be related to the observed vitamin E-related decrease in oxygen consumption and hydrogen peroxide levels in neutrophils phagocytizing bacteria and to the partial inhibition of glucose oxidation in such cells [374–376].

Resistance to infection was increased in laboratory and farm animals which were fed with higher than normal levels of vitamin E. Decreased mortality and enhanced recovery was observed in rats infected with *Mycoplasma pulmonas* [377], in mice infected with *Diplococcus pneumoniae* [373], in chicks infected with *Escherichia coli* [378], in turkeys infected with *Histamonas meleagridis* [379] or in lambs infected with *Chlamydia* [380]. In some of these studies the effects on survival were shown to be associated with effects on antibody production or phagocytosis. In humans, Chavance *et al.* [381] found a statistically significant correlation between high vitamin levels and low number of infections in 100 healthy subjects over 60 years old.

Prostaglandin synthesis was diminished in lymphoid cells of infected animals fed with vitamin E [382,383]. Since increased local concentrations of prostaglandins may be immunosuppressive [149, 384], the beneficial effect of vitamin E on host resistance to infection may be related in part to the prevention of infection-induced increase in tissue prostaglandins [384].

Transplanted tumours grow faster in vitamin E-deficient mice. This was not accompanied by a change in the ability of splenic natural killer cells to lyse tumour cells *in vitro* [385]. The mechanism of this effect awaits further elucidation.

Autoimmune manifestations were effectively controlled in vitamin E-fed NZB mice [386] and probably also in humans [387].

Three types of interactions were specifically studied in relation to the interaction of vitamin E with other nutrients: with PUFA, vitamin C and selenium.

1 PUFA are more liable to peroxidation than saturated fatty acids. Peroxidation metabolites of fatty acids decrease membrane fluidity and immune response, probably as inter-related phenomena [349,389]. Indeed, vitamin E deficiency augmented immunosuppression caused by a high PUFA diet, whereas higher than normal levels of vitamin E in the diet could partially overcome this suppression [389]. Vitamin E can alleviate chronic inflammatory damage to arthritic joints, which was shown to be associated with the generation of free radicals from lipid peroxidation [390]. In addition, it can reduce inflammatory prostaglandin (e.g. prostaglandin E_2) production, and this effect may be synergistic with that of indomethacin or aspirin in enhancing lymphocyte PR [367,391].

2 The interaction of vitamins C and E was studied in guinea pigs. The best responses to T- and B-cell mitogens were achieved in animals fed with high levels of both vitamins [392]. *In vitro* and *in vivo* studies suggest that vitamin C can help maintain

vitamin E levels.

3 The interaction of selenium and vitamin E is discussed in the section on selenium.

Minerals

Minerals serve key roles in cell function, as constituents of metalloenzymes, as components of cell excitation signal transduction, and in other vital cellular processes. These functions are important also to the proper activity of the immune system. Divalent cations are essential for cell membrane complement, kinin and coagulation system functions. Iron is important for all oxidative functions in every cell. In contrast, sodium chloride, potassium and phosphorus do not seem to have a unique or independent effect on the immune system.

The minerals which were found to be most important for the proper functioning of the immune system include calcium, magnesium, selenium, iron and zinc. Another group of minerals is of less fundamental importance: cobalt, manganese, copper, cadmium and sodium. A few other minerals (mercury, lead, chromium, silicon, platinum, gallium, gold, titanium, aluminium, thorium-vanadium and titanium) have only few reports on their interaction with the immune system. A review on the role of minerals in immunobiology was published recently [12].

Calcium

The major portion of calcium is in bone. However, the small quantity of ionized calcium in body fluids and cells is essential for the functional integrity of nerve and muscle (where it has a major influence on excitability), for integrity of cell membrane, for blood coagulation and as a secondary messenger in the cells. It is mainly the last-mentioned activity which is important for proper immune function.

T lymphocytes can be activated independently of antigen or mitogen stimulation by simultaneous treatment of the cells with calcium ionophores and phorbol esters. Calcium ionophores allow calcium to cross the cell membrane, increasing the intracellular concentration of calcium. The increased calcium then activates the calcium-binding regulatory protein calmodulin. Calmodulin is a heat-stable relatively acidic small protein with an unusually high content of aspartic and glutamic acids. Each calmodulin molecule binds four calcium ions and the complex is able now to interact with receptor sites on enzymes, including kinases and other cellular proteins. That such calcium fluxes are physiologically relevant to the growth of T cells is further indicated by the recent findings that activation of T cells by antigens opens up calcium channels in the cell membrane [393]. Also, when lymphocytes are stimulated *in vitro* by PHA, they normally accumulate calcium ions from the surrounding medium in amounts which can be quantitated by the use of ^{45}Ca [394]. Lipoproteins which inhibit PHA-stimulated lymphocyte PR diminish the uptake of radiolabelled calcium by the stimulated cells. A correlation exists between the ability of various types of lipoproteins to inhibit ^{45}Ca uptake and their ability to inhibit PHA-induced PR.

The generation of oxygen radicals and degranulation in activated human neutrophils is dependent on mobilization of intracellular calcium ions.

Magnesium

Magnesium is a cofactor in all enzymes involved in phosphate transfer reactions that utilize adenosine triphosphate and other nucleotide triphosphates as substrates. An enormous list of enzymes (e.g. phosphatases and pyrophosphatases) is influenced by this ion. It also plays a vital role in the reversible association of intracellular particles and in the binding of macromolecules to subcellular organelles. For example, the binding of messenger RNA to ribosomes is magnesium-dependent, as is the functional integrity of ribosomal subunits. It is also essential for neurochemical transmissions and muscular excitability.

Magnesium deficiency may occur in chronic gastrointestinal disturbances, alcoholism and haemodialysis and is characterized by changes in skeletal and cardiac muscles and typical nephrocalcinosis.

The effect of magnesium deficiency on the immune system was studied mainly on mice and rats who were kept on diets moderately deficient in magnesium for extended periods of time. Several profound changes occur in such animals, which have not hitherto been observed in humans.

1 Humoral immunity is impaired, as expressed by the minimal appearance of splenic plaque-forming cells and specific antibodies in response to immunization with sheep RBC [395–397], or by depressed serum levels of IgG and IgA [395,398]. The last phenomenon was not confirmed by other investigators [396,397].

2 CMI was impaired by magnesium deficiency, as judged by the diminished ability to be immunized by live lymphoma cells [397] or to develop experimental allergic encephalomyelitis after inoculation with brain tissue antigen [397]. Resistance to infections was also reduced [397]. Interestingly, magnesium deficiency caused marked thymic hyperplasia, in contrast to the frequently occurring thymic atrophy in many nutrient deficiencies.

3 Persistent leukocytosis which may transform into myelogenous leukaemia or malignant lymphoma [397,399–401]. The leukocytosis included an increase in neutrophil, mononuclear cells and particularly (up to 10-fold) in eosinophils [400]. The eosinophils were present in massive amounts both in blood and in several tissues, including lymph nodes and lungs. If leukocytosis persisted uncorrected by magnesium supplementation, rats developed malignant lymphoma in 20% of cases within 8–24 weeks of initiation of a low-magnesium diet, and leukaemia in another 5% within 28–60 weeks. Both diseases could be transplanted to other animals. Moreover, magnesium-deficient rats were more susceptible to develop lymphoma from transplanted cells [402].

4 Mast cells underwent extensive changes in magnesium-deficient rats, including massive degranulation, decreased histamine content in the cells and increased excretion in the urine [400,401,403]. The distribution of mast cells in tissues was found to be abnormal [400,404].

Iron

The body store of iron is divided between iron-containing compounds that are essential and those in which excess iron is held in storage. Haemoglobin dominates the essential fraction, followed by myoglobin and a variety of haem and non-haem iron-dependent enzymes. Ferritin is the storage protein in the reticuloendothelial system and hepatocytes, and transferrin is the carrier protein in plasma. Iron deficiency is a most frequent single micronutrient deficiency and is likely to occur in the absence of any other accompanying form of malnutrition.

Both iron deficiency and its excess may profoundly affect immune functions and other host defence mechanisms. Most of the studies were done in humans.

Lymphocytes and lymphoid tissues are changed during iron-deficiency anaemia. Total lymphocyte numbers have been found to be reduced, with vacuolar changes in their mitochondria. These changes were reversed within 4 weeks by iron therapy [405,406]. Similar changes were found in iron-deficient animals [407,408].

Changes in humoral immunity have been reported in animal but not in clinical studies. In rats, a decrease in antibody production after immunization with tetanus toxoid was proportional to the decline in iron intake [409]. In contrast, no abnormalities have been found in serum immunoglobulin concentrations [410,411], in salivary IgA values [412] or in antibody response to vaccination with tetanus toxoid, in association with iron deficiency. Complement levels were also normal [410].

CMI was assessed by several types of assays in iron-deficient patients.

1 Studies on PR to mitogens or antigens do not agree with each other. Several reports show a decreased response to PHA or to antigens like tuberculin or *Candida* [405,406,411–413] which could be corrected by iron therapy. Other studies failed to confirm these observations, and did not find changes in PR in such patients [414]. This controversy may be related to differences in various variables, such as other nutritional deficiencies, *in vitro* assay conditions, severity of anaemia and infection. It should be mentioned, however, that in iron-deficient mice, PR and interleukin-2 production induced by Con A were significantly reduced, and correlated with parameters of iron status (haemoglobin, haematocrit and liver iron stores) [415].

2 CTL activity was diminished in iron-deficient mice [416]. However, the ability to reject allogeneic bone marrow cells was not modified by a combination of iron deficiency and irradiation in rats [417]. Both stimulated and unstimulated natural killer cell activity was reduced in iron-deficient rats [418].

3 DTH response to recall antigens was impaired in patients with iron deficiency according to some reports [405,410,419], with the exception of one [255]. This may be related to diminished inflammatory response [420] and MIF production [413,419]. Primary sensitization with dinitrofluorobenzene in iron-deficient mice resulted in a minimal inflammatory response [421].

Phagocytic cell functions are impaired in iron deficiency; the main defect is in bactericidal activity [410,412], which may be attributed to impaired myeloperoxidase activity in the phagocytic cells. Other metalloenzymes of phagocytic cells may also be defective in such patients. In addition, hypersegmentation of neutrophil nuclei was observed [422].

Susceptibility to infection was increased in conditions of either iron deficiency or excess. In iron deficiency, increased susceptibility to infection is related to impaired immune and phagocytic functions. This was demonstrated in iron-deficient rats intestinally infected by *Salmonella typhimurium* [423]. In iron excess the increased susceptibility to infection can be attributed to increased availability of iron to bacteria. Iron is essential for optimal bacterial growth and for the production and release of exotoxins. Normally, all iron in the body is sequestered in cells or bound with high affinity to carrier molecules and thus it is not available for the invading bacteria [424,425]. In case of iron excess, the binding capacity of transferrin becomes saturated and free iron becomes available for uptake by micro-organisms, allowing their rapid growth with resultant septic consequences [424–427]. Indeed, African children with kwashiorkor, treated with a high-protein diet, vitamins and iron, died because of acute overwhelming bacterial sepsis [428]. Sepsis and death were correlated with low transferrin levels in blood. In other studies on African patients, malarial attacks were found to occur more frequently after initiation of iron therapy [427] or when serum iron values rose rapidly to oversaturation levels with change in diet [429]. Similarly, symptomatic activation of latent malaria, brucellosis or tuberculosis took place 2 weeks after initiation of iron therapy in iron-deficient Somali nomads. However, if the refeeding programme did not include iron, the incidence of infections was much lower. The correlation between the saturation of iron-carrying molecules (transferrin, lactoferrin) and susceptibility to infection is supported by additional studies in experimental animals [424,426,429,430] and on the bacteriostatic effects of human milk [426]. It should be noted, however, that iron-dependent increased virulence of micro-organisms is not the only pathogenic mechanism caused by iron excess. The refeeding of a malnourished subject using many nutrients, including iron, allows him or her to develop better an immuno-inflammatory response to a pre-existing latent infection, thus producing symptomatic disease. The interaction of nutrients with host defence mechanisms in a starved subject is as yet not thoroughly understood.

Zinc

Zinc is closely associated with a large variety of proteins and enzymes and is essential for either the catalytic function and/or the structural integrity of the molecule. In addition to its critical role in the mechanism of action of more than 100 metalloenzymes, zinc increases the activities of many other enzymes. By being an essential part of enzymes involved in nucleic acid and protein synthesis and consequently cell division, zinc may be especially important for rapidly replicating cell systems and during development. Since the immune system depends on the rapid proliferation of cells in order to be effective, zinc deficiency profoundly impairs immune functions. Zinc also stabilizes cell membranes and protects them from peroxidative damage. In addition, zinc is essential for the activity of several hormones, including the thymic hormone thymulin. Zinc deficiency has been observed or experimentally produced in a large variety of animal species and in humans. In contrast to iron, zinc cannot be stored in the body and therefore zinc deficiency is produced easily and quickly. The syndrome is characterized by a failure to grow, anorexia, testicular atrophy, skin lesions and susceptibility to infections. In humans the deficiency may be from dietary causes, gastrointestinal problems, infectious diseases, certain drugs or alcohol abuse and liver or renal diseases. However, the most dramatic examples of zinc deficiency are two 'experiments of nature'—one in animals, the other in humans. The animal disorder was described in a mutant cattle

(A46 mutant of Dutch Fresian type) [431,432]. The human disorder is called acrodermatitis enterohepatica (AE) [433]. Both have an inherited inability to absorb zinc properly. A few weeks after birth the animals or the infants started to be lethargic with growth arrest, skin lesions and extreme susceptibility to infection, which is the usual cause of early death. The immunological and other abnormalities could be completely corrected by adequate amounts of zinc, given either orally or parenterally. These disorders have provided evidence that adequate supplies of zinc are essential to the development and maintenance of a healthy immune system, particularly its cell-mediated arm, as will be detailed below.

The study of the immunological consequences of zinc deficiency was based on these inherited disorders and on experimental and clinical zinc deficiencies. Patients suffering from iatrogenic zinc deficiency because of inadequate total parenteral nutrition are of special interest because these patients are not simultaneously deficient in protein or calories [434].

Lymphoid tissue cellularity is profoundly diminished by zinc deficiency; severe cases of deficiency may result in complete atrophy of the thymus, spleen and lymph nodes, particularly of T-dependent areas. It should be mentioned that the observed thymic atrophy was accompanied by decreased production of thymic hormones [435], particularly thymopoietin [436] and thymulin [437]. Thymulin was shown to be a zinc-dependent hormone. The changes can be completely reversed by zinc supplementation [438]. No marked lymphopenia was observed in one study, but proportions of lymphoid cell subpopulations were changed with an increased percentage of large immature or Fc receptor-positive cells and decreased T cells [439]. In another study, a more severe lymphopenia was noticed in zinc-deficient mice, attributable to reduced bone marrow lymphopoiesis. This was correlated with increased glucocorticoid levels in these mice [440]. Abnormal migration of circulating lymphocytes was also reported [438].

Humoral immunity was only marginally affected, if at all. In the inherited zinc deficiency in cattle, IgM and IgG, but not IgA, levels were increased. Early antibody response to tetanus toxoid was normal but late response was diminished [441]. In

AE patients immunoglobulin levels were either normal or deficient [442–444]. In experimental zinc deficiency, a diminished number of splenic plaque-forming cells responding to sheep RBC immunization was found [437,438,445,446]. Zinc supplementation may cause a rebound to greater than normal antibody response [447]. The *in vitro* addition of supplemental zinc to antibody-forming cultures of cells from aged mice caused a pronounced improvement in the ability to synthesize specific antibody [448]. The addition of zinc at varying times during the culture period suggests that zinc affects early events in the activation of antibody-forming cells [449], an effect which is dependent on the production of non-dialysable factors, including interleukin-1 and -4 [450,451].

CMI was profoundly diminished by zinc deficiency, as judged by the poor DTH response to skin tests with DNCB or other antigens [84,452] and by markedly diminished PR to mitogens or antigens *in vitro* [435,436,453,454]. The zinc dependence of DTH response was elegantly demonstrated in a study [455] on children with moderate zinc deficiency on whom identical skin tests were performed on both arms of each child; one arm was topically treated by 1% zinc sulphate ointment, the other arm by placebo ointment. DHT reactions were significantly greater in the zinc-treated arm, indicating that local absorption of zinc is sufficient to restore local CMI in the deficient children. Topical application was ineffective in severe zinc deficiency. Moreover zinc also had a strong *in vitro* effect on human lymphocyte receptors (e.g. it enhanced the ability of peripheral blood lymphocytes to form rosettes with sheep RBC [456] and on PR of human lymphocytes with or without the addition of PHA [457–460]. In animals, a narrow *in vitro* concentration range of zinc chloride (10 µm in hamsters, 50 µm in guinea pigs) was shown to be optimal for PR to Con A using lymph node cells [461]. Zinc supplementation of *in vitro* cultures of murine thymocytes enhances their response to suboptimal concentrations of PHA and prime thymocytes to respond to interleukin-1 in the absence of PHA. It affects early stages of PR [462]. In addition, zinc-deficient animals exhibited reduced natural killer cell activity, a depressed allogeneic cytotoxic T-cell response to EL-4 tumour cells after *in vivo* immunization [445,463] and defective T-cell

helper function [445,446,463].

Phagocytic cell functions were also impaired by zinc deficiency, including phagocytosis, bactericidal capacity, chemotaxis and migratory activity. This was accompanied by biochemical changes measured by diminished oxygen consumption and inhibition of membrane fluidity. Correction of some of these abnormalities could be accomplished by *in vitro* zinc supplementation [464–468]. It has been suggested that zinc regulates macrophage functions through a direct effect on the plasma membrane [465,468] and through its need for enzymes involved in phagocytic activity.

The relationship between zinc deficiency and PCM is evident in several studies [469]. Anorexia, a consistent finding in AE, may lead to PCM. PCM patients, in turn, are almost always found with low blood levels of zinc [469], not only because of low intake but also because of diarrhoea, infections and the low plasma protein levels (e.g. albumin, transferrin) needed for zinc transport.

Dietary zinc deficiency appears to be responsible, at least in part, for the immunodeficiency that is so regularly associated with certain human cancers [470].

Copper

Copper is a constituent and essential nutrient of most, if not all, animals and plants and its deficiency can lead to severe derangement of growth and metabolism. It is associated with a large number of cuproenzymes and copper-containing proteins, e.g. ceruloplasmin, the copper transport protein in the plasma, or cytochrome oxidase, the terminal oxidase of the electron transport chain from which adenosine triphosphate is synthesized.

Copper deficiency results in anaemia, skeletal, vascular, dermal and central nervous system disorders. An excess of zinc in the diet may cause copper deficiency because of competition in the intestinal mucosa on same carrier molecule. The Menkes kinky hair syndrome is an inherited disease with defective copper metabolism and low copper concentrations in the blood [471].

Immunological studies on an infant suffering from Menkes kinky hair syndrome were generally normal, short of poor IgM to IgG conversion in secondary antibody response [471]. Indeed, copper-deficient mice had a reduced antibody response to immunization with sheep RBC [472,473]. The initiation and maintenance of CMI to leukaemia cells was severely impaired in copper-deficient mice [474]. Other characteristics of copper-deficient mice include reduction in thymus weight, in the presence of normal plasma corticosterone levels [475], a decrease in PR to PHA and Con A and in interleukin-2 production and an increase in interleukin-1 production [476,477], a reduced production of IgG, but not IgM [478] in the face of an increased absolute and relative percentage of B cells [479]. Copper-deficient rats had an impaired phagocytic function [90]. *In vitro* addition of copper (50 μmol/l) to dog granulocyte cultures improved their phagocytic activity and oxygen uptake [480].

Susceptibility to infection was increased by copper deficiency [481], as well as by copper excess [482,483]. Infection is the usual cause of death in Menkes kinky hair syndrome [471].

Selenium

The physical and chemical properties of selenium closely resemble those of sulphur. It is a component of several enzymes, in particular those related to redox reactions. Moreover, vitamin E and selenium have a mutually sparing action, suggesting that both serve as anti-oxidants. Indeed, selenium was found to be an integral part of glutathione peroxidase which protects cells from oxidative damage.

Both selenium deficiency and excess were found to have deleterious effects on several body systems, including the immune system. Antibody response to sheep RBC was diminished under both conditions, but was increased by the administration of an optimal selenium dose [484,485]. A similar observation was made regarding the immune response to *Plasmodium berghei* vaccination in mice [486]; an optimal selenium dose which is in fact in modest excess enhanced the acquisition of immunity and recovery from the subsequent challenge from the parasite. Immunosuppression in selenium-deficient dogs was more pronounced when they were fed diets rich in PUFA, but could be corrected by vitamin E [487].

The bactericidal activity of neutrophils against yeast, but not phagocytic function, was impaired by selenium deficiency [488]. Glutathione peroxidase activity in such neutrophils was low.

Selenium and vitamin E have a synergistic effect. The combined deficiency of both had severely depressed mitogen responses, more than with each deficiency alone, whereas combined supplementation with both agents enhanced T-lymphocyte responses above those seen with either nutrient alone [489]. Deficiency of both led to reduced glutathione reductase activity in plasma, to be restored by adding either one of them to the diet [490]. However, selenium cannot substitute for vitamin E in the enhancement of T- and B-cell responses [491].

Cadmium

Cadmium is needed in ultratrace amounts. It is known to be a part of a metallothionein. Its physiological function is unknown, although it was shown that cadmium can activate a number of enzymes in a non-specific manner. Exposure to excess amounts is toxic to lungs and kidneys.

The effects of cadmium on the immune system were studied primarily using subtoxic doses in water or feed of animals.

Antibody response to pseudorabies vaccine in rabbits [492] or sheep RBC in mice [492,493] was diminished; the immunosuppressive effects persisted for months after elimination of cadmium from the diet. A single dose of cadmium could also change antibody production depending on its dose, route of administration and timing in relation to antigen [494].

CMI was also inhibited by prolonged subtoxic cadmium feeding of mice, as judged by PR to mitogens [495] and by DTH to sheep RBC [496].

Phagocytic cell functions were studied with conflicting results. Stimulation [497] or inhibition [498] or no effect were reported depending on dose, exposure time, species and assay conditions.

Conclusions

An attempt has been made to condense into one chapter a comprehensive updated picture of the impact of nutrition on the immune system. Obviously, any such summary cannot be complete and reflects the writer's bias. The main message is, however, clear—nutrition, being the most important environmental factor interacting with our body, has a profound influence on the way our immune system and other defence mechanisms function. This major effect can be related to both under- and over-nutrition and to either multinutrient or certain specific single-nutrient deficiencies or excesses. It results not only in measurable effects on various immune functions, assayed *in vivo* or *in vitro*, but also on important disease processes, such as infections, cancer and autoimmune disorders. The effects of nutrition on the immune system cover virtually all aspects of the immune system, its organs and cellular elements, its development and differentiation, the production of its soluble constituents (immunoglobulins, lymphokines, complement proteins and other immune mediators) and the development of a humoral or cellular immune response to specific antigens. Single nutrients have specific effects on certain aspects of this picture. These paramount effects are easily conceivable if one bears in mind the extreme sensitivity of the immune system to various perturbations. Indeed this sensitivity can be utilized as a tool for the assessment of nutritional status, in addition to other criteria (e.g. clinical, anthropometric, haematological, biochemical) already employed for this purpose.

Most of the studies done until now describe phenomena; only few have made an attempt to elucidate the mechanism of the effects of certain nutrients on the immune system. Even at the phenomonological descriptive level we still miss a lot of information on many nutrients and their impact on the immune system and disease-related processes. However, today we should take advantage of our deeper understanding of the way the immune system functions in order to analyse the interaction of single nutrients and specific immune functions.

Nutrition is related to immunotoxicology in two ways:

1 Nutritional status changes the vulnerability of the immune system to the effects of drugs and xenobiotics [2].

2 Food in general and processed food in particular may contain harmful ingredients (e.g. remnants of fungicides, insecticides etc., artificial colours and flavouring materials, preservatives, emulsifiers and other chemicals used in the food industry), which may cause gradual accumulative damage to the immune system.

In summary, to achieve the proper optimal function of the immune system, food should include appropriate constituents and amounts and should be prepared properly. Properly designed nutritional intervention is important not only in the renourishment of subjects with severe malnutrition, but also in cases of immune-related diseases or when medical intervention is contemplated (e.g. operation, immunization and particularly total parenteral feeding). Non-nutritional, potentially immunotoxic food additives should be eliminated or kept to an unavoidable minimum.

References

1 Jackson CM. *The Effect of Inanition and Malnutrition upon Growth and Structure.* Philadelphia: Blackiston's Son, 1925.
2 Shoham J. Vulnerability to toxic or therapeutic immunomodulation—as two complementary aspects of age and nutrition dependent immunodeficiency. In: Berlin A, Dean J, Draper MH, Smith EMB, Spreafico F, eds. *Immunotoxicology.* Dordrecht: Martinus Nijhoff, 1987:389–410.
3 Shils ME, Young VR. *Modern Nutrition in Health and Disease.* Philadelphia: Lea & Febiger, 1988.
4 Nielsen FH. Ultratrace elements in nutrition. *Annu Rev Nutr* 1984; 4:21–41.
5 Beisel WR. Single nutrients and immunity. *Am J Clin Nutr* 1982; 35:417–69.
6 Gurr MI. The role of lipids in the regulation of the immune system. *Progr Lipid Res* 1983; 22:257–87.
7 McMurray DN. Cell-mediated immunity in nutritional deficiency. *Progr Food Nutr Sci* 1984; 8:193–228.
8 Johnston DV, Marshall LA. Dietary fat, prostaglandins and the immune response. *Progr Food Nutr Sci* 1984; 8:3–25.
9 Panush RS, Delafuente JC. Vitamins and immunocompetence. *World Rev Nutr Diet* 1985; 45:97–132.
10 Chandra S, Chandra RK. Nutrition, immune response and outcome. *Progr Food Nutr Sci* 1986; 10:1–65.
11 Bendich A, Chandra RK, eds. Micronutrients and immune functions. *Ann NY Acad Sci* 1989:in press.
12 Spallholz JE, Stewart JR. Advances in the role of minerals in immunobiology. *Biol Trace Elements Res* 1989; 19:129–51.
13 Keusch GT, Farthing MJG. Nutrition and infection.

Annu Rev Nutr 1986; 6:131–54.

14 Chandra RK. Nutrition, immunity and infection: present knowledge and future directions. *Lancet* 1983; i: 688–91.

15 Shive W, Shive-Matthews K. Nutritional requirements for growth of human lymphocytes. *Annu Rev Nutr* 1988; 8:81–97.

16 Stinnet JD. *Nutrition and the Immune Response.* Boca Raton: CRC Press, 1983.

17 Gershwin ME, Beach RS, Hurley LS. *Nutrition and Immunity.* London: Academic Press, 1985.

18 Suskind RM. Malnutrition and the immune response. In: Suskind RM, ed. *Textbook of Pediatric Nutrition.* New York: Raven Press, 1981:241–62.

19 Beatty DW, Dowdle EB. The effects of kwashiorkor serum on lymphocyte transformation *in vitro. Clin Exp Immunol* 1978; 32:134–43.

20 Bell RG, Turner KJ, Gracey MJ. Serum and small intestinal immunoglobulin levels in malnourished children. *Am J Clin Nutr* 1976; 29:392–7.

21 Bhaskaram C, Reddy V. Cell mediated immunity in protein calory malnutrition. *J Trop Pediatr Environ Child Hlth* 1974; 20:284–6.

22 Chandra RK. Immunocompetence in undernutrition. *J Pediatr* 1972; 81:1194–200.

23 Chandra RK. Serum thymic hormone activity in protein-energy malnutrition. *Clin Exp Immunol* 1979; 38:228–30.

24 Chandra RK, Gupta S, Singh H. Inducer and suppressor T cell subsets in protein energy malnutrition. Analysis by monoclonal antibodies. *Nutr Res* 1982; 2:21–6.

25 Chandra RK, Chandra S, Gupta S. Antibody affinity and immune complexes after immunization with tetanus toxoid in protein-energy malnutrition. *Am J Clin Nutr* 1984; 40:131–4.

26 Douglas SD, Schopfer K. Phagocytic function in protein-calorie malnutrition. *Clin Exp Immunol* 1974; 17:121–6.

27 Drabik M, Pasulka P, LoPreste G, Moldawer L, Dinarello C. *In vitro* measurement of lymphocyte activating factor in hospitalized PCM patients. *J Leuk Biol* 1985; 37:698–9.

28 Freyer EA, Chabes A, Poemape O. Abnormal Rebuck skin window response in kwashiorkor. *J Pediatr* 1973; 82:523–4.

29 Grace HJ, Armstrong D, Smythe PM. Reduced lymphocyte transformation in protein calorie malnutrition. *S Afr Med J* 1972; 46:402–3.

30 Harland PS. Tuberculin reactions in malnourished children. *Lancet* 1965; ii:719–21.

31 Heresi GP, Laitra MT, Schlesinger L. Leukocyte migration inhibition factor in marasmic children. *Am J Clin Nutr* 1981; 34:909–13.

32 Jose DG, Shelton M, Tauro GP, Belbin R, Hosking CS. Deficiency of immunological and phagocytic function in aboriginal children with protein-calorie malnutrition. *Med J Aust* 1975; 2:699–705.

33 Koster F, Gaffer A, Jackson TM. Recovery of cellular immune competence during treatment of protein-calorie malnutrition. *Am J Clin Nutr* 1981; 34:887–91.

34 Lal N, Bazaz-Malik G, Sehgal H. Profile of T and B lymphocytes in malnourished children. *Ind J Med Res* 1980; 71:576–88.

35 Linn BS. Outcomes of older and younger malnourished and well nourished patients 1 year after hospitalization. *Am J Clin Nutr* 1984; 39:66–73.

36 Lloyd AVC. Tuberculin test in children with malnutrition. *Br Med J* 1960; 3:529–31.

37 Munoz C, Heresi G, Arevalo M, Saitua MT, Schlesinger L. Impaired lymphoproliferative response to alloantigens and PHA in marasmic infants. *Nutr Res* 1983; 3:181–7.

38 Neumann CG, Lawlor GJ, Steihm ER. Immunological responses in malnourished children. *Am J Clin Nutr* 1975; 28:89–91.

39 Pertschuck MJ, Crosby LO, Barol L, Multon JL. Immunocompetence in anorexia nervosa. *Am J Clin Nutr* 1982; 35:968–72.

40 Akpom CA, Warren KS. The inhibition of granuloma formation around *Schistosoma mansoni* eggs. VI. Protein, calorie, vitamin deficiency. *Am J Pathol* 1975; 79:435–50.

41 Chandra RK, Sharma S, Bhujwala RA. Effect of acute and chronic starvation on plaque forming cell response in mice. *Ind J Med Res* 1973; 61:93–7.

42 Heresi G, Chandra RK. Effects of severe calorie restriction on thymic factor activity and lymphocyte stimulation response in rats. *J Nutr* 1980; 110:1888–93.

43 Hoffman-Goetz L, Bell RC, Keir R. Effect of protein malnutrition and interleukin 1 on *in vitro* rabbit lymphocyte mitogenesis. *Nutr Res* 1985; 4:769–80.

44 Jose DJ, Good RA. Absence of enhancing antibody in cell mediated immunity to tumour heterografts in protein deficient rats. *Nature* 1971; 231:323–5.

45 Lopez V, Davis SD, Smith NJ. Studies in infantile marasmus IV. Impairment of immunological responses in the marasmic pig. *Pediatr Res* 1972; 6:779–82.

46 McMurray DN, Yetley EA. Immune responses in malnourished guinea pigs. *J Nutr* 1982; 112:167–74.

47 Quazz ST, Mamattah JHK, Ashcroft T, McFarlane H. The development and nature of immune deficit in primates in response to malnutrition. *Am J Exp Pathol* 1981; 62:452–60.

48 Sakamoto M. The sequence of recovery of the com-

plement system and PHA skin reactivity in malnutrition. *Nutr Res* 1982; 2:137–45.

49 Miller RM, Schook LB, Nelson RA. Lymphocyte proliferation and polymorphonuclear phagocytic function in dormant-fasted and non dormant fed black bears. *FASEB J* 1989; 3:A666.

50 Watts T. Thymus weights in malnourished children. *J Pediatr* 1969; 15:155–8.

51 Smythe PM, Schonland M, Breston-Stiles GG, Coovadia HM, Grace HJ. Thymolymphatic deficiency and depression of cell mediated immunity in protein calorie malnutrition. *Lancet* 1971; ii:939–43.

52 Chandra RK. Rosette forming T lymphocytes and cell mediated immunity in malnutrition. *Br Med J* 1974; 3:608–9.

53 Chandra RK. Numerical and functional deficiency in T helper cells in protein energy malnutrition. *Clin Exp Immunol* 1983; 51:126–32.

54 Chandra RK. T and B lymphocyte subpopulations and leukocyte terminal deoxynucleotidyl transferase in energy-protein malnutrition. *Acta Paediatr Scand* 1979; 68:841–5.

55 Olusi SO, Thurman GB, Goldstein AL. Effect of thymosin on T-lymphocyte rosette formation in children with kwashiorkor. *Clin Immunol Immunopathol* 1980; 15:687–91.

56 Zaman S, Jackson T. Effect of thymopoietin on rosette formation *in vitro* in malnutrition. *Clin Exp Immunol* 1980; 39:354–7.

57 Chandra RK. Cell mediated immunity in nutritional imbalance. *Fed Proc* 1980; 39:3088–92.

58 Chandra RK. *Immunology of Nutritional Disorders.* London: Arnold, 1980.

59 Chandra RK. Reduced secretory antibody response to live attenuated measles and polio virus vaccines in malnourished children. *Br Med J* 1975; 2:583–5.

60 Chandra RK. Serum complement and immunoconglutinin in malnutrition. *Arch Dis Child* 1975; 50:225–9.

61 Haller L, Zubler RH, Lambert PH. Plasma levels of complement components and complement hemolytic activity in protein energy malnutrition. *Clin Exp Immunol* 1978; 34:248–52.

62 Abbassy AS, Badr El-din NK, Hassan AI. Studies of cell mediated immunity and allergy in protein-energy malnutrition. I. Cell mediated delayed hypersensitivity. *J Trop Med Hyg* 1974; 77:13–17.

63 Edelman R, Suskind R, Olson RE, Sirisinha S. Mechanisms of defective delayed cutaneous hypersensitivity in children with protein-calorie malnutrition. *Lancet* 1973; ii:506–8.

64 Beatty DW, Dowdle EB. Deficiency in kwashiorkor serum of factors required for optimal lymphocyte transformation *in vitro*. *Clin Exp Immunol* 1979;

35:435–42.

65 Heyworth B, Moore DL, Brown J. Depression of lymphocyte response to PHA in the presence of plasma from children with acute protein energy malnutrition. *Clin Exp Immunol* 1975; 22:72–7.

66 Schlesinger L, Ohlbaum A, Grez L, Stekel A. Decreased interferon production by leukocytes in marasmus. *Am J Clin Nutr* 1974; 29:758–61.

67 Chandra RK, Chandra S, Ghai OI. Chemotaxis, random mobility and mobilization of polymorphonuclear leucocytes on malnutrition. *J Clin Pathol* 1976; 29:224–7.

68 Kelley RE, Boehm K, Storm MS, Gadd MA, Hansbrough IF, Tonks MT. Determination of phagocytosis and stimulated oxidative burst activity in neutrophils obtained from protein malnourished rats. *FASEB J* 1989; 3:A664.

69 Beisel WR. Effects of infection on nutritional status and immunity. *Fed Proc* 1980; 39:3105–8.

70 Chandra RK. Fetal malnutrition and postnatal immunocompetence. *Am J Dis Child* 1975; 129:450–4.

71 Chandra RK. Immunological consequences of malnutrition including fetal growth retardation. In: Hambreaus L, Hanson LA, McFarlane F, eds. *Food and Immunology.* Almquist & Wiksell, 1977:58–67.

72 Chandra RK, Mutzumura T. Ontogenetic development of immune system and effects of fetal growth retardation. *J Perinat Med* 1979; 7:279–90.

73 Chandra RK. Immunocompetence in low birth weight infants after intrauterine malnutrition. *Lancet* 1974; ii:1393–5.

74 Kelley RE, Storm MC. Effect of nitrogen and calorie intake on recovery of delayed hypersensitivity response in malnourished rats. *FASEB J* 1988; 2:A436.

75 McGee DW, McMurray DN. Short term renourishment of severely malnourished mice induces an enhanced rebound of the immune response after oral immunization. *Nutr Res* 1988; 8:1207–12.

76 Kramer TR, Singkamani R, Yuttabootr Y. Cellular immunity in formerly malnourished children of northern Thailand. *FASEB J* 1989; 3:A664.

77 Price P, Bell RG. The response of protein-deficient mice to tetanus toxoid. *Immunol* 1977; 32:65–74.

78 Price P. Responses to PVP and pneumococcal polysaccharide in protein deficient mice. *Immunol* 1978; 34:87–96.

79 Aschkenasy A. Protein deprivation induces a premitotic block on the lymphocytes of rats and primarily suppressor cortisone-sensitive cells. *Nutr Rep Int* 1978; 18:177–85.

80 Bell RG, Hazell LA, Price P. Influence of dietary protein restriction on immune competence. II. Effect on lymphoid tissue. *Clin Exp Immunol* 1976; 26:314–26.

81 McMurray DN, Carlomagno MA, Mintzer CL, Tetzlaff CL. *Mycobacterium bovis* BCG vaccine fails to protect protein deficient guinea pigs against respiratory challenge with virulent *Mycobacterium tuberculosis*. *Infect Immun* 1985; 50:555–9.

82 Cohen MK, Bartow RA, Mintzer CL, McMurray DN. Effects of diet and genetics on *Mycobacterium bovis* BCG vaccine efficacy in inbred guinea pigs. *Infect Immun* 1987; 55:314–19.

83 McMurray DN, Bartow RA, Mintzer CL. Impact of protein malnutrition on exogenous reinfection with *Mycobacterium tuberculosis. Infect Immun* 1989; 57:1746–9.

84 Coghlan LG, Carlomagno MA, McMurray DN. Effect of protein and zinc deficiencies on vaccine efficacy in guinea pigs following pulmonary infection with *Listeria. Med Microbiol Immunol* 1988; 177:255–63.

85 McGee DW, McMurray DN. The effect of protein malnutrition on the IgA immune response in mice. *Immunol* 1988; 63:25–9.

86 McGee DW, McMurray DN. Protein malnutrition reduces the IgA immune response to oral antigen by altering B-cell and suppressor T-cell functions. *Immunol* 1988; 64:697–702.

87 Petro T, Peterson D, Schwartz K. Mixed lymphocyte reactions and intradermal tumour growths using alterations in dietary protein levels. *FASEB J* 1989; 3:A664.

88 Fernandes G, Friend P, Yunis EJ, Good RA. Influence of protein restriction on immune functions in NZB mice. *J Immunol* 1976; 116:782–9.

89 Fernandes G, Friend P, Yunis EJ, Good RA. Influence of dietary restriction on immunologic function and renal disease in (NZB x NZW) F$_1$ mice. *Proc Natl Acad Sci* 1978; 75:1500–4.

90 Gross RL, Newberne PM. Role of nutrition in immunologic function. *Physiol Rev* 198; 60:188–302.

91 Kenney MA, McGee JL, Piedad-Pascual F. Dietary amino acids and immune response in rats. *J Nutr* 1970; 100:1063–72.

92 Gershoff SN, Gill TJ, Simonian SJ, Steinberg AI. Some effects of amino acid deficiencies on antibody formation in the rat. *J Nutr* 1968; 95:184–90.

93 Coovadia HM, Soothill JF. The effect of amino acid restricted diets on the clearance of ^{125}I-labelled PVP in mice. *Clin Exp Immunol* 1976; 26:562–7.

94 Bowman LA, Nockels CF. L-Tryptophan decreases broiler chick mortality to *E. coli. FASEB J* 1989; 3:A666.

95 Norris J, Meadows G, Massey L, Bergland D, Starkey J, Sylvester D, Liu SY. Increased natural killer cells in humans fed a tyrosine and phenylalanine restricted formula diet. *FASEB J* 1988; 2:A435.

96 Parker N, Goodrum KJ. Arginine enhancement of a

97 Parker N, Goodrum KJ. Arginine suppression of thymocyte mitogenesis. *FASEB J* 1988; 2:A435.

98 Jose DJ, Good RA. Quantitative effects of nutritional essential amino acid deficiency upon immune response to tumors in mice. *J Exp Med* 1973; 137:1–9.

99 Chevalier PH, Aschkenasy A. Hematological and immunological effects of excess dietary leucine in the young rat. *Am J Clin Nutr* 1977; 30:1645–54.

100 Aschkenasy A. Prevention of immunodepressive effects of excess dietary leucine by isoleucine and valine in the rat. *J Nutr* 1979; 109:1214–22.

101 Dubois EL. *Lupus Erythematosus.* Los Angeles: University of South California Press, 1974.

102 Gardner MB, Ihle JN, Pillorisetty RJ, Talal N, Dubois EL, Levy JA. Type C virus expression and host response in diet cured NZB/W mice. *Nature* 1977; 268:341–3.

103 Batsford S, Schwerdtfeger M, Rohrbach R, Cambiaso C, Kluthe R. Synthetic amino acid diet prolongs survival in autoimmune murine disease. *Clin Nephrol* 1984; 21:60–9.

104 Elliot RB, Martin JM. Dietary protein: a trigger of insulin-dependent diabetes in the BB rat? *Diabetologia* 1984; 26:297–303.

105 Bardana EJ, Malinow MR, Houghton DC. Diet induced systemic lupus erythematosus in primates. *Am J Kidney Dis* 1982; 1:345–52.

106 Bardana EJ, Malinow MR, Craig S, McLaughlin P. Cross reacting antibody to alfalfa seed and DNA. *J Allergy Clin Immunol* 1983; 71:102–11.

107 Roberts JL, Hayashi JA. Exacerbation of SLE associated with alfalfa ingestion. *Lancet* 1983; i:1361–3.

108 Reidenberg M, Durant P, Harris R, De Boccardo G, Lahita R, Steizel KH. Lupus erythematosus-like disease due to hydrazine. *Am J Med* 1983; 75:365–74.

109 Teppo AM, Maury CPJ. Antibodies to gliadin, gluten and reticulin glycoprotein in rheumatoid diseases: elevated levels in Sjogren's syndrome. *Clin Exp Immunol* 1984; 57:73–80.

110 Plotz P. Autoantibodies are anti-idiotypes to antiviral antibodies. *Lancet* 1983; ii:824–6.

111 Cooke A, Lydyard PM, Roitt IM. Mechanisms of autoimmunity: a role for cross reactive idiotypes. *Immunol Today* 1983; 4:170–3.

112 Cooke A, Lydyard PM, Roitt IM. Autoimmunity and idiotypes. *Lancet* 1984; i:723–6.

113 Welsh CJR, Hanglow AC, Conn P, Barker THW, Coombs RRA. Early rheumatoid-like lesions in rabbits drinking cows' milk. I. Joint pathology. *Int Arch Allergy Appl Immunol* 1985; 78:145–51.

114 Hanglow AC, Welsh CJR, Conn P, Coombs RRA. Early rheumatoid-like lesions in rabbits drinking

cows' milk. II. Antibody response to bovine serum proteins. *Int Arch Allergy Appl Immunol* 1985; 78:152–9.

115 Trail KN, Wick G. Lipids and lymphocyte function. *Immunol Today* 1984; 5:70–6.

116 Goodwin JS, Webb DR. Regulation of the immune response by prostaglandins. *Clin Immunol Immunopathol* 1980; 15:106–22.

117 Goldyne ME, Stobo JD. Immunoregulatory role of prostaglandins and related lipids. *CRC Crit Rev Immunol* 1981; 189–223.

118 Wardle EN. Immunosuppression by fatty acids. *Lancet* 1976; ii:423–4.

119 Hirata F, Axelrod J. Phospholipid methylation and biological signal transmission. *Science* 1980; 209:1082–90.

120 Dawson RMC. Phospholipid structure as a modulator of intracellular turnover. *J Am Oil Chem Soc* 1982; 59:401–6.

121 Ferber E, Resch K. Structure and physiologic role of lipids in the lymphocyte membrane. In: Marchalonis JJ, ed. *Lymphocyte Structure and Function.* New York: Marcel Dekker, 1977; 593–625.

122 Ferber E, Kroner E, Schmidt B, Fischer H, Peskar BA, Anders C. Dynamic of membrane fatty acids during lymphocyte stimulation by mitogens. In: Katz M, Kuksis A, eds. *Membrane Fluidity: Biophysical Techniques in Cellular Recognition.* Clifton NJ: Humana Press, 1980:239–63.

123 Chandra RK. Cell mediated immunity in genetically obese (C57B1/6J ob/ob) mice. *Am J Clin Nutr* 1980; 13–16.

124 Erickson KL, McNeill CJ, Gershwin ME, Ossmann JB. Influence of dietary fat concentration and saturation on immune ontogeny in mice. *J Nutr* 1980; 110:1555–72.

125 Meade CJ. How arachidonic acid depresses thymic weight. *Int Arch Allergy Appl Immunol* 1979; 59:432–6.

126 Di Luzio NR, Wooles WR. Depression of phagocytic activity and immune response by methyl-palmitate. *Am J Physiol* 1969; 206:939–43.

127 De Wille JW, Fraker PJ, Romsos DR. Effects of essential fatty acid deficiency and various levels of dietary PUFA on humoral immunity in mice. *J Nutr* 1979; 109:1018–27.

128 Ring J, Seifert J, Mertin J, Brendel W. Prolongation of skin allografts in rats by treatment with linoleic acid. *Lancet* 1974; ii:1331.

129 Mertin J. Effect of PUFA on skin allograft survival and primary and secondary cytotoxic response in mice. *Transplant* 1976; 21:1–4.

130 Mertin J, Hughes D, Shenton BK, Dickinson JP. In vitro inhibition by unsaturated fatty acids of the PPD

and PHA induced lymphocyte response. *Klin Wochenschr* 1974; 52:248–50.

131 Mertin J, Hughes D. Specific inhibitory action of PUFA on lymphocyte transformation induced by PHA and PPD. *Int Arch Allergy Appl Immunol* 1975; 48:203–10.

132 Mertin J, Hunt R. Influence of PUFA on survival of skin allografts and tumor incidence in mice. *Proc Natl Acad Sci* 1976; 73:928–31.

133 Meade CJ, Mertin J. The mechanism of immunoinhibition by arachidonic and linoleic acids. *Int Arch Allergy Appl Immunol* 1976; 51:2–24.

134 Thomas IK, Erickson KL. Dietary fatty acid modulation of murine T cell responses *in vitro. J Nutr* 1985; 115:1528–34.

135 Selivonchick DP, Johnston PV. Fat deficiency in rats during development of central nervous system and susceptibility to experimental allergic encephalomyelitis. *J Nutr* 1975; 105:288–300.

136 Weston PG, Johnston PV. Cerebral prostaglandin synthesis during the dietary and pathological stresses of essential fatty acid deficiency and experimental allergic encephalomyelitis. *Lipids* 1978; 13:408–14.

137 Meade CJ, Mertin J. The mechanism of immunoinhibition by arachidonic and linoleic acid: effects on the lymphoid and reticuloendothelial systems. *Int Arch Allergy Appl Immunol* 1976; 2:501–2.

138 Frost P, Frost H, Hollander D. Non effect of PUFA on thoracic duct cell and lymph output in rats. *Lancet* 1978; ii:382.

139 Thomas IK, Erickson KL. Lipid modulation of mammary tumor cell cytolysis. Direct influence of dietary fats on the effector component of cell mediated cytotoxicity. *J Natl Cancer Inst* 1985; 74:675–80.

140 Uldall PR, Wilkinson R, McHugh MI. Linoleic acid and transplantation. *Lancet* 1975; ii:128–9.

141 McHugh MI, Wilkinson R, Elliott RW. Immunosuppression with PUFA in renal transplantion. *Transplant* 1977; 24:263–7.

142 Clausen J, Moller J. Allergic encephalomyelitis induced by brain antigen after deficiency in PUFA during myelination. *Acta Neurol Scand* 1967; 43:375–88.

143 Levine S, Sowinski R. Effect of essential fatty acid deficiency on experimental allergic encephalomyelitis in rats. *J Nutr* 1980; 110:891–6.

144 Marshall LA, Johnston PV. The influence of dietary essential fatty acids on rat immunocompetent cell prostaglandin synthesis and mitogen induced blastogenesis. *J Nutr* 1985; 115:1572–80.

145 Berken A, Benacerraf B. Depression of reticuloendothelial system phagocytic function by ingested lipids. *Proc Soc Exp Biol Med* 1968; 128:793–5.

146 Nordenstrom J, Jarstrand C, Wiernik A. Decreased

chemotactic and random migration of leukocytes during intralipid infusion. *Am J Clin Nutr* 1979; 32:2416–22.

147 Hawley HP, Gordon GB. The effects of long chain free fatty acids on human neutrophil function and structure. *Lab Invest* 1976; 34:216–22.

148 Kowolenko M, Tracy J, Lawrence DA. Lipid modulation of bone marrow cell responsiveness to CSF-1. *FASEB J* 1989; 3:A665.

149 Field EJ, Shenton BK. Inhibition of lymphocyte response to stimulants by unsaturated fatty acids and prostaglandins. *Lancet* 1974; ii:725.

150 Frost P, Hollander D, Chen J. Effect of PUFA on lymphoid cell survival *in vitro*. *Lancet* 1977; ii:410.

151 Tonkin CH, Brostoff J. Do fatty acids exert a specific effect on human lymphocyte transformation *in vitro*? *Int Arch Allergy Appl Immunol* 1978; 57:171–6.

152 Magnum LJ, Johnston PV. Effect of dietary provided linoleic and α-linolenic acid on the function of rat peritoneal macrophages. *Nutr Res* 1986; 6:287–93.

153 Schnieder E, Dy M. The role of arginase in the immune response. *Immunol Today* 1985; 6:136–40.

154 Oropeza-Rendon RL, Cremel G, Ernst M, Fischer H. Does PGE_1 induce modifications at the membrane level of bone macrophages? A fluorescence study. *Prostaglandins* 1980; 20:909–22.

155 Murphy RC, Pickett WC, Culp BR, Lands WEM. Tetraene and pentaene leukotrienes. Selective production from murine mastocytoma cells after dietary manipulation. *Prostaglandin* 1981; 22:613–23.

156 Leitch AG, Lee TH, Ringel EW, Prickett JD, Robinson DR. Immunologically induced generation of tetraene and pentaene leukotrienes in the peritoneal cavities of menhaden fed rats. *J Immunol* 1984; 132:2559–65.

157 Lee TH, Hoover RL, Williams JD, Sperling RI. Effect of dietary enrichment with eicosapentanoic and docoshexaenoic acids on *in vitro* neutrophil and monocyte leukotriene generation and neutrophil function. *N Engl J Med* 1985; 312:1217–24.

158 Newberne PM. Effect of overnutrition on resistance of dogs to distemper virus. *Fed Proc* 1966; 25:1701–10.

159 Fiser RH, Rollins JB, Beisel WR. Decreased resistance against infection by canine hepatitis in dogs fed a high fat ratio. *Am J Vet Res* 1972; 33:713–19.

160 Hedgecock LW. Effect of dietary fatty acids and protein intake on experimental tuberculosis. *J Bacteriol* 1955; 70:415–20.

161 Levy JA, Ibrahim AB, Shirai T, Ohta K, Nagasawa R, Yoshida H, Estes J, Gardner M. Dietary fat affects immune response, production of antiviral factors and immune complex disease in NZB/NZW mice. *Proc Natl Acad Sci* 1982; 79:1974–80.

162 Fernandes G, Alfonso RA, Tanaka T, Tahler HT, Yunis EJ, Good RA. Influence of diet on vascular lesions in autoimmune prone mice. *Proc Natl Acad Sci* 1983; 80:874–8.

163 Kelley VE, Izui S. Enriched lipid diet accelerates lupus nephritis in NZB x W mice. *Am J Pathol* 1985; 111:288–99.

164 Morrow WJW, Ohashi Y, Hall J, Pribnow J, Hirose S, Shirai T, Levy JA. Dietary fat and immune function. I. Antibody responses, lymphocyte and accessory cell function in (NZB/NZW) F_1 mice. *J Immunol* 1985; 135:3857–63.

165 Yumura W, Hattori S, Morrow WJW, Mayes DC, Levy JA, Shirai T. Dietary fat and immune function. II. Effect on immune complex nephritis in (NZB/NZW) F_1 mice. *J Immunol* 1985; 135:3864–9.

166 Fernandes G. Role of nutrition and hyperglycemia on immunity and on the development of renal and cardiovascular disease in autoimmune prone mice. *Fed Proc* 1983; 42:1212.

167 Hurd ER, Johnston JM, Okita JR, MacDonald PC, Ziff M, Gilliam JN. Prevention of glomerulonephritis and prolonged survival in (NZB/NZW) F_1 hybrid mice fed fatty acid deficient diet. *J Clin Invest* 1981; 67:476–83.

168 Prickett JD, Robinson OR, Steinberg AD. Dietary enrichment with PUFA eicosapentanoic acid prevents proteinuria and prolongs survival in B/W mice. *J Clin Invest* 1981; 68:556–64.

169 Prickett JD, Robinson OR, Steinberg AD. Effects of dietary enrichment with eicosapentanoic acid upon autoimmune nephritis in female B/W mice. *Arthr Rheumat* 1983; 26:133–40.

170 Kelley VE, Ferretti A, Izui S, Strom TB. A fish oil diet rich in eicosapentanoic acid reduces cyclooxygenase metabolites and suppresses lupus in MRL/lpr mice. *J Immunol* 1985; 134:1914–19.

171 Leslie CA, Gonnerman WA, Ullman MD, Hayes KC, Franzblau C, Cathcart ES. Dietary fish oil modulates macrophage fatty acids and decreases arthritis susceptibility in mice. *J Exp Med* 1985; 162:1336–49.

172 Panush RS, Carter RL, Katz P, Kowsari B, Longeley S, Finnie S. Diet therapy for rheumatoid arthritis. *Arthr Rheum* 1983; 26:457–62.

173 Kremer J, Bigaubette J, Michalek AV. Effects of manipulation of dietary fatty acids on clinical manifestations of rheumatoid arthritis. *Lancet* 1985; i:700–2.

174 Birtwistle S, McEwen LM. Dietary fatty acids and rheumatoid arthritis. *Lancet* 1985; i:700–2.

175 Curtiss LK, Edington TS. Regulatory serum lipoproteins: regulation of lymphocyte stimulation by a species of low density lipoprotein. *J Immunol* 1976; 116:1452–9.

176 Carroll KK. The role of dietary fats in carcinogenesis.

In: Perkins EG, Visek WJ, eds. *Dietary Fat and Health.* Monograph 10. Champaign, IL: American Oil Chemical Society, 1983; 710–72.

177 Carroll KK. Role of lipids in tumorigenesis. *J Am Oil Chem Soc* 1984; 61:1888–91.

178 Clinton SK, Imrey PB, Alster JM, Simon J. The combined effect of dietary protein and fat on 7,12-dimethyl benz(a)anthracene-induced breast cancer in rats. *J Nutr* 1984; 114:1213–23.

179 Erickson KL, Thomas IK. Susceptibility of mammary tumor cells to complement-mediated cytotoxicity after *in vitro* or *in vivo* fatty acid manipulation. *J Natl Cancer Inst* 1985; 75:333–40.

180 Kollmorgen GM, King MM, Kosanke SD, Do C. Influence of dietary fat and indomethacin on the growth of transplantable mammary tumors in rats. *Cancer Res* 1983; 43:4714–19.

181 Helyor L, Sherman AR, Layman O, Yedinak R. Effect of dietary fat level and exercise training on natural killer cell activity in DMBA treated rats. *FASEB J* 1988; 2:A435.

182 Karmali RA, Marsh, Fuchs C. Effect of omega-3 fatty acids on growth of a rat mammary tumor. *J Natl Cancer Inst* 1984; 73:457–61.

183 Carroll KK, Braden LM. Dietary PUFA in relation to mammary carcinogenesis. *J Am Oil Chem Soc* 1985; 62:640.

184 Jurkowski JJ, Cave WT. Dietary effects of menhaden oil on the growth and membrane composition of rat mammary tumors. *J Natl Cancer Inst* 1985; 74:1145–50.

185 Schlager SI, Ohanian SH. A role for the fatty acid composition of complex cellular lipids in the susceptibility of tumor cells to humoral killing. *J Immunol* 1979; 123:146–52.

186 Yoo TJ, Chin HC, Spector AA. Effect of fatty acid modifications of cultured hepatoma cells on susceptibility to complement mediated cytolysis. *Cancer Res* 1980; 40:1084–8.

187 Gill R, Clark W. Membrane–structure–function relationships in cell mediated cytolysis. *J Immunol* 1980; 125:689–95.

188 Bialick R, Gill R, Berke G, Clark WR. Modulation of cell-mediated cytotoxicity function after alteration of fatty acid composition *in vitro*. *J Immunol* 1984; 132:81–7.

189 Parkar RS, Lala PK. Changes in the host natural killer cell population in mice during tumor development. *Cell Immunol* 1985; 93:265–79.

190 Fulton AM. *In vivo* effects of indomethacin on the growth of murine mammary tumors. *Cancer Res* 1984; 45:4779–84.

191 Fulton AM, Heppner GH. Relationships of prostaglandin E and natural killer sensitivity to metastatic potential in murine mammary adenocarcinoma. *Cancer Res* 1985; 45:4779–84.

192 Fiser RH, Denniston JC, McGann VG. Altered immune functions in hypercholesterolemic monkeys. *Infect Immun* 1973; 8:105–9.

193 Kos WL, Loria RM, Snodgrass MJ. Inhibition of host resistance by nutritional hypercholesterolemia. *Infect Immun* 1979; 26:658–67.

194 Klufred DM, Allison MJ, Gerszten E, Dalton HP. Alterations of host defenses paralleling cholesterol induced atherogenesis. II. Immunologic studies in rabbits. *J Med* 1979; 10:49–64.

195 Chassin MR, Bruger M. Effect of induced hypercholesterolemia on antibody response in rabbits. *Proc Soc Exp Biol Med* 1939; 42:457–9.

196 Heiniger HJ, Brunner KT, Grottini JC. Cholesterol is a critical cellular component of T-lymphocyte cytotoxicity. *Proc Natl Acad Sci* 1978; 75:5683–7.

197 Chen SS-H. Requirement of cholesterol for successful blastogenesis in mitogen stimulated lymphocytes. *Fed Proc* 1978; 37:377.

198 Dewey K, Nuzum F. The effect of cholesterol on phagocytosis. *J Infect Dis* 1914; 15:472–82.

199 Di Luzio NR. Employment of lipids in the measurement and modification of cellular and humoral immune responses. *Adv Lipid Res* 1972; 10:43–88.

200 Chapman HA, Hibbs JB. Modulation of macrophage tumoricidal capability by components of normal serum. *Science* 1977; 197:282–5.

201 Edgington TS, Curtiss LK. Lipoprotein regulation of immune cell functions. In: Perkins EG, Visek WJ, eds. *Dietary Fats and Health.* Monograph 10. Champaign, IL: American Oil Chemical Society, 1983:901–18.

202 Eshel I, Savion N, Shoham J. Analysis of thymic stromal cell subpopulations grown *in vitro* on extracellular matrix in defined medium. I. Growth conditions and morphology of murine thymic epithelial and mesenchymal cells. *J Immunol* 1990; in press.

203 Eshel I, Savion N, Shoham J. Analysis of thymic stromal cell subpopulations grown *in vitro* on extracellular matrix in defined medium. II. Cytokine activities in murine thymic epithelial and mesenchymal cells culture supernatants. *J Immunol* 1990; in press.

204 Morse JH, Witte LD, Goodman DS. Inhibition of lymphocyte proliferation stimulated by lectins and allogeneic cells by normal plasma lipoproteins. *J Exp Med* 1977; 146:1791–803.

205 Hui DY, Harmony JAK, Innerarity TL, Makley RW. Immunoregulatory plasma lipoproteins. Role of apoprotein E and B. *J Biol Chem* 1980; 255:11775–81.

206 Harmoni JAK, Hui DY. Inhibition by membrane bound LDL of the primary inductive events of mitogen stimulated lymphocyte activation. *Cancer Res* 1981; 41:3799–802.

207 Chisari FV. Modulation of the immune response by human plasma VLDL. *Cell Immunol* 1980; 52:223–8.

208 Hsu KH, Ghanta VK, Hiramolo RN. Immunosuppressive effects of mouse serum lipoproteins. I *In vitro* studies. *J Immunol* 1981; 126:1909–13.

209 Curtiss LK, Forte TM, Davis PA. Cord blood plasma lipoprotein inhibits mitogen stimulated lymphocyte proliferation. *J Immunol* 1984; 133:1379–83.

210 Cramer W, Drew AH, Mattram JC. On the function of the lymphocyte and of lymphoid tissue in nutrition. *Lancet* 1921; ii:1202–8.

211 Pruzansky J, Axelrod AE. Antibody production to diphtheria toxoid in vitamin deficiency states. *Proc Soc Exp Biol Med* 1955; 89:323–5.

212 Axelrod AE. Immune processes in vitamin deficiency states. *Am J Clin Nutr* 1971; 24:265–71.

213 Axelrod AE. Role of the B vitamins in the immune response. *Adv Exp Med Biol* 1981; 135:93–106.

214 Anderson R, Jones PT. Increased leucoattractant binding and reversible inhibition of neutrophil motility mediated by the peroxidase/H_2O_2/halde system. *Clin Exp Immunol* 1982; 47:487–96.

215 Anderson R, Van Rensburg CEJ, Eftydus H, Joone G. Further on erythromycin effects on cellular immune functions *in vitro* and *in vivo*. *J Antimicrob Chemother* 1982; 10:409–17.

216 Jones PT, Anderson R. Oxidative inhibition of PMN leucocyte motility. *Int J Immunopharmacol* 1983; 5:377–89.

217 Szutz P, Katona A, Ilyes M, Szabo I, Csato M. Correction of defective chemotaxis with thiamine in Schwachman-Diamond syndrome. *Lancet* 1984; i:1072–3.

218 Goodwin JS, Gorry PJ. Relationship between megadose vitamin supplementation and immunological function in healthy elderly population. *Clin Exp Immunol* 1983; 51:647–53.

219 Wertman K, Crisley FD, Sarandria JL. Complement fixing murine typhus antibodies in vitamin deficiency states. III. Riboflavin and folic acid deficiencies. *Proc Soc Exp Biol Med* 1952; 80:404–6.

220 Cook ME, Springer WT. Effect of reovirus infection and dietary levels of selected vitamins on immunocompetence of chickens. *Avian Dis* 1983; 27:367–77.

221 Saiki I, Tono-oka S, Azumi I. Adjuvant and mitogenic activities of niacin derivatives and their NAD analogs. *Int J Vit Nutr Res* 1981; 51:239–46.

222 Bochette-Egly C, Ittel ME, Bilen J, Mandel P. Effect of nicotinamide on RNA and DNA synthesis and on poly (ADP-ribose) polymerase activity in normal and phytohemagglutinin stimulated human lymphocytes. *FEBS Lett* 1980; 120:7–11.

223 Beisel WR, Edelman R, Nauss K, Suskind RM. Single nutrient effects on immunological functions. *JAMA* 1981; 254:53–8.

224 Axelrod AE, Trakatellis AC. Relationship of pyridoxine to immunological phenomena. *Vit Horm* 1964; 22:591–607.

225 Stoerk HL, Zucker TF. Nutritional effects on the development and atrophy of the thymus. *Proc Soc Exp Biol Med* 1944; 56:151–3.

226 Davis SD, Nelson T, Shepard TH. Teratogenicity of vitamin B_6 deficiency. *Science* 1970; 169:1329–30.

227 Axelrod AE, Hopper S, Long DA. Effects of pyridoxine deficiency upon circulating antibody formation and skin hypersensitivity reactions to diphtheria toxoid in guinea pigs. *J Nutr* 1961; 74:58–64.

228 Blalock TL, Thaxton JP, Garlich JD. Humoral immunity in chicks experiencing marginal vitamin B-6 deficiency. *J Nutr* 1984; 114:312–22.

229 Hodges RE, Bean WB, Ohlson MA, Bleiler RE. Factors affecting human antibody response. IV. Pyridoxine deficiency. *Am J Clin Nutr* 1962; 11:180–6.

230 Hodges RE, Bean WB, Ohlson MA, Bleiler RE. Factors affecting human antibody response. V. Combined deficiencies of pantothenic acid and pyridoxine. *Am J Clin Nutr* 1962; 11:188–99.

231 Trakatellis AC, Slinebring WR, Axelrod AE. Studies on systemic reactivity to purified protein derivative (PPD) and endotoxin. I. Systemic reactivity to PPD in pyridoxine-deficient guinea pigs. *J Immunol* 1963; 91:39–45.

232 Axelrod AE, Trakatallis AC, Bloch H, Slinebring WR. Effect of pyridoxine deficiency on DTH in guinea pigs. *J Nutr* 1963; 79:161–5.

233 Trakatellis AC, Axelrod AE. Effect of pyridoxine deficiency on the induction of immune tolerance in mice. *Proc Soc Exp Biol Med* 1969; 132:46–9.

234 Ha C, Miller LT, Kerkvliet NI. The effects of vitamin B_6 deficiency on cytotoxic immune responses of T cells, antibodies and natural killer cells and phagocytosis by macrophages. *Cell Immunol* 1984; 85:318–29.

235 Chandra RK, Heresi G, Au B. Serum thymic factor activity in deficiency of calories, zinc, vitamin A and pyridoxine. *Clin Exp Immunol* 1980; 42:332–5.

236 Casciato DA, McAdam LP, Kopple JD, Bluestone R. Immunologic abnormalities in hemodialysis patients. Improvement after pyridoxine therapy. *Nephron* 1984; 38:9–16.

237 Fisher B, Axelrod AE, Fisher ER, Lee SH, Calvanese N. The favorable effect of pyridoxine deficiency on skin homograft survival. *Surgery (St Louis)* 1985; 44:149–67.

238 Robson LC, Schwartz MR. Vitamin B_6 deficiency and the lymphoid system. I. Effects on cellular immunity and *in vitro* incorporation of ^{3}H-uridine by small lymphocytes. *Cell Immunol* 1975; 16:135–44.

239 Robson LC, Schwartz MR. Vitamin B_6 deficiency and

the lymphoid system. II. Effects of vitamin B$_6$ *in utero* on the immunocompetence of the offspring. *Cell Immunol* 1975; 16:145–62.

240 Stinebring WR, Trakatellis AC, Axelrod AE. Studies on systemic reactivity to PPD and endotoxin II. Systemic reactivity to endotoxin in pyridoxine deficient guinea pigs and its relationship to systemic reactivity to PPD. *J Immunol* 1963; 91:46–9.

241 Moriguchi S, Kishino Y. Phagocytosis of alveolar macrophages of pyridoxine deficient rats. *J Nutr* 1984; 114:888–93.

242 Ha C, Kerkvliet NI, Miller LT. The effects of vitamin B$_6$ deficiency on host susceptibility to Molony sarcoma virus induced tumor growth in mice. *J Nutr* 1984; 114:938–45.

243 Prasad R, Rao YVBG, Sindhu RK, Subrahmanyam DF. Effect of pyridoxine deficiency on *Litomosoides carini* infection in albino rats. *Trans R Soc Trop Med Hyg* 1980; 74:459–62.

244 Panda B, Combs JF. Impaired antibody production in chicks fed diets low in vitamin A, pantothenic acid or riboflavin. *Proc Soc Exp Biol Med* 1963; 113:530–4.

245 Lederer WH, Kumar M, Axelrod AE. Effects of pantothenic acid deficiency on cellular antibody synthesis in rats. *J Nutr* 1975; 105:17–25.

246 Hodges RE, Bean WB, Ohlson MA, Bleiler RE. Factors affecting human response. III Immunologic responses of men deficient in pantothenic acid. *Am J Clin Nutr* 1962; 11:85–93.

247 Kumar M, Axelrod AE. Cellular antibody synthesis in thiamine, riboflavin, biotin and folic acid-deficient rats. *Proc Soc Exp Biol Med* 1978; 157:421–3.

248 Petrelli F, Moretti, Companati G. Studies on the relationship between biotin and behaviour of B and T lymphocytes in the guinea pigs. *Experientia* 1981; 37:1204–6.

249 Rabin BS. Inhibition of experimentally induced autoimmunity in rats by biotin deficiency. *J Nutr* 1983; 113:2316–22.

250 Cowan MJ, Wara DW, Packman S. Multiple biotin dependent carboxylase deficiencies associated with defects in T and B cell immunity. *Lancet* 1979; ii:115–18.

251 Fischer A, Munnich A, Sandubray JM, Mamas S. Biotin responsive immunoregulatory dysfunction in multiple carboxylase deficiency. *J Clin Immunol* 1982; 2:35–8.

252 Petrelli F, Moretti P, Sciaresi P, Dalur AM. The effect of biotin on the formation of different types of E-rosettes by human lymphocytes. *J Leuk Biol* 1985; 37:503–9.

253 Williams EAJ, Gross RL, Newberne PM. Effect of folate deficiency on the cell mediated immune responses in rats. *Nutr Rep Int* 1975; 12:137–48.

254 Turk JL. Cytology of the induction of hypersensitivity. *Br Med Bull* 1967; 23:3–8.

255 Gross RL, Reid JVO, Newberne PM. Depressed CMI in megaloblastic anemia due to folic acid deficiency. *Am J Clin Nutr* 1975; 28:225–32.

256 Kaplan SS, Basford RE. Effect of vitamin B$_{12}$ and folic acid deficiencies on neutrophil function. *Blood* 1976; 47:801–5.

257 Youinou PY, Garre MA, Menez JF, Bales JM. Folic acid deficiency and neutrophil dysfunction. *Am J Med* 1982; 73:652–7.

258 Garre MA, Youinou PY, Morin JF, Vaurette DE. Folic acid deficiency in patients under intensive care. *Crit Care Med* 1981; 9:219.

259 Skacel PO, Cjamarin I. Impaired chemiluminescence and bactericidal killing neutrophils from patients with severe cobalamine deficiency. *Br J Haematol* 1983; 55:203–15.

260 Nelson JD, Haltalin KC. Effect of neonatal folic acid deprivation on later growth and susceptibility to *Shigella* infection in the guinea pig. *Am J Clin Nutr* 1972; 25:992–6.

261 Morrey JD, Sidewell RW, Noble RL, Barnett BB, Mahoney AW. Effects of folic acid malnutrition on rotaviral infection in mice. *Proc Soc Exp Biol Med* 1984; 176:77–83.

262 MacCuish AC, Urbaniak SJ, Goldstone AH, Irvine WJ. PHA responsiveness and subpopulations of circulating lymphocytes in pernicious anemia. *Blood* 1974; 44:849–55.

263 Tai C, McGuigan JE. Immunologic studies in pernicious anemia. *Blood* 1969; 34:63–71.

264 Das KC, Herbert V. The lymphocyte as a marker of past nutritional status. *Br J Haematol* 1978; 38:219–33.

265 Sekane T, Takada S, Kotani H, Tsunematsu T. Effect of methyl-B$_{12}$ on the *in vitro* immune functions of human T-lymphocytes. *J Clin Immunol* 1982; 2:101–9.

266 Takimoto G, Yoshimatsu K, Isomura J, Ikeda T. The modulation of murine immune responses by methyl B$_{12}$. *Int J Tissue React* 1982; 4:95–101.

267 Haurami FI, Kauh YS, Abboud EM. Methylcobalamin corrects the deleterious effect of nitrous oxide on thymidilate synthetase. *Mol Cell Biochem* 1984; 65:153–7.

268 Seger R, Frater N, Schroeder M, Hitzig WH. Granulocyte dysfunction in transcobalamin II deficiency responding to leucovorin. *J Inherit Metab Dis* 1980; 3:3–9.

269 Katka K. Immune functions in pernicious anemia before and during treatment with vitamin B$_{12}$. *Scand J Haematol* 1984; 32:76–82.

270 Thomaskuthy KG, Lee CM. Interaction of nutrition

and infection. Effect of vitamin B$_{12}$ deficiency on resistance to *Trypanosoma lewisi. J Natl Med Assoc* 1985; 77:289–99.

271 Tolbert BM. Ascorbic acid metabolism and physiological function. *Int J Vit Nutr Res* 1979; 19 (suppl): 127–42.

272 Wilson CW. Clinical pharmacological aspects of ascorbic acid. *Ann NY Acad Sci* 1975; 258:355–76.

273 Pauling L. *Vitamin C and the Common Cold.* San Francisco: WH Freeman, 1970.

274 Vilter RW, Woolford RM, Spies TD. Severe scurvy. A clinical and hematological study. *J Lab Clin Med* 1976; 31:609–30.

275 Kumar M, Axelrod AE. Circulating antibody formation in scorbutic guinea pigs. *J Nutr* 1969; 98:41–4.

276 Prinz W, Bortz R, Hersch M, Gilich G. Vitamin C and the humoral immune response. *Int J Vit Nutr Res* 1979; 19 (suppl): 25–34.

277 Prinz W, Bloch G, Milchell G. A systemic study of the effect of vitamin C supplementation on the humoral immune response in ascorbate dependent mammals. *Int J Vit Nutr Res* 1980; 50:294–300.

278 McCorkle F, Taylor R, Stinson R, Day EJ, Glick B. The effects of a megalevel vitamin C on the immune response of the chicken. *Poult Sci* 1980; 59:1324–7.

279 Panush RS, Delafuerte JC, Katz P, Johnson J. Modulation of certain immunologic response by vitamin C III. Potentiation of *in vitro* and *in vivo* lymphocyte responses. *Int J Vit Nutr Res* 1982; 23:35–47.

280 Thomas WR, Holt PG. Vitamin C and immunity an assessment of the evidence. *Clip Exp Immunol* 1978; 32:370–9.

281 Anderson R, Oosthuizen R, Maritz R, Theron A. The effects of increasing weekly doses of ascorbate on certain cellular and humoral immune functions in normal volunteers. *Am J Clin Nutr* 1980; 33:71–6.

282 Johnston CS. Effect of vitamin C supplementation on complement component C1q. Concentration in the plasma of men and women. *FASEB J* 1988; 2:A435.

283 Mueller PS, Keis MW, Alvord EC, Show CM. Prevention of EAE by vitamin C deprivation. *J Exp Med* 1962; 111:329–38.

284 Mueller PS, Kies MW. Suppression of tuberculin reaction in the scorbutic guinea pigs. *Nature* 1962; 195:813.

285 Kalden JR, Guthy EA. Prolonged skin allograft survival in vitamin C deficient guinea pigs. *Eur Surg Res* 1972; 4:114–19.

286 Zweiman B, Schoenwetter WF, Hildreth EA. The effect of the scorbutic state of tuberculin hypersensitivity in the guinea pig. *J Immunol* 1966; 96:296–300.

287 Zweiman B, Schoenwetter WF, Hildreth EA. The effect of the scorbutic state of tuberculin hypersensitivity on the guinea pig. *J Immunol* 1966; 96;672–5.

288 Hsu CK. Vitamin C and immune responses in rhesus monkeys. *Fed Proc* 1977; 36:1177.

289 Anthony LE, Kurahara CG, Taylor KB. Immunocompetence and ascorbic acid deficiency in guinea pig. *Fed Proc* 1978; 37:931.

290 Fraser RC, Pavlovic S, Kurahara CG, Murata A. The effect of variations in vitamin C intake on the cellular immune response of guinea pigs. *Am J Clin Nutr* 1980; 33:839–47.

291 Seigel BV, Morton JI. Vitamin C and the immune response. *Experientia* 1977; 33:393–5.

292 Munster AM, Loadholdt CB, Barnes MA. The effect of antibiotics on CMI. *Surgery (St Louis)* 1977; 81:692–5.

293 Ramierez I, Riebie E, Waag YM, Van Eys J. Effect of ascorbic acid *in vitro* on lymphocyte reactivity to mitogens. *J Nutr* 1980; 110:2207–15.

294 Manzella JP, Roberts NJ. Human macrophage and lymphocyte responses to mitogen stimulation after exposure to influenza virus, ascorbic acid and hyperthermia. *J Immunol* 1979; 123:1940–4.

295 Panush RS, Katz P, Powell G, Somberg L. Immunopharmacologic effects of vitamin C. IV Perturbation of mononuclear cell cyclic nucleotides. *Int J Vit Nutr Res* 1983; 53:61–7.

296 Atkinson JP, Weiss A, Ho M, Kelly J, Parker CW. Effects of ascorbate on cyclic nucleotide metabolism in human lymphocytes. *J Cycl Nucl Res* 1979; 5:107–23.

297 Pickert WC, Austen KF, Goetzl EJ. Inhibition by non steroidal antiinflammatory agents of the ascorbate induced elevations of platelet cGMP levels. *J Cycl Nucl Res* 1979; 5:197–209.

298 Kay NE, Holloway DE, Hutton SW, Bona ND, Duane WC. Human T-cell function in experimental ascorbic acid deficiency and spontaneous scurvy. *Am J Clin Nutr* 1982; 36:127–30.

299 Moser R, Weber F. Uptake of ascorbic acid by human granulocytes. *Int J Vit Nutr Res* 1983; 54:47–55.

300 Stankova L, Gerhardt NB, Nagel L, Bigley RH. Ascorbate and phagocytic dysfunction. *Infect Immun* 1975; 12:252–6.

301 Nungester WJ, Ames AM. The relationship between ascorbic acid and phagocytic activity. *J Infect Dis* 1948; 83:50–4.

302 Cooper MR, McCall CE, DeChatelet LR. Stimulation of leukocyte hexose monophosphate shunt activity by ascorbic acid. *Infect Immun* 1971; 3:851–3.

303 Sandler JA, Jullin JI, Vaughan M. Effects of serotonin carbamylcholine and ascorbic acid on leucocyte cGMP and chemotaxis. *J Cell Biol* 1975; 67:480–4.

304 Ganguly R, Duriecix MF, Waldman RH. Macrophage function in vitamin C deficient guinea pigs. *Am J Clin Nutr* 1976; 29:762–5.

305 Goetzl EJ, Wasserman SI, Gigli I, Austen KF. Enhancement of random migration and chemotactic responses of human leukocytes by ascorbic acid. *J Clin Invest* 1974; 53:813.

306 Anderson R. Effects of ascorbate on normal and abnormal leucocyte functions. *Int J Vit Nutr Res* 1982; 23 (suppl): 23–34.

307 Anderson R, Lukey PT, Theron AJ, Dippenaar U. Ascorbate and cysteine mediated selective neutralization of extracellular oxidants during N-formyl peptide activation of human phagocytes. *Agents Actions* 1987; 20:77–81.

308 Boxer LA, Watanabe AM, Rister M, Besch HR. Correction of leucocyte function in Chediak-Higashi syndrome by ascorbate. *N Engl J Med* 1976; 295:1041–5.

309 Weening RS, Schoorel EP, Roos D. Effect of ascorbate on abnormal neutrophil, platelet and lymphocyte function in a patient with Chediak-Higashi syndrome. *Blood* 1981; 57:856–65.

310 Gallin JI, Elin RJ, Hubert RT, Fanci AS. Efficacy of ascorbic acid in Chediak-Higashi syndrome: studies on humans and mice. *Blood* 1979; 53:226–34.

311 Anderson R, Theron A. Effects of ascorbate on leucocytes. III *in vitro* and *in vivo* stimulation of abnormal neutrophil motility by ascorbate. *S Afr Med J* 1979; 56:429–33.

312 Rebora A, Dallegri F, Patrone F. Neutrophil dysfunction and repeated infections: influence of levamisole and ascorbic acid. *Br J Dermatol* 1980; 21:49–56.

313 Hitchcock M. Effect of variation in endogenous levels of ascorbic acid on the *in vitro* immunological release of histamine and slow reacting substances of anaphylaxis from actively sensitized guinea pig lung fragments. *Br J Pharmacol* 1980; 11:539–43.

314 Alvares RG, Mesa MG. Ascorbic acid and pyridoxine in experimental anaphylaxis. *Agents Actions* 1981; 11:89–93.

315 Zuskin E, Lewis AJ, Bouhuys A. Inhibition of histamine induced airway constriction by ascorbic acid. *J Allergy Clin Immunol* 1973; 51:218–26.

316 Ogilacy CS, DuBois AB, Douglas JS. Effects of ascorbic acid and indomethacin on airways of healthy subjects with or without inferred bronchoconstriction. *J Allergy Clin Immunol* 1981; 67:363–9.

317 Kordansky DW, Rosenthal RR, Norman PS. The effect of vitamin C on antigen induced bronchospasm. *J Allergy Clin Immunol* 1979; 63:61–4.

318 Fortner BR, Danziger RC, Rabinowitz PS, Nelson HS. The effect of ascorbic acid on cutaneous and nasal response to histamine and allergen. *J Allergy Clin Immunol* 1982; 69:484–8.

319 Siegel BV. Enhancement of interferon production by Poly IC in mouse cultures by ascorbic acid. *Nature* 1975; 254:431–2.

320 Dahl H, Degre M. The effect of ascorbic acid on production of human interferon and the antiviral activity *in vitro*. *Acta Pathol Microbiol Scand* 1976; 84B:280–4.

321 Siegel BV, Morton JI. Vitamin C, interferon and the immune response. *Int J Vit Nutr Res* 1977; 16 (suppl): 245–65.

322 Dieter MP. Further studies on the relationship between vitamin C and thymic humoral factor. *Proc Soc Exp Biol Med* 1971; 136:316–22.

323 Chalmers TC. Effects of ascorbic acid on the common cold. An evaluation of the evidence. *Am J Med* 1975; 58:532–6.

324 Editorial. Ascorbic acid: immunological effects and hazards. *Lancet* 1979; i:308.

325 Editorial. Vitamin C and the common cold. *Br Med J* 1976; i:606–7.

326 Krishnan S, Bhuyan UN, Talwar GP. Effect of vitamin A and PCM on immune responses. *Immunol* 1974; 27:383–92.

327 Passtiempo AMG, Taylor CE, Ross AC. Effects of early stages of vitamin A deficiency on the immune response to *S. pneumonia*. *FASEB J* 1989; 3:A663.

328 Bruns NJ, Webb KE, Edgert KD, Veil HP. Humoral immunity in vitamin A deficient and vitamin A repleted lambs. *FASEB J* 1989; 3:A663.

329 Cohen BE, Cohen IK. Vitamin A: adjuvant and steroid antagonist in the immune response. *J Immunol* 1973; 111:1376–80.

330 Jurin M, Tannock IF. Influence of vitamin A on immunological response. *Immunol* 1972; 23:283–7.

331 Brown KH, Rajan MM, Chakraborty J, Aziz KMA. Failure of large dose of vitamin A to enhance the antibody response to tetanus toxoid in children. *Am J Clin Nutr* 1980; 33:212–17.

332 Bryant RL, Barnett JB. The adjuvant effect of retinol on IgE production in mice. *Fed Proc* 1978; 37:1490.

333 Medawar PB, Hunt R. Anti-cancer actions of retinoids. *Immunol* 1981; 42:349–53.

334 Nauss KM, Mark DA, Suskind RM. The effect of vitamin A deficiency on the *in vitro* cellular immune response of rats. *J Nutr* 1979; 109:1815–23.

335 Levis WR, Emden RG. Enhancing effect of vitamin A on *in vitro* antigen stimulated lymphocyte proliferation. *Proc Am Assoc Cancer Res* 1976; 17:112A.

336 Cohen BE, Gill G, Cullen PR, Morris PJ. Reversal of postoperative immunosuppression in man by vitamin A. *Surg Gyn Obstet* 1979; 149:658–62.

337 Cohen BE, Elin RJ. Vitamin A induced nonspecific resistance to infection. *J Infect Dis* 1974; 129:597–600.

338 Gershwin ME, Lentz DR, Beach RS, Hurley LS. Nutritional factors and autoimmunity. IV. Dietary

vitamin A deprivation induces a selective increase in IgM autoantibodies and hypergammaglobulinemia in NZB mice. *J Immunol* 1984; 133:222–8.

339 Felix EL, Loyd B, Cohen MH. Inhibition of the growth and development of a transplantable human melanoma by vitamin A. *Science* 1975; 189:886–9.

340 Bollag W. Effects of vitamin A on transplantable and chemically induced tumors. *Cancer Chemother Rep* 1971; 55:53–8.

341 Dennert G, Lotan R. Effects of retinoic acid on the immune system: stimulation of T killer cell induction. *Eur J Immunol* 1978; 8:23–9.

342 Newberne PM, Suphakarn V. Preventive role of vitamin A in colon carcinogenesis in rats. *Cancer* 1977; 40:2553–6.

343 Olson JA. The biological role of vitamin A in maintaining epithelial tissues. *Isr J Med Sci* 1972; 8:1170–8.

344 Darip MD, Sirisinha S, Lamb AJ. Effect of vitamin A deficiency on susceptibility of rats to *Angiostrongylus cantonesis*. *Proc Soc Exp Biol Med* 1979; 161:600–4.

345 Mohanram M, Reddy V, Mishra S. Lysozyme activity in plasma and leucocytes in malnourished children. *Br J Nutr* 1974; 32:313–16.

346 Bang FB, Bang BG, Foard M. Acute Newcastle viral infection of upper respiratory tract of the chicken. II. The effects of diets deficient in vitamin A on the pathogenesis of the infection. *Am J Pathol* 1975; 78:417–26.

347 Sepe SM, Clark RA. Oxidant membrane injury by the neutrophil myeloperoxidase system. II. Injury by stimulated neutrophils and protection by lipid-soluble antioxidants. *J Immunol* 1985; 134:1896–901.

348 Alexander M, Newmark H, Miller RG. Oral beta carotene can increase the number of OKT4 + cells in human blood. *Immunol Lett* 1985; 9:221–4.

349 Meade CJ, Mertin J. Fatty acids and immunity. *Adv Lipid Res* 1978; 16:127–65.

350 Bendich A, Sapiro SS. Effect of beta carotene and cathaxanthin on the immune responses of the rat. *J Nutr* 1986; 116:2254–62.

351 Seifter E, Rettura G, Padawer J, Stratford F, Goodwin P, Levenson SM. Regression of C₃H BA mouse tumor due to x-ray therapy combined with supplemental β-carotene or vitamin A. *J Natl Cancer Inst* 1983; 71:409–17.

352 Leslee CA, Dubey TP. Carotene and NK cell activity. *Fed Proc* 1982; 41:331.

353 Schwartz JL, Suda D, Light G. Beta carotene is associated with the regression of hamster buccal pouch carcinoma and the induction of tumor necrosis factor in macrophages. *Biochem Biophys Res Commun* 1986; 136:1130–5.

354 Schwartz JL, Shklar G. Regression of experimental hamster cancer by beta carotene and algae extracts. *J Oral Maxillofac Surg* 1987; 45:510–15.

355 Schwartz JL, Shklar G. Regression of experimental oral carcinoma by local injection of beta carotene and canthaxanthin. *Nutr Cancer* 1988; 11:35–42.

356 Shklar G, Schwartz J. Tumor necrosis factor in experimental cancer. Regression with α-tocopherol, β-carotene and algae extract. *Eur J Cancer Clin Oncol* 1988; 24:839–50.

357 Ludorici PP, Axelrod AE. Circulating antibodies in vitamin deficiency states. *Proc Soc Exp Biol Med* 1951; 77:526–30.

358 Miller ER, Ullrey DE, Vincent BH, Hoefer JA. Deficiencies of magnesium and vitamin D and antibody production and hematology of the baby pig. *J Anim Sci* 1963; 22:1127.

359 Halliwell B, Gutteridge JMC (eds). *Free Radicals in Biology and Medicine.* Oxford: Clarendon Press, 1985:206–45.

360 Wagner DDM, Barton GW, Ingold KU, Locke S. Quantitative measurement of the total peroxyl radical trapping antioxidant capability of human plasma by controlled peroxidation. *FEBS Lett* 1985; 187:33–7.

361 Tengerdy RT, Mathias MM, Nockels CF. Effect of vitamin E on immunity and disease resistance. In: Prasad KN, ed. *Vitamins, Nutrition and Cancer.* Basle: Karger, 1984:123–33.

362 Barber TL, Nockels CF, Jochim MM. Vitamin E enhancement of Venezuelan equine encephalomyelitis antibody response in guinea pigs. *Am J Vet Res* 1977; 38:731–4.

363 Bendich A, Gabriel E, Machlin LJ. Dietary vitamin E requirement for optimum immune responses in the rat. *J Nutr* 1986; 116:675–81.

364 Bendich A, Gabriel E, Machlin LJ. Effect of dietary level of vitamin E on the immune system of the spontaneously hypertensive and normotensive Wistar Kyoto rat. *J Nutr* 1983; 113:1920–6.

365 Corwin LM, Gordon RK. Vitamin E and immune regulation. *Ann NY Acad Sci* 1982; 393:437–51.

366 Corwin LM, Shloss J. Influence of vitamin E on the mitogenic response of murine lymphoid cells. *J Nutr* 1980; 110:910–23.

367 Meydani SN, Barklund MP, Liu M. Effect of vitamin E supplementation on immune responsiveness of healthy elderly subjects. *FASEB J* 1983; 3:A1057.

368 Prasad JS. Effect of vitamin E supplementation on leucocyte function. *Am J Clin Nutr* 1980; 33:606–8.

369 Hamilton PD, Carey FJ, Fitch CD. Reduced inflammatory response with vitamin E deficiency. *Clin Res* 1977; 25:A618.

370 Warshawer D, Goldstein E, Hoeprich PD, Lippert W. Effect of vitamin E and ozone on pulmonary antibacterial defense mechanisms. *J Lab Clin Med* 1974;

83:228–40.

371 Gebremichael A, Levy EM, Corwin LM. Adherent cell requirement for the effect of vitamin E on antibody synthesis. *J Nutr* 1984; 114:1297–305.

372 Harris RE, Boxer LA, Baehner RL. Consequences of vitamin E deficiency on the phagocyte and oxidative function of the rat PMN leukocyte. *Blood* 1980; 55:338–43.

373 Heinzerling RH, Tengerdy RP, Wick LL, Lucker DC. Vitamin E protects mice against *Diplococcus pneumoniae* type I infection. *Infect Immun* 1974; 10:1292–5.

374 Baehner RL, Boxer LA, Allen JM, Davis J. Autooxidation as a basis for altered function by PMN leukocytes. *Blood* 1977; 50:327–35.

375 Repine JE, Rao G, Beall GD, White GG. Inhibition of human neutrophil oxidative metabolism and degranulation *in vitro* by nitroblue tetrazolium and vitamin E. *Am J Pathol* 1978; 90:659–74.

376 Butterick CJ, Baehner RL, Boxer LA, Jersild RA. Vitamin E—a selective inhibitor of the NADPH oxidoreductase enzyme system in human granulocytes. *Am J Pathol* 1983; 112:287–93.

377 Tredton HW, Whitchair CK, Langham RF. Influence of vitamins A and E on gnotobiotic and conventionally maintained rats exposed to mycoplasma pulmonis. *J Am Vet Med Assoc* 1973; 163:605–12.

378 Tengerdy RP. Vitamin E or vitamin A protects chickens against. *E. coli* infection. *Poult Sci* 1975; 54:1292–6.

379 Schildknecht EG, Squibb RL. The effect of vitamins A, E and K on experimentally induced histomoniasis on turkeys. *Parasitol* 1979; 78:19–31.

380 Stephens LC, McChesney AE, Nockels CF. Improved recovery of vitamin C-treated lambs that have been experimentally infected with intratracheal chlamydia. *Br Vet J* 1979; 135:291–3.

381 Chavance M, Brubacher G, Herbeth B, Vernhes G. Immunological and nutritional status among the elderly. In: de Weck AL. ed. *Lymphoid Cell Functions in Aging.* Rijswijk: Eurage, 1984:231–7.

382 Meydani SN, Meydani M, Verdon CP, Blumberg JB, Hayes KC. PGE$_2$ control of vitamin E enhanced immunity in old mice. *Fed Proc* 1984; 43:478.

383 Lawrence LM, Mathias MM, Nockels CF, Tengerdy RP. The effect of vitamin E on prostaglandin levels in the immune organs of chicks during the course of an *E. coli* infection. *Nutr Res* 1985; 5:497–509.

384 Pelus LM, Strausser HR. Prostaglandins and the immune response. *Life Sci* 1977; 20:903–14.

385 Kurek MP, Corwin LM. Vitamin E protection against tumor formation by transplanted murine sarcoma cells. *Nutr Cancer* 1982; 4:128–39.

386 Harman D. Free radical theory of aging: beneficial effects of antioxidants on the life span of NZB mice.

Age 1980; 3:64–75.

387 Mihan R, Ayres S. Lupus erythematosus and vitamin E: an effective and non-toxic therapy. *Cutis* 1979; 23:49–58.

388 Erickson KL, Adams DA, McNeill CJ. Dietary lipid modulation of immune responsiveness. *Lipids* 1983; 18:468–74.

389 Bendich A, Gabriel E, Machlin LJ. Effect of dietary PUFA and vitamin E on T and B cell mitogen responses. *Fed Proc* 1985; 44:934.

390 Dillard CJ, Kunert KJ, Tappel AL. Lipid peroxidation during chronic inflammation induced in rats by Freund's adjuvant: effect of vitamin E as measured by expred pentane. *Res Commun Chem Pathol Pharmacol* 1982; 37:143–6.

391 Deshago RD, Ewel C, Londono S, Metzger Z, Hoffeld JT, Oppenheim JJ. Evidence for the involvement of monocyte derived toxic oxygen metabolites in the lymphocyte dysfunction of Hodgkin's disease. *Clin Exp Immunol* 1981; 46:313–20.

392 Bendich A, D'Apolito P, Gabriel E, Machlin LJ. Interaction of dietary vitamin C and vitamin E on guinea immune responses to mitogens. *J Nutr* 1984; 114:1588–93.

393 Truneh A, Albert F, Goldstein P, Schmidt-Cerhulst AM. Early steps of lymphocyte activation bypassed by synergy between calcium ionophores and phorbol ester. *Nature* 1985; 313:318–20.

394 Hui DY, Berebitsky GL, Harmony JAK. Mitogen stimulated calcium ion accumulation by lymphocytes. Influence of plasma lipoproteins. *J Biol Chem* 1979; 254:4666–73.

395 Elin RJ. The effect of magnesium deficiency in mice on serum immunoglobulin concentrations and antibody plaque forming cells. *Proc Soc Exp Biol Med* 1975; 148:620–4.

396 McCoy JH, Kenney MA. Depressed immune response in the magnesium deficient rat. *J Nutr* 1975; 105:791–7.

397 Hass GM, McCreary PA, Laing GH, Galt RM. Lymphoproliferative and immunologic aspects of magnesium deficiency. In: Cantin M, Seelig M, eds. *Magnesium in Health and Disease.* Jamaica: Spectrum, 1980:185–200.

398 Alcock NW, Shils ME. Serum immunoglobulin G in the magnesium depleted rat. *Proc Soc Exp Biol Med* 1974; 145:855–8.

399 Kashiwa HK, Hungerford GF. Blood leukocyte response in rats fed a magnesium deficient diet. *Proc Soc Exp Biol Med* 1958; 99; 441–3.

400 Hungerford GF, Karson EF. The eosinophilia of magnesium deficiency. *Blood* 1960; 16:1642–50.

401 McCreary PA, Battifora HA, Hahneman BM. Leukocytosis, bone marrow hypoplasia and leukemia in

chronic magnesium deficiency in the rat. *Blood* 1967; 29:683–90.

402 McCreary PA, Laing G, Hass G. Susceptibility of normal and magnesium deficient rats to weekly sub-tumorigenic doses of liver lymphoma cells. *Am J Pathol* 1973; 70:89a–90a.

403 Kreuter SL, Schwartz R. Blood and mast cell histamine levels in magnesium deficient rats. *J Nutr* 1980; 110:851–8.

404 Bois P. Effect of magnesium deficiency on mast cells and urinary histamine in rats. *Br J Exp Pathol* 1963; 44:151–5.

405 Bhaskaram C, Reddy V. Cell mediated immunity in iron and vitamin deficient children. *Br Med J* 1975; 3:522.

406 Bhaskaram C, Siva Prasad J. Anemia and immune response. *Lancet* 1977; i:1000.

407 Rothembacher H, Sherman AR. Target organ pathology in iron deficient suckling rats. *J Nutr* 1980; 110:1648–54.

408 Baliga BS, Kuvibidila S, Tygart S, Suskind RM. Effect of dietary iron on T cell membrane proteins. *Clin Res* 1981; 29:622A.

409 Nalder BN, Mahoney AW, Ramakrishnan R, Hendricks DG. Sensitivity of the immunological response to the nutritional status of rats. *J Nutr* 1972; 102:535–42.

410 Chandra RK, Saraya AK. Impaired immunocompetence associated with iron deficiency. *J Pediatr* 1975; 86:899–902.

411 Sawitsky B, Kanter R, Sawitsky A. Lymphocyte response to phytomitogens in iron deficiency. *Am J Med Sci* 1976; 272:153–60.

412 MacDougal LG, Anderson A, MacNab GM, Katz J. The immune response in iron deficient children. *J Pediatr* 1975; 86:833–43.

413 Joynson DHM, Jacobs A, Murray Walker D, Dolby AE. Defect of CMI in patients with iron deficiency anemia. *Lancet* 1972; ii:1058–9.

414 Kulapongs P, Vithayasai S, Suskind R, Olson RE. CMI, phagocytosis and killing function in children with severe iron deficiency anemia. *Lancet* 1974; ii:689–91.

415 Kuvibidila S, Murthy KK, Suskind RM. Iron deficiency and interleukin-2 production in murine spleen cells. *FASEB J* 1989; 3:A664.

416 Baliga BS, Kuvividila S, Suskind RM. The cytotoxic capacity of spleen and peritoneal cells from iron deficient animals. *Fed Proc* 1981; 40:A918.

417 Rodday P, Bennett M, Vitale JJ. Delayed erythropoiesis in irradiated rats grafted with syngeneic marrow of cytotoxic drugs and iron deficient anemia. *Blood* 1976; 48:435–47.

418 Helyar L, Sherman AR. Interleukin-2 production and responsiveness by rat leucocytes during iron deficiency. *FASEB J* 1989; 3:A665.

419 Jacobs A, Joynson DHM. Lymphocyte function and iron deficient anemia. *Lancet* 1974; ii:844.

420 Strauss RG. Iron deficiency, infections, and immune functions, a reassessment. *Am J Clin Nutr* 1978; 31:660–6.

421 Kuvibidila S, Baliga BS, Suskind RM. Effect of iron deficiency on DTH. *Fed Proc* 1981; 40:A918.

422 Beard MEJ, Weintraub LR. Hypersegmented neutrophilic granulocytes in iron deficiency anemia. *Br J Haematol* 1969; 16:161–3.

423 Baggs RB, Miller SA. Defect in resistance to *Salmonella typhimurium* in iron deficient rats. *J Infect Dis* 1974; 130:409–11.

424 Bullen JJ, Rogers HJ, Griffiths E. Role of iron in bacterial infections. *Curr Topics Microbiol Immunol* 1978; 80:1–30.

425 Weinberg ED. Nutritional immunity. Host's attempt to withhold iron from microbiol invaders. *JAMA* 1975; 231:39–41.

426 Bullen JJ, Armstrong JA. The role of lactoferrin in the bactericidal function of PMN leukocytes. *Immunol* 1979; 36:781–91.

427 Masawe AEJ, Muindi JM, Swai GBR. Infections in iron deficiency and other types of anemia in the tropics. *Lancet* 1974; ii:314–16.

428 McFarlane H, Reddy S, Adcock KJ. Immunity, transferrin and survival in kwashiorkor. *Br Med J* 1970; 4:268–70.

429 Murray MJ, Murray AB. Refeeding, malaria and hyperferraemia. *Lancet* 1975; i:653–4.

430 Kochan I, Wasynczuk J, McCabe MA. Effect of injected iron and siderophores on infections in normal and immune mice. *Infect Immun* 1978; 22:560–7.

431 Andersen E, Basse A, Brummerstedt E, Flagstad T. Zinc and the immune system in cattle. *Lancet* 1973; i:839–40.

432 Weismann K, Flagstad T. Hereditary zinc deficiency in cattle; an animal parallel to acrodermatitis enterotrepatica. *Acta Dermatol Venereol (Stockholm)* 1976; 56:151–4.

433 Danbolt N, Closs K. Acrodermatitis enterohepatica. *Acta Dermatol Venereol* 1942; 23:127–69.

434 Holbrook IB, Milewski PJ, Clark C, Shipley K. Low serum zinc and long term intravenous feeding. *Am J Clin Nutr* 1980; 33:1891–2.

435 Good RA, West A, Fernandes G. Nutritional modulation of immune response. *Fed Proc* 1980; 39:3098–104.

436 Cunningham-Rundles C, Cunningham-Rundles S, Genrofolo J. Increased T lymphocyte function and thymopoietin following zinc repletion in man. *Fed Proc* 1979; 38:1222.

437 Iwata T, Incefy GS, Tanaka T. Low levels of serum thymic factor (FTS) in zinc deficient A/Jax mice. *Fed Proc* 1978; 37:1827.

438 Frost P, Chen JC, Rabbani I, Smith J, Prasad AS. The effect of zinc deficiency on the immune response. In: Brewer GJ, Prasad AS, eds. *Zinc Metabolism: Current Aspects in Health and Disease.* New York: Alan R Liss, 1977:143–50.

439 Nash L, Iwata T, Fernandes G, Good RA, Incefy GS. Effect of zinc deficiency on autologous rosette forming cells. *Cell Immunol* 1979; 48:238–43.

440 Garvy B, King L, Fraker P. Relationships between zinc deficiency, lymphopenia and B-cell lymphopoiesis. *FASEB J* 1989; 3:A1057.

441 Brummerstedt E, Andersen E, Basse A, Flagstad T. Lethal trait A46 in cattle: immunological investigations. *Nord Vet Med* 1974; 26:279–93.

442 Idress ZH, der Kaloustian VM. Acrodermatitis enterohepatica. *Clin Pediatr* 1973; 12:393–5.

443 Julius R, Schulkind M, Sprinkle T, Rennert O. Acrodermatitis enterohepatica with immune deficiency. *J Pediatr* 1973; 83:1007–11.

444 Rass RF, Johnston RB, Cooper MD. Agammaglobulinemia with B lymphocytes in a neonate with acrodermatitis enterohepatica. *Am J Dis Child* 1974; 128:251–3.

445 Fernandes G, Nair M, Onoe K, Tanaka T, Floyd R, Good RA. Impairment of CMI functions by dietary zinc deficiency in mice. *Proc Natl Acad Sci* 1979; 76:457–61.

446 Fraker PJ, Haas SM, Luecke RW. Effect of zinc deficiency on the immune response of the young adult A/J mouse. *J Nutr* 1977; 107:1889–95.

447 Zwickl CM, Fraker PJ. Restoration of the antibody mediated response of zinc/calorie deficient neonatal mice, *Immunol Commun* 1980; 9:611–26.

448 Winchurch RA. The role of zinc in regulating immune responses in the aged. *FASEB J* 1989; 3:A1057.

449 Winchurch RA, Thomas DJ, Adler WH, Lindsay TJ. Supplemental zinc restores antibody formation in cultures of aged spleen cells. *J Immunol* 1984; 133:569–71.

450 Winchurch RA, Togo J, Adler WH. Supplemental zinc (Zn⁺) restores antibody formation in cultures of aged spleen cells. II. Effects on mediator production. *Eur J Immunol* 1987; 17:127–32.

451 Winchurch RA, Togo J, Adler WH. Supplemental zinc (Zn⁺) restores antibody formation in cultures of aged spleen cells. III. Impairment of IL-2 mediated responses. *Clin Immunol Immunopathol* 1988; 49:215–22.

452 Brummerstedt E, Basse A, Flagstad T, Andersen E. Animal model of human disease. Acrodermatitis enterohepatica. Zinc malabsorption. *Am J Pathol* 1977;

87:725–8.

453 van Gool JD, Went K. Acrodermatitis enterohepatica and cellular immune deficiency. *Lancet* 1976; i:1085.

454 Gross RL, Osdin N, Fong L, Newberne PM. Depressed immunological function in zinc-deprived rats as measured by mitogen response of spleen, thymus and peripheral blood. *Am J Clin Nutr* 1979; 32:1260–5.

455 Golden MHN, Golden BE, Harband PSEG, Jackson AA. Zinc and immunocompetence in PCM. *Lancet* 1978; i:1226–8.

456 McMahon L, Montgomery J, Guschewsky A, Woods AH, Zukoski CF. *In vitro* effects of ZnCl on E rosette formation by lymphocytes from cancer patients and normal subjects. *Immunol Commun* 1976; 5:53–7.

457 Alford RH. Metal cation requirements for PHA transformation of human peripheral blood lymphocytes. *J Immunol* 1970; 104:698–703.

458 Berger NA, Skinner AM. Characterization of lymphocyte transformation induced by zinc ions. *J Cell Biol* 1974; 61:45–55.

459 Gallagher K, Matarazzo W, Gray I. Trace metal modification of lymphocyte transformation *in vitro, Fed Proc* 1978; 37:377.

460 Hart DA. Augmentation of zinc ion stimulation of lymphoid cells by calcium and lithium. *Exp Cell Res* 1979; 121:419–25.

461 Hart DA. Effect of zinc chloride on hamster lymphoid cells: mitogenicity and differential enhancement of lipopolysaccharide stimulation of lymphocytes. *Infect Immun* 1978; 19:457–61.

462 Winchurch RA. Activation of thymocyte responses to IL-1 by zinc. *Clin Immunol Immunopathol* 1988; 47:174–80.

463 Chandra RK, Au B. Single nutrient deficiency and CMI responses. I. Zinc. *Am J Clin Nutr* 1980; 33:736–8.

464 Briggs WA, Pederson M, Mahajan S. Mononuclear and PMN cell function in zinc deficient hemodialysis patients. *Am J Clin Nutr* 1981; 34:628.

465 Chvapil M. Effect of zinc on cells and biomembranes. *Med Clin N Am* 1976; 60:799–812.

466 Weston WL, Huff JC, Humbert JR. Zinc correction of defective chemotaxis in acrodermatitis enterohepathica. *Arch Dermatol* 1977; 113:422–5.

467 Stankova L, Drach GW, Hicks T, Zukoski CF, Chvapil M. Regulation of some functions of granulocytes by zinc of the prostatic fluid and tissue. *J Lab Clin Med* 1976; 88:640–8.

468 Chvapil M, Stankoua L, Bernhard DS, Weldy PL, Carlson EC, Campbell JB. Effect of zinc on peritoneal macrophages *in vitro. Infect Immun* 1977; 16:367–73.

469 Golden BE, Golden MHN. Plasma zinc and the clinical features of malnutrition. *Am J Clin Nutr* 1979;

32:2490–4.

470 Garofalo JA, Erlandson E, Strong E, Lesser M, Gerold F, Spiro R, Schwartz M, Good RA. Serum zinc, serum copper and the Cu/Zn ratio in patients with epidermoid cancers of the head and neck. *J Surg Oncol* 1980; 15:381–6.

471 Sullivan JL, Ochs HD. Copper deficiency and the immune system. *Lancet* 1978; ii:686.

472 Lukasewycz OA, Prohaska JR. Dietary copper deficiency suppresses the immune response of C58 mice. *Fed Proc* 1981; 40:918.

473 Prohaska JR, Lukasewycz OA. Copper deficiency suppresses the immune response of mice. *Science* 1981; 213:559–61.

474 Lukasewycz OA, Prohaska JR. Immunization against transplantable leukemia impaired in copper deficient mice. *J Natl Cancer Inst* 1982; 69:489–93.

475 Prohaska JR, Olson MC, Lukasewycz OA. Copper deficient mice have small thymus glands but normal plasma corticosterone levels. *FASEB J* 1989; 3:A1057.

476 Lukasewycz OA, Prohaska JR. Lymphocytes from copper deficient mice exhibit decreased mitogen reactivity. *Nutr Res* 1983; 3:335–41.

477 Lukasewycz OA, Prohaska JR. Increased IL-1 and decreased IL-2 production in copper deficient mice. *FASEB J* 1989; 3:A665.

478 Lukasewycz OA, Kolquist KL, Prohaska JR. Modulation in immunoglobulin isotype production in copper deficient mice. *FASEB J* 1988; 2:A436.

479 Lukasewycz OA, Prohaska JR, Meyer SG, Schmidtke JR. Alterations in lymphocyte subpopulations in copper deficient mice. *Infect Immun* 1985; 48:644–7.

480 Chvapil M, Stankova L, Zukoski C. Inhibition of some functions of PMN leukocytes by *in vitro* zinc. *J Lab Clin Med* 1977; 89; 135–46.

481 Newberne PM, Hunt CE, Young VR. The role of diet and the reticuloendothelial system in the response of rats to *Salmonella typhimurium* infection. *Br J Exp Pathol* 1968; 49:448–57.

482 Vaughn VJ, Weinberg ED. *Candida albicans* dimorphism and virulence: role of copper. *Mycophatol* 1978; 64:39–42.

483 Hill CH. Influence of time of exposure to high levels of minerals on the susceptibility of chicks to *Salmonella gallinarium. J Nutr* 1980; 110:433–6.

484 Spallholz JE, Martin JL, Gerlach ML, Heinzerling RH. Immunologic responses of mice fed diets supplemented with selenite selenium. *Proc Soc Exp Biol Med* 1973; 143:685–9.

485 Spallholz JE, Martin JL, Gerlach ML, Heinzerling RH. Injectable selenium: effect on primary immune response of mice. *Proc Soc Exp Biol Med* 1975; 148:37–40.

486 Desowitz RS, Barnwell JW. Effect of selenium on vaccine induced immunity of Swiss Webster mice against malaria. *Infect Immun* 1980; 27:87–9.

487 Sheffy BE, Schultz RD. Influence of vitamin E and selenium on immune response mechanisms. *Fed Proc* 1979; 38:2139–43.

488 Boyne R, Arthur JR. Alterations of neutrophil function in selenium-deficient cattle. *J Comp Pathol* 1979; 89:151–8.

489 Eskew ML, Scholz RW, Reddy CC, Todhunter DA, Zarkower A. Effects of vitamin E and selenium deficiencies on rat immune function. *Immunol* 1985; 54:173–80.

490 Dreizen S. Nutrition and the immune response. *Int J Vit Nutr Res* 1979; 49:220–8.

491 Bendich A, Gabriel E, Machlin LJ. Depression of rat and guinea pig lymphocyte blastogenic responses by vitamin E deficiency. *Ann NY Acad Sci* 1984; 435:382–4.

492 Koller LD. Immunosuppression produced by lead, cadmium and mercury. *Am J Vet Res* 1973; 34:1457–8.

493 Koller LD, Brawner JA. Decreased B lymphocyte response after exposure to lead and cadmium. *Toxicol Appl Pharmacol* 1977; 42:621–4.

494 Koller LD, Exon JH, Roan JG. Humoral antibody response in mice after single dose exposure to lead or cadmium. *Proc Soc Exp Biol Med* 1976; 151:339–42.

495 Gaworski CL, Sharma RP. The effects of heavy metals on ³H-thymidine uptake in lymphocytes. *Toxicol Appl Pharmacol* 1978; 46:305–13.

496 Muller S, Gilbert KE, Krause C. Effects of cadmium on the immune system of mice. *Experientia* 1977; 35:909–10.

497 Koller LD, Roan JG. Effects of lead and cadmium on mouse peritoneal macrophages. *J Reticuloendothel Soc* 1977; 24:7–12.

498 Loose LD, Silkworth JB, Simpson DW. Influence of cadmium on phagocytic and microbicidal activity. *Infect Immun* 1978; 22:378–81.

10

Psychoneuroimmunology: interaction between the immune system, endocrine system and central nervous system

BRIAN E. LEONARD

Introduction

Awareness of a possible relationship between melancholia and malignant disease reaches back to the second century, when Galen commented that melancholic women were more prone to cancer than those of sanguine temperament. In more recent times, anecdotal reports have suggested that stress might influence the immune response and thereby render the individual more susceptible to infectious disease and cancer [1].

In the last decade, interest in the interconnection between the immune system and mental illness has achieved considerable prominence, largely as a result of a series of controlled studies showing that malignant disease is often heralded by severe depression that is not apparently related to brain damage and antedating the discovery of the malignancy [2, 3]. More recently, the discovery that human immunodeficiency virus infection can result in dementia in those patients who recover from the various infections that are generally fatal further suggests that the immune system may play a direct role in altering brain function. This link between the brain and the immune system forms the basis of psychoimmunology, a term introduced by Solomon and Moos [4] to integrate stress, emotions, immunological dysfunction and physical and mental disease. Increasing evidence linking the nervous and immune systems has led to the discipline of psychoneuroimmunology, which has resulted in the publication of several monographs [5, 6], international symposia and the launching of *International Journal on Brain, Behaviour and Immunity* in 1987. The present review will attempt to summarize the experimental and clinical evidence, indicating how stress may modify the activity of different components of the immune system.

Control of the immune system by the nervous system

There is increasing evidence to show that the central nervous system controls the activities of the immune system in a way somewhat similar to how it controls the endocrine system; the interaction between the immune system and the brain is largely dependent on negative feedback mechanisms. As it is well established that the response of an animal to any form of stress usually involves a mobilization of both the pituitary–adrenal axis and the immune system, it is clearly important to consider the mechanisms whereby the brain can modulate the activities of these systems.

There are two main regulatory processes involving the immune system—those dependent on the presence of a specific antigen and those which are independent of antigen. It appears that only the latter type of immune response is clearly modulated by the nervous system. This interconnection between the nervous system and the immune system is brought about directly via neuronal connections to the immune-related organs and to the vascular system and indirectly through the endocrine system and by feedback regulation from target organs. A summary of the interactions between the brain and the immune system is shown in Fig. 10.1.

In addition to the thymosins that are produced by the thymus gland and play a role in the immune process, it has been shown that activated lymphocytes produce adrenocorticotrophic hormone (ACTH), γ-endorphin, thyroid-stimulating hormone and human chorionic gonadotropin-like peptides [7,8]. This could be a mechanism whereby lymphocytes may serve to activate endocrine function. Conversely the endocrine system can modify immune function due to the presence of specific endocrine receptors located on T and B cells. Thus glucocorticoids suppress the activity of thymus-dependent immune responses, including the production of lymphokines by T cells and antibodies by B cells [9]. Besides steroids, insulin [10], prolactin [11], vasopressin [12] and the endogenous opioids [13,14] have been shown to alter immune responses, at least *in vitro*; these changes would appear to be regulated by the substances acting at specific receptor sites on the lymphocyte membrane.

The autonomic nervous system is also important in modifying the activity of the immune system. Neuronal projections originating in the central nervous system innervate the bone marrow and the thymus.

Neurotransmitters and the immune system

Several neurotransmitter systems have been suggested as modulating the immune system, both within the central nervous system and in the autonomic nervous system. A brief overview only will be presented here. Those interested in a more extensive account are referred to articles by Hall and Goodstein [15] and Felten and-Overhage [16].

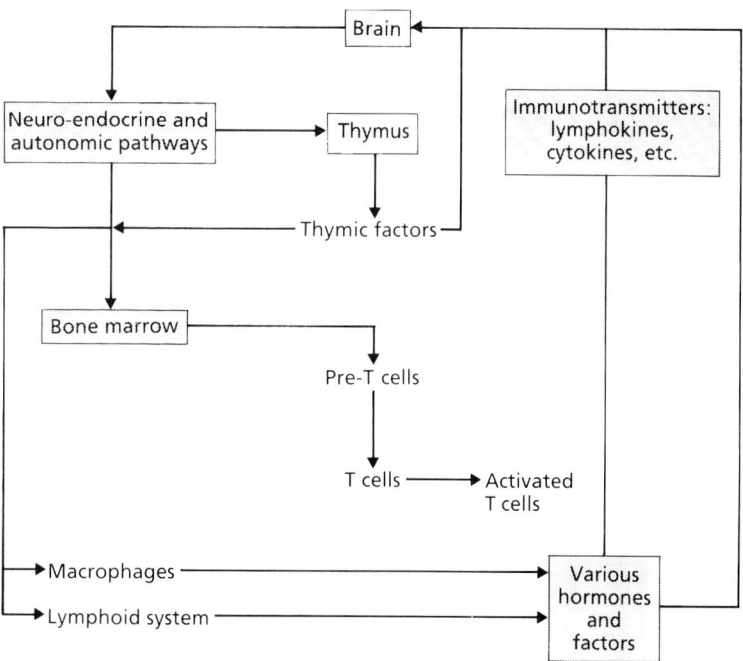

Fig. 10.1 Summary of pathways postulated to be involved in the interactions between the nervous and immune systems.

Serotonin

While the direct effects of serotonin upon the immune system have not been systematically investigated, indirect evidence suggests that serotonin exerts a net inhibitory influence over immunogenesis. This conclusion is based on the investigation of Devoino and colleagues [17] and Idova and Devoino [18] who demonstrated that an inverse relationship exists between brain serotonin concentrations and antibody synthesis.

Dopamine

The central dopaminergic system appears to exert a net stimulatory influence over the immune system, a conclusion which is based on changes in the immune system of patients suffering from such neurological diseases as parkinsonism [19].

Noradrenaline and adrenaline

Both of these catecholamines have been implicated as immunomodulators; most of the evidence suggests that their effects are modulated by changes in the autonomic nervous system. Thus adrenergic fibres have been identified in the interlocular septa of the rat thymus [19], while during the course of the immune response the spleen concentration of noradrenaline has been shown to decrease significantly [20]. Although changes in the vasculature might be associated with the alterations in the catecholamines, the presence of physiologically active β-adrenoceptors on T, B cells and macrophages [21] suggests that these catecholamines may exert a direct effect on the immune system.

Acetylcholine

Several investigators have reported the presence of acetylcholine receptors in thymus tissue [22–24] and have suggested that nicotinic receptors occur on thymocytes [22–24]. Cholinergic stimulation has been shown to stimulate the formation of cyclic guanosine monophosphate in such cells which can result in lymphocyte activation [21].

Opioids

Exposure to stress can cause the release of opioidpeptides from both central and peripheral sites and there is considerable experimental evidence to suggest that the opioids can alter the percentage of T cells forming active rosettes, the reactivity of T cells to mitogenic stimulation and the cytotoxic activity of natural killer cells [24]. In addition to these effects of opioids on the immune system, which have been observed *in vivo* and *in vitro* , opioid receptors have been identified on granulocytes, monocytes, lymphocytes and the terminal complexes of complement [25]. While the precise mechanism whereby endogenous opioid peptides mediate the suppression on natural killer cell activity is unclear, Shavit and co-workers [25] have hypothesized that this may occur due to a suppression of interferon which normally induces and augments natural killer cell activity.

The effects of a number of neurotransmitters on the cellular components of the immune response are summarized in Table 10.1.

Stress, conditioning and immune function

Ader [26] demonstrated that the immunosuppressive effect of cyclophosphamide can be simulated by a neutral stimulus in rodents providing the administration of the drug is initially paired with that neutral stimulus. This important finding suggests that the neutral, or conditioned, stimulus is capable of causing the secretion of endogenous immunosuppressive agents.

Table 10.1 Effect of some neurotransmitters on the cellular component of the immune response

Neurotransmitter	B-cell response	T-cell response	Macrophages
Serotonin—increased	–	0	0
Dopamine—increased	–	+	+
β-Adrenergic stimulation	–	–	–
α-Adrenergic stimulation	+	+	0
Cholinergic stimulation	+	+	0
Morphine	0	–	0
Encephalins	0	+	0

– , Decreased response; + , increased response; 0, no data available.

Stressful stimuli have been utilized experimentally as a means of inducing both analgesia and immunosuppression, which have been shown to cause enhanced tumour growth [27]. The link between analgesia and immunosuppression induced by severe stress would appear to involve both opioid and non-opioid mechanisms; the pituitary–adrenal axis appears to play a prominent role in the adaptation to severe stress. Thus hypophysectomy attenuates the opioid component of stress analgesia, an effect which could be attributed to a reduction in the secretion of both the pituitary and adrenal opioids [28]; adrenalectomy was also shown to produce a marked reduction in opioid-dependent stress analgesia.

The connection between severe stress, immunosuppression and the susceptibility to cancer induction has been experimentally investigated by Shavit and co-workers [25]. These investigators studied the development of ascites tumours in rats subjected to inescapable and escapable forms of foot-shock. It appears that inescapable shock produces both opioid-mediated analgesia and the suppression of natural killer cell activity whereas escapable footshock results in non-opioid analgesia and the absence of immunosuppression. The results of this study showed that tumour growth only occurred in those rats subject to the opioid-mediated foot-shock, an effect that could be blocked by the opioid antagonist naltrexone. In addition to the endogenous opioids that may play a role in immunosuppression, it seems likely that ACTH and the glucocorticoids also have an important role; increased corticosterone has been shown to facilitate tumour growth [29]. Prolactin, which is released in response to stress, also has tumour-promoting properties. Thus it would appear that stress may or may not adversely affect the response of the immune system to tumour cells depending on the nature of the stress and the consequent changes in the concentrations of the various hormones and immunotransmitters that may activate or suppress the immune system.

Glucocorticoids have long been known to play a crucial role in immune function. These hormones are secreted by the adrenal cortex in response to the stimulation of ACTH which is released from the pituitary under the control of the hypothalamic corticotropin-releasing factor; β-endorphin is usually co-released with ACTH. The circulating glucocorti-

coids can regulate their further release by activating specific steroid receptors in the brain; the hippocampus, septum and corticomedial amygdala are known to have a high density of corticosterone receptor for example. There is experimental evidence to show that prolonged elevation of corticosterase levels leads to a reduction (down-regulation) of these receptors in the hippocampus, thereby reducing the hippocampal control of the pituitary–adrenal stress response [30]. If the plasma corticosterone concentration is elevated for a prolonged period (e.g. 12 weeks), hippocampal neurons are lost, the effect being most marked in the CA2 and CA3 regions of Ammon's horn [31].

The precise relevance of these experimental findings to pathological states in humans is subject to conjecture. Nevertheless, it is well known that the hypersecretion of glucocorticoids is a common component of severe psychiatric illness. Glucocorticoid hypersecretion is frequently used as a diagnostic marker of endogenous depression: a substantial proportion of untreated depressives fail to show an attenuation of the elevated cortisol levels in response to a challenge with 1 mg dexamethasone. This forms the basis of the dexamethasone suppression test [32] and may provide a link between changes in the immune system, with the possibility of an increased incidence of cancers, and chronic immune-based diseases and changes in central nervous system function which may be manifest in alterations in the emotional state. The connection between psychiatric illness and changes in immune function will be considered later in this chapter.

A variety of stressors has been found to alter humoral immune responses in animals. Thus Rasmussen *et al.* [33] reported that the stress of passive avoidance learning in mice decreased the susceptibility of the animals to passive anaphylaxis, while others showed that the production of specific antibodies could be suppressed by exposing the animals to such environmental stressors as noise, bright light and adverse housing conditions [34,35]. Solomon *et al.* [36] showed that both primary and secondary antibody responses could be suppressed but some environmental stressors, such as repeated low-voltage electric shocks, enhanced the antibody response. Such findings have led to the suggestion that acute exposure to a stressor can suppress humoral immune responses, while repeated exposure to the same stressor can result in immunological adaptation and even enhanced responsiveness [37].

The experimental findings of Laudenslager *et al.* [38] may be particularly pertinent to the immunological abnormalities reported to occur in humans subjected to severe mental stress. These investigators reported that stress-induced suppression of lymphocyte stimulation may be related to the psychological state of the animal. Thus in rats, mitogen-stimulated lymphocyte division was suppressed in rats exposed to inescapable, uncontrollable electric shocks to the tail for 80 min followed 24 h later by several minutes of tail shock. Animals receiving the same total number of shocks but able to terminate the shock did not show a decreased lymphocyte response to the mitogens. Such findings are consistent with the hypothesis that the ability to cope with a stressor protects against its noxious effects.

In a more recent commentary, Maier and Laudenslager [39] considered the numerous factors that lead to a profound variation in the effect of different types of stressor on components of the immune response. There is evidence for example that mitogen proliferation is highly variable even under standardized experimental conditions [40], so that even when a stressor has a profound effect on lymphocyte proliferation, the detection of the effect may be difficult when it is superimposed on even larger individual differences that exist with regard to mitogen proliferation. A further complication relates to the fact that the studies are conducted in *in vitro* systems in which the lymphocytes are removed from the normal neuroendocrine and neural environments. The relationship of *in vitro* assays to the functioning of the immune system *in vivo* is far from understood. Thus the lymphocyte population found in the blood represents only a small portion of the total pool of lymphocytes found in the body [41]; lymphocytes maintain a dynamic relationship between the blood, bone marrow, lymph nodes, thymus and spleen which may be differentially affected by a stressor [42]. This could mean that different populations of cells may be sampled from one experiment to the next, thereby creating a difficulty in replicating the results. Furthermore, stress can alter the circadian pattern of adrenocorticoid secretions, possibly shifting the circadian pattern of lymphocyte subsets at a particular sampling site [42]. Despite such variations, it would appear that the effects of inescapable foot-shock on lymphocyte mitogenesis are robust and repeatable.

The effect of stress on the immune system is not always immunosuppressive even though most experimental studies show evidence that this is the case. Thus the influence of the stressor depends not only on the characteristics of the stressor (its nature, duration and frequency for example), but also the precise time at which it is applied to the animal in relation to the activity of the immune system [43,44]. It has been found for example that stressors can increase the host resistance to pathogenic organisms [45] and enhance the activity of the immune system. In support of this view, Croiset [46] demonstrated that exposure of rats to a single foot-shock or habituation to the passive avoidance apparatus increased the proliferative response after mitogenic stimulation *in vitro* and also the ability to generate a primary antibody response *in vivo* after immunization with sheep red blood cells.

Many of the experimental studies that have been cited in this review may be criticized because stressors such as electric shock are completely unnatural to the experimental animal. It appears that familiarity with the nature of the stressor is not of major importance however as social stressors also have a profound influence on the immune system. Thus dominance in rats or mice is accompanied by enhanced cellular [47] and humoral [35] immune responses. Depressed immunocompetence has also been shown to occur when fully weaned infant monkeys are separated from their mothers for periods of several days [48].

Despite the marked changes that can occur in different aspects of the immune system following exposure to different types of stressor, it is still not certain that the resistance of the host to infectious and neoplastic diseases is inevitably decreased [49]. Nevertheless, several important aspects of cellular immune function, including natural killer cell lysis, inhibition of mitogen-stimulated proliferative response to mitogens and production of interferon-γ are inhibited by most forms of stress [50,51]. Even relatively mild stress (e.g. examination stress in university students) can lead to significant increases in antibody titres to herpes viruses [52]. The effect of stress on the development of acquired immune deficiency syndrome in infected individuals is further evidence to suggest that, in most cases, stress results in a suppression of the most important aspects of the immune system, which is instrumental in the full expression of the disease [53].

In humans, probably one of the most potentially stressful and frequently occurring events that has been associated with increased mortality is conjugal bereavement. Schleifer and co-workers [54] investigated the effect of bereavement on immunity in a prospective longitudinal study of spouses of women with advanced breast cancer. They found that mitogen-stimulated lymphocyte response in the men was significantly lower during the first 2 months following the death of wives than it was in the period before the death. In most cases, the lymphocyte response normalized later in the years following the death. Whether such stress-induced mitogen responses are related to the onset or course of physical illness following stressful life events remains to be established. Such factors as changes in nutrition, physical activity, sleep and use of drugs are known to influence lymphocyte function and may complicate the interpretation of such results [55]. Other studies have shown that bereaved subjects show a depression of mood which occasionally leads to a pattern of symptoms that resemble a major depressive disorder [56]. As there is clinical evidence to show that major depressive states result in reduced lymphocyte response to mitogens [57] and viruses [58], it is possible that a stress-induced depression may be causally related to the abnormal lymphocyte function.

Changes in the immune system in psychiatric illness: depressive illness

Abnormal functioning of the immune system in patients with psychiatric illness was proposed as long ago as the second century when Galen observed that cancer occurred more frequently in women of melancholic than in those with a sanguine temperament. Anecdotal reports of a possible connection between stress, psychiatric illness and cancer have frequently appeared in the medical literature since that time. In 1759 Guy [59], for example, noted that melancholic women were prone to breast cancer, observations that were repeated by Paget in 1863 [60] and Parker in 1865 [61]. However no assumptions can be drawn from such reports regarding a causal association between melancholia and cancer. Most of the more recent studies for example have the disadvantage of being retrospective and based on patients with diagnosed cancer [62,63]. It would be anticipated that a patient's attitude and emotional state might profoundly affect the progress of the disease once cancer has been diagnosed. Nevertheless, there is some evidence that an abnormal mental state may precede the establishment of cancer. Thus Kerr *et al.* [64], in a 4-year follow-up of patients with a primary diagnosis of affective disorder, reported a higher than expected mortality from cancer among men who had been treated for first attacks of depression. Similarly Varsanis *et al.* [65], in a 6-year follow-up of psychiatric patients, found a high incidence of malignant disease in 24 patients who had suffered from affective psychoses while Whitlock and Siskind [3] studied 39 male and 90 female depressives who were over 40 years of age and found that the deaths in the male patients from cancer over a period of 4 years following the psychiatric diagnosis was significantly higher than expected. It may be concluded from such studies that malignant disease may be heralded by severe depressive illness, not related to gross brain damage and antedating the diagnosis of the malignancy.

The possible mechanism whereby this may occur has been postulated by Brown and Paraskevas [66] who speculated that antibodies against a protein released from the cancer cells could bind to central serotonin receptors and block them. Such primary antibodies could stimulate the production of anti-idiotypic antibodies, thereby acting as an alternative receptor for serotonin and so reducing its synaptic availability. Such a hypothesis is based on the assumption that the primary defect in central neurotransmission in depression is in the serotonergic system and that antibodies to myelin basic protein or tumour basic protein selectively block those subtypes of serotonin receptor that are primarily involved in central serotonergic transmission.

The past 20 years have seen a broad interest in the role of the hypothalamic–pituitary–adrenal axis in the psychobiology of the affective disorders [32]. In the depressed patient, there is usually an increase in cortisol levels in the plasma, cerebrospinal fluid and urine compound to normal controls [67,68]. Other abnormalities in the functioning of the pituitary–adrenal axis include a disruption of the circadian pattern of cortisol secretion [69] and an insensitivity of the secretion of cortisol to suppression by glucocorticoids such as dexamethasone [32]; this forms the basis of the dexamethasone suppression test which is still widely used as a biochemical marker of major depression.

One of the major consequences of hypercortisolaemia is a suppression in immune function [70]. Impaired immunity has been reported to occur in depressed patients [50] so that it may be speculated that the reduction in the immune function is primarily a reflection of the hypercortisolaemia. However the relationship between the immune system and the pituitary adrenal axis would not appear to be so simple. Kronfol and co-workers [57], for example, studied the lymphocyte response to mitogen stimulation (a correlate of cell-mediated immunity according to Oppenheim *et al.* [71]) in groups of depressed patients who had either elevated urinary free cortisol or normal cortisol levels. The results of this study showed that the lymphocyte mitogen response was significantly suppressed in all the depressed patients relative to their controls but that there was no relationship between the altered immune competence and the elevated free urinary cortisol levels. The results of this study emphasize the complexity of the relationship between the immune response and the endocrine system. Other studies have shown that the number of peripheral T cells was decreased among ambulatory depressed patients but not in those with schizophrenia [51]. Experimental studies suggest that such changes in lymphocyte function are associated with enhanced endogenous opioid activity [72], although other naturally occurring neuropeptides such as neurotensin, vasoactive intestinal peptide, substance P, somatostatin and bombesin have also been implicated in the diminished lymphocyte responsiveness [73]. Chang [72] has suggested that the effect of neuropeptides on the immune system is indirect and operates through the hypothalamic–hypophyseal pathway; the hypothalamus probably controls a T-cell-inducing factor.

Another approach to an assessment of immune function in depressed patients has been to determine changes in neutrophil phagocytosis before and following treatment. The advantage of this approach is that it gives a direct functional measure of an important immune mechanism. Furthermore, the changes in phagocytosis would not appear to be affected by plasma cortisol or by the antidepressant used to treat the patient. Using this approach, we have shown that the phagocytosis response is significantly impaired in depressed patients but normalizes following affective treatment; those failing to respond to treatment continue to show a diminished response [74]. Thus it appears that changed neutrophil phagocytosis may be a state rather than a trait marker of depression. More recent studies have revealed that only patients suffering from panic disorder show similar abnormal neutrophil responses: those with schizophrenia, Alzheimer's disease, alcoholism, mania and anxiety states did not differ from controls. It is not without interest that the olfactory bulbectomized rat model of depression also exhibits a defective neutrophil phagocytosis which is partly normalized by chronic antidepressant treatment [75].

Recently, we have been attempting to determine the nature of the factors responsible for the subnormal phagocytic response in depressed patients. It would not appear to be associated with the immunoglobulins, plasma calcium or complement but there is increasing evidence that elevated plasma prostaglandins (prostaglandin E_2?) may be responsible [74]. Such a possibility is supported by the findings of Calabrese *et al.* [76] who discovered that prostaglandin E_1 and E_2 concentrations were raised in depressed patients. These investigators have hypothesized that abnormalities in cellular immunity found in depressed patients may be directly associated with enhanced synthesis of prostaglandins of the E series. Of course it remains to be proven that such changes are relevant to the psychiatric symptoms of the disease and the action of antidepressants on the brain.

There is convincing evidence that immunoregulation is mediated by the central and peripheral sympathetic system [77,78] and that prostaglandins of the E series can modulate central neurotransmitter release, possibly by affecting calcium flux [79,80]. Further support for the hypothesis linking an abnormality in prostaglandin E_2 and depression is provided by the finding that lithium [81], monoamine oxidase inhibitors [81,82] and tricyclic antidepressants inhibit the synthesis of these neurotransmodulators. Clearly, more detailed studies must be undertaken to validate this hypothesis but it is appealing in that it serves to link proven biochemical changes in depressed patients with the delay in the onset of action of antidepressants and the alteration in cellular immunity.

Beside polymorphoneutrophils exhibiting abnormal phagocytosis in patients suffering from depression and panic attack, monocytes also exhibit abnormal phagocytosis in these and other psychiatric disorders. In a recent study, McAdams and Leonard (unpublished) found that the phagocytic response of monocytes was significantly elevated in depressed, manic and schizophrenic patients (but not in those with severe mental handicap), before they exhibited a response to treatment. Following effective treatment however, the activity of the monocytes in the depressed patients returned to control values whereas those with mania or schizophrenia did not show a normalization of their monocyte phagocytic response despite a marked improvement in their mood state. These results suggest that enhanced monocyte phagocytosis could be a trait characteristic of mania and schizophrenia. It is not without interest that the monocytes are a source of both interleukins and prostaglandins which act as immunotransmitters and thereby play a role in modulating the activities of other cellular components of the immune system. The relationship between these cellular components and the different types of psychiatric illness will be the subject of further investigation.

Changes in the immune system in psychiatric illness: schizophrenia

Evidence suggesting an abnormality in immune function in those subject to severe stress or suffering from depression largely relates to an abnormality in polymorphoneutrophil function. Such abnormalities do not appear to occur in schizophrenia [74]. Possibly because of its well established genetic component, many aspects of the immune system would appear to be deranged in schizophrenic

patients. Thus abnormalities in the concentrations of serum immunoglobulins and deficiencies in immune responsiveness have been reported to occur in such patients [83].

Several investigators have reported a generalized increase in the immunoglobulins in both acute and chronic schizophrenics [84,85], although other investigators have not been able to confirm this [86]. Perhaps it is of greater interest to note that antibrain antibodies have been detected in schizophrenic patients [87]. Fessel isolated a factor from the serum of schizophrenic patients that produced catatonia and an abnormal electroencephalogram pattern when injected intravenously into monkeys or human volunteers; the electroencephalogram changes were similar to those seen in schizophrenic patients. The serum protein causing these abnormalities was termed taraxein. These findings were confirmed by some researchers [88,89] but not all [90,91] using the more reliable radioimmunoassay method. (Baron *et al.* [92] and Pandey *et al.* [93]) have found an increased prevalence of antibrain antibodies in schizophrenics compared to controls. However, in an extensive study of antibrain antibodies in 69 schizophrenics and 58 controls, de Lisi *et al.* [86] have shown that if antibrain antibodies play any role in psychiatric disorders, they are non-specific and only present in a small percentage of patients.

Allergic reactions entail disordered immune functioning and controversy exists regarding allergies to various food substances and the incidence of schizophrenia. Some studies have suggested that schizophrenics have an increased incidence of allergies in childhood, especially involving an intolerance to wheat gluten [94]. However, there are few adequately controlled studies to show that food allergies play any role in the aetiology of schizophrenia and, to date, there is little unequivocal evidence to support the view that allergies play a causal role in this illness.

Vartanian *et al.* [95] have produced evidence to suggest that there are at least two genetically determined components in those at risk from schizophrenia. One of these components facilitates a decrease in suppressor cells while the other promotes the accumulation of antithymic immunoglobulins. The consequences of the resultant imbalance between the helper and suppressor mechanism which arises from these immune malfunctions are the occurrence of specific antitissue antibodies, the formation of which is normally controlled by a balance between helper and suppressor mechanisms. Kolyaskina *et al.* [96] have illustrated diagrammatically how changes in immune function may ultimately result in brain damage which causes schizophrenia (Fig. 10.2).

The role of infection

There have been several suggestions whereby the negative symptoms of schizophrenia could represent an autoimmune encephalitis-like syndrome in which a viral infection, for example, could initiate an autoimmune response against dopaminergic pathways. One possibility is that dopamine receptor-stimulating antibodies could be produced as part of the pathological processes that have a high affinity for the dopamine autoreceptors and thereby decrease the release of the neurotransmitter in specific dopaminergic pathways. Such views form the basis of the hypothesis advanced by Knight [97] and lend support to the scheme postulated by Kolyaskina and colleagues [96]. However, it must be emphasized that the clinical data upon which many of these speculations are based have been obtained from patients on prolonged treatment with neuroleptics. These drugs are known to modify the immune system [98] which could increase the vulnerability of

the patient to viral infections [99]. It may be speculated that an inherited primary defect in the immune system could initiate schizophrenia by stimulating the production of antibrain antibodies or by increasing the vulnerability of the patient to a viral infection. Alternatively, a primary defect in central neurotransmitter metabolism, possibly involving dopamine, may cause the immune abnormalities which have been described. In this case it may be argued that the immune changes are an epiphenomenon of the disease and not necessarily the primary cause.

Conclusions

It seems probable that some disturbances in immune function do occur in mental illness and are not artefacts of medication or the effects of institutionalization. The known effects of the neuroendocrine system on the immune response, and the recent evidence that receptor sites for neurotransmitters and neuroendocrine factor occur on lymphocytes and macrophages, support the hypothesis that immunological abnormalities may assist in precipitating the symptoms of anxiety, depression and schizophrenia. Nevertheless, the nature of specific immunological disturbances which underlies these diseases remains elusive. Clearly more evidence is required, based on adequately controlled studies,

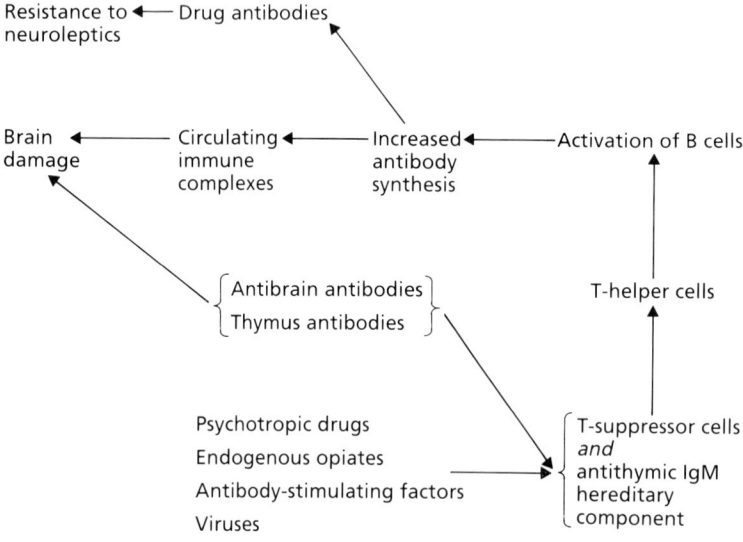

Fig. 10.2 Connection between possible immune mechanisms and the aetiology of schizophrenia. After [96].

before one can conclude with any certainty that immune incompetence is a causal factor in mental disorder.

References

1 Kowal SJ. Emotion as a cause of cancer: eighteenth and nineteenth century contributions. *Psychoanal Rev* 1955; 42:217–27.

2 Whitlock FA. Suicide, cancer and depression. *Br J Psychiat* 1978: 132:269–74.

3 Whitlock FA, Siskind M. Depression and cancer: a follow-up study. *Psychol Med* 1979: 9:747–52.

4 Solomon GF, Moos RH. Emotions, immunity and disease: a speculative theoretical integration. *Arch Gen Psychiatr* 1964; 11:657–74.

5 Ader R. *Psychoneuroimmunology.* New York: Academic Press, 1988.

6 Kurstak E, Lipowski ZJ, Morozov PV. (eds) *Viruses, Immunity and Mental Disorders.* New York: Plenum Medical, 1987.

7 Smith EM, Blalock JE. Human lymphocytes production of corticotropin and endorphin-like substances: association with leukocyte interferon. *Proc Natl Acad Sci (USA)* 1981; 78:7530–5.

8 Blalock JE. The immune system as a sensory organ. *J Immunol* 1984; 132:1067–70.

9 Munck A, Guyre PM, Holbrook NJ. Physiological functions of glucocorticoids in stress and their relation in pharmacological actions. *Endocrinol Rev* 1984; 5:25–44.

10 Strom TB, Bangs JD. Human serum-free mixed lymphocytes response: the stereospecific effect of insulin and its potentiation by transferrin. *J Immunol* 1982; 128:1555–9.

11 Spangelo BL, Hall NR, Goldstein AL. Evidence that prolactin is an immunomodulatory hormone. In: MacLeod RM, Thorner MO, Scapagnini U, eds. *Prolactin, Basic and Clinical Correlates.* Padova: Liviana Press, 1985; 343–9.

12 Johnson HM, Farraar WL, Torres BA. Vasopressin replacement of interleukin 2 requirement for gamma interferon production: lymphokine activity of a neuroendocrine hormone. *J Immunol* 1982; 129:983–6.

13 Wybran J. Enkephalins and endorphins: activation molecules for the immune system and natural killer cell activity. *Neuropeptides* 1985; 5:371–4.

14 Wybran J. Enkephalins and endorphins as modifiers of the immune system: present and future. *Fed Proc* 1985; 44:92–4.

15 Hall NR, Goldstein AL. Neurotransmitters and the immune system. In: Ader R, ed. *Psychoneuroimmunology.* New York: Academic Press, 1981; 521–43.

16 Felten DL, Overhage JM. Noradrenergic sympathetic innervation of lymphoid tissue in the rat appendix: further evidence for a link between the nervous and immune systems. *Brain Res* 1981; 7:595–612.

17 Devoino LV, Ermerina OFN. The role of the hypothalamo-pituitary system in the mechanism of action of reserpine and 5–hydroxytryptophan on antibody production. *Neuropharmacol* 1970; 9:67–72.

18 Idova GV, Devoino LV. Dynamics of formation of M and G antibodies in mice after administration of serotonin and its precursor 5–hydroxytryptophan. *Bull Exp Biol Med* 1972; 73:294–6.

19 Fujiwara M, Murgobayashi T, Kitamura J. Histochemical demonstrations of monoamines in the thymus of rats. *J Progr Neuropathol* 1976; 3:1–50.

20 Besedovsky HD, Sorkin E. Network of immune neuroendocrine interactions. *Clin Exp Immunol* 1977; 27:1–12.

21 Bourne HR, Lichtenstein LM. Modulation of inflammation and immunity by cyclic AMP. *Science* 1974; 184:19–28.

22 Lindstrom JM, Lennon VA. Experimental autoimmune myasthenia gravis and myasthenia gravis: biochemical and immunochemical aspects. *Ann N Y Acad Sci* 1976; 274:254–74.

23 Engel WK, Trotter JL. Thymic epithelial cell contains acetylcholine receptor. *Lancet* 1977; i:1310.

24 Singh U, Owen JJT. Studies on the maturation of thymus stem cells. The effects of catecholamines, histamine and peptide hormones on the expression of T–cell alloantigens. *Eur J Immunol* 1976; 6:559–62.

25 Shavit Y, Terman GW, Martin FC, Lewis JW, Liebeskind JC, Gale RP. Stress, opioid peptides, the immune system and cancer. *J Immunol* 1985; 135:834–7.

26 Ader R. Behaviourally conditioned modulation of immunity. In: Guillemin R, Cohn M, Melnechuk T. eds. *Neural Modulation of Immunity.* New York: Raven Press, 1985.

27 Terman GW, Shavit Y, Lewis JW, Cannon JJ, Liebeskind JC. Intrinsic mechanisms of pain inhibition: activation by stress. *Science* 1984; 226:1270–7.

28 Shavit YM, Lewis JW, Terman GW, Gale RP, Liebeskind JC. Opioid peptides mediate the suppression effect of stress on natural killer cell cytotoxicity. *Science* 1984; 232:188–91.

29 Sapolsky RM, Donnelly T. Vulnerability to stress-induced tumour growth increases with age in rats: role of glucocorticoids. *Endocrinol* 1985; 117:662–5.

30 Sapolsky RM, Krey LC, McEwen BS. The adrenocortical stress response in the aged male rat: impairment of recovery from stress. *Exp Gerontol* 1983; 18:55–64.

31 Sapolsky RM. A mechanism of glucocorticoid toxicity in the hippocampus: increased neuronal vulnerability to metabolic insults. *J Neurosci* 1985; 5:1228–32.

32 Carroll BJ. The dexamethasone suppression test for melancholia. *Br J Psychiatr* 1982; 140:292–304.

33 Rasmussen AF, Spencer ET, Marsh JT. Decrease in susceptibility of mice to passive anaphylaxis following avoidance learning stress. *Proc Soc Exp Biol Med* 1959; 100:878–86.

34 Hill CW, Greer WE, Felsenfeld O. Psychological stress, early response to foreign protein and blood cortisol in vervets. *Psychosom Med* 1967; 29:279–84.

35 Vessey SH. Effects of grouping on levels of circulating antibodies in mice. *Proc Assoc Biol* 1964; 1215:252–8.

36 Solomon GF, Allansmith M, McClellan B, Ankraut A. Immunoglobulins in psychiatric patients. *Arch Gen Psychiatr* 1969; 20:272–7.

37 Gisler RH. Stress and the humoral regulation of the immune response in mice. *Psychother Psychosom* 1974; 23:197–210.

38 Laudenslager ML, Ryan SM, Drugan RC, Hyson RL, Maier SF. Coping and immunosuppression; inescapable but not escapable shock suppresses lymphocyte proliferation. *Science* 1983; 24:568–70.

39 Maier SF, Laudenslager ML. Inescapable shock, shock controllability and mitogen stimulated lymphocyte proliferation. *Brain Behav Immun* 1988; 2:87–91.

40 Dorey F, Zighelboim J. Immunologic variable in a healthy population. *Clin Immunol Immunopathol* 1980; 16:406–15.

41 Butcher EC. The regulation of lymphocyte traffic. *Curr Top Microbiol Immunol* 1986; 128:85–122.

42 Cohen JJ, Crnic LS. Behaviour, stress and lymphocyte recirculation. In: Cooper EL, ed. *Stress, Aging and Immunity.* New York: Dekker, 1984.

43 Lysle DT, Lyte M, Fowler H, Rabin BS. Shock-induced modulation of lymphocyte reactivity; suppression, habituation and recovery. *Life Sci* 1987; 41:1805–14.

44 Sklar L, Bruto V, Anisman H. Adaptation to the tumour-enhancing effects of stress. *Psychol Med* 1981; 43:331–42.

45 Gross WB, Siegel PB. Effect of social stress and steroids on antibody production. *Avian Dis* 1972; 17:807–15.

46 Croiset G, Heijnen CJ, Vekldhuis D, de Wied D, Ballieux RE. Modulation of the immune response by emotional stress. *Life Sci* 1987; 40:775–82.

47 Raab A, Dantzer R, Michand B, Mormede P, Taghzouti H, Simon H, Le Moal M. *Physiol Behav* 1986; 36:223–328.

48 Coe CL, Wiener SG, Rosenberg LT, Levine S. In: Reite M, Field T, eds. *The Psychobiology of Attachment and Separation.* New York: Academic Press, 1985; 163–200.

49 Dantzer R, Kelley KW. Stress and immunity: an integrated view of relationships between the brain and the immune system. *Life Sci* 1989; 44:1995–2008.

50 Schleifer S, Keller S, Meyerson A, Raskin M, Davis K, Stein M. Lymphocyte function in major depressive disorder. *Arch Gen Psychiatr* 1984; 41:484–6.

51 Schleifer SJ, Keller SE, Siris SG, Davis KL, Stein M. Depression and immunity. *Arch Gen Psychiatr* 1985; 42:129–33.

52 Glaser R, Kiecolt-Glaser JK, Speicher CE, Holliday JE. Stress, loneliness and changes in herpes virus latency. *J Behav Med* 1985; 8:249–60.

53 Glaser R, Kiecolt-Glaser J. Stress-associated depression in cellular immunity: implications for acquired immune deficiency syndrome (AIDS). *Brain Behav Immun* 1987; 1:107–12.

54 Schleifer SJ, Keller SE Camerino M, Thomton CJ, Stein M. Suppression of lymphocyte stimulation following bereavement. *JAMA* 1983; 250:374–7.

55 Bistrain BR, Blackburn GL, Serimshaw NS. Cellular immunity in semistarved states in hospitalized adults. *Am J Psychiatr* 1975; 28:1148–55.

56 Clayton PJ, Halikes JA, Maurcie WL. The depression of widowhood. *Br J Psychiatr* 1972; 120:71–80.

57 Kronfol Z, House JD, Silva J, Greden J, Carroll BJ. Depression, urinary free cortisol excretion and lymphocyte function. *Br J Psychiatr* 1986; 148:70–3.

58 Cappel RF, Gregoire LT, Sprecher S. Antibody and cell mediated immunity to herpes simplex virus in psychotic depression. *J Clin Psychiatr* 1978; 39:266–72.

59 Guy R. *An Essay on Scirrous Tumours and Cancer.* London: J and A Churchill, 1759.

60 Paget J. *Lectures on Surgical Pathology* (Rev. and Ed. W. Turner). London: Longman Green, 1863.

61 Parker W. *Cancer: A Study of 397 Cases of Cancer of the Female Breast.* New York: G.P. Putman, 1865.

62 Surawicz FG, Brightwell DR, Weitzel DW, Ekkehard O. Cancer, emotions and mental illness: the present state of understanding. *J Psychiatr* 1976; 133:1306–9.

63 Watson CG, Schuld D. Psychosomatic factors in the aetiology of neoplasms. *J Consult Clin Pathol* 1977; 45:455–64.

64 Kerr TA, Schapira K, Roth M. The relationship between premature death and affective disorder. *Br J Psychiatr* 1969; 115:1277–82.

65 Varsanis J, Zuckhowski T, Maini KK. Survival rates of deaths in geriatric psychiatric patients: a six year follow-up. *Can Psychiatr Assoc J* 1972; 7:17–22.

66 Brown JH, Paraskevas F. Cancer and depression: cancer presenting with depressive illness. An autoimmune disease? *Br J Psychiatr* 1982; 141:227–32.

67 Carroll BJ, Curtis GC, Mendels J. Cerebrospinal fluid and plasma free cortisol levels in depression. *Psychol Med* 1976; 6:235–44.

68 Carroll BJ, Davis BM, Mendels J, Sugerman A. Urinary free cortisol excretion in depression. *Psychol Med* 1976; 6:43–50.

69 Sachar E, Hellman L, Roffwarg H. Disrupted 24 hour

patterns of cortisol secretion in psychotic depression. *Arch Gen Psychiatr* 1973; 28:19–24.

70 Dougherty T, Berliner M, Schneebeli G. Hormonal control of lymphatic structure and function. *Ann N Y Acad Sci* 1964; 113:825–43.

71 Oppenheim J, Dougherty S, Chen S. Use of lymphocyte transformation to assess clinical disorders. In: Vyas G, Stites D, Brecher G, eds. *Laboratory Diagnosis of Immunological Disorders*. New York: Grune and Stratton, 1975.

72 Chang KJ. Opioid peptides have actions on the immune system. *Trends Neurosci* 1984; 7:234–5.

73 Morley JE, Kay N. Neuropeptides as modulators of immune function. *Psychopharmacol Bull* 1986; 22:1089–92.

74 O'Neill B, Leonard BE. Abnormal zymosan induced neutrophil chemiluminescence as a marker of depression. *J Affect Dis* 1990; 19:265–72.

75 O'Neill B, O'Connor WT, Leonard BE. Depressed neutrophil phagocytosis in the rat following olfactory bulbectomy reversed by chronic desipramine treatment. *Med Sci Res* 1987; 15:267–8.

76 Calabrese J, Skwerer RG, Bara B, Geilledge AD, Valenzuela R, Butkus A, Subichin S, Krupp NE. Depression, immunocompetence and prostaglandins of the E series. *Psychiatr Res* 1986; 17:44–7.

77 Besedovsky HO, Del Rey A, Sorkin E, Da Prada M, Keller HA. Immunoregulation mediated by the sympathetic nervous system. *Cell Immunol* 1979; 48:346–55.

78 Besedovsky HP, Del Rey A, Sorkin E, Da Prada M, Burri R, Honegger C. The immune response evokes changes in brain noradrenergic neurons. *Science* 1983; 221:564–5.

79 Hedqvist P. Effects of prostaglandins on autonomic neurotransmission. In: Karin SMM, ed. *Prostaglandins: Physiological, Pharmacological and Pathological Aspects*. Lancaster: MTP Press, 1976.

80 Manku MS, Mtabaji PP, Horrobin DF. Effects of prostaglandins on baseline pressure and responses to noradrenaline in a perfused rat mesenteric artery preparation: PGEI as an antagonist of PGE2. *Prostaglandins* 1977; 3:701–7.

81 Lee RD. The influence of psychotropic drugs on prostaglandin biosynthesis. *Prostaglandins* 1973; 5:63–70.

82 Hong SL, Carty T, Deykin D. Tranylcypromine and 15-hydroperoxy arachidonate affect arachidonic acid release in addition to inhibition of prostacyclin synthesis in calf aortic endothelial cells. *J Biol Chem* 1980; 225:9538–41.

83 Solomon GF. Immunologic abnormalities in mental illness. In: Ader R, ed. *Psychoneuroimmunology*. New York: Academic Press, 1981: 259–77.

84 Amkraut A, Solomon GF, Allan-Smith M, McClellan

B, Rappaport M. Immunoglobulins and improvement in acute schizophrenic reactions. *Arch Gen Psychiatr* 1973; 28:673–7.

85 Domino EF, Krasuse RR, Thiessen MM, Batsakis JG. Blood protein fraction comparisons of normal and schizophrenic patients. *Arch Gen Psychiatr* 1975; 32:717–21.

86 De Lisi LE, Neckers LM, Weinberger DR, Potkin SG, Shilling D, Wyatt RJ. Abnormal immune function in schizophrenic patients. *J Psychiatr* 1987; 139:513–18.

87 Fessel WJ. Autoimmunity and mental illness: preliminary report. *Arch Gen Psychiatr* 1962; 6:320–3.

88 Heath RG, Krupp IM, Byers LW, Liljevist JI. Schizophrenia as an immunological disorder. II. Effects of serum protein fractions on brain function. *Arch Gen Psychiatr* 1967; 16:10–23.

89 Heath RG, Krupp IM, Byers LW, an Liljekvist JI. Schizophrenia as an immunological disorder. III Effects of antimonkey and antihuman brain antibody on brain function. *Arch Gen Psychiatr* 1967; 16:24–33.

90 Logan DG, Deodhan SD. Schizophrenia, an immunologic disorder? *JAMA* 1970; 212:173–704.

91 Whitlingham S, Mackay IR, Jones IH, Davis B. Absence of brain antibodies in patients with schizophrenia. *Br Med J* 1968; 1:347–8.

92 Baron M, Stern M, Anair R, Witz IP. Tissue binding factor in schizophrenic sera. A clinical and genetic study. *Biol Psychiatr* 1977; 12:199–212.

93 Pandey RS, Gupta AK, Chaturvedi VC. Autoimmune models of schizophrenia with special reference to antibrain antibodies. *Biol Psychiatr* 1981; 16:1123–36.

94 Dohan FC, Harper EH, Clark MH, Rodringe RB, Zigas V. Is schizophrenia rare as grain is rare? *Biol Psychiatr* 1984; 19:385–99.

95 Vartanian ME, Kolyaskina GI, Lozovsky DV. Aspects of humoral and cellular immunity in schizophrenia. In: Bergsma D, Goldstein AL, eds. *Neurochemical and Immunological Components of Schizophrenia*. vol. 18. New York: Alan Liss, 1978:339–58.

96 Kolyaskina GI, Sekirina TP, Zozulya AA, Kushner SG. Immunologic studies in schizophrenia. In: Kurstak E, Lipowsi AJ, Morozov PV, eds. *Viruses, Immunity and Mental Disorder*. New York: Plenum, 1987:285–94.

97 Knight JG. Dopamine receptor-stimulating autoantibodies: a possible cause of schizophrenia. *Lancet* 1982; iv:173–1076.

98 Ferguson RM, Schmidtke JR, Simmons, RL. Effects of psychoactive drugs on *in vitro* lymphocyte activation. In: Bergsma D, Goldstein AL, eds. *Neurochemical and Immunological Components of Schizophrenia*. New York: Alan Liss, 1978:379–402.

99 Morozov PV (ed.) *Research on the Viral Hypothesis of Mental Disorders*. vol. 12, Basel: Karger, 1983:1–175.

Part III
Specific examples relating to the immunotoxic/health effects of chemicals

11
Mineral dusts: asbestos, silica and others

KLARA MILLER

Introduction

Mankind is continually exposed to an increasing number of atmospheric and industrial dusts and particles. The fate of inhaled particles or fibres is dependent on their size and shape. Fibres are defined as being of a length greater than 5 μm and having a length:breadth ratio of at least 3 : 1. There is no upper limit for the length of a fibre, but a maximum diameter of 3 μm is defined. Large particles or fibres which are carried into the mammalian respiratory tract are usually deposited on the muco-ciliary epithelium lining the upper airways, including the trachea, bronchi and bronchioles. These particles are subsequently eliminated by ciliary mucus transport to the pharynx.

Particles less than 7 μm in diameter and fibres less than 3 μm in diameter penetrate the lower respiratory tract in varying degrees, and as many as 50% of particles approaching 1 μm in size may reach the alveolar spaces of the lung distal to the terminal bronchioles. It is in these alveolar spaces that the free-lying pulmonary alveolar macrophage plays a key role in host defences. By virtue of its phagocytic activity, this cell constitutes an essential first line of pulmonary defence against inhaled particles.

Many mineral dusts which are taken up by the macrophages, such as carbon particles, are innocuous and may remain in the macrophages more or less indefinitely. The effects of other mineral dusts, however—notably quartz and asbestos—may be fibrogenic and—in the case of asbestiform fibres—carcinogenic. Whilst it is generally acknowledged that macrophages play a fundamental role in the pathogenesis of dust diseases, little is known of the sequence of events following phagocytosis of these mineral dusts by the alveolar macrophage or the possible contribution of the immune system to the development of fibrosis. Industrial exposure to such mineral dusts may serve to illustrate two basic questions of conceptual and practical importance:

1 Are there occupational exposures which can alter the immune status of the host and thus result in enhanced risk of specific disease?

2 After exposure has induced disease, can immune factors play a role in inducing changes not usually caused by the disease itself?

Asbestos

Inhalation of asbestos fibres is associated with a variety of diseases, including pleural plaques and interstitial fibrosis of the lung parenchyma, as well as the development of bronchogenic carcinomas and mesotheliomas of the pleura or peritoneum. The molecular and cellular mechanisms associated with both the fibrogenic and carcinogenic effects of asbestiform fibres have not yet been established, although a number of studies have demonstrated that the length, diameter and physicochemical characteristics of fibres as well as durability in the lung are important determinants of their ability to induce disease. Changes in the immune status of asbestos-exposed populations have also been documented and these may well play a role in the pathogenesis of disease.

Clinical studies

Many studies of workers with long-term occupational exposure to asbestos have shown alterations of cellular and humoral immune responses in individual subjects (Table 11.1). Humoral immune function has been evaluated largely by measurement of autoantibodies and immunoglobulin types. Increased prevalence of autoantibodies, including antinuclear antibodies (ANA), rheumatoid factor (RF) and other antibodies to tissue have been reported, primarily in subjects with asbestosis [1–3], although two other studies found no change in ANA with asbestosis [4,5]. Those with elevated anti-idiotypic antibodies were more likely to have ANA. The results of these later studies do not indicate a specific effect of asbestos, although they suggest a general increase in humoral immunity.

Measurement of immunoglobulins themselves also indicates augmented humoral immune function. Most studies show increased levels of immunoglobulin M (IgM), IgG, IgA and IgE, although not all studies found increases in all immunoglobulin classes [2,6,7]. These increases appear to be of polyclonal origin, suggesting diffuse rather than specific immune stimulation and could be related to the adjuvant-like action ascribed to asbestos [8]. The complement system also appears to be affected. One study found increased levels of components C3 and C4 in subjects with asbestosis [6]; others have shown that several types of asbestos fibres could activate the alternative complement pathway *in vitro* [9,10]. Thus complement may participate in the inflammatory response caused by asbestos exposure.

With regard to neoplasia, one report has described three patients with B-lymphocyte-related neoplasia, all of whom had coexistent asbestos-related disease [11]. The authors speculated that the apparent B-cell stimulation in asbestos exposure could be the cause of the lymphoproliferative disorder but there is at present little evidence to support this hypothesis.

Impaired cell-mediated immunity after asbestos exposure has been reported in most studies although results are not uniform. Delayed hypersensitivity skin tests on patients with interstitial lung fibrosis showed significantly fewer patients had positive responses to the standard test antigens commonly used to assess immunological recall [12,13]. Studies on circulating T lymphocyte numbers and subpopulations have produced varying results, although these may be due to advances in identifying specific populations. Studies where T cells were enumerated using a specific marker found that the number and percentage of T cells decreased in asbestos-exposed subjects compared to controls, even after correction for age and smoking histories. The observation of a diminished ability to generate suppressor activity by lymphocytes obtained from asbestos-exposed subjects [14] suggests that a qualitative alteration of T-cell function also occurs. T-lymphocyte function has been evaluated primarily by mitogen (phytohaemagglutinin, PHA)-induced blast transformation assays, and the preponderance of evidence has demonstrated a significant impairment of responsiveness [15–17]. Possible explanations for this effect include a specific decrease in helper T cells or an effect of some other mononuclear cell involved in the PHA response [18]. Two studies have described decreased cytotoxic functions in lymphocytes obtained from subjects with asbestos exposure [12,19], raising the possibility of an immune alteration beyond the putative effect on suppressor cells.

Table 11.1 Alterations of cellular and humoral immune responses in populations occupationally exposed to asbestos

---

Depressed delayed type hypersensitivity (DTH) skin response

Decreases in total numbers of peripheral blood T lymphocytes

Diminished ability to generate suppressor cell activity *in vitro*

Reduced PHA-induced *in vitro* cytotoxic cell function

Reduced mitogen (PHA)-induced proliferation of lymphocytes

Increased levels of serum immunoglobulins

Increased prevalence of autoantibodies

Of particular interest here may be an incomplete study where difference in PHA-induced cytotoxic T-cell function was found in asbestos-exposed subjects with pleural plaques but no radiological evidence of parenchymal fibrosis [20]. In 16 out of 20 subjects the cytotoxic cell function was found to be markedly reduced compared to a group with similar exposure but no evidence of pleural reactions. A significant depression of lymphocyte responsiveness to PHA was also observed in these subjects. The finding that impaired T lymphocyte function is evident in some asbestos-exposed subjects with no evidence of fibrosis at the time of the sampling suggests that immune changes might be involved in the pathogenesis of disease. This impairment might relate to pre-existing asbestos-related cell alterations, or a depletion of functional helper T lymphocytes resulting from activation of the immune system by asbestos-exposed macrophages [21,22], and will be discussed later in this chapter.

With regard to neoplasia, two peer-reviewed studies have measured PHA responses in small groups of patients with mesothelioma [15,23]. In both studies, PHA response was normal, although in one of the studies [15] a patient with asbestosis and an associated bronchial carcinoma had depressed lymphocyte responses to PHA. Another group has reported some aberrations in both cell-mediated and humoral immunity in patients with mesothelioma as well as in asbestos workers with long-term exposure [24]. It should be remembered, however, that the immunological status of individuals with asbestos-related cancers has been described in a few, very limited studies [25]. The question therefore remains open as to whether there is any association between immune alterations and asbestos-associated malignancies and whether such alterations influence the rate of progression of the disease. The rest of this chapter will therefore consider the impact asbestos—as well as other mineral fibres—has on the immune system in relation to inflammatory and fibrogenic reactions only.

The role of macrophages

The location of alveolar macrophages means that they are one of the first cell types to encounter inhaled mineral fibres. The participation of mac-

rophages in both cell-mediated and humoral reactions clearly focuses attention on the macrophage as an immunoregulatory cell and also its potential role as an effector cell, directing the course of fibrogenesis through elaboration of various mediators.

Cellular events. Many investigators have made use of tissue and cell culture techniques to understand the biological effects of asbestos fibres at a cellular level. Allison and his co-workers [26] were perhaps the first to investigate the limits of the size of fibres that can be ingested by macrophages. Irrespective of the type of asbestos, short fibres were completely phagocytosed whereas long fibres were not. The cells attached or enveloped the ends of the latter but portions of the fibre remained outside the wall. Under these conditions, after fusion of lysosomes with the phagosomes, the lysosomal enzymes would have a route to the cell exterior along the partially phagocytosed fibre so that selective release of enzymes rather than cell death would ensue. (Partial ingestion of fibres could also lead to continual release of free radicals, possibly leading to non-enzymatic activation of carcinogens—a hypothesis outside the remit of this chapter.) The observations suggested that lysosomal enzymes themselves, or some other factor released from damaged macrophages with similar kinetics, could be responsible for the fibrogenic activity of mineral dusts. For example, the release of proteases could lead to the cleavage of plasma proteins such as fibronectin or generate peptides with growth factor-like activities [27].

The studies described above were primarily concerned with a connection between macrophage toxicity and fibrosis and have led to the practice of using the effects of fibres and other particulates on macrophages as an *in vitro* screen for fibrogenic dusts. This practice has been extended to the use of macrophage-like cell lines in place of primary macrophages. However, a common problem with such studies has been that, while stimulating one activity, asbestos types such as chrysotile or amphibole asbestos have differing cytotoxic or sublethal effects on macrophages *in vitro*, making the interpretation of results extremely difficult [28].

Some *in vitro* studies have been concerned with macrophage function more specifically related to its immunoregulatory role. Chrysotile asbestos has been shown to induce macrophages to release prostaglandin E_2 in one study [29], whereas another study found stimulated prostaglandin production in cocultures of fibroblasts and macrophages treated with crocidolite [30]. Both silica and fibrous dust cause the release of metabolites of arachidonic acid and in the case of fibres, activity is dependent on fibre length [31]. The interest in the context of immunoregulatory mechanism is the known effect prostaglandins have on T suppressor cells [32].

More recently interest in growth factors and lymphokines has led to the investigation of the role of these agents in the development of fibrosis. Tumour necrosis factor (TNF), a substance which may enhance the activation of polymorphonuclear neutrophils [33], has been shown to be secreted in significantly increased quantities after exposure of rat alveolar macrophages to chrysotile in a dose- and time-dependent manner. In contrast, latex beads at the same mass concentration were inactive in stimulating secretion of TNF [34]. Asbestos fibres also stimulate the release of interleukin-1 in several *in vitro* studies [35]. Both of these cytokines are capable of stimulating fibroblasts and it is possible that some of the early observations on 'the fibrogenic factor' could have been due to the release of these or other growth factors. It is important to keep in mind, however, that although asbestos fibres cause a number of short-term effects on isolated cells *in vitro*, many of the cellular responses may be different in the whole animal. Factors such as mediators are perhaps best studied after *in vivo* exposure.

The role of complement in macrophage responses to fibres. The mechanism whereby pulmonary alveolar macrophages are attracted to the sites of asbestos fibre deposition has recently been clarified in a number of studies on rats and mice. They are based on the hypothesis that macrophages are attracted to sites of asbestos deposition by a chemotactic factor activated by the inhaled fibres on alveolar surfaces, and supported by *in vitro* experiments demonstrating that asbestos fibres activate the alternative complement pathway in serum [10]. In these studies a series of *in vitro* experiments was undertaken incubating chrysotile asbestos fibres with rat serum or unexposed lavaged proteins as a first step. Incubation produced an enhanced pulmonary macro-

phage chemotactic response compared to controls, demonstrating that pulmonary macrophages respond to asbestos-activated chemoattractants. This finding was confirmed *in vivo* where it was demonstrated that fluids lavaged from the lung of asbestos-exposed rats contained enhanced chemotactic activity for macrophages, which was detected in the molecular weight range of $C5_a$ [36]. Later studies in which congenic strains of complement-deficient mice or decomplemented rats were exposed to chrysotile asbestos for brief periods showed that the number of macrophages that had accumulated at sites of fibre deposition were significantly depressed compared to normal animals [37].

Furthermore, time-course studies conclusively demonstrated that the chemoattractant generation preceded the macrophage migration response and that macrophage phagocytosis of inhaled asbestos fibres was reduced in complement-deficient animals. Other mineral fibres including crocidolite fibres and glass fibres have also been shown significantly to activate complement in rat serum and in lung fluids, and it was concluded that activation of complement by inorganic mineral dusts facilitates lung clearance of inhaled materials by providing a mechanism through which free-lying alveolar macrophages can detect and phagocytose particulates on alveolar surfaces [38]. Whether or not complement mechanisms are involved in asbestos-induced inflammatory responses in experimental animals or humans remains to be determined.

Immunoregulatory effects in experimental animals

Several animal species (mice, rats, guinea pigs and sheep) have been used successfully in studying inflammatory fibrotic reactions to various types of asbestos. These *in vivo* studies suggest an intricate series of cellular events which are involved in asbestos-associated disease. Many of the biological responses involve interactions between cells of the immune system and target cells of disease. Inhalation of asbestos has also been shown to confer antigenic properties on the macrophage leading to the presence of activated lymphocytes in the exposed animal.

In all published studies phagocytosis of asbestos fibres has been reported to induce greater membrane ruffling in the alveolar macrophages. Moreover, after prolonged exposure alveolar macrophages will become bi- or multi-nucleated due to fusion of cells or inability of a dividing cell to undergo mitosis [8]. Longer fibres are not completely engulfed by phagocytic cells, possibly resulting in lysosomal enzyme release from phagolysosomes and secretion of various cytokines. These cytokines may affect the proliferation of fibroblasts, thereby increasing collagen deposition, a hallmark of the fibrotic process [39].

In a number of investigations on rats, alveolar macrophages isolated from crocidolite-exposed rats showed increased percentages of cells forming rosettes with sensitized sheep red blood cells as well as an elevation in the number of red blood cells making up the rosette [40], compared to the patterns observed in controls. Further experiments demonstrated that crocidolite exposure also led alveolar macrophages to exhibit significantly increased levels of immune adherence activity as compared with control cells, indicating that deposition of complement components on the macrophages had occurred *in vivo* [41]. This was postulated to be evidence of a humoral immune response directed against altered or newly expressed membrane determinants on macrophages and a consequence of prolonged asbestos phagocytosis. Such alterations would be consistent with the ability of macrophages that move into the pulmonary interstitium or migrate into the lymphatics to interact with lymphocytes circulating to the lung, giving rise to systemically sensitized lymphocytes. To test this postulate experiments were performed wherein macrophages from asbestos-exposed rats were co-cultured *in vitro* with autologous T lymphocytes or with T lymphocytes obtained from control rats [21,42].

Two separate asbestos-related effects, both dependent on surface membrane changes, were observed. The first phenomenon was observed in co-cultures of exposed macrophages with control lymphocytes. In these cultures prolonged binding of lymphocytes to macrophages occurred followed by a blastogenic response. Both binding and proliferation could be abolished by treatment of the asbestos-exposed macrophages with L-cysteine which would reduce or block stimulating oxidized surface glycoproteins. This effect is similar to alveolar membrane peroxi-dation, and provides a functional correlate of the adjuvant-like morphological response described earlier.

The second asbestos-related phenomenon was noted in co-cultures of macrophages and lymphocytes obtained from exposed animals. In this system, the induction of proliferation of lymphocytes was not abolished by treatment with L-cysteine and required major histocompatibility complex-linked restriction between the interacting macrophages and lymphocytes. Hence the stimulatory effect could have been caused by cell-bound alloantigen or expression of antigen-like molecules. Since splenic lymphocytes were used the findings are consistent with systemic immune recognition.

The nature of the proliferating T cell remains to be determined but other studies have provided additional evidence for the antigen-like elaboration of stimulatory factors after asbestos inhalation. Supernatants from co-cultures of immune splenic lymphocytes and alveolar macrophages obtained from rats exposed to chrysotile or crocidolite *in vivo* contained greater interleukin-1 and -2 activity than controls [43]. Other studies also indicate that the cytokine produced by macrophages after exposure to asbestos mediates the growth and proliferation of endothelial, epithelial and mesenchymal cells. For example, groups with conditioned medium from alveolar macrophages of chrysotile-exposed sheep with asbestosis have been shown to stimulate incorporation of tritiated thymidine in human embryonic lung fibroblasts (WI-38 cells) [44]. Thus immunological mechanisms are operative in the development of asbestos-associated disease and, in particular, play a significant role in the pulmonary macrophage response to inhaled fibres.

Man-made mineral fibres

Another group of fibrous materials of concern are the man-made mineral fibres (MMMF). These include fibres made from borosilicate or calcium aluminium silicate glasses, rock and slag wools which are amorphous glassy fibres made from molten slags or natural rocks such as basalt and ceramic fibres. The ceramic fibres which, among other uses, are used to line industrial furnaces are made from aluminosilicate minerals such as kaolin.

Table 11.2 Effect of crocidolite asbestos or glass fibre inhalation on the ability of rat alveolar macrophages to bind sensitized sheep erythrocytes (EA rosette formation)

Macrophages	Rosetting (%)	Number of erythrocytes/rosette
Control	60 ± 8	4 ± 3.1
Crocidolite	75 ± 10	9 ± 4.8***
Glass fibre	92 ± 8	16 ± 6.9***

*** $P<0.001$.

Not surprisingly, fewer epidemiological studies exist on workers exposed to MMMF compared to asbestos [45] and those have been concerned mainly with cancer incidence and in particular with lung cancer mortality. There are no data linking MMMF exposure to increased mesothelioma incidence. There are also no published studies on the immune status of workers exposed to MMMF fibres, although it should be borne in mind that the better a substitute mimics the physical and chemical properties of asbestos, the closer the ill-effects on the immune system are likely to be.

There is some evidence from animal studies that inhalation of glass fibres of the same dimensions as crocidolite asbestos over 6 months produced changes in alveolar macrophage topography and function similar to those already demonstrated following asbestos inhalation [46]. In this study macrophage populations varied in size from 10 to 40 μm and showed an enhanced ability to spread across a glass substrate. An increase in the percentage of cells forming erythrocyte antibody (EA) rosettes as well as an increased avidity of Fc receptors when compared to control macrophages was observed (Table 11.2).

Interest in growth factors and cytokines, as mentioned earlier, has led to the investigation of the effect of MMMF on rat alveolar macrophages after short-term inhalation exposure to low concentrations of refractory ceramic fibres [47] (Fig. 11.1). In macrophages recovered by bronchoalveolar lavage increases in both Fc and major histocompatibility complex class II expression were evident compared to controls. No increase in interleukin-1 and fibronectin gene expression, compared to controls, was evident when messenger RNA was extracted immediately after lavage. However, when the cells were cultured overnight and then stimulated with lipopolysaccharide interleukin-1β transcription was significantly increased when compared to controls, thus indicating that fibre exposure had resulted in priming macrophages for a considerable length of time [48]. Whether these early events could lead to alterations in systemic immune parameters remains to be elucidated.

Quartz

Many mineral dusts, not just fibres, stimulate a severe reaction in the lung when inhaled in sufficient

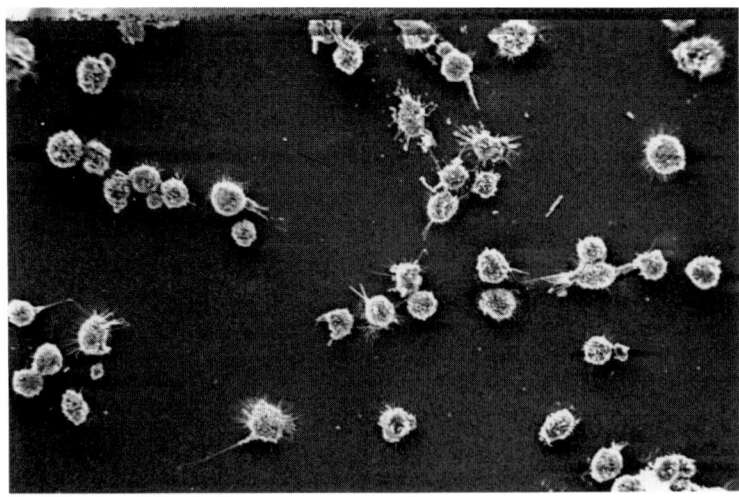

Fig. 11.1 Scanning electron micrograph of rat alveolar macrophages obtained 180 days after a 5-day exposure to refractory ceramic fibres (12.5 μg ml^{-1}). Original magnification × 900.

quantity and there is conflicting evidence whether they do so by a common mechanism. Indeed some experimental work has provided evidence that quartz (crystalline silica) and crocidolite asbestos cause fibrosis by quite different mechanisms [40,49]. To some extent this observation is supported by the dissimilar nature and distribution of the lesions seen in silicosis and asbestosis. Silicosis is characterized at first by the deposition of concentric nodules in the hilar lymph nodes, and as these lymph nodes become fibrosed nodules of concentric fibrosis appear within the lung; these may then coalesce to form conglomerate areas. Asbestosis is a chronic inflammatory reaction in the terminal bronchioles and alveoli of the lung with considerable fibrosis leading to distortion and eventual obliteration of the alveoli. Perhaps the most important difference, however, lies in the situation that whilst both dusts are fibrogenic there is no conclusive pathological and epidemiological evidence of a relationship between quartz exposure and the development of neoplasms (although there are a few reports of an excess death rate from lung cancer among silicosis and coal workers) [50].

Both quartz and fibres are phagocytosed by pulmonary macrophages after entering the lung and it may be that the sequence of events following phagocytosis differs markedly. Indeed, unlike asbestos, particulate silica has the property of damaging the structural integrity of the macrophage phagolysosomal membrane through the interaction of similar groups with membrane lipoproteins or phosphate esters, resulting in lysis of the macrophage and release of quartz particles in the lumen. In silicosis, therefore, the primary lesion stems basically from injury to alveolar macrophages and may be compounded by other phagocytic cells being recruited into the bronchoalveolar spaces. Experimental studies have demonstrated that alveolar macrophages under these circumstances produce a quartz-induced macrophage chemotactic factor for many months after cessation of dust exposure, suggesting that such a factor might be responsible for providing a large and continuous supply of macrophages to the lung [51]. Quartz probably exerts its effects on the macrophage function that ingests it by altering their function while they are alive rather than by disrupting them. Under these sublethal conditions it is

known also to have an adjuvant-like effect [52] and to induce the secretion of several potentially fibrogenic cytokines such as interleukin-1 and TNF-α. Very recent evidence has demonstrated that production of TNF plays an important part in the development of silica-induced pulmonary fibrosis [53].

Silicotic lesions are also frequently observed in hilar lymph nodes of individuals after chronic exposure to silica in industry and in experimental studies. This is due to free quartz particles in the lymphatics reaching the lymph nodes where they are engulfed by macrophages, or to quartz-laden macrophages transported from the lung via the lymphatics to the lymph nodes [54]. Examination of these regional thoracic nodes showed both a fibroblast connective tissue reaction and the aggregation of plasmacytoid lymphocytes and plasma cells in close opposition to macrophages [55], suggesting an activation of lymphocytes and ensuing humoral immune response. Little work, however, has been done to try to correlate the site and mode of particle deposition with the subsequent immune response in lymphatic tissue associated with the respiratory tract.

Immunological factors have been incriminated in the pathogenesis of silicosis [56]. Many investigators have demonstrated an increased prevalence of autoantibodies and autoimmune diseases in silicotic patients [57]. Later studies however have shown little correlation between the aberrant humoral immune responses and progression of disease [58]. This suggests that autoantibody formation and immune complexes are not directly responsible for the lung changes in silicosis. On the other hand, the increased prevalence of autoantibodies, elevation of serum immunoglobulin levels and the presence of immune complexes all support the postulate of B-lymphocyte hyperactivity in silicotic patients. This could be secondary to direct polyclonal B-cell stimulation by silica particles or B-cell stimulation by degradation products of cytokines released during silica–macrophage interactions. Increased levels of serum-complemented components [59] and of serum lysozyme have also been reported in silicotic subjects, which again points to increased macrophage numbers and/or activity [60]. Hypothetically, macrophages with adjuvant-like properties could influence and activate lymphocytes whilst also generating fibroblast proliferation factors; these lymphocytes would then feed back to amplify the response by stimulating the same or other recruited macrophages. Once stimulated, the pro-inflammatory cycle could proceed non-specifically and without antigen direction.

Coal-mine dust

Exposure to coal-mine dust may cause simple coal-worker's pneumoconiosis (CWP), characterized radiologically by the appearance of small opacities in the lung. It is associated with minimal respiratory impairment, and there is no evidence that CWP progresses in the absence of exposure [61]. Miners and ex-miners with simple pneumoconiosis survive as well as those with no radiological change [62]. However, a subgroup of those with categories 2 and 3 simple pneumoconiosis (more widespread small opacities) are at risk of developing progressive massive fibrosis (PMF), associated with impaired lung function and premature death. PMF is not related to exposure but represents an 'attack' on well developed simple pneumoconiosis. Furthermore, PMF may develop after cessation of exposure, and at present there is no way of detecting whether a miner is going to develop PMF after leaving the industry.

Effects of coal dust on the immune system

It must be emphasized that simple pneumoconiosis is related to the degree of exposure, whereas PMF is not related to the degree of exposure, although it occurs mainly in the heavily exposed. At one time PMF was considered to represent tuberculosis superimposed on silicosis [63] but more recent studies do not provide any evidence that PMF is related to present or previous mycobacterial infection. There is also no support for the suggestion that quartz dust is a factory in the aetiology of PMF [64] and no evidence has been found of any association between the attack rate of PMF and age, energy expenditure at work, body type and smoking habits. The question therefore arises whether immunological factors favour the development of the disease in some miners but not in others.

A number of studies have been carried out on the immunology of CPW. An increase in IgA levels has been reported and several clinical studies have shown significantly higher mean concentrations of IgA and

IgG than controls [65]. However, few significant differences in serum immunoglobulin levels were noted among the subtypes of pneumoconiosis, including PMF. Other investigators found a greater percentage of coal miners with CPW and PMF had ANA when compared to coal miners without pneumoconiosis [66]. Later studies also found ANA and RF in a large proportion of miners with pneumoconiosis but have been unable to detect any serological differences between CPW and PMF [67,68].

Few investigators have looked at parameters of cell-mediated immunity. One study however [69] estimated T- and B-lymphocyte numbers and the percentage was compared with the pneumoconiosis category, age and smoking habits in 324 men. A significant decrease in the proportion of T lymphocytes able to form spontaneous rosettes with sheep red blood cells on resuspension after 4°C overnight incubation (O/N T cells) was found in men with PMF compared to other groups. This decrease in O/N rosettes, believed to identify cells with suppressor function, may be of fundamental importance. Further studies to evaluate cell-mediated immune responses are clearly needed, but these preliminary results indicate that a qualitative loss of T-lymphocyte function occurs only in PMF. Recent studies on retired coal miners by a French group [70] have also demonstrated differences in alveolar macrophage secretion of pro-inflammatory cytokines such as interleukin-1 and TNF between patients with simple pneumoconiosis or PMF, supporting the concept that alveolar macrophages play a key role in the development of fibrotic lung disease.

Ideally, comparisons could be made among subjects with varying degrees of exposure and radiological changes. All one can say at present is that what is necessary for PMF is an appreciable dust burden plus another factor yet unknown. It may be an impaired balance of the helper/suppressor feedback loop, mediated by factors released as a consequence of coal dust—macrophage interactions in susceptible individuals.

References

1 Turner-Warwick M, Parkes WR. Circulating rheumatoid and anti-nuclear factors in asbestos workers. *Br Med J* 1970; 3:492–5.

2 Kagan E, Solomon A, Cochrane JC, Kuba P, Rocks PH, Webster I. Immunological studies of patients with asbestosis. II. Studies of circulating lymphoid numbers and humoral immunity. *Clin Exp Immunol* 1977; 28:268–75.

3 Lange A. An epidemiological survey of immunological abnormalities in asbestos workers. I. Nonorgan- and organ-specific autoantibodies. *Environ Res* 1980; 22:162–75.

4 Doll NJ, Diem JE, Jones RN, Rodriquez H, Bozellia BE, Stankus RP, Weill H, Salvaggio JE. Humoral immunologic abnormalities in workers exposed to asbestos cement dust. *J Allergy Clin Immunol* 1983; 72:509–12.

5 Lange A. Anergy and auto-immunity in asbestos-exposed people. *Arch Immunol Ther Exp* 1982; 30:211–18.

6 Huuskone MS, Rasanen YA, Harkonen H, Asp S. Asbestos exposure as a cause of immunological stimulation. *Scand J Resp Dis* 1978; 59:326–32.

7 Lange A. An epidemiological survey of immunological abnormalities in asbestos workers. II. Serum immunoglobulin levels. *Environ Res* 1980; 22:176–83.

8 Miller K, Kagan E. The *in vivo* effects of asbestos on macrophage membrane structure and population characteristics of macrophages. *J Reticuloendothel Soc* 1976; 20:159–71.

9 Wilson MR, Caumer HR, Salvaggio JR. Activation of the alternative complement pathway and generation of chemotactic factors by asbestos. *J Allergy Clin Immunol* 1977; 60:218–22.

10 Saint-Remy JMR, Cole P. Interaction of chrysotile asbestos fibres with the complement system. *Immunol* 1980; 41:431–7.

11 Kagan E, Jacobson RJ. Lymphoid and plasma cell malignancies: asbestos-related disorders of long latency. *Am J Clin Pathol* 1983; 80:14–20.

12 Kagan E, Solomon A, Cochrane JC, Beissner EK, Gluckman J, Rocks PH, Webster I. Immunological studies of patients with asbestosis. I. Studies of cell mediated immunity. *Clin Exp Immunol* 1977; 28:261–7.

13 Lange A, Sibinski G, Garncarek D. The follow-up study of skin reactivity to recall antigens and E- and EAC-RFC profiles in blood in asbestos workers. *Immunobiol* 1980; 157:1–11.

14 Goumer HR, Doll NJ, Karmal J, Schuyler M, Salvaggio JE. Diminished suppression cell function in patients with asbestosis. *Clin Exp Immunol* 1981; 44:108–16.

15 Haslam PL, Lukozak A, Merchant JA, Turner-Warwick M. Lymphocyte responses to phytohaemagglutinin in patients with asbestosis and pleural mesothelioma. *Clin Exp Immunol* 1978; 31:178–88.

16 Campbell MJ, Wagner MMF, Scott MP, Brown DG. Sequential immunological studies in an asbestos exposed population. II. Factors affecting lymphocyte function. *Clin Exp Immunol* 1980; 39:276–81.

17 DeSahzo RD, Nordberg BA, Baser Y, Bozelka B, Weill H, Salvaggio J. Analysis of depressed cell-mediated immunity in asbestos workers. *J Allergy Clin Immunol* 1983; 71:418–24.

18 Tsang PH, Chu FN, Fischbein A, Bekesi JG. Impairments in functional subsets of T-suppressor (CD8) lymphocytes, monocytes and natural killer cells among asbestos-exposed workers. *Clin Immunol Immunopathol* 1988; 47:323–32.

19 Ginns LC, Ryu JH, Rogo PR, Sprince NL, Oliver LC, Larsson CJ. Natural killer cell activity in smokers and workers. *Am Rev Resp Dis* 1985; 131:831–4.

20 Miller K, Brown RC. The immune system and asbestos-associated disease. In: Dean JH, Munson A, Luster M, eds. *Toxicology of the Immune System.* New York: Raven Press, 1985:429–40.

21 Miller K, Weintraub Z, Kagan E. Manifestations of cellular immunity in the rat after prolonged asbestos inhalation. I. Physical interactions between alveolar macrophage and splenic lymphocytes. *J Immunol* 1979; 123:1029–38.

22 Gellert AP, Macey MG, Uthayakumor S, Newland AC, Rudd RM. Lymphocyte sub-populations in bronchoalveolar lavage fluid in asbestos workers. *Am Rev Resp Dis* 1985; 132:824–8.

23 Wagner MMF, Campbell MJ, Edwards RE. Sequential immunological studies on an asbestos-exposed population. I. Factors affecting peripheral blood leucocytes and T lymphocytes. *Clin Exp Immunol* 1979; 38:323–31.

24 Lew F, Tsang P, Holland JF, Warner N, Selikoff IF, Bekesi JG. High frequency of immune dysfunction in asbestos workers and in patients with malignant mesothelioma. *J Clin Immunol* 1986; 6:225–33.

25 World Health Organisation. Asbestos and other mineral fibres. Environmental Health Criteria No. 53. *International Programme on Chemical Safety.* WHO, 1986: 120.

26 Allison HC, Clark IA, Davies P. Cellular interactions in fibrogenesis. *Ann Rheum Dis* 1977; 36 (suppl):8–11.

27 Rom WN, Basset P, Gills GA, Nukiwa T, Trapnell BC, Crystal RG. Alveolar macrophages release an insulin-like growth factor I-type molecular. *J Clin Invest* 1988; 82:1685.

28 Miller K. The effects of asbestos on macrophage. *CRC Crit Rev Toxicol* 1978; 5:319–54.

29 Sirois P, Rola-Pleszczynski M, Begin R. Phospholipase A activity and prostaglandin synthesis from alveolar macrophages exposed to asbestos. *Prostag Med* 1980; 5:31–7.

30 Goldstein RH, Miller K, Glaseroth J, Linscott R,

Snider GL, Franzblau C, Polgar P. Influence of asbestos fibers on collagen and prostaglandin production in fibroblast and macrophage co-cultures. *J Lab Clin Med* 1982; 100:778–85.

31 Forget G, Lacroix MJ, Brown RC, Evans PH, Sirois P. Response of perfused alveolar macrophages to glass fibres; effect of exposure duration and fiber length. *Environ Res* 1986; 32:124–35.

32 Nicklin S, Shand FL. Abrogation of suppressor cell function by inhibitors of prostaglandin synthesis. *Int J Immunopharmacol* 1982; 4:407–14.

33 Tsujimoto M, Yokota S, Vilcek B, Weissman G. Tumour necrosis factor provokes superoxide generation from neutrophils. *Biochem Biophys Res Commun* 1986; 137:1094–7.

34 Dubois CM, Bissonette E, Rola-Pleszczynski M. Asbestos fibres and silica particles stimulate rat alveolar macrophages to release tumor necrosis factor: autoregulatory role of leukotriene B4. *Am Rev Resp Dis* 1989; 139:1257–62.

35 Tert MM, Kumar RR, Bennett R, Brody AR, Luster MI, Rosenthal GJ. Secretion of hydrogen peroxide (H$_2$O$_2$), interleukin 1 (IL-1) and tumor necrosis factor (TNF) by rat alveolar macrophages following asbestos exposure. *Toxicol* 1988; 8:197A.

36 Warheit DB, George G, Hill LH, Snyderman R, Brody AR. Inhaled asbestos activates a complement-dependent chemo-attractant for macrophages. *Lab Invest* 1985; 52:505–14.

37 Warheit DB, Hill LH, George G, Brody AR. Time course of chemotactic factor generation and the corresponding macrophage response to asbestos inhalation. *Am Rev Resp Dis* 1986; 134:128–33.

38 Warheit DB, Overby LH, George G, Brody AR. Pulmonary macrophages are attracted to inhaled particles through complement activation. *Exp Lung Res* 1988; 4:51–66.

39 King RJ, Jones MB, Minoo P. Regulations of lung cell proliferation by polypeptide growth factors. *Am J Physiol (Lung Cell Mol Physiol)* 1989; 257:1–23.

40 Miller K. Alterations in surface-related phenomena of alveolar macrophages following inhalation of crocidolite asbestos and quartz dusts. *Environ Res* 1979; 29:152–8.

41 Miller K, Kagan E. Immune adherance reactivity of rat alveolar macrophages following inhalation of crocidolite asbestos. *Clin Exp Immunol* 1977; 29:152–8.

42 Miller K, Kagan E. Manifestations of cellular immunity in the rat after prolonged asbestos inhalation. II. Alveolar macrophage-induced splenic lymphocyte proliferation. *Environ Res* 1981; 26:182–94.

43 Hartmann DP, Georgian MM, Oghiso Y, Kagan E. Enhanced interleukin activity following asbestos inhalation. *Clin Exp Immunol* 1984; 55:643–50.

44 Lemaise I, Beaudoin H, Masse H, Grondin C. Alveolar macrophage stimulation of lung fibroblast growth in asbestos-induced pulmonary fibrosis. *Am J Pathol* 1986; 122:201–8.

45 Mossman BT. Carcinogenic potential of asbestos and non-asbestos fibres. *Environ Sci Hlth* 1988; C6:151–95.

46 Miller K. The *in vivo* effects of glass fibres on alveolar macrophage membrane characteristics. In: Wagner JC, ed. *Biological Effects of Mineral Fibres*. Scientific Publication 30. Lyon: IARC, 1980:459–65.

47 Miller K, Lawrence F, Riley AR. Consequences of MMMF inhalation on lung and pleural cavity cell populations. In: Mossman BT, Begin RO, eds. *Effects of Mineral Dusts on Cells*. Nato ASI series H30. Berlin: Springer Verlag, 1989: 321–8.

48 Miller K, Hudspith BH, Meredith C. Rat pleural cell populations: effects on cytokine mRNA expression and population characteristics. In: Brown RC, Hoskins J, Johnson N, eds. *Mechanisms in Fibre Carcinogenesis* Nato ASI series. Plenum Press, 1991 (in press).

49 Miller K, Webster I, Handfield RIM, Skikne MI. Ultrastructure of the lung in the rat following exposure to crocidolite asbestos and quartz. *J Pathol* 1978; 124:39–44.

50 Heppleston AG. Silica pneumoconiosis and carcinoma of the lung. *Am J Ind Med* 1985; 7:285–94.

51 Miller K, Calverley A, Kagan E. Evidence of a quartz-induced chemotactic factor for guinea pig alveolar macrophages. *Environ Res* 1980; 22:31–9.

52 Munder PG, Modofell M, Ferber E, Fischer H. The relationship between macrophages and adjuvant activity. In: van Furth R, ed. *Mononuclear Phagocytes*. Oxford: Blackwell, 1970:445–60.

53 Piquet PF, Collart MA, Grav GE, Sappina AP, Vassalli P. Requirement of tumour necrosis factor for development of silica-induced pulmonary fibrosis. *Nature* 1990; 344:245–7.

54 Kaltreider HB. Expression of immune mechanisms in the lung. *Am Rev Resp Dis* 1976; 113:347–79.

55 Klempman S, Miller K. The *in vivo* effects of quartz on rat thoracic lymph nodes. *Br J Exp Pathol* 1977; 58:557–64.

56 Vigliani EC, Permis B. Immunological aspects of silicosis. *Adv Tuberc Res* 1973; 12:643–65.

57 Ziekind M, Jones RN, Weill N. Silicosis. *Am Rev Resp Dis* 1976; 113:643–65.

58 Doll NJ, Stankins RP, Hughes J, Weill H, Gupton RC, Rodriquez M, Jones RN, Alspangh MA, Salvaggio JE. Immune complexes and autoantibodies in silicosis. *J Allergy Clin Immunol* 1981; 68:281–5.

59 Miller K. Complement factors in workers exposed to silica. *Br J Ind Med* 1983; 40:111–12.

60 Koskinen H, Nordman H, Froseth B. Serum lysozyme concentration in silicosis patients and workers exposed

to silic dust. *Eur J Resp Dis* 1984; 65:481–5.

61 Cochrane AI, Haley TJL, Moore F, Hole D. The mortality of men in the Rhondaa Fach 1950–1970. *Br J Ind Med* 1979; 36:15–22.

62 Cochrane AI. The attack rate of progressive massive fibrosis. *Br J Ind Med* 1962; 19:51–64.

63 Gough J. Fibrosis in coal workers. *Arch Environ Hlth* 1968; 17:836–43.

64 McLintock JS, Rae S, Jacobsen M. The attack rate of progressive massive fibrosis in British coal miners. In: Walton WH, ed. *Inhaled Particles III.* Old Woking: Unwin, 1971: 933–52.

65 Hahon N, Morgan WKC, Petersen M. Serum immunoglobulin levels in coal worker's pneumoconiosis. *Ann Occup Hyg* 1980; 23:165–74.

66 Lippman M, Eckert HL, Hahan N. Circulating antinuclear and rheumatoid factors in coal miners. A prevalence study in Pennsylvania and West Virginia. *Ann Intern Med* 1973; 79:807–11.

67 Pearson DJ, Mentneck MS, Elliot JA, Price CD, Taylor G, Major PC. Serological changes in pneumoconiosis and progressive massive fibrosis of coal workers. *Am Rev Resp Dis* 1981; 124:696–9.

68 Boyd JE, Robertson MD, Davis JMG. Autoantibodies in coal miners: their relationship to the development of progressive massive fibrosis. *Am J Ind Med* 1982; 3:201–8.

69 Robertson MD, Boyd JE, Fernie JH, Davis JMG. Some immunological studies on coal workers with and without pneumoconiosis. *Am J Ind Med* 1983; 4:467–76.

70 Lasalle P, Gosset P, Aerts C, Benhamour M, Fortin F, Wallaert B, Tonnel AB, Voisin C. Alveolar macrophages secretory dysfunctions in coal workers pneumoconiosis. Comparison between simple pneumoconiosis and progressive massive fibrosis. In: Mossman BT, Begin RO, eds. *Effects of Mineral Dusts on Cells.* NATO 131 Series. Berlin: Springer-Verlag, 1989:65–71.

12

Occupational asthma and allergic reactions to inhaled compounds

MERYL H. KAROL

Introduction

The current industrial setting provides diverse opportunities for chemical exposures. Many exposures have resulted in allergic sensitization. The objective of this review is to present factors which have a major impact on the development of sensitization; factors associated with chemical agents and worksites, as well as those inherent to the workers.

The incidence of occupational allergic sensitization is estimated to be from 5 to 45 or 50% [1]. The disparity can be attributed in part to inclusion of certain industries and to industrial facilities in some underdeveloped countries. However, a significant problem in estimating the extent of sensitization lies with current diagnostic procedures. These procedures will be discussed and suggestions made for improved practices.

Agents capable of causing occupational sensitization comprise a diverse group of substances. As seen in Table 12.1, this includes biologically derived materials, such as plant and animal products, drugs, and chemicals both organic and inorganic in nature. The allergens are frequently classified as high versus low molecular weight agents with the size cut-off being 1000 Da. This classification serves to distinguish those which are complete antigens (high molecular weight) from those which are haptens (low molecular weight) and are incapable alone of inducing an immune response.

Among the list of chemical allergens, isocyanates and acid anhydrides appear prominent. Symptoms associated with respiratory sensitization to these chemicals include chest tightness, cough, bronchospasm, bronchitis, fever, malaise, weakness. Of interest with isocyanates is the observation that some isocyanates have been associated with respiratory tract sensitization, whereas others have been linked to dermal manifestations. For example, toluene diisocyanate (TDI) is potent as a pulmonary sensitizer having a permissable exposure limit (PEL) of 20 p.p.b. and a threshold limit value (TLV) of 5 p.p.b. [3]. There are few, if any, case reports of rash or other dermal lesions associated with occupational TDI exposure. By contrast, dicyclohexylmethane 4,4'-diisocyanate (HMDI) is recognized for potency as a dermal sensitizer [4,5], even though the chemical is heated during use and therefore is present in the workplace atmosphere, and available for inhalation exposure.

Some general features of chemical sensitizers can be recognized. The chemicals display ability to react with nucleophiles. In so doing, covalent linkages are formed, predominantly with serum proteins, and the

Table 12.1 Causes of occupational asthma

Grains, flour, plants and gum	*Fungi*	*Chemicals*
Buckwheat	*Alternaria*	Azodicarbonamide
Castor beans	*Aspergillus* sp.	Chloramine T
Cinnamon	*Cladosporium*	Cyanoacrylate
Coriander	*Didymella exitialis*	Dimethyl ethanolamine
Green coffee beans	*Merulius lacrymans*	Diphenylmethane
Gum acacia	Mushrooms	diisocyanate
Gum tragacanth	*Verticillim*	Ethylenediamine
Hops		Furfuryl alcohol
Mace	*Biotechnology plants/microbiological*	Glutaraldehyde
Maiko	*contamination*	Hexachlorophene
Rye	*Aspergillus niger*	Hexahydrophthalic anhydride
Sunflower pollen	*Candida*	Hexamethylene diisocyanate
Tamarind seeds	Contaminated humidifiers	Maleic anhydride
Tea	Oil mists	Methyl methacrylate
Tobacco		Paraphenylene diamine
Weeping fig pollen	*Woods*	Persulphates
Wheat	Abiruana	Phthalic anhydride
	African maple (*Obeche*)	Tannic acid
Arthropods	African zebrawood	Tetrachlorophthalic anhydride
Bee moths	California redwood	Tetrazine
Beetles (*Coleoptera*)	Cedar of Lebanon	Toluene diisocyanate
Blowflies	Cocabolla	Triethylene tetramine
Carmine	Eastern white cedar	Trimellitic anhydride
Crickets	Iroko	
Fruitflies	Kejaat	*Solder fluxes*
Grain storage mite	Mahogany	Aminoethylethanolamine
Grain weevil	*Mansonia*	Colophony
Honeybee body	Oak	Polyether alcohol-polypropylene
Housefly maggot	Pulverized fuel ash	glycol
Locusts	Ramin	
Mexican bean weevil	South African boxwood	*Reactive dyes*
River flies	*Tanganyiks aningre*	Cibachrome brilliant scarlet
Screw worm fly	Walnut	Drimaren brilliant yellow
Silkworms	Western red cedar	Henna
		Levafix brilliant yellow
Laboratory and other animals	*Enzymes*	
Cow dander	Alpha-amylase	*Drugs*
Guinea pigs	*Bacillus subtilis*	Alginates
Mice	Bromelin	Amprolium hydrochloride
Monkey dander	Cellulase	Cephalosporins
Pigs	Flaviastase	Cimetidine
Rabbits	Papain	Dichloramine
Rats	Trypsin	Gentian powder
Sea squirts		Isphaghula
	Metals	Methyldopa
Crustaceans etc.	Aluminium fluoride (or sodium	Penicillin
Hoya	fluoride)	Piperazine
King crabs	Chromates	Pituitary extracts
Oysters	Cobalt	Psyllium
Pearl shell dust	Nickel sulphate	Salbutamol intermediate
Prawns	Platinum salts	Sulphathiazole
Snow crabs	Vanadium	Tetracyclines

Adapted from [2].

chemical–protein conjugates become immunogenic.

Other interactions of low molecular weight chemicals with biomolecules also result in immunogenicity of the chemical hapten. The nickel and platinum salts are examples of chemicals which appear to react through non-covalent means with host biomacromolecules. Evidence for immunogenicity of such conjugates has been obtained from detection of immunoglobulin E (IgE) antibodies in sensitized workers reactive with platinum–serum albumin complexes [6].

Penicillin is representative of a further type of chemical allergen (discussed in Chapter 15). Such chemicals become reactive under physiological conditions. With penicillin, the β-lactam ring spontaneously opens, and its carbonyl moiety forms an amide linkage largely with ε amino groups of adjacent proteins [7]. Approximately 5% of the penicillin molecules administered to humans become covalently bound to protein [7]. The route of administration influences sensitization. For penicillin, intravenous administration has been found to produce fewer positive cases when compared with intramuscular administration.

Agents of larger-size molecular weight are complete antigens and function as sensitizers without need of reaction with carrier biomolecules. The active component can be a protein, polysaccharide or gum. The latter is exemplified by the bulk laxative, psyllium [8]. Some of the most potent allergens are proteolytic enzymes, for example, subtilisin which currently has the lowest ceiling limit of any industrial chemical, $0.06\ \mu g\ m^{-3}$ [3].

Classification of allergic reactions

Although allergens comprise a diverse group of materials with greatly differing size and functionalities, the clinical reactions to all allergens have been classified successfully into only four types [9]. This classification scheme is presented in Table 12.2.

The type I reactions are characterized by rapid onset, i.e. within 1 h of contact with the allergen. The reactions are mediated by pharmacologically active molecules released from mast cells or basophils as a result of allergen cross-linking cytotrophic antibody on the surface of these cells. Mediators (including histamine and heparin) are released from the cells causing smooth muscle contraction and dilatation of capillaries. Degranulation also results in release of factors chemotactic for eosinophils and neutrophils.

The type I reactions appear to be additionally responsible for late-onset responses. Reaction of

Type	Mechanism	Symptoms
I	Release of pharmacologically active mediators from mast cells/basophils as a result of allergen reacting with cytotrophic antibody	Shock, bronchial asthma, pulmonary oedema, urticaria
II	Antibody reacting with cell constituent or haptenated cell results in cell destruction via complement or antibody-dependent cell-mediated cytotoxicity	Haemolytic anaemia, purpura, granulocytopenia
III	Antigen reaction with antibody results in microprecipitates, complement activation and local inflammation	Vascular thrombosis, haemorrhage, local necrosis, nephritis
IV	Sensitized T cells release lymphokines or become cytotoxic	Contact dermatitis

Table 12.2 Classification of allergic reactions

Summarized from [9].

cytotrophic antibody with chemical allergen leads not only to release of preformed mediators, but to synthesis of other factors as well, the latter including leukotrienes, prostaglandins and thromboxanes. These mediators are instrumental in establishment of an inflammatory reaction, thus providing a late-onset phase to the allergic response. The time of onset of the late phase can vary from 1 to 18 h (or more) following the chemical exposure. Examples of late-phase responses in an animal model and in a sensitized worker are shown in Fig. 12.1. The response of the sensitized guinea pig to inhalation challenge with an MDI aerosol was characterized by an increase in breathing rate (and not shown is a decrease in tidal volume). Responses were noted at 9.5 (minor response) and 11 h (major response) following challenge. The response of a sensitized worker to inhalation challenge with TDI was indicated by a decrease in forced expiratory volume in 1 s (FEV_1). In both the animal and human cases, isolated late-onset responses were observed which were not preceded by immediate-onset responses.

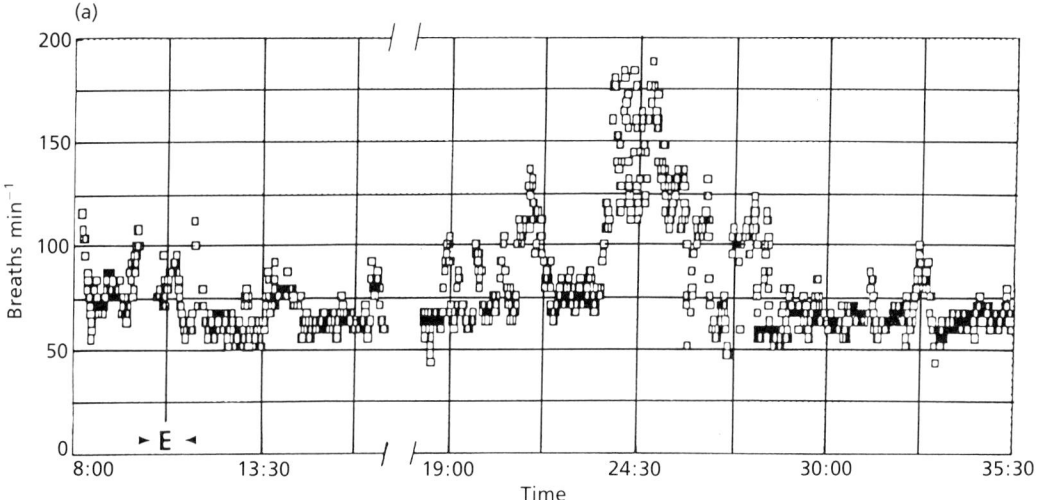

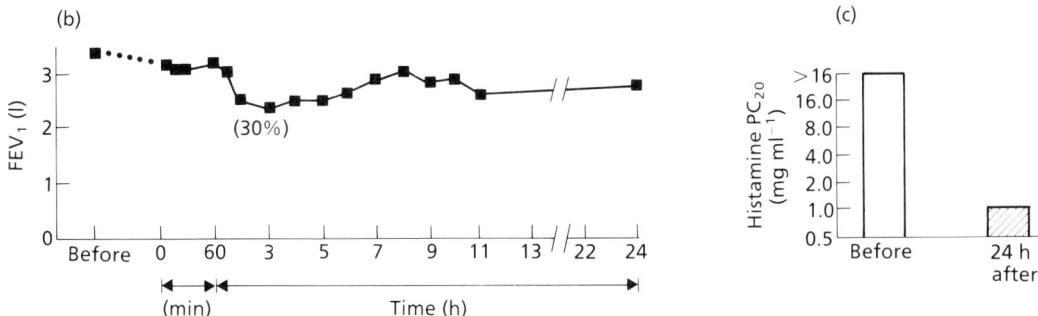

Fig. 12.1 (a) Late-onset response in a guinea pig sensitized to diphenylmethane-4,4'-diisocyanate. The animal received inhalation challenge at 10:00 h (E) with an MDI aerosol. Responses are apparent at 21:15 and 24:15 h. (b) Forced expiratory volume in 1 s (FEV_1) in a subject who received bronchial inhalation challenge with 20 p.p.m. TDI for 60 min. The 30% decrease in FEV_1 occurred more than 1 h after the exposure ended. (c) Histamine responsiveness (PC_{20}) before and 24 h after the challenge indicated increased airway responsiveness following the response to TDI. Modified from [10, 11].

Isolated late-onset responses are typically observed with low molecular weight.

The type II allergic response is an antibody-dependent cytotoxic reaction typified by haemolytic anaemia and granulocytopenia. These responses are caused by IgG or IgM antibody reacting with the chemical bound to a cell surface component. Activation of complement may ensue with eventual lysis of the cell. Cytotoxicity may also occur via phagocytic and non-phagocytic myeloid cells. Examples of allergens which have been associated with type II reactions include penicillin and trimellitic anhydride.

Type III reactions are characterized clinically by vascular thrombosis and haemorrhage. They are mediated by reaction of antibody with antigen, resulting in formation of microprecipitates. Cytotoxic lesions result from subsequent activation of complement and local inflammation. This type of reaction is most frequently observed with the large molecular weight occupational allergens, such as those associated with fungi, plants and other biological materials. Type III reactions require substantial quantities of antibody to provide immune complex lattice formation.

The type IV reaction is typified by contact dermatitis and is the only type of allergic response which is mediated by cells rather than by antibodies. The inflammatory responses result from release of lymphokines from activated T lymphocytes. The reactions are characterized by a late onset (24–72 h) and can be passively transferred using cells. Contact dermatitis from penicillin has been attributed to a type IV reaction [7], as has chronic beryllium disease [12] which is caused by the inhalation of beryllium fumes or dust.

The classification described above has been very successful in describing the clinical reactions of sensitization. However, it should not be assumed that one type exists to the exclusion of others. For example, it is unusual to identify IgE antibodies (suggesting a type I response) without observing the presence of antibodies of other classes. Similarly, the presence of sensitized T lymphocytes is often accompanied by that of antibodies. In addition, the detection of antibodies or sensitized T lymphocytes need not imply disease or abnormal response. The presence of these immunological components signifies exposure to the particular agent.

Occupational asthma versus respiratory tract sensitivity

The definition of occupational asthma has undergone revision in recent years. It has traditionally been defined as reversible airways obstruction resulting from occupational exposure [13]. However, since this definition does not connote chronic aspects of the disease, the definition has been modified [14]. Asthma is currently considered a chronic inflammatory disease of the airways which involves many interacting cells. The response is characterized by infiltration of eosinophils and lymphocytes and shedding of airway epithelial cells. A variety of inflammatory mediators are released which activate target cells in the airways. The resulting response consists of airway constriction, mucus hypersecretion, stimulation of neural reflexes and microvascular leakage. It is the eosinophilic infiltration which differentiates asthma from other inflammatory states of the airways. For this reason a current conception of asthma is chronic eosinophilic bronchitis.

The other characteristic feature of asthma is the presence of airway hyper-responsiveness (AHR). AHR can be defined as an exaggerated bronchoconstrictive reaction upon exposure to an amount of non-specific stimulus which would not provoke a response in normal individuals. Although its cause is uncertain, it has been proposed that AHR may relate to mediators released by eosinophils.

Sensitization may result in acute bronchospasm or development of allergic asthma; the distinction is that of isolated reactions versus chronic airway disease. Much information regarding development of the acute response has been obtained from animal models. The models have been invaluable in identifying exposure factors conducive to development of allergic sensitization and pharmacological mediators of response. By contrast, there has been little success in the development of animal models reflective of the asthmatic state. For this reason, care must be exercised in extrapolating principles and conclusions regarding allergic sensitization which have been obtained from animal models of the acute response, to those operative in allergic asthma. Recent progress in the development of an animal model reflective of asthma deserves note. Ishida and co-workers [15] achieved AHR to acetylcholine in guinea pigs, which persisted for several days after the antigen challenge. Their hypothesis was that repeated mediator release in the lung was necessary for the development of chronic airway disease. Guinea pigs were sensitized to ovalbumin in the presence of heat-killed *Bordetella pertussis*, and challenged by inhalation of ovalbumin twice weekly for 4–6 weeks. The repeated inhalation challenges were required for development of AHR. Sensitization itself, without evoking responses, was not sufficient. Eosinophilia in the airway epithelium was also noted although epithelial damage was not apparent. This model represents an exciting beginning for study of allergic asthma and, as such, holds promise for elucidation of factors contributing to development of chronic airway disease and AHR.

Factors associated with development of allergic sensitization and asthma

With the above caveat regarding distinctions between acute episodes of airway limitation and occupational asthma, considerable information has been obtained from both clinical and animal studies regarding factors which influence sensitization. Animal models which utilize exposure conditions that simulate occupational settings have revealed basic principles governing sensitization resulting from chemical exposure. Some of these concepts are discussed below.

The factors which affect development of allergic sensitization can be broadly divided into two categories: those related to the agent and the mode of exposure, and those related to the subject and susceptibility to response.

Factors related to the sensitizing agent

Irritation. Airway reactions to chemical allergens may be more complex than those to other large molecular weight inhalant materials since chemicals may be irritants as well as allergens. As irritants they may cause airway constriction, pulmonary oedema and epithelial damage, reactions which are also typical of allergic responses.

Accidental exposure of individuals to high levels of chemical irritants has been found to result in chemical pneumonitis. Brooks and colleagues [16] described airway disease as a result of such high exposures. Histologically, this was distinguished from sensitization by detection of plasma cells and lymphocytes in the bronchial mucosa as opposed to the eosinophils usually found in asthmatic patients.

The suggestion has been made that asthma is a result of bronchial epithelial inflammation. In support of this idea, cigarette smoking was reported to predispose to sensitization as evidenced by increased levels of IgE and skin-test results in smokers as compared with non-smokers [17]. Evidence for predisposition to asthma is less clear. Inflammation is known to play an important role in the development of AHR, an important feature of asthma. Agents which cause airway inflammation, i.e. ozone, TDI, have been shown to cause increased airways responsiveness. Yet asthma can develop in the absence of irritant exposure. It has been suggested that different types of inflammation are produced by allergens as compared with irritants; the former produces eosinophilic inflammation, the latter, neutrophilic response [18]. The relationship between irritation and asthma appears to be complex and in need of further clarification.

Information regarding the relationship between irritation and acute manifestation of respiratory sensitization has been obtained from animal models of chemical exposure. In a guinea pig model [19], proteins with irritative properties (proteolytic enzymes such as subtilisin) have been found to be potent respiratory sensitizers [20], as have non-irritating proteins such as ovalbumin [21]. Regarding sensitization from chemicals, concentration–response data were obtained for both respiratory sensitization [22] and respiratory irritation [23] from TDI. The concentration required for sensitization of guinea pigs was 0.25 p.p.m., while that required for irritation was 0.18 p.p.m. In this model, sensitization to TDI required exposure to an irritating concentration. Using the same model and employing formaldehyde (a potent dermal sensitizer) as the agent, 4 p.p.m. resulted in respiratory irritation. However, no respiratory tract sensitization was produced even after repeated exposure to concentrations of 6 and 10 p.p.m. formaldehyde [24].

It is apparent that the relationship between respiratory irritation and sensitization is not clear. Until more data are available and understanding increases, it appears prudent to use the irritation concentration as a guide for concentrations not to be exceeded to protect against sensitization.

Exposure concentration. In both clinical and experimental studies, the airborne exposure concentration of an agent has been found to exert a profound influence on sensitization. A clear indication of the importance of this factor is the reported decrease in the number of cases of TDI sensitization coincident with the lowering of occupational TDI exposure levels [3]. A decrease in the average amount of TDI in the workplace environment was accompanied by a decrease in the number of reported cases of sensitization (Table 12.3).

These data were reinforced by data from Brooks [25] in which increased occurrence of respiratory disease, encompassing occupational asthma, bronchitis and reduced lung function, was detected only in those isocyanate workers who had frequent exposure to spills (implying exposure to high isocyanate concentrations). Similarly, in a study of western red cedar wood workers, a significant association was detected between dust concentration and the prevalence rate of occupational asthma [25]. The chemical within wood dust believed responsible for the majority of asthmatic reactions is the 422 Da compound plicatic acid.

Animal data have demonstrated more directly the relationship between exposure concentration and respiratory sensitization. As summarized in Table 12.4, exposure of guinea pigs to monitored concentrations of TDI vapour (on 5 consecutive days) led to development of pulmonary sensitization. A threshold concentration of 0.25 p.p.m. was necessary since animals exposed to lesser TDI concentrations (0.02 or 0.12 p.p.m.) did not become sensitized [22]. Similarly, in studies utilizing subtilisin, exposure to a threshold concentration of 150 µg m^{-3} was observed to be required for sensitization. Exposure to lesser concentrations for 6-h time periods was not effective in producing sensitization even after repeated exposures [20]. The conclusion drawn from the animal studies is that prolonged low-level exposure to potent respiratory sensitizers is not sufficient to effect sensitization.

Table 12.3 Reduction of air-borne toluene diisocyanate (TDI) levels

Year	Sensitivity cases	Average TDI concentration (p.p.b.)
1956*	1	60
1957	4	60
1958	3	60
1959	3	60
1960	1	60
1961	2	60
1962	3	60
1963	1	60
1964	3	60
1965	1	60
1966	1	60
1967	1	60
1968	1	60
1969	2	60
1970	1	<50
1971	2	<50
1972	0	<20
1973	0	<20
1974	0	< 4

*Start-up.
From [3].

Exposure frequency. Although it is commonly believed that increased frequency of exposure to an allergen enhances the likelihood of sensitization, there is little evidence to support this concept. A direct test of the influence of exposure frequency on sensitization was performed using an animal model [20]. Results indicated that the incidence and degree of respiratory sensitization were equivalent in guinea pigs whether exposed to subtilisin on one occasion for 20 min or on 5 consecutive days for 20 min each day. Moreover, exposure repeatedly given on 85 days to atmospheres of the allergen maintained below a previously determined threshold concentration for sensitization (based on a 5-day exposure protocol) failed to induce respiratory sensitization.

The effect of exposure frequency on development of sensitization was also examined using guinea pigs exposed to TDI [22]. The data presented in Table 12.5 demonstrate that exposure on 70 days to 20 p.p.b. TDI (a concentration found to be below

Table 12.4 Concentration-dependent respiratory sensitization to inhaled allergenic compounds

Agent	Species	Concentration required for sensitization	Reference
Toluene diisocyanate	Guinea pig	$\geqslant 0.25$ p.p.m. (1.8 mg m^{-3})	[22]
Subtilisin	Guinea pig	$\geqslant 150$ μg m^{-3}	[20]

Table 12.5 Effect of repeated exposure to toluene diisocyanate (TDI) on the development of sensitization in guinea pigs

Agent	Concentration of TDI	Number of exposures	Sensitization rate (% of responders)	Total TDI exposure (p.p.m. h^{-1})
TDI	1.6	2	13	9.6
TDI	0.61	5	25	9.2
TDI	0.02	70	0	8.7

Data from [22].

the threshold concentration for acute sensitization) did not produce sensitization. In the same study, exposure on 5 days to 0.61 p.p.m. TDI or exposure on 2 days to 1.6 p.p.m. TDI resulted in pulmonary sensitization, with the 5-day exposure regimen being more effective than the 2-day schedule.

Route of exposure. One of the findings to emerge from animal studies which has broad implications for establishment of a proper industrial TLV was the recognition that respiratory sensitization could result from non-respiratory exposure to the allergen. Intraperitoneal [8,21] or topical [26] exposure of guinea pigs to allergens resulted in sensitization of the respiratory tract. Moreover, fatal respiratory anaphylaxis frequently occurred upon the initial bronchial provocation challenge of guinea pigs which had received 1 mg ovalbumin administered intraperitoneally 14 days previously. The responses of intraperitoneally injected animals to the first ovalbumin inhalation exposure were consistently more severe than were those evoked subsequently by repeated inhalation challenge [21].

The studies demonstrating the ability of dermal exposure to induce respiratory tract sensitivity utilized guinea pigs exposed to TDI [26]. Animals received 25 µl TDI (1–100%) applied to an area of 25 cm on the dorsal skin. (Measurements of the air-borne concentration of TDI, resulting from vaporization from the skin site, near the breathing zone of the guinea pigs, indicated negligible amounts.) The limited dermal exposures resulted in respiratory tract sensitization. Animals underwent typical respiratory hypersensitivity reactions upon

initial inhalation challenge. Additionally, the dermal exposure was shown to result in production of TDI-specific antibodies (including IgE) which were detected in the circulation.

Extrapolating from the above results to occupational sensitization, it is apparent that exposure to a quantity of chemical allergen, which is sufficient to result in production of cytotrophic antibody and allow for its distribution from local lymphoid tissue, can result in respiratory tract sensitization, irrespective of the exposure route. Consequently, controlling exposure to an occupational agent must include more than controlling the air-borne concentration.

Host-related factors

In addition to factors related to the agent, development of respiratory tract sensitization is dependent upon subject-related factors. The latter are considered below.

Atopy. The association of atopy with occupational asthma has received considerable attention. Atopy is the tendency to develop IgE antibodies to environmental allergens as a result of sensitization in which entry of allergen is across mucosal surfaces [27]. The prevalence of atopy in the population (assessed from positive responses to skin-prick tests with a panel of environmental allergens) is estimated to be 30–50%. Approximately one-half of atopic subjects demonstrate symptoms consistent with allergy [27].

In certain industries atopy may be a risk factor for sensitization. As seen in Table 12.6, in industries (such as bakeries) employing high molecular weight

Agent	Atopy (%)	Positive skin test to responsible allergens (%)	Immediate	Late	Biphasic
High molecular weight					
Flour	83	91	100	0	0
Animal dander	80	86	40	0	60
Detergent enzymes	63	88	0	0	100
Low molecular weight					
Toluene diisocyanate	25	0	32	43	25
Western red cedar	25	0	7	44	49
Platinum salt	6	63	70	10	20
Tetrachlorophthalic anhydride	14	100	0	50	50

Table 12.6 Clinical features of patients with occupational asthma

Modified from [17].

allergens, atopics appear to have an increased risk of developing occupational asthma [17]. In other industries there does not appear to be this association. Examples of the latter include industries utilizing low molecular weight allergens such as isocyanates and western red cedar. The reason for this distinction is unknown.

Airway responsiveness (AR). Constriction of the airways is a physiological process dependent upon numerous factors including mechanical factors, cells, nerves, mediators and the level of lung function. Hyper-responsiveness occurs in about 20% of the population, many of whom do not have asthma [11]. However, it is a characteristic of those with asthma. Almost all patients with symptomatic occupational asthma have hyper-responsive airways.

The suggestion has been made that AHR should be used to predict likely development of occupational asthma. However, there is no evidence that AHR predisposes to occupational asthma. Rather, AHR usually develops as a result of exposure. An example of this occurrence is seen in the lower part of Fig. 12.1. Histamine responsiveness of the sensitized subject was at a normal level (> 16 mg ml^{-1}) prior to the TDI bronchial challenge. After the response to challenge, AR had increased [11]. Accordingly, the finding of normal AHR in a subject should not preclude the diagnosis of occupational asthma, just as the presence of AHR should not define occupational asthma [11].

Pre-existing airway disease. It has been been suggested that one reason for the varied responses of workers upon chemical exposure may be the presence in some of pre-existing airway disease [28]. In an investigation of possible mechanisms underlying TDI asthma, Patterson and colleagues [28] found it helpful to consider the possibility of pre-existing disease. Patterns of response were clarified by establishing the following categories:

1 TDI asthma. These individuals did not have asthma prior to TDI exposure. Their symptoms were markedly reduced or absent when TDI exposure was avoided. In almost all cases specific IgE antibodies were detected in the sera, providing evidence for immunological involvement.

2 Chronic respiratory disease. These individuals had chronic respiratory disease (including asthma) prior to the TDI exposure. TDI may have contributed to the symptoms through irritant or immunological means. Symptoms usually persisted after removal from TDI exposure.

3 Development of asthma coincident with TDI exposure. These individuals developed asthma unrelated to TDI exposure, although TDI may have exacerbated symptoms by acting as an irritant. In these subjects, too, symptoms persisted after exposure terminated.

4 Irritant-induced respiratory disease. In these subjects respiratory reactions occurred as a result of the toxic, irritant or inflammatory properties of TDI. These exposures may result in chemical pneumonitis. Immunological involvement is not implied.

It is apparent that many factors contribute to an individual's susceptibility to developing occupational allergic sensitivity and asthma. As indicated above, these factors include atopy, AHR, pre-existing airway disease and irritant exposures. However, the conclusion of most studies of sensitization is that the *level of exposure* has the greatest influence on sensitization. If exposure is reduced, sensitization is less likely to occur.

Diagnosis of allergic sensitization

The diagnosis of sensitivity to a particular agent requires establishment of a relationship between the specific allergen and a sensitization response to the agent. Three methods are available for diagnosis: specific inhalation challenge, skin-testing, and *in vitro* serology.

Bronchial provocation challenge (BPC), frequently referred to as the 'gold standard' for diagnosis [29] would appear to be the preferred method to detect sensitization (and asthma) to a specific agent. This method requires generation of the agent and close control of exposure atmospheres. To allow detection of both early- and late-onset allergic reactions, it additionally requires frequent measurement of pulmonary function in test subjects and close medical surveillance in case of severe reactions. An accepted minimum indication of response to BPC is a 20% decrease in FEV_1 (see Fig. 12.1).

Although BPC provides a direct demonstration of the existence of specific respiratory sensitization, it is infrequently employed. Few facilities have the capability to generate and continuously monitor atmospheres of occupational allergens. For example, to assess pulmonary sensitivity to TDI, the chemical must be vaporized and atmospheres maintained below the 20 p.p.b. TLV. Exposure to higher concentrations would present the risk to the subject of respiratory irritation, chemical pneumonitis and possibly sensitization. Other drawbacks include the possible induction of a late-phase reaction which may persist for days after challenge, and an increase in AR which may also persist for days or weeks [29].

Bronchial provocation testing is typically used when other methods have failed to provide information relative to specific sensitization. A detailed occupational history, physical examination, immu-nological studies and pulmonary function tests are recommended prior to consideration of BPC [29].

Skin-testing

Skin-testing has been used to assist in diagnosis of specific allergen sensitivity. Two tests are in general use, the prick test and the intradermal test [30]. In the prick test, a drop of allergen solution is placed on the subject's skin. A needle is placed in the solution and the skin is gently pricked. The intradermal test utilizes intradermal injection of 20–50 µl of antigen solution. For chemical allergens, a conjugate of the chemical must be made by coupling it to a protein (usually serum albumin). The conjugate is used for administration. A positive result is a wheal-and-flare response.

Problems may be encountered with these tests. Difficulties may arise in patients having atopy or eczema. Additionally, appropriate composition of the chemical conjugates is essential for proper testing. (This will be discussed below regarding serological testing.) The major disadvantage of the method, however, is the poor correspondence of skin-test results with the presence of pulmonary sensitivity to chemicals [17]. However, some enthusiasm has been given to the combined use of skin tests and assessment of AR as an indication of likelihood of pulmonary responsiveness upon contact with a specific allergen [31].

Radioallergosorbent test (RAST)

A number of *in vitro* assays have been developed for detection and quantification of antibodies directed toward specific allergens. *In vitro* assays offer the advantage of avoiding deliberate exposure of the individual to the allergen. Accordingly, they present no danger of eliciting severe adverse reactions, and medical personnel need not be assigned for extended periods of time to monitor responses.

The greatest interest lies in detection of specific IgE antibodies. The procedure most frequently employed is RAST, first developed by Wide and co-workers [32]. The method, as illustrated in Fig. 12.2, involves detection of IgE antibodies specific to the allergen through use of a radiolabelled second antibody (either rabbit or monoclonal anti-human

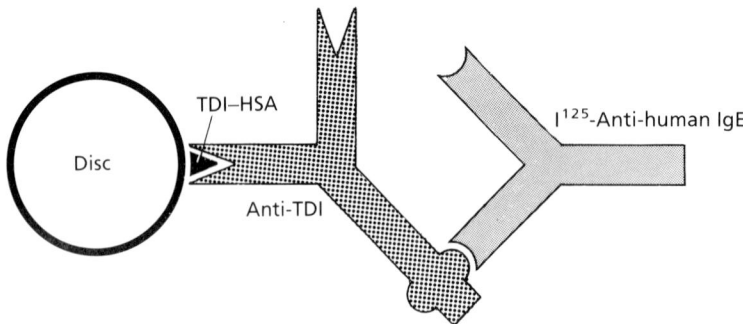

Fig. 12.2 Diagram of the detection of IgE antibody by radioallergosorbent test (RAST). Immunoglobulin E (IgE) antibodies in a serum sample which are specific for toluene diisocyanate (TDI) will bind to TDI epitopes on the disc. Bound IgE is detected by subsequent exposure of the disc to I^{125}-labelled antibody to human IgE.

IgE). Recently, variations of the method have been developed which utilize alternative second antibody indicator systems such as enzyme or fluorescent-labelled reagents.

Problems may be encountered using RAST. False-negative values may result from the presence in the sera of high titres of other classes of specific antibody. Such antibodies may block IgE from reacting with allergen on the disc or block assess of anti-IgE reagents. False-positive results may occur when sera contain large amounts of total IgE (IgE not specific to the particular allergen of interest). These problems can be overcome, in the first instance, by modification of the methodology to that of an antigen capture mode, and in the second, by performing specific RAST inhibition tests.

Whereas RAST has been highly successful in detecting IgE antibody to high molecular weight (non-haptenic) occupational allergens, it has been considerably less successful with low molecular weight allergens. As a result, many clinicians have reluctantly concluded that such sensitization may not be IgE-mediated. However, as discussed below, problems have been identified recently which may have contributed to the negative serology.

Characterization of chemical–protein antigens

RAST testing for IgE to chemical allergens requires immobilization of the allergen on to cellulose discs, followed by reaction of the chemical ligand with hapten-specific IgE antibody. As shown in Table 12.7, detection of hapten-specific antibody is dependent upon the composition of the conjugate antigen. RAST values were substantially greater when the serum from the sensitized subject was tested using a conjugate antigen which contained 35 mol MDI per mol serum albumin (MDI_{35}-HSA) as opposed to using the conjugate composed of 4 mol MDI per mol protein (MDI_4-HSA). Similarly, using the guinea pig animal model and enzyme-linked immunosorbent assay (ELISA), greater titres of antibody to MDI were detected with conjugates having high hapten substitution as compared with those having fewer MDI haptenic groups (Fig. 12.3). No antibodies were detected to the protein alone (HSA). Based on these findings, it would be expected that sera with low quantities of antibody may provide false-negative results if improper hapten–conjugate antigens are employed.

The Committee on Occupational Lung Disease of

Human sera	Total IgE (iu mT^{-1})	NC RAST titre* (net c.p.m.)	
		MDI_4-HSA	MDI_{35}-HSA
Control patient	170	0	0
Exposed worker[†]	120	228	1208

Table 12.7 Detection of immunoglobulin E (IgE) antibodies to diphenylmethane-4,4'- diisocyanate (MDI) using MDI–serum albumin conjugate antigens

*Nitrocellulose (NC) discs were used in the radioallergosorbent test (RAST).
[†]The serum was from a subject with clinical evidence of MDI pulmonary sensitivity. The control subject had a comparable level of total IgE in the serum but had not been exposed to MDI.

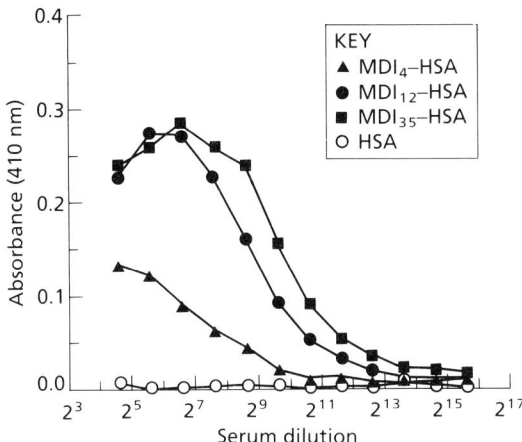

Fig. 12.3 Enzyme-linked immunosorbent assay (ELISA) for detection of antibody to MDI. The titre of antibody in serum obtained from a guinea pig exposed to MDI was dependent upon the composition of the MDI–protein conjugate used for assay. The greatest titre was obtained using MDI_{35}-HSA (unpublished data).

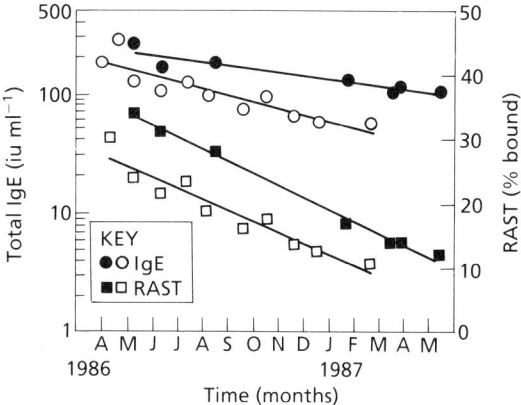

Fig. 12.4 Decline in IgE response following removal from exposure. The total IgE and antigen-specific IgE (RAST) titres were measured in serum samples from 2 workers taken at intervals following removal from exposure. Open symbols, worker sensitized to MDI [34]; closed symbols, worker sensitized to psyllium.

the American Academy of Allergy and Immunology has recommended guidelines for the preparation and characterization of antigens to be used for the diagnosis of occupational immunological lung disease caused by reactive low molecular weight chemicals [33]. The guidelines include determination of the ratio of chemical ligand bound per molecule carrier protein, and immunological characterization of chemical–protein conjugates. The latter would require positive reference sera and RAST inhibition assays. Adherence to these recommendations should resolve many of the current difficulties in assessing results from immunological assays.

Time of testing. Another factor which may have contributed to the infrequent detection of IgE antibodies in workers sensitized to certain chemicals is the short half-life (2.3 days) of IgE in the blood. The persistence of several IgE responses was recently studied and is presented in Fig. 12.4. One subject (signified by open symbols) was sensitized to MDI; the other (closed symbols) to the bulk laxative, psyllium. In each, decline in antigen-specific (squares) and in total IgE titre with time was apparent. The titres declined steadily following removal from exposure. Calculation of the half-lives of each of the IgE responses yielded values of 6.2 months for MDI-specific IgE,

7.7 months for psyllium IgE, 6.4 months for total IgE of the MDI workers and 11.6 months for total IgE of the psyllium worker.

The implication of these findings for diagnosis is considerable. Had RAST testing been performed 1 year after symptomatic exposure, false-negative results might have been obtained. From both animal and clinical data, it appears that the optimal time for taking sera for antibody determination is 3–4 weeks following exposure. Caution must be applied when testing sera from workers with historical indication of workplace sensitivity.

Dot-binding assay. Modifications of RAST have been developed which have some distinct benefits. Grunewalder and Karol [35] tested nitrocellulose as an alternative to cellulose-based RAST. The advantages of the nitrocellulose system are apparent from Table 12.8. The high binding capacity of nitrocellulose allowed for considerable reduction in the amount of chemical–protein conjugate required for each assay. This is an important advantage when considering the time and effort required for production, analysis and testing of each batch of chemical–protein conjugate.

A recent modification of nitrocellulose-based assays has been the use of dot-binding for adherence of

Procedure	Nitrocellulose	Cellulose
Chemical activation of disc	None	Cyanogen bromide
Optimal antigen concentration	0.001–0.1%	1%
Binding of antigen to disc	2 h, 37°C	6 h, ambient temp.
Reaction of antigen with serum	2 h 37°C	16 h, ambient temp.
Reaction with second antibody	16 h, ambient temp.	16 h, ambient temp.
Storage of discs	Dry at ambient temp.	In buffer at 10°C

Table 12.8 Comparison of methodology for radioallergosorbent test (RAST) using nitrocellulose versus paper discs

From [35].

antigen to discs. This procedure allows separate application of several antigens on to distinct sites of one nitrocellulose disc. It is possible then to detect antibodies to a variety of allergens using a single disc and a minimum volume of serum (usually 50 μl or less). For isocyanate assays, this arrangement would allow detection of possible cross-reactions of antibodies with related isocyanates.

Conclusions

It is clear that development of allergic (and asthmatic) responses to inhaled chemicals is a function of the agent, and conditions of exposure to the agent, as well as being a function of the susceptibility of the individual at the time. Elucidation of factors contributing to each component is an ongoing effort.

The true incidence of occupational asthma and lung sensitivity is unknown. Questions remain regarding the mechanisms of the disease, diagnostic methodology and long-term outcome. However, in recent years, there has been substantial progress toward gaining understanding in each of these areas. It is expected that with further efforts to control occupational exposures and with technological developments in diagnostic methodology, the trend in future years will be toward a decreased incidence of occupational disease.

Acknowledgements

The author thanks colleagues and students for contributions to the studies described. The author additionally acknowledges Gloria Curtis for preparing the manuscript and the National Institute of Environmental Health Sciences for support under grant no. ES01532.

References

1 Chan-Yeung M, Lam S. Occupational asthma. *Am Rev Resp Dis* 1986; 133:686–703.
2 Burge PS. Occupational asthma. In: Barnes PJ, Rodger IW, Thomson NC, eds. *Asthma: Basic Mechanisms and Clinical Management.* San Diego: Academic Press, 1988; 465–82.
3 *Documentation of the Threshold Limit Values and Biological Exposure Indices.* 5th ed. Amer Conf Govt Ind Hyg Inc., Cincinnati, OH: 1986; 580–5.
4 Stadler JC, Karol MH. Use of dose-response data to compare the skin sensitizing abilities of dicyclohexylmethane-4,4'-diisocyanate and picryl chloride in two animal species. *Toxicol Appl Pharmacol* 1985; 78:445–50.
5 Emmett EA. Allergic contact dermatitis in polyurethane plastic moulders. *J Occup Med* 1976; 18:802–4.
6 Cromwell O, Pepys J, Parish WE, Hughes EG. Specific IgE antibodies to platinum salts in sensitized workers. *Clin Allergy* 1979; 9:109–17.
7 Weiss ME, Atkinson NF. Immediate hypersensitivity reactions to penicillin and related antibiotics. *Clin Allergy* 1988; 18:515–40.
8 Gauss WF, Alarie JP, Karol MH. Experimental assessment of the allergenicity of a psyllium-containing laxative. *Allergy* 1985; 40:535–9.
9 Coombs RRA, Gell PGH. Classification of allergic reactions responsible for clinical hypersensitivity disease. In: Gell PGH, Coombs RRA, Lachmann PJ, eds. *Clinical Aspects of Immunology.* Oxford: Blackwell Scientific Publications, 1975:761–81.
10 Griffiths-Johnson D, Spear K, Jin R, Karol MH. Late-onset pulmonary responses in guinea pigs sensitized by inhalation of diphenylmethane-4,4'-diisocyanate (MDI). *Toxicologist* 1990; 10:222.
11 Graneck BJ, Durham SR, Newman-Taylor AJ. Late asthmatic reactions and changes in histamine responsiveness provoked by occupational agents. *Bull Eur Physiopathol Resp* 1988; 23:577–81.
12 Newman LS, Kreiss K, King TE Jr, Seay S, Campbell PA. Pathologic and immunologic alterations in early stages of beryllium disease. *Am Rev Resp Dis* 1989;

139:1479–86.

13 Pepys J, Turner-Warwick M. The lung in allergic disease. In: Gell PGH, Coombs RRA, Lachman PJ, eds. *Clinical Aspects of Immunology.* Oxford: Blackwell Scientific Publications, 1975; 1241–68.

14 Barnes PJ. Our changing understanding of asthma. *Resp Med* 1989; 83:17–23.

15 Ishida K, Kelly LJ, Thomson RJ, Beattie LL, Schellenberg RR. Repeated antigen challenge induces airway hyperresponsiveness with tissue eosinophilia in guinea pigs. *J Appl Physiol* 1989; 67:1133–9.

16 Brooks SM, Weiss MA, Bernstein IL. Reactive airways dysfunction syndrome. *J Occup Med* 1985; 27:473–6.

17 Vedal S, Chan-Yeung M. Airway responsiveness and atopy in occupational airway disease. In: Weiss ST, Sparrow D, eds. *Airway Responsiveness and Atopy in the Development of Chronic Lung Disease.* New York: Raven Press, 1989; 271–92.

18 Barnes PJ, Rodger IW, Thomson NC. Pathogenesis of asthma. In: Barnes PJ, Rodger IW, Thomson NC, eds. *Asthma: Basic Mechanisms and Clinical Management.* San Diego: Academic Press, 1988; 415–44.

19 Karol MH. The development of an animal model for TDI asthma. *Bull Eur Physiopathol Resp* 1988; 23:571–6.

20 Thorne PS, Hillebrand J, Magreni C, Riley EJ, Karol MH. Experimental sensitization to subtilisin. I. Production of immediate- and late-onset pulmonary reactions. *Toxicol Appl Pharmacol* 1986; 86:112–23.

21 Karol MH, Hillebrand J, Thorne PS. Characteristics of weekly pulmonary hypersensitivity responses elicited in the guinea pig by inhalation of ovalbumin aerosols. *Toxicol Appl Pharmacol* 1989; 100:234–46.

22 Karol MH. Concentration-dependent immunologic response to toluene diisocyanate (TDI) following inhalation exposure. *Toxicol Appl Pharmacol* 1983; 68:229–41.

23 Karol MH, Dixon C, Brady M, Alarie Y. Immunologic sensitization and pulmonary hypersensitivity by repeated inhalation of aromatic isocyanates. *Toxicol Appl Pharmacol* 1980; 53:260–70.

24 Lee HK, Alarie Y, Karol MH. Induction of formalde-hyde sensitivity in guinea pigs. *Toxicol Appl Pharmacol* 1984; 75:147–55.

25 Brooks SM. The evaluation of occupational airways disease in the laboratory and workplace. *J Allergy Clin Immunol* 1982; 70:56–66.

26 Karol MH, Hauth BA, Riley EJ, Magreni CM. Dermal contact with toluene diisocyanate (TDI) produces respiratory tract hypersensitivity in guinea pigs. *Toxicol Appl Pharmacol* 1981; 58:221–30.

27 Cockcroft DW. Allergens. In: Barnes PJ, Rodger IW, Thomson NC, eds. *Asthma: Basic Mechanisms and Clinical Management.* San Diego: Academic Press, 1988:445–64.

28 Patterson R, Hargreave FE, Grammer LC, Harris KE, Dolovich J. Toluene diisocyanate respiratory reactions. I. Reassessment of the problem. *Int Arch Allergy Appl Immunol* 1987; 84:93–100.

29 Bernstein DI, Cohn JR. Guidelines for the diagnosis and evaluation of occupational immunologic lung disease: preface. *J Allergy Clin Immunol* 1989; 84:791–3.

30 Grammer LC, Patterson R, Zeiss CR. Guidelines for the immunologic evaluation of occupational lung disease. *J Allergy Clin Immunol* 1989; 84:805–14.

31 Karol MH, Thorne PS. Pulmonary hypersensitivity and hyperreactivity: implications for assessing allergic responses. In: Gardner DE, Crapo JD, Massaro EJ, eds. *Toxicology of the Lung.* New York: Raven Press, 1988; 427–48.

32 Wide L, Bennich H, Johansson SGO. Diagnosis of allergy by an *in vitro* test for allergen antibodies. *Lancet* 1967; ii:1105–7.

33 Bernstein DI, Zeiss CR. Guidelines for preparation and characterization of chemical-protein conjugate antigens. *J Allergy Clin Immunol* 1989; 84:820–2.

34 Karol MH, Jin R, Rubanoff B. Clinical and experimental evaluation of isocyanate lung injury. *Comments Toxicol* 1989; 3:117–30.

35 Grunewalder E, Karol MH. Nitrocellulose-based RAST to detect IgE antibodies in workers hypersensitive to diphenylmethane-4,4'-diisocyanate. *Allergy* 1986; 41:203–9.

13
The toxic effects of polychlorinated biphenyls

TEE-PING LEE

Introduction

Polychlorinated biphenyls (PCBs) are a group of chemicals having the structure generalized in Fig. 13.1, in which X denotes the positions that may be occupied by either chlorine or hydrogen atoms. PCBs are inert chemicals that are resistant to biological and chemical degradation. PCBs have many desirable physical and chemical properties, such as low volatility and water solubility, thermo-stability and non-flammability, high dielectric constant, general compatibility with other halogenated hydrocarbons, and solubility in most organic solvents. In addition, physical states of PCBs may vary with different degrees of chlorination. PCB mixtures, depending on the chlorine contents, may exist as mobile oil, viscous resin or solid. For these reasons, PCBs have been used in a broad spectrum of

applications. The major areas of utility include dielectric fluid, heat exchangers, paints and printing inks, and pesticide extender [1,2]. PCBs have been available commercially for 50 years and are marketed under a number of trade names such as Aroclor, Clophen, Phenoclor, and Kaneclor. These chemicals are sold and used as a mixture of homologues. In addition, the mixture may contain polychlorinated dibenzofurans. The current uses of PCBs have been curtailed and the production of these chemicals was stopped during the 1970s. Significant quantities of PCBs are still employed as dielectric fluids in older transformers and capacitors [2,3].

PCBs are inert lipid-soluble molecules and tend to accumulate in food chains. The presence of these chemicals has been detected in various biological samples, including human tissues [4,5]. In general, the accumulation of PCBs and other halogenated hydrocarbons in most tissues correlates with the lipid content of target tissues. Thus, various adipose tissues have the highest concentration of halogenated hydrocarbons in animals [2,6,7].

The retention time of PCBs in human and animal bodies is long and varies with different types of isomers. As a general rule, homologues with a higher chlorine content are more difficult to metabolize and remain in the body for a longer period of time,

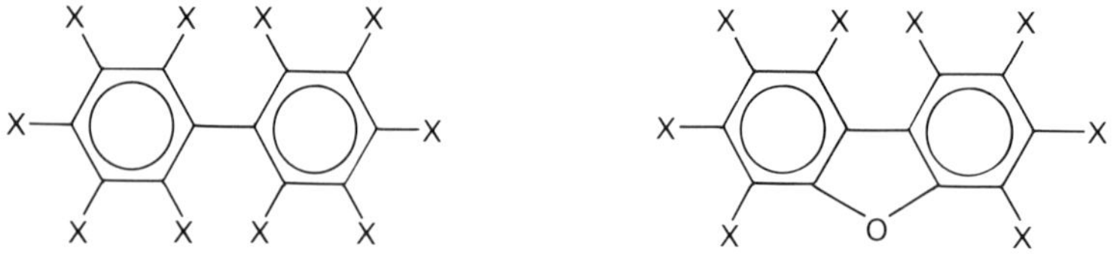

Fig. 13.1 Structure of polychlorinated biphenyls (PCBs) and polychlorinated dibenzofurans (PCDFs).

whereas the homologues with fewer chlorine atoms are readily metabolized and excreted. For instance, the biological half-lives of 2,4,4′-tri-,2,4,5, 4′-tetra and 2,4,5,2′,4′,5′,-hexachlorobiphenyl were estimated to be 3.0, 8.4 and 27.5 years respectively [8,9]. PCBs may be excreted as unchanged molecules or metabolized derivatives, such as hydroxy- or methoxy-derivatives [2,6]. The major route of excretion is through bile and the gastrointestinal tract. Small amounts of PCB may be excreted through urine.

There have been several reports concerning the toxic effects of PCBs in association with occupational exposure due to dermal contact with these chemicals [2,7,10–15]. In addition, there have been two major outbreaks of poisonings due to the consumption of PCB-contaminated rice bran oil. The first such incident occurred in Japan in 1968. The disease was termed *yusho* [6]. More than 1600 victims have been identified. The second incident occurred in western central Taiwan in 1979 [16–18]: more than 2000 victims were claimed. The disease associated with PCB poisoning in Taiwan has been termed *yu-cheng*, which in Chinese means oil disease [19]. In the case of *yusho*, the source of the contamination was due to the use of PCBs as heat exchanger in the manufacturing of rice bran oil [6]. The PCB concentrations in the contaminated oil were about 1000 p.p.m. in the Japanese [20] and 50–300 p.p.m. in the Taiwanese samples [18,21].

The onset of clinical symptoms following the consumption of the contaminated oil varied from less than 1 month to 6 months. At the time of the onset of clinical symptoms, blood PCB concentrations in *yu-cheng* patients ranged from 7 to 460 p.p.b. [17,22]. No comparative data were available for *yusho* patients.

Symptoms associated with PCB poisoning

The most prominent symptoms associated with *yu-cheng* or *yusho* patients are ocular and dermal abnormalities such as swelling of the eyelids and meibomian glands, hypersecretion of cheese-like material from the eyes, hyperpigmentation of the skin and mucosal membrane, acne-like eruptions, and enlargement of the hair follicles [6,22]. Patients also displayed signs of neuropathy such as numbness in the limbs, headache, fatigue, and slowing of the nerve-conducting velocity [6,17,23]. Laboratory tests showed increased serum triglyceride concentration and increased serum aspartate aminotransferase (SAST or SGOT) and alanine aminotransferase (SALT or SGPT) activities. These data suggest abnormal hepatic functions [6,16,17,24], blood urea nitrogen (BUN) concentration and lactate dehydrogenase (LDH) activities were normal. The symptoms associated with *yu-cheng* were persistent for long periods of time. For instance, in a special clinic designated for *yu-cheng* patients, at a follow-up study of the patients 8–17 months later, only 38% of the patients had improved. The majority of the patients had the same (54%) or exacerbated (8%) condition [25]. A detailed description of the clinical symptoms and laboratory findings associated with PCB poisoning has been reviewed by Lu and Wong [25]. In addition, children born to poisoned mothers had lower birthweights [26] and abnormalities of gingiva, skin, nails, teeth and lung [2,27]. The excretion of porphyrin was elevated [28].

The symptoms associated with workers who have had occupational exposure to PCBs due to dermal contact are not as devastating as those who have suffered oral PCB poisoning [29,30]. In one study involving over 300 capacitor manufacturing workers, most of whom had been employed over 10 years, the only visible sign of abnormality was skin rash in 39% of the workers. The lesions usually disappear after discontinuation of PCB-handling.

The prevailing symptoms suffered by the majority of orally PCB-poisoned patients, such as hyperpigmentation, abnormal eye discharge, and abnormal liver function, were rare among workers exposed to PCBs [10,30]. While the route of poisoning (oral versus dermal) and the difference in dosage (large amount over a relatively short period of time in the case of oral poisoning versus low dosage over a long period of time in the case of dermal exposure) may be significant factors, the blood PCB concentration found in these workers appears to be higher than that found in *yu-cheng* patients. Recent evidence has suggested that the difference in the chemical compositions rather than the blood concentration of PCBs may play an important role in the development of the symptoms.

PCBs are known to contain different mixtures of homologues and various toxic impurities such as polychlorinated dibenzofurans (PCDFs) and polychlorinated naphthalenes [6,31–33]. Some of the impurities have been shown to be more toxic than the corresponding PCBs. Therefore, the discrepancy observed between oral and dermal PCB poisonings may be due to the quality of the PCBs involved.

Immune suppression associated with PCB poisoning

In animal experiments, exposure to PCBs by feeding, injection or dermal application has been shown to cause immune suppression [2,32–38]. The toxic effects include suppression of antibody response, atrophy of the cortex of the thymus, reduction in the number of germinal centres in the spleen and lymph nodes, and reduction in the number of circulating leucocytes and lymphocytes [2,34,39,40]. In addition, PCB-treated animals were more susceptible to hepatitis virus [41], *Plasmodium berghei* [42], *Salmonella typhimurium*, and endotoxins [43].

Yusho and *yu-cheng* patients also showed signs of immune suppression such as persistent skin infection, bronchitis-like respiratory symptoms [6,16] and a moderate decrease in immunoglobulin concentrations, especially immunoglobulin M (IgM) and IgA fractions. The concentrations of IgG appeared to be normal [44] (Table 13.1). It has been reported that serum IgA and IgM concentrations were decreased while IgG concentrations were increased 2 years after the 1968 outbreak of *yusho* but were generally in the normal range by 1972 [6].

Table 13.1 Serum immunoglobulin concentrations (mean ± s.d.)

Subjects	IgG (mg%)	IgA (mg%)	IgM (mg%)
Normal (n = 23)	1377 ± 214	245 ± 70	173 ± 48
Yu-cheng (n = 30)	1469 ± 566	185 ± 88	105 ± 58
t-test	NS	$P < 0.01$	$P < 0.001$

NS, Not significant.
Adapted from [44].

In animal studies, feeding PCBs led to decreased immunoglobulin concentrations in mice [42], monkeys [43], and other animal species [45,46]. In mice both primary and secondary antibody responses to sheep red blood cells and the memory cell functions are inhibited. The B lymphocytes are the source of immunoglobulins. The diminished antibody production in PCB-poisoned animals may be attributed to the reduction in the number of B cells [2,40]. In *yu-cheng* patients, however, the number of B cells was not significantly affected (Table 13.2).

The functions of B cells are regulated by various types of T cells. It has been shown that a subpopulation of T cells (T helper cells) collaborates with B cells in antibody production, whereas another subpopulation of T cells (T suppressor cells) suppresses this activity [47]. PCB poisoning appears to affect helper T cells but not suppressor T cells (Table 13.2). At the present time, it is not known whether the decreased IgM and IgA concentrations found in *yu-cheng* patients are due to decreased helper T cells or a decreased number of IgM- and IgA-producing B cells.

In a similar incidence, Michigan farmers who consumed dairy products contaminated with polybrominated biphenyls (PBBs) had increased IgG and IgA concentrations [48]. The numbers of T and B cells were decreased [48–50]. Landrigan *et al.* [51], on the other hand, found no significant differences in lymphocyte numbers or functions between PBB-exposed residents and normal controls. Enhanced release of IgG was found in lymphocyte cultures obtained from PBB-exposed farmers. The observation suggested that PBB caused a non-specific activation of B lymphocytes [52].

The initial haematological studies of the *yu-cheng* patients showed that the total white blood cell counts were increased. The distribution of the major types of white blood cells (e.g. neutrophils, lymphocytes, monocytes, and basophils) was not significantly altered [16]. When the patients were given a subcutaneous injection of a solution containing streptokinase and streptodornase, about 40% of the patients had a positive response. On the other hand, of the normal, healthy volunteers tested, 80% had a positive response [16,53]. Delayed hypersensitivity response is an indicator of cellular immune function. The result suggests an impaired cellular immunity.

Table 13.2 Enumeration of lymphocyte subpopulations (mean ± s.d.)

Subjects	Total lymphocytes (cells mm^{-3})	Total T cells (%)*	Active T cells (%)*	Suppressor T cells (%)†	Helper T cells (%)†	B cells (%)
Normal (n = 23)	3005 ± 971	63.3 ± 9.5	22.1 ± 4.4	24.9 ± 8.7	36.9 ± 12.1	26.6 ± 6.1
Yu-cheng (n = 30)	3103 ± 908	41.7 ± 16.3	11.3 ± 6.7	22.2 ± 8.7	21.6 ± 6.9	28.0 ± 7.1
t-test	NS	P < 0.001	P < 0.001	NS	P < 0.001	NS

*Calculated as % of lymphocytes; †calculated as % of T cells.
NS, Not significant.
Adapted from [44].

Similar observations have been reported in animal studies. Feeding PCBs to guinea pigs [54,55] and rabbits caused a decreased hypersensitivity response to tuberculin.

Ocular and dermal symptoms were the most prominent feature of *yu-cheng* patients. When the patients were graded according to the severity of these symptoms, it was found that the symptoms, plasma PCB concentrations, and the depression of the delayed-type hypersensitivity responses were all correlated (Table 13.3). Exceptions do exist: there were a few patients whose blood PCB concentrations were low (below 10 p.p.b.) and yet who showed severe ocular and dermal abnormalities. Conversely, there were patients whose blood PCB concentrations were high (over 60 p.p.b.) and yet who had very mild symptoms [53].

It has been suggested that the percentage of the active, but not total, T-cell rosette formation is an indicator of cellular immunity [56]. In *yu-cheng* patients, the size of the induration following strepto-kinase and streptodornase injections correlated with the percentage of active T cells [53]. Similar to the delayed hypersensitivity response, the percentage of the active T cells was negatively correlated with blood PCB concentration [44]. The data suggested that PCB poisoning caused abnormal cellular immune function by inhibiting active T cells.

The expression of E rosettes, which is used to enumerate T cells and active T cells, requires intact metabolic pathways for glycolysis, protein and nucleic acid synthesis [57]. In addition, the regulation of intracellular cyclic nucleotide concentrations by hor-

Table 13.3 Correlation between ocular and dermal lesions, delayed-type skin hypersensitivity response, and blood polychlorinated biphenyl (PCB) concentrations (mean ± s.d.)

Severity of lesions	Patients with positive skin reaction (%)	Diameter of induration (cm)	Blood PBC concentration (p.p.b.)
Grade I	90	2.63 ± 0.80	34 ± 5
Grade II	50	1.23 ± 1.21	37 ± 5
Grade III	18	0.38 ± 0.26	54 ± 20
Grade IV	0	0.10 ± 0.22	61 ± 28

Adapted from [53].
Grading of ocular and dermal symptoms:
Grade I: Ocular signs (hypersecretion, swelling of eyelids and meibomian glands) and pigmentary changes on mucosa and skin without developing follicular lesion.
Grade II: Localized comedones and accentuation of hair follicles.
Grade III: Localized acne-like inflamed lesions with or without external genital cysts.
Grade IV: The most prominent cutaneous lesions with generalized acneiform or keratoic follicular eruptions, frequently associated with secondary bacterial infections.

mones and pharmacological agents may modulate the expression of E rosettes [57–59]. Therefore, it is not clear whether the decreased T cells found in *yu-cheng* patients was due to the alteration of cellular function or to the actual decrease of cell numbers.

Effects of PCB on phagocytes

Phagocytic cells, polymorphonuclear leucocytes (PMNs) and monocytes, possess surface receptors for the Fc portion of IgG and complements C3 and C4. It has been suggested that the complement receptors may be primarily involved in the attachment, whereas the participation of Fc receptors is required for inducing the mechanism of phagocytosis [60,61]. When PMNs are separated into two populations based on the presence of Fc receptors, the cells bearing Fc receptors appear to have a stronger adherence to nylon wool and higher chemotactic, phagocytic, and bactericidal capacities [62]. The maturation of promonocytes to monocytes and then to macrophages is associated with the increased percentages of cells bearing complement and Fc receptors [63]. Among the peripheral blood monocytes, the activity of antibody-dependent cellular toxicity is associated with monocytes bearing Fc receptors [63]. Thus, the expression of Fc and complement receptors may be associated with cellular activities.

The mean percentages of PMNs and monocytes bearing Fc receptors and complement receptors were lower in samples obtained from *yu-cheng* patients when compared to samples obtained from normal, healthy volunteers [64] (Table 13.4). The observed decreased percentage of receptor-bearing cells may suggest impairment of cellular function and, consequently, increased incidence of infections. The mechanism responsible for the decreased percentage of receptor-bearing cells is not known; however, it

Table 13.4 Percentage of phagocytes bearing Fc and complement receptors (mean ± s.d.)

Subjects	Phagocytes	Cells with Fc receptors (%)	Cells with complement receptors (%)
Normal (n = 23)	PMNs	69 ± 12	68 ± 13
Yu-cheng (n = 30)	PMNs	44 ± 15	43 ± 14
t-test		P < 0.001	P < 0.001
Normal	Monocytes	50 ± 11	51 ± 8
Yu-cheng	Monocytes	38 ± 14	38 ± 12
t-test		P < 0.005	P < 0.005

Adapted from [64]. PMNs, Polymorphonucleocytes.

could be due to alteration of cell subpopulations, or to direct PCB toxicity on target cells.

Toxic effects of PCBs on phagocytic cells of experimental animals have been reported. Loose *et al.* [42] and Thomas and Hinsdill [43] have found that the exposure of mice to PCBs enhanced susceptibility to endotoxin shock. The major pathway for endotoxin detoxification is through a macrophage-dependent process [65]. The increased susceptibility may suggest impaired macrophage functions. In addition, after PCB poisoning, the ability of the animal to clear the injected micro-organisms was diminished [43]. PCB poisoning in humans [66] and experimental animals [2,34] is associated with increased incidences of infection. Phagocytic cells, PMNs and monocytes are responsible for the elimination of the invading micro-organisms. Decreased numbers of phagocytic cells or defects in cell functions may cause the host to be more susceptible to invading micro-organisms.

In vitro lymphocyte function

The lymphocytes obtained from *yu-cheng* patients showed an enhanced spontaneous proliferation when analysed on the third day in culture. The increased rate of proliferation returned to normal after 5 days. Cellular response to phytohaemagglutinin was enhanced, while responses to concanavalin A and pokeweed mitogen were normal. The response to purified protein-derivative of tuberculin was significantly increased on the 7th day of culture but not on the 5th day of culture [25]. The significance of these observations is not clear.

Causal agents for PCB poisoning

Initially, the presence of PCBs in rice oil was considered as the causal agent for various clinical symptoms associated with PCB poisoning. Several years later, however, the toxic oil samples from Japan [20,67] and Taiwan [21] were found also to contain polychlorinated dibenzofurans (PCDFs) and polychlorinated quarterphenyls (PCQs). It has been well documented that the toxicity of PCDFs was much higher than that of PCBs [32,37,68,69]. Thus, PCDFs instead of PCBs have been suspected as the causal agents for *yu-cheng* and *yusho*.

Recent developments in chromatographic technology have permitted the separation and purification of PCBs, PCDFs and PCQs from crude PCB mixtures. By feeding animals with a diet containing PCBs, PCDFs or PCQs singly or in combination, Kunita *et al.* [67] were able to demonstrate that a significant decrease of thymic weight was observed in rats feeding on a PCDF-containing diet (0.01 mg rat^{-1} day^{-1}). PCBs or PCQs (1 g rat^{-1} day^{-1}) alone did not cause a decrease in thymic weight. PCBs, PCDFs and PCQs were all effective in increasing liver weight. Experiments with monkeys also showed that a PCDF-containing diet caused dermal abnormalities similar to those of *yusho* (e.g. acne, pigmentation and oedema of the lips and eyelids). These observations suggested that PCDFs were the main causal agents in the pathogenesis of oral PCB poisoning. It should be noted, however, that halogenated hydrocarbons may act synergistically or antagonistically towards one another [70,71]. The toxic oil contains various isomers and congeners of halogenated hydrocarbons. The exact mechanism of how each individual chemical contributes to the disease has yet to be resolved.

Treatment of PCB poisoning

At the present time, the management of PCB victims is limited to symptomatic medication such as analgesics, sedatives, control of infections and supportive therapy for the general condition. The use of cholestyramine or a diet with a high fibre content to interfere with the reabsorption of PCBs and/or their metabolites has been unsuccessful [25]. A fasting therapy, however, has been claimed to be effective in relieving some of the symptoms such as headache, lumbago, coughing and acneiform eruptions. Blood PCB concentrations, however, were elevated during and shortly after ($5–7$ days) fasting [72]. The effects of fasting on the immune function were not reported.

In animal studies, limiting the food intake to 50% of their mean *ad libitum* level facilitates the excretion of the injected hexachlorobiphenyl [73]. It appears that the beneficial effects of fasting may be due to its ability to facilitate the release of PCBs and other halogenated hydrocarbons from target organs and adipose tissues and subsequent excretion of these halogenated hydrocarbons and their metabolites through bile.

Conclusions

Halogenated hydrocarbons cause various biological responses in animals. At the present time, it is not clear whether the observed immune suppression following PCB (or PCDF) poisoning is due directly to toxic effects of these chemicals or is the indirect result of toxicity to other tissues. Abnormalities in hepatic, neural, and endocrinological functions as the result of PCB poisoning could lead to irregular metabolism of steroids, hormones, biogenic amines, and vitamins [2,69]. Steroids, hormones, biogenic amines, and vitamins affect various tissue functions, including those of the lymphoid system. Thus, the toxicity to other tissues may indirectly contribute to the immune suppressions observed. In this regard, it is important to note that in animal experiments, the hepatic abnormalities appeared to precede immune dysfunction.

PCBs added *in vitro* affect various aspects of leucocyte functions (e.g. lymphocyte mitogenic responses, neutrophil β-glucuronidase release) and lymphocyte metabolism (e.g. glycolysis, glucose uptake, and intracellular adenosine triphosphate concentration) [74–77]. In addition, various enzymes, especially sodium, potassium-adenosine triphosphatase [2] and protein kinase C [78], are affected by PCBs. These results suggest that PCBs could affect leucocytes directly.

The clinical symptoms associated with PCB poisoning are complicated. It is reasonable to assume that PCBs affect the immune system both directly and indirectly. At the present time there is no effective treatment for PCB poisoning. Continuing research using *in vivo* animal models as well as *in vitro* leucocyte culture studies may help to clarify the mechanism of abnormalities. Hopefully, the data obtained may help to design an effective treatment of the disease.

References

1 Cleseri LS. Case history: PCBs in the Hudson river. In: Guthrie FE, Perry JJ, eds. *Introduction to Environmental Toxicology*, New York: Elsevier North Holland,

1980:227–35.

2 Fishbein L. Toxicity of chlorinated biphenyls. *Annu Rev Pharmacol* 1974; 14:139–56.

3 Kimbrough R. Human health effects of PCBs and PBBs. *Annu Rev Pharmacol Toxicol* 1987; 27:87–111.

4 Nelson N. Polychlorinated biphenyls: environmental impact. *Environ Res* 1972; 5:253–362.

5 Zitco V, Choi PMK. PCB and other industrial halogenated hydrocarbons in the environment. In: *Fisheries Research Board of Canada Technical Report*, 272:2–54.

6 Higuchi K. (ed.) *PCB Poisoning and Pollution.* New York: Academic Press, 1976.

7 Buckley JL, (ed.) *National Conference on Polychlorinated Biphenyls.* Washington DC: Environmental Protection Agency, 1976.

8 Yakushiji T, Watanabe I, Kuwabara K, Yoshida S, Koyama K, Kunita N. Levels of PCBs and organochlorine pesticides in human milk and blood collected in Osaka prefecture from 1972 to 1977. *Int Arch Occup Environ Hlth* 1979; 43:1–15.

9 Yakushiji T, Watanabe I, Kuwabara K, Tanaka R, Kashimoto T, Kunita N, Hara I. Rate of decrease and half life of PCBs in the blood of mothers and their children occupationally exposed to PCBs. *Arch Environ Toxicol* 1984; 13:341–5.

10 Fischbein A, Wolff M, Lilis R, Thornton J, Selikoff IJ. Clinical findings among PCB–exposed capacitor manufacturing workers. *Ann N Y Acad Sci* 1979; 320:703–15.

11 Meigs J, Albom J, Kartin BL. Chloracne from an unusual exposure to Aroclor. *J A M A* 1954; 154:1417–18.

12 Ouw KH, Simpson GR, Siyali DS. The use and health effects of Aroclor 1242. *Arch Environ Hlth* 1976; 31:189–94.

13 Schwartz L. Dermatitis from synthetic resins and waxes. *Am J Public Hlth* 1936; 26:586–92.

14 Schwartz L. An outbreak of halowax acne among electricians. *J A M A* 1942; 122:158–61.

15 Warshaw R, Fischbein A, Thornton J, Miller A, Selikoff IJ. Decrease in vital capacity in PCB-exposed workers in a capacitor manufacturing facility. *Ann N Y Acad Sci* 1979; 320:277–83.

16 Chang KJ, Chen JS, Huang PC, Tung TA. Study of patients with PCB-poisoning. *J Formosan Med Assoc* 1980; 79:304–13.

17 Wong CK. (ed.) PCB poisoning. *Clin Med (Taipei)* 1981; 7:1–100.

18 Hsu S, Ma C, Hsu S, Wu S, Hsu N, Yeh C. Discovery and epidemiology of PCB poisoning in Taiwan. *Am J Ind Med* 1984; 5:71–9.

19 Chang KJ, Lu FJ, Tung TC, Lee TP. Studies of patients with PCB-poisoning. *Res Commun Chem Pathol Pharmacol* 1980; 30:547–54.

20 Masuda Y, Yoshimura H. Polychlorinated biphenyls and dibenzofurans in patients with Yusho and their toxicological significance. *Am J Ind Med* 1984; 5:31–44.

21 Chen P, Luo M, Wong C, Chen C. PCBs, PCDFs and PCQs in the toxic rice bran oil and PCBs in the blood of patients with PCB poisoning in Taiwan. *Am J Ind Med* 1984; 5:133–45.

22 Lee YY, Wong PN, Lu YC, Sun CC, Wu YC, Lin RY, Jee SH, Ng KY, Yeh HP. An outbreak of PCB poisoning. *J Dermatol (Tokyo)* 1980; 7:435–41.

23 Chen RC, Chang YC, Tung TC, Chang KC. *Proc Natl Sci Council (Taiwan)* 1983; 7:87–91.

24 Hirayama C. Hepatocellular dysfunction in patients with PCB poisoning. *Fukoka Acta Med* 1979; 70:238–45.

25 Lu Y, Wong P. Dermatological, medical and laboratory findings of patients in Taiwan and their treatments. *Am J Ind Med* 1984; 5:81–115.

26 Sunahara G, Nelson K, Wong T, Lucier G. Decreased human birth weights after *in utero* exposure to PCBs and PCDFs. *Mol Pharmacol* 1987; 32:572–8.

27 Rogan W, Gladen B, Hung K, Koong S, Shih L, Taylor J, Wu Y, Yang D, Ragan N, Hsu C. Congenital poisoning by PCBs and their contaminants in Taiwan. *Science* 1988; 241:334–6.

28 Gladen BC, Rogan WJ, Ragan NB, Spierto FW. Urinary porphyrins in children exposed transplacentally to polyhalogenated aromatics in Taiwan. *Arch Environ Hlth* 1988; 43:54–8.

29 Emmett E, Maroni M, Schmith J, Levin B, Jefferys J. Studies of transformer repair workers exposed to PCBs. *Am J Ind Med* 1988; 13:415-27.

30 Takamatsu M, Oki M, Maeda K, Inoue Y, Hirayama H, Yoshizuka K. PCBs in blood of workers exposed to PCBs and their health status. *Am J Ind Med* 1984; 5:59-68.

31 Bowes G, Mulvihill M, Simoneit B, Burlingame A, Risebrough R. Identification of chlorinated dibenzofurans in American PCBs. *Nature (Lond)* 1975; 256:305–7.

32 Safe S. PCBs and PBBs: biochemistry, toxicology and mechanism of action. *CRC Crit Rev Toxicol* 1984; 13:319-95.

33 Vos JG, Koeman JH. Comparative toxicology study with PCBs in chickens. *Toxicol Appl Pharmacol* 1970; 17:656–68.

34 Allen JR. Response of the non-human primate to PCB exposure. *Fed Proc* 1975; 34:1675–9.

35 Subba Rao DS, Glick B. Pesticide effects on the immune responses of chicken lymphocytes. *Proc Soc Exp Biol Med* 1977; 154:27–9.

36 Vos JG. Toxicology of PCBs for mammals and for

birds. *Environ Hlth Perspect* 1972; 1:105–17.

37 Vos JG, Koeman JH, Van der Mass HL, ten Noever de Brauw MC, de Vos RH. Identification and toxicological evaluation of chlorinated dibenzofuran and chlorinated napthalene in PCBs. *Food Cosmet Toxicol* 1970; 8:625–33.

38 Wasserman M, Wasserman D, Gershon A, Zellermayer L. Effect of organochlorine insecticides on body defense systems. *Ann N Y Acad Sci* 1969; 160:393–401.

39 Flick DF, O'Dell R, Childs V. Studies of the chick edema disease. *Poult Sci* 1965; 44:1460–5.

40 Vos J, Faith R, Luster M. Immune alterations. In: Kimbrough R, ed. *Halogenated Biphenyls, Terphenyls, Napthalenes, Dibenzodioxins and Related Products.* New York: Elsevier North Holland Biomedical Press, 1980:241–66.

41 Friend M, Trainer D. PCB: interaction with duck hepatitis virus. *Science* 1970; 170:1314–16.

42 Loose L, Silkworth J, Pittman K, Benitz K, Mueller W. Impaired host resistance to endotoxin and malaria in PCB-treated mice. *Infect Immun* 1978; 20:30–5.

43 Thomas PT, Hinsdill RD. Effects of PCBs on the immune responses of rhesus monkeys and mice. *Toxicol Appl Pharmacol* 1978; 44:41–51.

44 Chang KJ, Hsieh KH, Lee TP, Tang SY, Tung TC. Immunologic evaluation of patients with PCB-poisoning: determination of lymphocyte subpopulations. *Toxicol Appl Pharmacol* 1981; 61:58–63.

45 Koller LD, Thigpen JE. Reduction of antibodies to pseudorabies virus in PCB exposed rabbits. *Am J Vet Res* 1973; 34:1065–6.

46 Vos JG, DeRoij T. Immunosuppressive activity of a PCB preparation on the humoral immune response in guinea pig. *Toxicol Appl Pharmacol* 1972; 21:549–55.

47 Moretta L, Webb S, Grossi C, Lydyard P, Cooper M. Functional analysis of two human T-cell subpopulations. *J Exp Med* 1977; 146:184–200.

48 Bekesi J, Roboz J, Fischbein A, Mason P. Immunotoxicology: environmental contamination by PBBs and immune dysfunction among residents of the state of Michigan. *Cancer Detect Prev Suppl* 1987; 1:29–37.

49 Bekesi JG, Holland J, Anderson H, Fischbein A, Rom W, Wolfe M, Selikoff I. Lymphocyte function of Michigan dairy farmers exposed to PBBs. *Science* 1978; 199:1207–9.

50 Bekesi JG, Anderson HA, Roboz JP, Roboz J, Fischbein A, Selikoff IJ, Holland JF. Immunologic dysfunction among PBB-exposed Michigan dairy farmers. *Ann N Y Acad Sci* 1979; 320:717–28.

51 Landrigan P, Wilcox K, Silva J Jr, Humphrey H, Kauffman C. Cohort study of Michigan residents exposed to PBBs. *Ann N Y Acad Sci* 1979; 320:284–94.

52 Lipson S. Effect of PCBs on the growth and maturation of human peripheral blood lymphocytes. *Clin Immunol Immunopathol* 1987; 43:65–72.

53 Chang KJ, Hsieh KH, Tang TY, Tung TA, Lee TP. Immunologic evaluation of patients with PCB-poisoning: evaluation of delayed-type skin hypersensitive response and its relation to clinical studies. *J Toxicol Environ Hlth* 1982; 9:217–23.

54 Vos JG, Van Driel-Grootenhuis L. PCB-induced suppression of the humoral and cell-mediated immunity in guinea pigs. *Sci Total Environ* 1972; 1:289–302.

55 Street J, Sharma R. Alteration of induced cellular and humoral responses by pesticides and chemicals of environmental concern. *Toxicol Appl Pharmacol* 1975; 32:587–602.

56 Wybran J, Fudenberg H. Thymus derived rosette forming cells in various human disease states. *J Clin Invest* 1973; 52:1026–32.

57 Chisari F, Edgington T. Human T-lymphocyte E-rosette function. *J Exp Med* 1974; 140:1122–6.

58 Galant SP, Remo R. Beta-adrenergic inhibition of human T-lymphocyte rosettes. *J Immunol* 1975; 114:512–13.

59 Grieco M, Siegel J, Goel Z. Modulation of human T-lymphocyte rosette formation by autonomic agonists and cyclic nucleotides. *J Allergy Clin Immunol* 1976; 58:149–59.

60 Mantovani B. Different roles of IgG and complement receptors in phagocytosis by PMNs. *J Immunol* 1975; 115:15–17.

61 Ross G, Medof M. Membrane complement receptors specific for bound fragments of C3. *Adv Immunol* 1985; 37:217–67.

62 Klempner M, Gallin J. Separation and functional characterization of human neutrophil subpopulations. *Blood* 1978; 51:659–69.

63 Cline M, Lehren R, Territo M, Gold D. Monocytes and macrophages. *Ann Intern Med* 1978; 88:78–88.

64 Chang KJ, Hsieh KH, Lee TP, Tung TA. Immunologic evaluation of patients with PCB-poisoning: determination of phagocytic Fc and complement receptors. *Environ Res* 1982; 28:329–34.

65 Braude A, Carey F, Zalesky M. Studies with radioactive endotoxin. *J Clin Invest* 1955; 34:858–66.

66 Shigematsu N, Ishimaru S, Saito R, Ikeda T, Matsuba K, Sugiyama K, Masuda T. Respiratory involvement in PCB-poisoning. *Environ Res* 1978; 16:92–100.

67 Kunita N, Kashimoto T, Miyata H, Fukushima S, Hori S, Obana H. Casual agents of Yusho. *Am J Ind Med* 1984; 5:45–58.

68 Goldstein J. The structure–activity relationship of halogenated biphenyls as enzyme inducers. *Ann N Y Acad Sci* 1979; 320:164–78.

69 Safe S. Comparative toxicology and mechanism of action of polychlorinated dibenzo-p-dioxins and dibenzofurans. *Ann Rev Pharmacol Toxicol* 1986; 26:371–99.

70 Bannister R, Safe S. Synergistic interactions of 2, 3, 7, 8-TCDD and 2, 2', 4, 4', 5, 5'-hexachlorobiphenyl in C57BL/6J and DBA/2J mice. *Toxicol* 1987; 44:159–69.

71 Bannister R, Davis D, Zacharewski T, Tizard I, Safe S. Aroclor 1254 as a 2, 3, 7, 8–TCDD antagonist. *Toxicol* 1987; 46:29–42.

72 Imamura M, Tung T. A trial of fasting cure for PCB-poisoned patients in Taiwan. *Am J Ind Med* 1984; 5:147–53.

73 Wyss P, Muhlebach S, Bickel M. Long term pharmacokinetics of 2, 2', 4, 4', 5, 5'-hexachlorobiphenyl in rats with constant adipose tissue mass. *Drug Metab Dispos* 1976; 14:361–5.

74 Lee TP, Moscati R, Park B. Effects of PCBs and pesticides on leukocyte function. *Res Commun Chem Toxicol Pharmacol* 1979; 23:597–609.

75 Lee TP, Park B. Biochemical basis of Aroclor 1254 and pesticide toxicity *in vitro. Res Commun Pathol Pharmacol* 1979; 25:597–605.

76 Lee TP, Park B. Effect of Aroclor 1254 on leukocyte glucose uptake. *J Toxicol Environ Hlth* 1980; 6:607–11.

77 Lee TP. The inhibition of PMN beta-glucuronidase release by Aroclor 1254. *Environ Res* 1981; 25:386–90.

78 Shukla R, Albro P. *In vitro* modulation of protein kinase C activity by environmental chemical pollutants. *Biochem Biophys Res Commun* 1987; 142:567–72.

14

Immunotoxic and other health effects of TCDD and toxic oils

P.K. RAY & A.K. PRASAD

Introduction

With the global increase in population, more particularly in developing countries of the world, the need for more food, shelter and other day-to-day necessities of life has become more intensely felt than ever in the past. This has resulted in launching and expansion of a wide variety of agricultural programmes and a multipronged strategy of industrial development which has taken place with great rapidity all over the world. The initial thrust of all these developmental programmes was one that held the prospect of food for all as a matter of immediate concern. After an appreciable breakthrough in the area, scientists the world over were seized with the problem of environmental pollution caused by the production and use of a wide variety of pesticides and chemical fertilizers. The introduction of heavy metals, polyaromatic hydrocarbons, oil and petroleum, noxious agents like 2, 3, 7, 8-tetrachlorodibenzo-p-dioxin (TCDD), volatile gases, solvents, colouring agents, dyes, food additives and a host of other pollutants came in the wake of heavy industrialization, new technology and the changed lifestyle of humans today. It will not go amiss to state here that more than 700 000 chemicals are already in the environment around us, to these, 1000–2000 new chemicals are being added every year [1].

We have published reports which include epidemiological surveys demonstrating that most of the chemicals with which our environment is replete today can cause different types of toxicities including immunotoxicity, resulting in altered immune function for the exposed individuals, who develop a state of either partial or complete immunosuppression [2,3]. Prolonged immunosuppression renders an individual extremely susceptible to various infections and even predisposes the host to develop cancer [2,4]. Impaired immune status not only weakens the ability of an individual to withstand infection but also decreases its ability to fight toxicosis caused by environmental toxicants [1,2]. Sometimes chronic exposure of even a very low concentration of drugs, biochemicals or toxicants may produce alterations in the immune system leading to immunotoxic signs or syndromes [5]. Measuring the immunotoxicity parameters, therefore, offers a sensitive tool to assess the toxicity potential of many toxicants [5,6].

All these details are discussed elsewhere in this book, so any elaboration here will be superfluous. In this chapter, we will discuss primarily the toxicological aspects of TCDD and some toxic oils, with particular reference to their immunotoxic potential. No attempt has been made to make this chapter acomprehensive one, but efforts were certainly made to collect the major information available in the literature.

The increased industrial production of phenoxy herbicides has exceeded all previous records because of their demand in agriculture. Much of the recent concern over the widespread use of 2,4,5-trichlorophenoxyacetate (2,4,5-T) and other phenoxy herbicides has centred around the presence of a toxic contaminant TCDD. TCDD is a strong teratogenic impurity (present in concentrations ranging from 0.5 to 1 p.p.m.) in commercial preparations of 2,4,5-T, silvex, 2,4,5-trichlorophenol (2,4,5-TCP) and pentachlorophenol [7].

This chapter describes acute and short-term toxicity, subacute and chronic toxicity, immunotoxicity, teratogenicity and the carcinogenicity of TCDD. It also delineates the hazards of human exposure to TCDD due to accidental spillage, such as took place in Missouri, Seveso and Arizona and the effects when TCDD was used deliberately as a warfare tool in South Vietnam by US armed forces.

Oils have a variety of uses in everyday life. Edible oils are used mostly as a cooking medium. Many of the essential oils have medicinal value apart from being commonly used as flavouring agents and perfumes. Petroleum fractions and mineral oils are used as illuminating fuel, car fuel, and cleaning and thinning agents for paints and lubricants [8].

The exposure to or ingestion of oils beyond a threshold concentration produces toxicity manifestations. This chapter deals with the toxicity manifestations of argemone, corn and kerosene oils, along with the description of accidental oil toxicity in Spain due to ingestion of denatured rape seed oil. The aetiology of the disease caused by this accidental oil toxicity is unknown and it has been termed toxic oil syndrome (TOS).

TCDD intoxication

Production of TCDD

As mentioned earlier, TCDD is a contaminant in commercial preparations of 2,4,5-T, silvex, 2,4,5-TCP and pentachlorophenol utilizing tri-, tetra- or penta-chlorophenols in the manufacturing process [7,9]. The structure of TCDD is shown in Fig. 14.1.

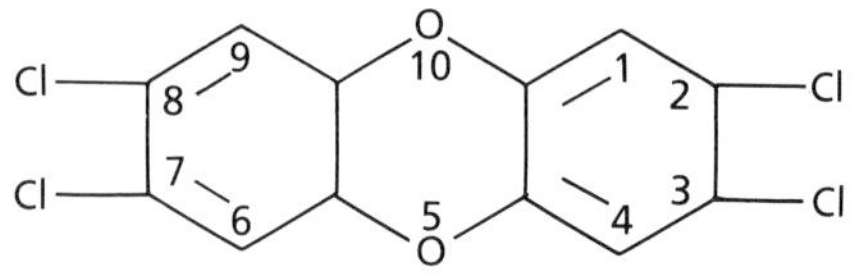

Fig. 14.1 Structure of 2,3,7,8-tetrachlorodibenzo-*p*-dioxin (TCDD).

TCDD is formed as a byproduct during the production of *n*-butyl ester of 2,4,5-T from sodium trichlorophenate when the latter is heated at a high temperature (more than 230°C) or at high alkalinity or pressure (Fig. 14.2) [7]. The structures of common phenoxy herbicides in which TCDD is present as a contaminant are shown in Fig. 14.3.

Experimental studies

Absorption, distribution and excretion of TCDD. Oral administration of a single dose of 50 μg ^{14}C TCDD to rats showed that approximately 30% was eliminated through faeces during the first 48 h [10]. The half-life for the disappearance of ^{14}C activity from the body was 17.4 ± 5.6 days. After this period the excretion rate of ^{14}C activity via faeces varied by 1–2% per day. ^{14}C TCDD was also absorbed in other body tissues and most of the activity was localized in liver and adipose tissues. Allen *et al.* [11] similarly treated Sprague-Dawley rats with a single intragastric dose of ^{14}C TCDD. The total amount of radioactivity in urine was 4.5% of the total dose. An appreciable percentage of the remaining radioactivity was localized in the liver and of this 90% was located in the microsomal fraction.

The tissue distribution and excretion of ^{14}C TCDD in guinea pigs following intraperitoneal injection of 2.0 μg kg^{-1} body weight of TCDD was investigated by Gasiewica and Neal [12]. The level of ^{14}C TCDD in liver increased to 3.23% on day 15. An increase in the level of TCDD was found in adrenals, kidneys and lungs, together with a significant increase in plasma albumin, total protein, iron, urea and cholesterol in TCDD-treated guinea pigs.

Thus the animal data indicate that the primary route of excretion of TCDD appears to be the faeces, with urinary excretion occurring at a much reduced

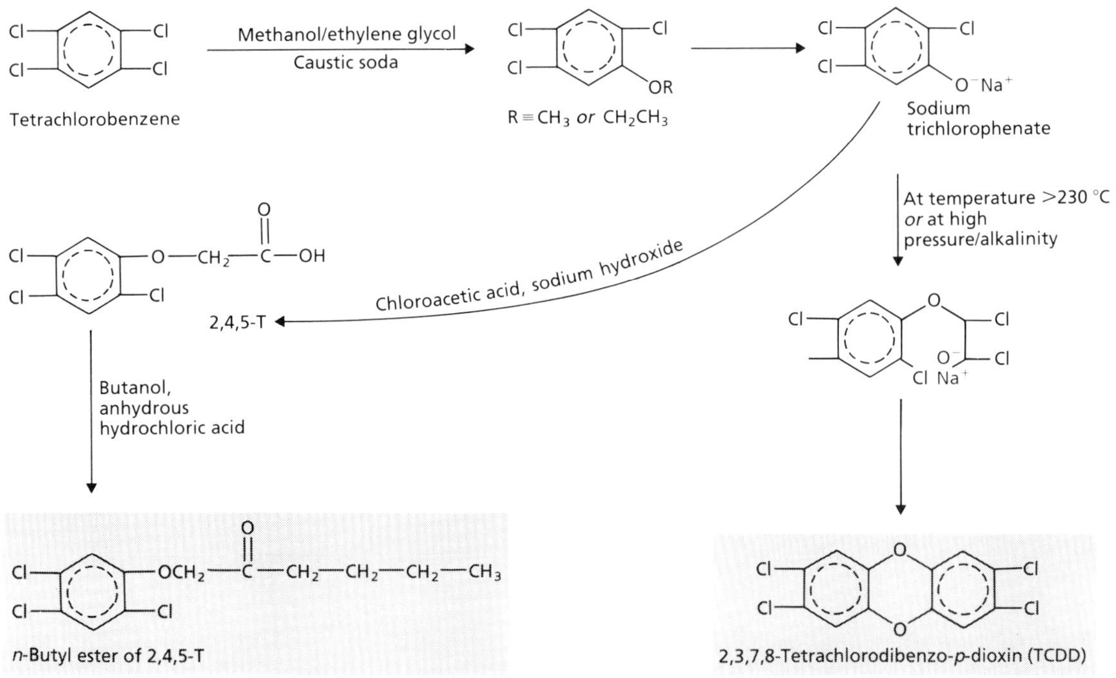

Fig. 14.2 Formation of TCDD as a byproduct during the commercial production of 2,4,5-T and its ester (modified from [33]).

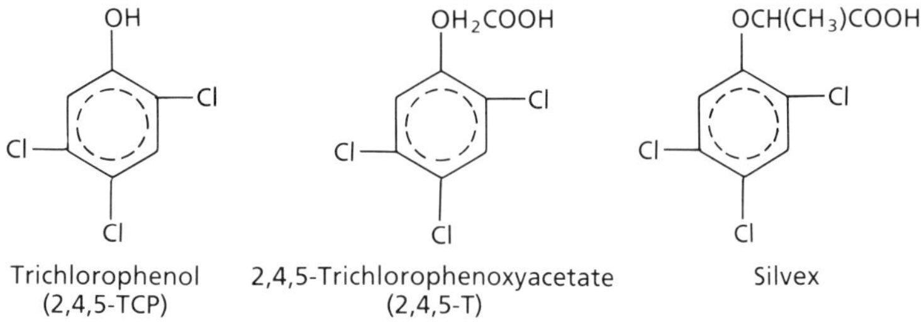

Fig. 14.3 Structure of some herbicides in which TCDD is present as a contaminant.

Trichlorophenol (2,4,5-TCP)   2,4,5-Trichlorophenoxyacetate (2,4,5-T)   Silvex

rate. Liver and adipose tissue accumulated about 10 times higher levels of TCDD compared to other body tissues.

Acute and short-term toxicity of TCDD. It has been reported that a single oral dose (0.6 μg kg^{-1} or 1 mg kg^{-1} body weight respectively) can prove fatal to guinea pigs and dogs [13,14]. TCDD causes liver cell necrosis, and the exposed individual dies of hepatotoxicity [14]. Experimental studies carried out by Cunningham *et al.* [15] showed that TCDD did not affect ^{3}H acetate incorporation in lipids metabolized in liver but caused alteration in fatty acid transport

across hepatocyte membrane. The storage of lipid reached its maximum 3 days after TCDD administration and subsequently there was increased protein biosynthesis, probably due to the induction of metabolizing enzymes.

Harris *et al.* [14], using rats and mice, observed that reduction in weight of the thymus was the most sensitive indicator of TCDD exposure, even at a very low dose at which there was no apparent toxic manifestation in terms of loss in body weight. However, it is highly probable that a reduction in thymus weight would almost always be associated with a reduction in the level of T lymphocytes. Therefore, both humoral and cell-mediated immune function of the host would be impaired, increasing the susceptibility of the host to infection and so reducing the longevity of the host.

Intradermal and intraperitoneal injection of TCDD resulted in dermatological abnormalities like alopecia and acne in rhesus monkeys [16].

Subacute and chronic toxicity potential. Subacute and chronic doses of TCDD have produced a wide variety of toxic effects including thymic atrophy, depletion of weights of lymphoid organs, hepatic necrosis, atrophy of adrenal zona glomerulosa and lesions in myocardium in the experimental animals like rabbits, guinea pigs and rats [17]. The main target organs affected by TCDD in rats, guinea pigs and mice appeared to be the liver and thymus.

Vos and Moore [18] investigated pre- and post-natal effects of TCDD in pregnant C57Bl/6 mice inoculated with 0–5 μg kg^{-1} body weight of TCDD on days 14 and 17 of gestation and post-natally on days 1, 8 and 15. These workers observed severe depletion of lymphocytes in thymic cortex, reduced weight of thymus and spleen, suppressed cell-mediated immune response and impaired allograft rejection in the offsprings of the TCDD-exposed mothers. It has been further reported that although low doses of TCDD did not produce pathological and/or clinical changes, yet they were sufficient to reduce the host's immune defence [19]. The oral administration of 1 μg TCDD kg^{-1} body weight to mice resulted in enhanced susceptibility and mortality due to *Salmonella* infection [19].

The oral administration of subacute doses of TCDD for 9 months to monkeys resulted in alopecia, thrombocytopenia, enlargement of the liver, haemorrhage, gastric hyperplasia, ulceration, hypocellularity of bone marrow lymphocytes and mortality due to severe pancytopenia [20].

Immunotoxic potential of TCDD. The immunotoxic effects of chronic and subacute doses of TCDD are apparent from thymic atrophy, suppressed cell-mediated immune response and necrosis of liver in rats, besides depletion of weights of lymphoid or-

gans, thymus atrophy and atrophy of adrenal zona glomerulosa in guinea pigs [18,21,22]. Detailed studies carried out by Vos and co-workers [18,23], testify strongly to the immunosuppressive property of TCDD.

The mode of action whereby TCDD affects the cells of the immune system is discussed in depth in Chapter 19.

Thigpen *et al.* [19] observed that minute quantities of TCDD, which did not show any apparent pathological or clinical changes, reduced significantly host resistance and immunological defence mechanisms. The group of mice fed with 1 μg kg^{-1} TCDD over 1–4 weeks showed enhanced susceptibility and mortality to *Salmonella* infection.

The autopsy of female rhesus monkeys, given a diet containing 500 mg TCDD for 9 months, revealed distinct hypocellularity of bone marrow and lymph nodes, leading finally to death due to severe pancytopenia [20].

Thus, a large number of studies have indicated that TCDD intoxication leads to degeneration of lymphoid organs and suppression of the host's immune response.

Carcinogenicity and tumorigenicity of TCDD. Van Miller *et al.* [24] investigated the effect of long-term (2 years) oral feeding of TCDD and the development of tumours in rats. Only 38% of animals were observed developing tumours after TCDD feeding, which included neoplastic nodules of liver, cholangiocarcinoma, carcinoma of the ear duct, kidney and bladder. Some animals showed retroperitoneal histiocytomas metastasizing to lung, kidney and liver.

A study of chronic TCDD exposure was carried out by Kociba *et al.* [25] on Sprague-Dawley rats. These workers fed the rats 0.001–1 μg kg^{-1} TCDD daily for 2 years. The group of animals fed with 0.01 μg TCDD kg^{-1} body weight showed hepatocellular carcinomas of liver, lung, hard palate and tongue.

Kouri *et al.* [26], while studying the mechanism of TCDD-induced carcinogenicity, found that TCDD is an indirect-acting weak carcinogen. In mice TCDD acted synergistically with methyl cholanthrene and enhanced tumour uptake. Aryl hydrocarbon hydroxylase (AHH) induction has been reported in human lymphocyte culture by TCDD [26].

Teratogenicity, fetotoxicity and embryotoxicity of TCDD. Several workers have reported that TCDD when administered in single or repeated low doses to different mammalian species can cause teratogenic changes as evident from an increase in frequency of cleft palate and renal abnormalities in the foetus [27,28]. TCDD caused renal hydronephrosis in pups through the mother's milk when foster mothers or nursing dams were orally administered TCDD (1–10 μg kg^{-1} body weight). The extent of hydronephrosis was proportional to the concentration of TCDD administered [29]. Becker [30] observed that low doses of TCDD ingestion (on days 13–15 of gestation) can cause fatty degeneration of liver in adult female rats and fatty inclusions were seen in the liver of embryos from TCDD-treated females.

TCDD has been found to be the most foetotoxic and teratogenic of several dioxin compounds given orally or subcutaneously to mice during 7–16 days of pregnancy. TCDD intoxication resulted in hydrocephalus, lack of eyelid formation (open eye) and clubfoot oedema following internal haemorrhages in foetuses of exposed mothers. Smith *et al.* [31] administered different amounts of TCDD through gavage to CF1 mice from day 6 to day 15 of pregnancy. The group of animals receiving 1 μg TCDD per kg body weight showed a significantly increased percentage of resorption sites per implantation site and litters of the treated mothers exhibited the formation of cleft palate and renal abnormalities.

The embryotoxic effects of TCDD have been studied in rats by Sparschu *et al.* [32]. These workers administered different amounts of TCDD to Sprague-Dawley rats on days 6–15 of gestation and observed a significant reduction in foetal weight, increased foetal mortality and internal haemorrhages.

TCDD disaster and human exposure

There are four well documented episodes of TCDD disasters which resulted in human exposure and are also suspected to have adversely affected the environment [33–35].

Vietnam episode. The use of herbicides as a modern warfare agent was first documented in 1962. The US military forces used phenoxy herbicides for forest defoliation and food crop destruction in Vietnam [33]. TCDD was released into the environment as an associated contaminant from the spray of herbicide orange in operation Ranch Hand in south Vietnam [33].

The release of TCDD into the environment from the herbicide orange, 2,4,5-T and silvex spray resulted in the mortality of fish in ponds and rivers and fowls in farmyards. Some cases of abortion and monster birth were also noticed in animals.

During the peak spray period (1968–1970) the number of stillbirths in the Tay Ninh hospital was reported to be twice the rate of the regions where there was no spray. Furthermore, teratogenic changes were observed at Saigon children's hospital where the incidences of spina bifida and pura cleft were significantly high during the time of heavy spray. The TCDD-exposed victims showed vomiting, nausea, dizziness and fatigue. Chloracne was also reported in many of the exposed victims. The average maximum TCDD exposure was about 6–25 mg per person. Interestingly, bioaccumulation of TCDD was found in crustacea, snails, fish and shellfish. Humans therefore could also be exposed through the food chain. There was marked variation in the ecology of the area where herbicide orange was sprayed. The leaves of the trees became yellow, shrivelled and dropped and the food crop withered, rotted and became inedible.

Missouri episode. As already described briefly, this incident occurred in May 1971 when a large amount of waste oil (motor salvage oil) was unwittingly contaminated with more than 330 mg kg^{-1} dioxin, which was spread as dust palliative at three horse arenas in eastern Missouri [34]. It was estimated that approximately 2000 gallons of salvaged motor oil was sprayed to prevent the dust problem. As a result, 54 of 57 horses died of dioxin toxicity characterized by skin lesions, severe weight loss and hepatotoxicity. Birds, dogs, cats, insects and rodents were also found dead around the area. A 6-year-old girl exposed to dioxin developed epistaxis, gastrointestinal disorders and severe haemorrhagic cystitis. Many other persons developed transient headache, nausea and dizziness. A large number of human victims were hospitalized for chloracne.

The laboratory analysis of soil samples from the affected arena showed the presence of 2,4,5-trichlorophenol and TCDD as possible toxic substances. The soil samples contained 33 μg TCDD per g of soil.

The soil sludge sprayed was collected from many industries and it was shown that dioxin had originated from hexachlorophene produced in the year 1970–1971. The producer contracted the disposal of TCDD to a chemical distributor, who subcontracted the salvage oil company that sprayed the horse arena. The fluid left in the storage tank at the salvage oil company showed 360–365 $\mu g\,g^{-1}$ TCDD. Hence the residues suspected to be those of TCDD and TCP collected by the salvage oil company from a hexachlorophene producer at South-west Missouri were thought to be responsible for all the catastrophe that had taken place.

Seveso explosion episode. An explosion occurred at a plant which was producing 2,4,5-trichlorophenol at Seveso in Italy [35]. The accident occurred on 10 July 1976 due to over-heating in the reaction vessel which resulted in the safety valve blowing away. The thick cloud of smoke and fumes released from the reactor was carried towards Seveso city. The smoke contained a high concentration of 2,4,5-trichlorophenol and TCDD.

The epidemiological survey showed that approximately 2000 people were exposed to dioxins: 300 of them suffered from skin disorders and 46 were hospitalized for severe medical problems. It was further found that more than 1000 animals were killed and an autopsy of a dead rabbit showed the presence of 255 mg TCDD g^{-1} liver tissue. The TCDD penetrated deep inside the soil, and the ecology of the surrounding area was also damaged significantly.

It has been reported [33] that birds, rabbits and chickens started dying 2–3 days after the accident. Some children and adults who were exposed to airborne dust consisting of reaction mixtures showed nausea along with swelling, redness and lesions in skin. In general the main toxicity symptoms included nausea, vomiting, headache and ultimate development of chloracne. A few exposed victims showed subclinical signs of impaired peripheral nervous system. The effects of TCDD released in the Seveso city explosion on pregnant women, the rate of abortions or stillbirths, the cancer incidences and immunotoxicity are not available in the literature.

Arizona episode. Human exposure to TCDD occurred at Globe, Arizona. The US forest service applied about 1656 kg of silvex and 54 kg of 2,4,5-T in Kellner Canyon–Russell Gulch Spray Project near Globe [33]. The harmful effects of the contaminant TCDD on the human population as well as on the ecology of the surrounding area became apparent immediately after the spraying.

Thus it can be concluded that TCDD present as contaminant in phenoxy herbicides can cause immunotoxicity, teratogenicity, and carcinogenicity during chronic and subacute exposure of experimental animals. There have been several disasters in which TCDD was released in the environment, causing human exposure. The data on the immunotoxic effects of TCDD on humans are not available, but on the basis of the data of experimental studies and in the opinion of the authors, it can be considered as a potent immunotoxic compound.

Toxic oil syndrome and oil toxicity

Toxic oil syndrome

In May 1981 a disease broke out in Madrid, Spain due to mass ingestion of illegally sold aniline adulterated rape seed oil. The aetiology of the disease was not known. However, because of its relationship with the ingestion of denatured rape seed oil, the disease was termed as 'aniline' toxic oil syndrome [36]. The withdrawal of rape seed oil from public use resulted in the disappearance of the acute phase of the disease. Between May 1981 and March 1984, 340 deaths and more than 20 000 cases were registered; at the height of the epidemic there were up to 600 hospital admissions every day.

The latency period from first ingestion of contaminated oil and the appearance of clinical symptoms varied and depended on the amount of oil absorbed and the frequency of ingestion. This latency period was about 1 week in the case of adults, whereas in children it was shorter.

The clinical symptoms during the acute phase of the disease included fever, respiratory dyspnoea, cough and exanthema. The other symptoms often seen in TOS included nausea, vomiting, headache, muscle pain and diarrhoea. Further examination showed the presence of non-cardiogenic pulmonary oedema, eosinophilia and increased levels of serum immunoglobulin E (IgE). Most of the cases of TOS mortality in the acute phase were due to respiratory failure. The patients showed skin changes like eczema patches and development of macules or papules. The immunological changes observed in acute-phase toxicity of TOS included increased serum IgE and the development of antinuclear/ antilymphocyte antibodies along with a reduced number of T lymphocytes leading to immunosuppression. Apparently TOS can cause autoimmune disorders producing antibodies against the self, thus inducing a life-threatening situation. Increased serum IgE levels are indicative of hypersensitivity reactions caused by TOS.

The immunological changes indicate alterations in the immune system and immunosuppression due to toxicity manifestations of TOS. A few patients showed clinical symptoms, such as pulmonary arterial hypertension, mesenteric thrombosis, myalgia, cramps and muscle weakness, thrombocytopenia, liver enzyme abnormalities and weight loss [36].

At first microbiological studies suggested that *Mycoplasma* infection in the oil could be the cause of the disease and raw oil was found to be more hazardous than the heated oil. The analysis of oil samples suggested that one or more components of the oil could be the cause of the syndrome, but as yet no specific component has been identified.

Subsequently the hunt for the causative agent focused on fatty acid anilides (FFAs), which were detected in significant amounts in suspected toxic oil samples. FAAs were shown to be immunogenic in rabbits [37] but all published reports on attempts to induce TOS-like lesions in experimental animals by the oral administration of either suspect oil or FAAs have failed. However, 1-phenyl-5-vinyl-2-imidazolidenethione (PVIZT), a phenlythiourea-derivative putatively produced following the interaction between aniline and certain isothiocyanites naturally occurring in industrial rape seed oil, has been shown to induce a local graft versus host reaction in a mouse assay system [38]. Although these observations clearly support the possibility that PVIZT or a similar compound may have the

potential to initiate an autoimmune response *in vivo* there is at present no explanation for the wide and diverse range of symptoms presented by the TOS patients.

As mentioned above, several important immunological features relevant to the present research proposal have been linked with TOS. Significantly raised IgE levels were noted in more than half of the early-phase patients yet other antibody isotypes remained within the control range [39,40]. Autoantibodies were also a commonly reported finding as characterized by an increased frequency of antinuclear, antipulmonary and antilymphocyte antibodies [41,42]. Perhaps more important, however, are the reports describing alterations in circulating T suppressor: T helper cell ratio [42,43]. These observations are clearly in accordance with the concept of toxin-induced immunodysfunction as manifested by the appearance of autoantibodies and significantly elevated IgE levels, two parameters that are usually maintained under strict suppressor cell control. The observation that the progressive multifocal lesions associated with TOS were similar to the pathological responses reported in graft versus host disease and certain drug or chemically induced autoallergic disease syndromes has led to the suggestion that TOS may have an autoallergic or graft versus host aetiology [44].

Argemone oil toxicity

Argemone oil is obtained from the seeds of *Argemonne mexicana* L. It is often used as an adulterant in edible oils such as mustard, sesame and groundnut oil in India and other tropical countries [45]. The consumption of argemone-contaminated oil, even for a short duration, results in diarrhoea, vomiting, erythema and breathlessness and swelling of the legs, together with glaucoma and cardiac arrest in extreme cases. The clinical symptoms following chronic ingestion of adulterated oil resemble those of dropsy [46]. The regular consumption of any edible oil contaminated with even as little as 0.1% of argemone oil may lead to epidemic dropsy. Other disorders like enlargement of the liver and respiratory distress may also be associated with argemone oil toxicity, leading to mortality due to cardiac arrest.

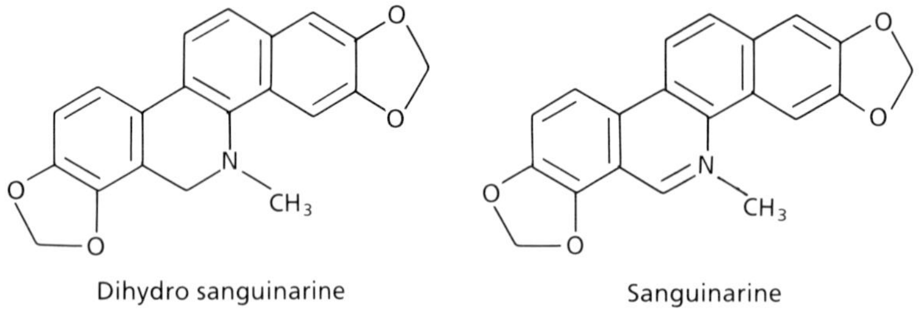

Dihydro sanguinarine   Sanguinarine

Fig. 14.4 Toxic alkaloids in argemone oil.

The toxicity of argemone oil is due to the presence of the physiologically active benzophenanthridine alkaloids, sanguinarine and dihydro sanguinarine [47] (Fig. 14.4). The histopathological investigations of argemone oil-intoxicated animals showed focal necrosis in liver together with vascular changes and a fatty liver [48].

Upreti *et al.* [49], while investigating the mechanism of argemone oil-induced toxicity, observed that intake of this oil can cause destruction of hepatic cytochrome P450 and inhibition of some monooxygenase activity as well as significant depletion of glutathione contents with a concomitant increase in microsomal lipid peroxidation. The same workers [50] have recently reported that hepatic microsomal as well as mitochondrial membrane is vulnerable to peroxidative attack and could be instrumental in causing hepatotoxicity symptoms observed in argemone oil-poisoning cases.

Corn oil

Corn oil is obtained from maize. It is a byproduct in wet milling of corn for the production of corn starch, corn syrup, glucose and dextrins etc. It has been reported that corn oil heated at 200°C for 2 h when fed to rats at a level of 20% in the diet caused growth retardation [51]. It has been further observed that larger dietary concentrations of corn oil inhibited the detoxification of hexabarbital and heptachlor by hepatic mixed function oxidases (MFO) enzymes [52]. Acute toxicity manifestations when sublethal doses of corn oil were taken in included diarrhoea, ataxia, loss in body weight, anorexia, and proteinuria. Death occurs due to respiratory failure with deep hypothermic coma [53]. A lethal oral-dose administration of corn oil produced local irritant inflammatory reactions in the tissues and the lining of the entire gastroenteral tract. Systemically, corn oil produced capillary venous congestion, sometimes with haemorrhage in many organs, such as the brain, heart, kidney, lung and liver.

Autopsy findings revealed that lethal oral doses of corn oil produced violent local irritant gastroenteritis which permitted the absorption of tiny droplets of corn oil in the blood stream and organs like the brain, kidney, lung. The animals fed with sublethal doses of corn oil also showed significantly reduced weight of organs like the liver, spleen and kidney.

The experimental work with mice has shown that animals fed with polyunsaturated fatty acids and 0.5% corn oil exhibited a reduced humoral immune response. Such animals after primary immunization with sheep red blood cells showed a lower number of IgM and IgG antigen-specific plaque-forming cells. Corn oil-fed animals also showed a decreased weight of spleen [54].

However, Barnett and Meena [55] have reported that cutaneous application of corn oil to suckling mice had no significant effect on cellular or humoral immunity. The antibody-secreting plaque-forming cells were non-significantly reduced.

Kerosene oil

Kerosene is one of several petroleum distillates obtained from the fractionation of crude petroleum oil. Recently there has been increasing concern over health hazards associated with petroleum products like kerosene and gasoline. Kerosene contains aliphatic, olefinic, naphthenic and polyaromatic hydrocarbons. It is commonly used as household burning oil in developing countries [56].

The major routes of kerosene exposure are through skin contact and inhalation. It has been reported that its prolonged skin contact may lead to the development of contact dermatitis and systemic toxic effects. At present relatively little is known about the toxicity manifestations of kerosene to other organs.

Rao *et al.* [57] have investigated the effect of repeated subcutaneous administration of kerosene oil to rats in order to study its toxic effects. These workers observed a significantly low lymphocyte count, increased weight of spleen and enlargement of lymph nodes (axial and popliteal) in exposed groups of rats. The histopathology of the spleen showed increased lymphopoiesis, but lymphoid follicles of white pulp were found to be depleted of their lymphocyte population. The red pulp showed signs of increased lymphoblastogenesis as well as mitotic figures, proplasmacytes and plasma cells. The thymus showed moderate atrophy of lobules, as was evident by a decrease in the density of cortical thymocytes. The histopathology of liver of kerosene-exposed rats exhibited characteristic changes of chronic venous congestion and necrosis of hepatocytes throughout the lobules. The adrenal glands showed moderate hypertrophy of the zona fasciculata together with prominent zona glomerulosa and zona veticularis of cortex.

These workers further observed an increase in DNA, RNA, protein and lipid contents in liver and spleen cells of kerosene oil-exposed rats. There was an increase in the activity of liver alkaline phosphatase and a decrease in benzo(a)pyrene hydroxylase, indicating the toxic effect of kerosene on hepatic metabolic machinery.

Upreti *et al.* [58] investigated the immunotoxic manifestations following repeated dermal exposure of mice to kerosene, simulating the actual human dermal exposure situation during occupational handling. The repeated dermal exposure to kerosene resulted in proliferation of stratum germinativum and oedema as well as infiltration of dermis, indicating its local irritant effect on skin. The kerosene-exposed mice showed a significant decrease in the weight of thymus, spleen, adrenal and abdominal lymph nodes. The thymus showed a marked reduction in cortical lymphocytes and loss of distinction between cortex and medulla. Bone marrow nucleated cell counts were also reduced in the group of mice exposed dermally to kerosene oil.

Thus it can be concluded that subcutaneous and dermal exposure to kerosene can lead to the toxicity of other organs of the body in addition to the skin, including the lymphoid organs resulting in immunotoxicity. This area needs extensive research, particularly in the case of occupational workers who face chronic exposure to kerosene oil.

Apart from the already mentioned toxicity of different oils, essential oils are also commonly used as flavouring agents, fragrances and perfumes. The immunotoxic manifestations of the essential oils are shown in Table 14.1.

Abrogation of toxicity of chemicals/toxicants by immunomodulation of host

Ray and colleagues [63,64] reported for the first time the abrogation of high-dose cyclophosphamide tox-

Table 14.1 Immunotoxicity of essential oils and flavouring agents

Name	Irritation	Sensitization/immunotoxic effect
Anise oil	Human—2%—no effect	Skin contact results in hypersensitivity reactions and erythema, vesiculation and scaling
Ginger oil	Rabbit—moderate	Use of cosmetics containing ginger oil may produce dermatitis
Spearmint oil	Rabbit—moderate Guinea pig—slight	Use of products containing spearmint oil (toothpaste) may lead to allergic stomatitis and dermatitis
Cinnamaldehyde	Human—8%—severe	Use in cosmetics may lead to the development of contact dermatitis

From [59–64].

icity by the administration of a multipotent immunostimulant, protein A of *Staphylococcus aureus* Cowan 1. Recent studies from our laboratory show that prior administration of protein A prevented carbon tetrachloride-induced hepatotoxicity, lymphoid organ toxicity and toxic insult to mixed-function oxidases [65,66,67]. The abrogation of cyclophosphamide and carbon tetrachloride-induced toxicity has been attributed to the ability of protein A to potentiate the reticuloendothelial system resulting in a quick removal of toxic metabolites from the body and accelerated repair and regeneration of depleted components [63,66].

Pandya *et al.* [68] from our laboratory have reported the reduction of toxicity induced by benzene using a synthetic immunostimulant and interferon-inducer polyinosinic polycytidilic acid (poly IC). These workers observed the restoration of superoxide dismutase and reversion of lipid peroxidation and hepatic necrosis induced by benzene following prior treatment with poly IC. The same workers further described the abrogation of the toxicity of benzene with a fungal interferon-inducer 6 mycelial fraction in acetone (6, MFA) [69].

Our observations [63–9] were supported by the findings from another laboratory, showing that the hepatotoxicity of acetaminophen has been found to be significantly reduced by stimulating the host with an immunomodulator and the interferon-inducer poly (rl-rc) [70].

Thus, a hypothesis (Ray's hypothesis) has emerged, primarily through our own studies and supported by others, that stimulation of the immune system (by immunomodulators) can reduce the toxicity of drugs and chemicals, probably due to increased and stimulated activity of the reticuloendothelial system for quick metabolism and removal of toxic metabolites from the body. The use of immunomodulators for immunopotentiation mediated by way of releasing lymphokines like γ-interferon, which may be responsible for the abrogation of toxicity rendered by drugs and chemicals can be considered as a newly emerging area of research interest throughout the world.

Finally it may be mentioned that host immunopotentiation by immunomodulators forms a very useful modality to abrogate the toxicity rendered by drugs and chemicals.

Conclusions

From the above description it can be concluded that TCDD exposure can cause a wide variety of toxicity manifestations including teratogenicity, foetotoxicity, immunotoxicity and carcinogenicity.

The toxicity rendered by toxic oils, oil adulterants and TOS can also lead to an impairment in immune status resulting in autoimmune disorders and immunosuppression.

A cautious and judicious use of phenoxy herbicides should be made and their indiscriminate use as chemical warfare agents must not be allowed. A control over the use of oil adulterants is also required.

Immunotoxicity evaluation of environmental toxicants is a relatively new developing area where much remains to be done. There is not much literature available on immunotoxicity of oils. We strongly suggest that there should be a comprehensive programme for immunotoxicity testing and the evaluation of different oils. Thereafter, the initial lead to reverse toxicity of chemicals and drugs by immunopotentiation of the host should be followed up enthusiastically.

Acknowledgements

The authors would like to thank Mr N. Garg for providing computer assistance.

References

1 Ray PK. Environmental toxicants, immunity infection and cancer. In: Hamig JP, Mhatre PM, Seth PR, Ray PK, eds. *Proceedings of the Indo-US Workshop on the Role of Predisposing Conditions of Health, Nutrition and Environment on Safety of Drugs and Chemicals.* Lucknow: ITRC, 1990 (in press).

2 Ray PK, Prasad AK. Environmental carcinogens and immune functions of the host. *J Sci Ind Res* 1987; 46:162–7.

3 Ray PK. Environmental toxicant induced immunosuppression and cancer: a great problem in the developing world. In: Ruchirawat M, Shank RC, eds. *Environmental Toxicity and Carcinogenesis*, Bangkok: Text and Journal Corporation, 1986:309–11.

4 Ray PK. Environmental pollution and cancer. *J Sci Ind Res* 1986; 45:370–1.

5 Ray PK, Saxena AK, Singh KP. Immunomodulation of

host as a predictive bioindicator of toxicity in the mammalian system. *Def Sci J* 1987; 37:245–55.

6 Ray PK, Singh KP. Immunotoxicologic studies and its potential. In: Mulky MJ, Srivastava HC, Vatsya B, eds. *Research in Industry.* New Delhi: Oxford and IBH, 1987:168–78.

7 Ahling BA, Lindskog B, Janssen B, Sundstrom G. Formation of polychlorinated dibenzo-*p*-dioxins and dibenzo furans during the composition of a 2,4,5-T formulation. *Chemosphere* 1977; 6:381–5.

8 Stockman MM. Syndrome of kerosene induced hemolysis. *Am J Dis Child* 1942; 74:32–44.

9 Young AL. The chlorinated dibenzo-*p*-dioxins. In: Borey RW, Young AL, eds. *The Science of 2,4,5-T and Associated Phenoxy Herbicides.* USA: John Wiley; 1980:133–205.

10 Piper WN, Rose JQ, Gehring PJ. Excretion and tissue distribution of TCDD in rat. *Adv Chem Ser* 1973; 120:85–91.

11 Allen JR, Van Miller JP, Norback DH. Tissue distribution excretion and biological effects of (^{14}C) TCDD in rats. *Food Cosmet Toxicol* 1975; 13:501–5.

12 Gasiewica TA, Neal RA. Tissue distribution and excretion of TCDD and effects upon clinical chemical parameters in the guinea pig. *Fed Proc* 1978; 37:501–4.

13 Schwetz BA, Norris JM, Sparschy GL, Rowe VK, Gehring PJ, Emerson JL, Gerbig CG. Toxicity of chlorinated dibenzo-*p*-dioxins. *Environ Hlth Perspect* 1973; 5:87–99.

14 Harris MW, Moore JG, Vos JG, Gupta BN. General biological effects of TCDD in laboratory animals. *Environ Hlth Perspect* 1973; 5:101–9.

15 Cunningham HM, Williams DT. Effect of TCDD on growth rate and synthesis of lipids and proteins in rats. *Bull Environ Contam Toxicol* 1972; 7:45–51.

16 Van Miller JP, Marlar RJ, Allen JR. Tissue distribution and excretion of tritiated TCDD in non-human primates and rats. *Food Cosmet Toxicol* 1976; 14:31–4.

17 Gupta BN, Vos JG, Moore JA, Zinkl JG, Bullock BC. Pathologic effects of TCDD in laboratory animals. *Environ Hlth Perspect* 1973; 5:125–40.

18 Vos JG, Moore JA. Suppression of cellular immunity in rats and mice by maternal treatment with 2,3,7,8-tetrachlorodibenzo-p-dioxin. *Int Arch Allergy Appl Immunol* 1974; 47:777–94.

19 Thigpen JE, Faith RE, McConnel EE, Moore JA. Increased susceptibility to bacterial infection as a sequela of exposure of TCDD. *Infect Immun* 1975; 12:1319–24.

20 Allen RR, Barsotti DA, Van Miller JP, Abrahamson LJ, Lalich JJ. Morphological changes in monkey consuming diet containing low levels of TCDD. *Food Cosmet Toxicol* 1977; 15:401–10.

21 Miller K. Various mechanisms in chemically induced injury. In: Gibson GG, Hubbard R, Park DV, eds. *Immunotoxicology.* London: Academic Press, 1983: 196–203.

22 Buu-Hoi NP, Chanh H, Saint-Ruf G. Organs as target of 'dioxin' (TCDD) intoxication. *Naturwissensch* 1972; 59:174–5.

23 Vos JG, Moore JA, Zinkl JG. Toxicity of TCDD in C57 Bl/6 mice. *Toxicol Appl Pharmacol* 1974; 29:229–41.

24 Van Miller JP, Lalich JJ, Allen JR. Increased incidence of neoplasma in rats exposed to low levels of TCDD. *Chemosphere* 1977; 9:537–44.

25 Kociba RJ, Keyes DG, Beyer JE *et al.* Results of two year chronic toxicity and oncogenicity study of TCDD in rats. *Toxicol Appl Pharmacol* 1978; 46:279–303.

26 Kouri RE, Salerno RA, Whitemire CE. Relationship between AHH inducibility and sensitivity to chemically induced subcutaneous sarcoma in various strains of mice. *J Natl Cancer Inst* 1973; 50:363–8.

27 Neubert D, Zens P, Rothenwallner A, Merker HJ. A survey of embryotoxic effect of TCDD in mammalian species. *Environ Hlth Perspect* 1973; 5:67–79.

28 Smith FA, Schewtz BA, Nitchke KD. Teratogenicity of 2,3,7,8-tetrachlorodibenzo-*p*-dioxin in CF-1 mice. *Toxicol Appl Pharmacol* 1976; 38:517–23.

29 Moore JA, Gupta BN, Zinkl JG, Vos JG. Postnatal effect of maternal exposure of TCDD. *Environ Hlth Perspect* 1973; 5:81–5.

30 Becker D. The effect of folate overdose and 2,3,7,8-tetrachlorodibenzo-*p*-dioxin (TCDD) on kidney and liver respectively of rat and mouse embryos. *Teratol* 1973; 8:215–19.

31 Smith FA, Scjwetz BA, Nitchke KD. Teratogenicity of 2, 3, 7, 8-tetrachlorodibenzo-p-dioxin in CF-1 mice. *Toxicol Appl Pharmacol* 1976; 38:517–23.

32 Sparschu GL, Dunn FL, Rowe VK. Study of the teratogenicity 2,3,7,8-tetrachlorodibenzo-*p*-dioxin in the rat. *Food Cosmet Toxicol* 1971; 9:405–12.

33 Young AL, Calcaqni JA, Thalkeon CE, Tremblay JW, eds. *The Toxicology, Environmental Fate and Human Risk of Herbicide Orange.* USAF OEHL Technical Report No. TR-78-92; 1978.

34 Carter CD, Kimbrough JA, Liddle RE, Cline MM, Zack WF Jr, Barthel RE, Phillips PE. Tetrachlorodibenzo: an accidental poisoning episode in horse arenas. *Science* 1975; 188:738–40.

35 Hay AWM. Tetrachlorodibenzo-p-dioxin release at Seveso. *Disasters* 1977; 1:289–304.

36 Philippe G, Stanislaw T, eds. Toxic oil syndrome—mass food poisoning in Spain. *Report on WHO Meeting.* Copenhagen: WHO Publication Office, 1984:1–92.

37 Marquez A, Larraga V, Diez JL, Amel C, Rodrigo J, Munoz E, Pestana A. Immunogenicity and the pathogenesis of the toxic oil syndrome. *Experentia* 1984; 40:977–80.

38 Kammuller ME, Pennicks, Seinen W. Spanish toxic oil syndrome and chemically-induced graft-versus-host like reactions. *Lancet* 1984; ii:805-6.

39 Tabuenca JH. Toxic allergic syndrome caused by the ingestion of rape seed oil denatured with aniline. *Lancet* 1981; ii:567–8.

40 Blanca M, Boulton P, Brostoff J. Toxic oil syndrome, clinical and immunological characteristics: a review. *Clin Allergy* 1984; 14:165–8.

41 Toxic Epidemic Syndrome Study Group. Toxic epidemic syndrome, Spain. 1981. *Lancet* 1982; ii:697–702.

42 Gomez-Reino JJ. Immune system disorders associated with adulterated cooking oil. In: Berlin A, Dean J, Draper MH, Smith EMR, Spreafico F, eds. *Immunotoxicology.* Dordrecht: Martinus Nijhoff, 1987:376–9.

43 Lahoz C, Tricas L, Vela C, Lauzurica P, Curbindo C, Garcia R. Hyper IgE, eosinophilia and immunological hyper-reactivity due to the ingestion of adulterated rape seed oil (toxic oil syndrome). *Eur J Resp Dis* 1983; 64(suppl):415–18.

44 Gleichmann H, Gleichmann E. GVHD: a model for Spanish toxic oil syndrome. *Lancet* 1984; i:1474.

45 Khanna SK, Singh GB. *Argemone mexicana* strikes again. *Sci Rep* 1983; 20:108–10.

46 Mohan M, Sood NN, Dayal Y, Bhatnagar S. Ocular and clinicoepidemiological study of epidemic. *Med Res* 1984; 80:449–56.

47 Sarkar SN. Isolation from argemone oil of dihydrosanguinarine and sanguinarine: toxicity of sanguinarien. *Nature* 1948; 162:265–6.

48 Chandra S, Mukherjee SK, Sethi NC. Effect of argemone oil feeding on blood biochemistry and tissue changes in albino rats. *Ind J Med Sci* 1972; 26:308–12.

49 Upreti KK, Das M, Khanna SK. Biochemical toxicology of argemone oil. Effect on hepatic xenobiotic metabolizing enzymes. *J Appl Toxicol* 1991 (in press).

50 Upreti KK, Das M, Khanna SK. Biochemical toxicology of argemone alkaloids. III. Effect on lipid peroxidation in different subcellular fraction of liver. *Toxicol Lett* 1988; 42:301–8.

51 Stecher PG, Windholz M, Leachy DS, Bolton DM, Eaton LG. *The Mercks Index. An Encyclopedia of Chemicals and Drugs.* 8th edn. Rahway, NJ: Meerderos, 1968.

52 Caster WO, Wade AE, Greene FE, Medows JS. Effect of different levels of corn oil on the rate of hexabarbital, heptachlor and aniline metabolism in the liver of male white rat. *Life Sci* 1970; 9:185–9.

53 Boyd EM, Boulanger MA, Carsky E. The acute oral toxicity of corn oil. *J Clin Pharmacol* 1969; 9:137–42.

54 Erickson KL, Adams DA, Scibenski RJ. Dietary fatty acid modulation of murine B-cell responsiveness. *J Nutr* 1986; 116:1830–40.

55 Barnett JB, Meena JH. The effect of precutaneously applied corn oil on the immune response of suckling mouse. *J Environ Pathol Toxicol Oncol* 1984; 5:353-6.

56 WHO. *Environmental Health Criteria 20: Selected Petroleum Products.* Geneva: World Health Organization, 1982:58–9.

57 Rao GS, Kannan K, Goel SK, Pandya KP, Shanker R. Subcutaneous kerosene toxicity in albino rats. *Environ Res* 1984; 35:516–30.

58 Upreti RK, Das M, Shanker R. Dermal exposure to kerosene. *Vet Hum Toxicol* 1989; 31:16–20.

59 Larsen WG. Perfume dermatitis. *Arch Dermatol* 1977; 113:623–8.

60 Rudzki E, Grzywazz, Brud WS. Sensitivity to 35 essential oils. *Contact Derm* 1976; 2:196–102.

61 *Clinical Toxicology of Commercial Products.* Gosselin RE (ed.) Baltimore: Williams & Wilkins, 1984.

62 Dannemen PJ, Booman KA, Dorsky J *et al.* Cinnamic aldehyde: a survey of consumer patch test sensitization. *Fd Chem Toxicol* 1983; 21:721–5.

63 Ray PK, Dohadwala M, Bandyopadhyay SK, Canchanapan P, Mc Laughlin D. Rescue of rats from large dose cyclophosphamide toxicity using protein A. *Cancer Chemother Pharmacol* 1985; 4:59–62.

64 Dohadwala M, Ray PK. *In vivo* protection by protein A of hepatic microsomal mixed function oxgenase system of cyclophosphamide treated rats. *Cancer Chemother Pharmacol* 1985; 14:135-8.

65 Singh KP, Saxena AK, Zaidi SIA, Dwivedi PD, Srivastava SP, Seth PK, Ray PK. Protection against carbon tetrachloride-induced hepatotoxicity by protein A. *J Appl Toxicol* 1988; 8:407–10.

66 Srivastava SP, Singh KP, Saxena AK, Seth PK, Ray PK. *In vivo* protection by protein A of hepatic microsomal mixed function oxidase system of CC14 administered rats. *Biochem Pharmacol* 1987; 36:4055–8.

67 Singh KP, Zaidi SIA, Raisuddin, Saxena AK, Dwivedi PD, Seth PK, Ray PK. Protection against carbon tetrachloride induced lymphoid organ toxicity in rats by protein A. *Toxicol Lett* 1990; 51: 339–51.

68 Pandya KP, Khan S, Umashanker A, Krishnamurthy R, Ray PK. Modulation of benzene toxicity by poly insoinic: polycytidilic acid—an interferon inducer. *Biochem Biophys Acta* 1989; 991:23–9.

69 Pandya KP, Shanker R, Gupta A, Khan WA, Ray PK. Modulation of benzene toxicity by an interferon inducer (6 MFA). *Toxicol* 1986; 39:291-305.

70 Renton KW, Dickson G. The prevention of acetaminophen-induced hepatotoxicity by interferon inducer poly (rl-rc). *Toxicol Appl Pharmacol* 1984; 72:40–5.

Part IV
Methods of assessing immunotoxic events in experimental systems

15

Hypersensitivity: adverse drug reactions

JANET M. DEWDNEY & ROBERT G. EDWARDS

Introduction

Drug hypersensitivity is the most readily recognized clinical manifestation of immunotoxicity in humans. The incidence of immunologically mediated adverse drug reactions is unknown and widely differing estimates have been made [1]. The true figure will not be known until accurate clinical diagnosis is possible. The problems associated with the diagnosis of drug hypersensitivity have been assessed previously [2]. In some situations, notably those involving multi-drug therapy, there is difficulty in establishing a causal relationship between drug administration and the adverse event. There is even more difficulty in establishing the underlying pathogenesis and without objective tests it is impossible to be certain that the reaction is a consequence of immune derangement. More often than not, the conclusion that an adverse drug reaction is of immunological aetiology is based on no more than presumptive logic involving past experience with the drug or drug class together with the clinical impression that the observed syndrome shares characteristic, though not specific, features with known immunologically driven reactions. Clearly this provides an inadequate database from which to try to assess the importance of immunotoxic phenomena in adverse drug reactions.

Preclinical assessment of the potential of drugs to give rise to hypersensitivity reactions in humans is no less difficult. The science of toxicology has developed along target-organ-specific lines and the immune system, although widely distributed throughout the body, can be regarded as an organ which is subject, like other organs in the body, to chemical-induced damage. Such damage might arise through direct toxic effects leading to generalized immune dysfunction. More relevant to the question of hypersensitivity adverse drug reactions, however, is immunotoxicity which is a consequence of interaction of the chemical agent with the immune system which leads to a specific immune response. In these circumstances, the initial target of the immunotoxic effects is more limited although the eventual consequences may affect many organs of the body. The manifestations of this type of immunotoxicity may be allergic drug reactions mediated through immunoglobulin E (IgE)-based mechanisms, antibody or immune complex-mediated tissue damage or cell-mediated reactions, including contact sensitization.

The clonal-specific immune response which underlies drug hypersensitivity differs significantly from direct organ-targeted immunotoxicity and the two represent fundamentally different challenges for the toxicologist. Strategies for immunotoxicology are being actively sought and several testing protocols have been published [3–7]. Bloom et al. [7] have drawn attention to the two main approaches which could be adopted. One strategy would be to determine whether a new chemical entity undergoing preclinical safety evaluation possessed the potential to exert an adverse effect on the immune system by introducing stand-alone studies for all new drugs. The alternative strategy is to integrate studies on the immune system into conventional repeat-dose toxicology studies [8,9] and to employ immune function testing directed towards clarifying the importance of any immune system changes noted. This problem-driven approach has much to recommend it as it allows selection of immunological tests most appropriate for investigation of an identified concern. Neither strategy, however, can currently be adopted to give risk-assessment data on drug hypersensitivity.

Discriminating predictive tests do not exist. Methods are available by which the ability of a drug or chemical to induce a specific immune response may be assessed and the structural determinants for some drug allergens are being established [10–14]. It is possible that studies of these kinds, backed by adequate clinical studies, might lead to a testing strategy for drug hypersensitivity but it seems likely that the low incidence and idiosyncratic nature of many of these reactions will impose severe constraints on predictive risk assessment. It is something of a paradox that we are least able to predict risks from animal studies for that category of adverse drug reaction deemed to be, in spite of diagnostic confusion, relatively common and of significant clinical concern.

It is not our intention in this chapter to catalogue hypersensitivity and autoimmune drug reactions. Several recent publications provide an invaluable source of such information [15,16]. Rather, it is our aim to draw attention to the issues which face immunotoxicologists charged with the task of developing risk-assessment strategies for drug hypersensitivity and to indicate some directions which might prove fruitful in the future. The focus of our review is classical drug allergy, that is, immediate hypersensitivity reactions mediated through IgE antibody. This type of reaction is of special concern. Clinical syndromes can be life-threatening and include anaphylaxis and severe urticarial or oedematous reactions, but because of the idiosyncratic nature of such reactions and their low incidence, the immunotoxicology challenge is immense.

Many other types of hypersensitivity tissue damage may be induced by drugs, including immune complex deposition, complement-mediated tissue damage and cell-mediated hypersensitivity. All by definition involve the induction by the drug, directly or indirectly, of an immune response specific for the drug itself, for a biotransformation product thereof, or for host tissue modified in some way by the drug to give rise to neo-antigens. Tissue damage induced by these pathways should be recognized in preclinical studies and trigger the need for immunological function testing. Advances are being made in histopathology techniques; these will improve the accuracy and sensitivity with which immune complex deposition or organ damage can be detected. Notable amongst these advances are the use of immunofluorescence and other cytofluorometric techniques; their use as part of conventional safety clearance programmes can be anticipated [8,17].

Cell-mediated immunity and its major clinical syndromes, contact sensitization and photoallergy, also require specific consideration. The predictive value of animal models is reasonably well accepted and the preclinical identification of potential contact drug allergens presents no major difficulties [18–20]. This topic is discussed in detail elsewhere in this publication.

Preclinical testing for hypersensitivity potential

The majority of drugs used in clinical practice are low molecular weight entities (<1000 Da) but recombinant DNA technology is making possible the therapeutic use of proteins heretofore unaccessible. These two drug groups represent fundamentally different challenges to the immunotoxicologist. Low molecular weight drugs are not, as such, recognized by the immune system and must conjugate *in vivo* to macromolecules to initiate antigen recognition and uptake. In contrast, proteins are intrinsically immunogenic and safety evaluation strategies appropriate to the one class may be of limited value for the other.

Low molecular weight drugs

Two general approaches to the introduction of a strategy for the preclinical assessment of potential drug allergens are being evaluated in different laboratories. One is based on the expectation that it will be possible to develop animal models which mimic clinical hypersensitivity reactions. The second is a mechanistic approach which assumes that all low molecular weight drug allergens possess certain chemical properties which can be evaluated to give an assessment of potential allergenicity.

Animal models. Animal models of hypersensitivity reactions, especially asthma and other respiratory disorders, exist and have been used in the evaluation of potential new drugs [21]. The application of these models to preclinical toxicological evaluation of allergenic potential, however, is not established, although the principle of using them for this purpose has been considered previously [22]. Most advances in this area are being made in relation to chemicals which cause occupational asthma. Detailed study of animal responses to toluene diisocyanate, a reactive chemical responsible for respiratory dysfunction in exposed workers, has been made and the role of the animal models for toxicological purposes discussed [23–25]. Botham *et al.* [26,27] have extended these studies and it is possible that models which predict the ability of chemicals to induce respiratory allergy may develop from these preliminary studies (see Chapter 12 for detailed discussion of occupational asthma). Gleichmann [28] and Kammüller and Seinen [29] have evaluated an animal model, the popliteal lymph node assay, which may be useful in predicting drugs likely to cause drug-induced autoimmunity but a substantial amount of validation and standardization work needs to be done before the predictive capability of the test can be accepted. Transgenic animals offer the prospect of modelling certain allergic and autoimmune conditions and these may become important in immunotoxicological strategies [30,31]. In the near future it is more likely that they will increase our knowledge of disease pathogenesis rather than play a role in the predictive assessment of risk.

It has been noted earlier that animal models exist which are of value in predicting the capability of a chemical or drug to cause contact sensitization and many of these are now included in regulatory guidelines [32]. This topic is dealt with elsewhere in this publication. However, we believe that these animal models may be valuable in the more general allergy risk assessment of new chemical entities, as discussed below.

Mechanistic approach. In contrast to the use of disease-oriented animal models, our overall strategy has been to approach the problem of the immunotoxicology of drug allergens from a different perspective. We are, thus, evaluating a mechanistic approach. Many of the determinants of an allergic response are beyond the reach of the immunotoxicologist, but central to the generation of such responses is an underlying immune response. Isotype specificity may be different and is to a large extent host-determined, but the drug must be capable of inducing an immune response if it is to act as an allergen. It has been recognized for many years that a key initial step in generating an immunogenic response to a low molecular substance is reaction between the chemical and protein carrier molecules and that further, there can be a close association between the ability of the chemical to form covalent bonds with macromolecules and contact sensitization induction in the guinea pig [33–35]. However, most drugs do not possess such intrinsic reactivity and a key issue in analysis of drug immunogenicity is to what extent the protein-reactive moiety is not the parent drug but a reactive metabolite of it formed during *in vivo* biotransformation processes.

Park *et al.* [36] in a review point out that whereas the role of chemically reactive metabolites in the induction of carcinogenesis is well recognized, their role in immunotoxicity is less understood. It seems likely that such metabolites will prove to be important not only as mediators of organ damage but also in the initiating events which lead to hypersensitivity. Critical also to understanding drug immunogenicity and antigenicity is consideration of the influence of hapten density, that is, the degree to which the drug is able to substitute in macromolecular carriers, the nature of the host-derived carrier itself and the biochemical stability of any conjugates formed [37–41].

The strategy we are investigating is based on these considerations and is outlined in Table 15.1. There is no possibility of such an approach being acceptable at the regulatory level at this time but it does provide a useful framework within which the problems of assessing the potential of a new chemical entity to cause hypersensitivity can be considered. We will describe our experiences to date using this approach. However, it is necessary to present a number of caveats. The majority of drugs being developed for clinical use will not possess intrinsic protein reactivity and methods must be developed which allow assessment of the reactivity of metabolic products arising from drug biotransformation. It is self-evident that immunogenicity and allergenicity, although both the consequence of the immunochemical properties of the initiating drug, cannot be equated. Allergenicity is considerably more restrictive, depending as it does on host-determined factors, and is not, at this time, able to be predicted from preclinical studies. Animal studies on immunogenicity can, however, provide a basis for assessing the potential of the drug to be an allergen.

It is equally self-evident that such studies must be carried out using the parent drug; the use of drug–protein conjugates, while of value in the development of appropriate assays, gives no information on the immunogenic potential of the drug.

Our use of guinea pig contact sensitization models requires comment. The use of these models to predict skin sensitization potential has received much attention [18–20,42]. In our experience, these models may also be of value in that, because high local concentration of drug can be achieved on the skin and because of the drug-metabolizing properties of skin [43], the model provides a means of detecting immune responses to the parent drug or metabolite in the absence of knowledge of the precise drug determinants involved.

Preliminary studies have been carried out to assess the value of this approach. Two structurally different compounds have been investigated—streptomycin and piperazine (Fig. 15.1).

Streptomycin is immunogenic in humans, can give rise to contact sensitization and has been associated with allergic drug reactions [44–47].

Piperazine, an anthelmintic drug, has been reported to induce occupational asthma and dermatitis in workers manufacturing the compound [48,49], and in nursing staff handling the drug [50]. More recently it has been noted that allergic asthma caused by piperazine can be associated with the presence of IgE antibody [51].

The results of our evaluation of these two drugs are summarized in Table 15.2. The predicted reactivity of the aldehyde group in streptomycin (Fig. 15.1a) was confirmed by *in vivo* studies and resulted in the subsequent immune responsiveness. Some comparative studies using dihydrostreptomycin, which does not contain a reactive aldehyde, and which has not been shown to be a drug allergen, confirmed the importance of this moiety in initiating the events leading to allergenicity.

Piperazine has no functional groups capable of reaction with nucleophiles (Fig. 15.1b) and no such reactivity was found *in vitro*. However, piperazine proved to be a potent contact sensitizer and to induce drug-related antibody, although further work is required to define fully the specificity of the antibody. We believe that these results underline the need for an *in vivo* evaluation for drug allergens, in which any immunogenic consequences of the formation of reactive metabolites from an unreactive parent drug can be determined.

1 Preliminary assessments	Are there any allergenicity indicators from preclinical toxicology, clinical reactions or drug class/structure considerations?	
2 Drug reactivity	Is the drug reactive with nucleophiles such as amino or thiol groups found on proteins?	
3 Immunogenicity	Does the drug immunize animals to give drug-related antibody?	
4 Contact sensitivity	Is the drug a contact sensitizer?	
5 Recommendations	What recommendations can be made resulting from points 1–4?	

Table 15.1 Strategy to investigate the potential allergenicity of drugs

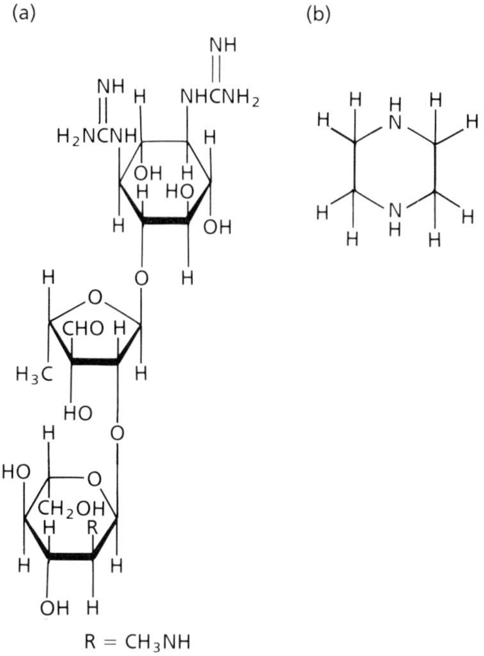

Fig. 15.1 Chemical structures of (a) streptomycin and (b) piperazine.

We have insufficient cumulative data at this stage to be confident about the impact results of these kinds should have had if they had been generated during the safety clearance programme of a new chemical entity. It is our current view that they should not have prevented progression of the drug to the clinic. However some potential warning signs had been identified. Clearly a drug with this profile would not be a suitable candidate for topical use in humans. A contained manufacturing process would have been recommended to ensure worker safety. Finally, immunological monitoring of early clinical trials would have been justified and any adverse drug reactions evaluated carefully for evidence of an immunological aetiology.

We challenged our strategic approach with a more daunting problem, comparative allergenicity within a class of compounds. Whilst the allergenicity of penicillins and cephalosporins has been studied extensively, the immunological properties of other β-lactam-containing drugs are less well investigated. Two such β-lactams are the clavams and the carbapenems, exemplified by potassium clavulanic acid and MM22383 respectively (Fig. 15.2 iii and ix). The studies undertaken on these two substances have been published [52] but the main findings are noted here as illustrative of some of the principles involved. In common with other β-lactam-containing compounds both had structural features which could lead to protein reactivity, a reactive carbonyl group, and both were shown in *in vitro* studies to interact with protein nucleophiles. However, *in vivo* studies showed that only MM22383 induced immunological responses, both antibody production and contact sensitization; clavulanic acid gave no detectable immune response (Table 15.3). These results are attributable to differences in degradation pathways for the two compounds. Based on studies by Pfaendler *et al.* [53], MM22383 would be expected to react with nucleophiles to give the

Table 15.2 Results of applying the allergenicity strategy to streptomycin and piperazine

Results for streptomycin	Strategy	Results for piperazine
Positive—reactive aldehyde group in structure	Preliminary assessments	Negative—no potentially reactive groups
Positive—reacts with thiol groups	Drug reactivity	Negative—unreactive with amino and thiol groups
Positive—streptomycin-specific antibody obtained	Immunogenicity	Positive—piperazine-related antibody obtained
Positive—14/20 animals sensitized	Contact sensitivity	Positive—17/18 animals sensitized
Streptomycin has allergenic potential	Recommendations	Piperazine has allergenic potential

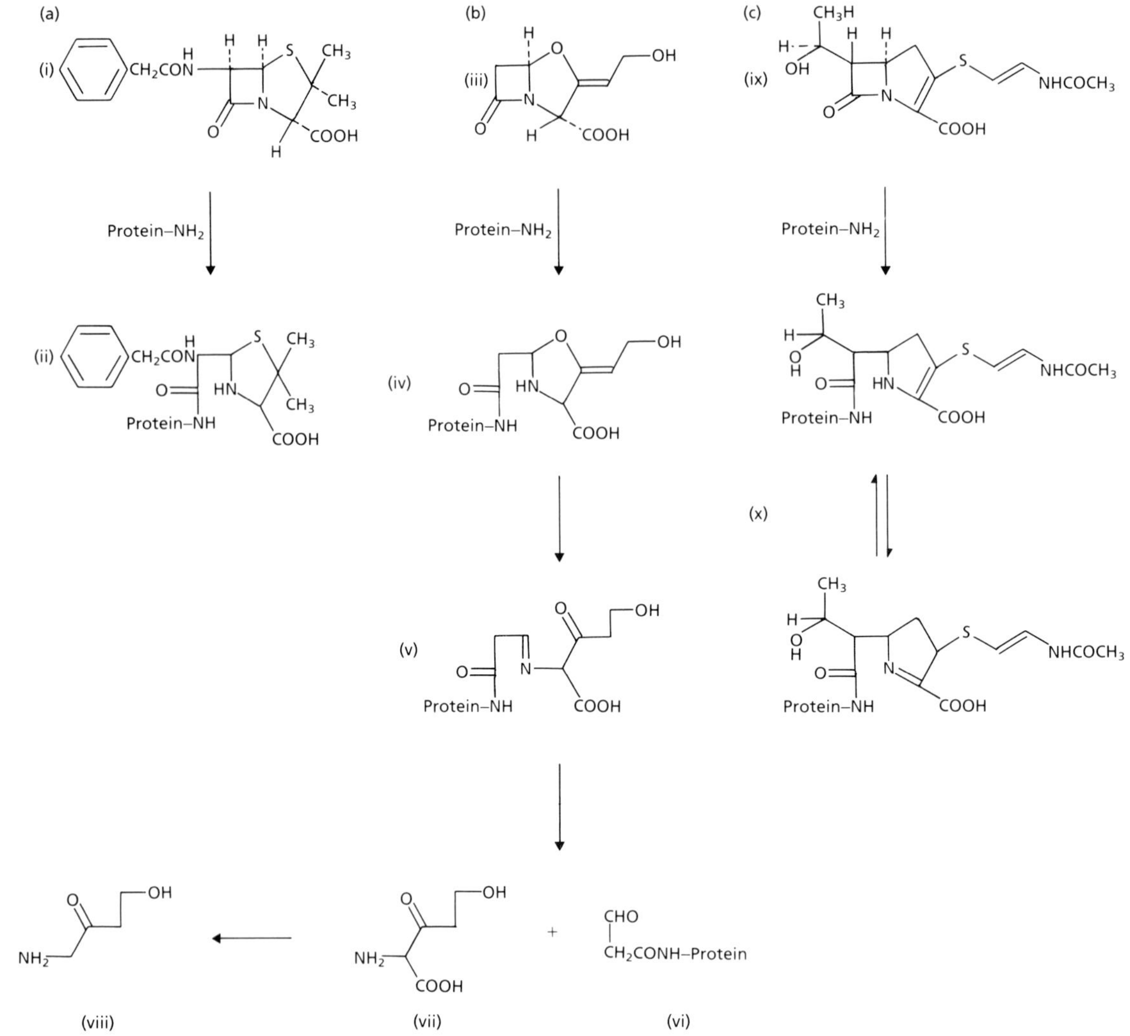

Fig. 15.2 Sequences for reaction of (a) benzyl penicillin; (b) clavulanic acid; and (c) MM22383 with protein amino groups.

relatively stable dihydrazole ring (Fig. 15.2x) analogous to the penicilloyl structure formed by penicillins (Fig. 15.2ii). Based on studies by Finn *et al.* [54] and Haginaka *et al.* [55], clavulanic acid would be expected to give a much more complex spectrum of products (Fig. 15.2b), resulting in heterogeneous conjugates with a number of haptenic determinants present. The resulting conjugates would be equivalent to sparsely substituted conjugates which are known to be poorly immunogenic [37,38]. The results suggest that in clinical use clavulanic acid is

likely to be less allergenic than many other β-lactam-containing drugs, and indicate that even within a drug class classically associated with drug allergy, differences in allergenic potential can be defined using the strategic approach outlined.

A further example illustrates the type of challenge likely to confront the immunotoxicologist developing predictive tests for drug allergenicity. In the above examples, the trigger which would alert the toxicologist to the need for immunotoxicity testing was structural features, that is, the presence of

Table 15.3 Results of applying the allergenicity strategy to clavulanic acid and MM22383

Results for clavulanic acid	Strategy	Results for MM22383
Positive—reactive β-lactam group in structure	Preliminary assessments	Positive—reactive β-lactam group in structure. Specific IgE antibody-mediated occupational allergy case
Positive—reacts with amino groups	Drug reactivity	Positive—reacts with amino groups
Negative—no clavulanic acid-specific antibody obtained	Immunogenicity	Positive—MM22383-specific antibody obtained
Negative—0/6 animals sensitized	Contact sensitivity	Positive—4/6 animals sensitized
Clavulanic acid has low allergenic potential	Recommendations	MM22383 has allergenic potential

potentially reactive groupings and extensive knowledge of the *β*-lactams as drug allergens.

It is equally important to be able to address the problem exemplified by two anti-depressant drugs, zimeldine and paroxetine. Zimeldine (zimelidine; Fig. 15.3) is a 5-hydroxytryptamine (5HT) uptake inhibitor with anti-depressant properties. It has been associated with adverse effects (influenza-like syndrome, Guillain–Barré-type neuropathy) which were considered immunological in nature [56]. Paroxetine (Fig. 15.3) is a novel 5HT uptake inhibitor with anti-depressant properties [57,58] and although it is structurally unrelated to zimeldine, it was felt prudent to investigate the allergenic potential of paroxetine [59]. The strategy in Table 15.1 formed the basis of the investigations and the results are shown in Table 15.4.

Neither paroxetine nor zimeldine would be predicted to react with protein-derived nucleophiles and the *in vitro* studies confirmed this. Paroxetine also failed to immunize rabbits and no antibody was detected in sera from treated patients or from rats treated with paroxetine for 1 year. Contact sensitivity studies with paroxetine were also negative and no antibody was detectable in the sera from these animals. Zimeldine was not so extensively studied for antibody induction but it was a contact sensitizer in guinea pigs, confirming previous studies in humans. Therefore in these studies zimeldine was shown to have allergenic potential through its contact-sensitizing ability, although the adverse reaction associated with its use was unrelated to this phenomenon. We predicted from these studies that paroxetine was unlikely to have allergenic effects.

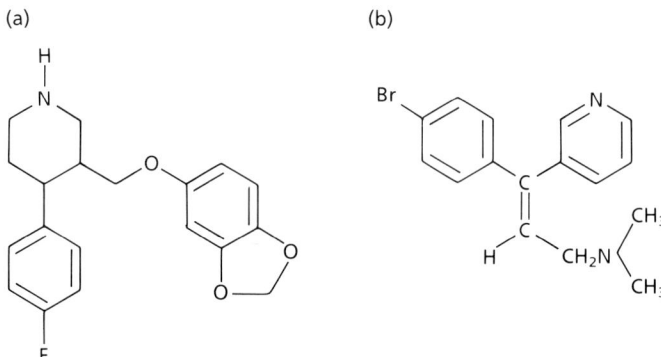

Fig. 15.3 Chemical structures of (a) paroxetine and (b) zimeldine.

Table 15.4 Results of applying the allergenicity strategy to zimeldine and paroxetine

Results for zimeldine	Strategy	Results for paroxetine
Positive—possible immune-mediated reactions in some patients, but no reactive groups in structure	Preliminary assessments	Negative—no preclinical or clinical problems, no reactive groups in structure
Negative—not reactive with amino or thiol groups	Drug reactivity	Negative—not reactive with amino or thiol groups
Not tested	Immunogenicity	Negative—no drug-specific/related antibody obtained
Positive—20/38 animals sensitized	Contact sensitivity	Negative—0/40 animals sensitized
Zimeldine has allergenic potential	Recommendations	Paroxetine unlikely to have allergenic potential

These preliminary studies and applications of a predictive strategy on several structurally diverse compounds suggest that it may be of value. However an omission amongst the tests is an *in vitro* assessment of the formation of reactive metabolites from drugs. Two papers [60,61] may provide the basis of such tests. Both methods employ glutathione to trap reactive metabolites formed after incubation of drug with microsomal fractions from rat liver. Mulder and Le [60] employed tritiated glutathione followed by high-performance liquid chromatography (HPLC) to identify new adducts, whereas Garle and Fry [61] measured loss of glutathione spectrophotometrically. These methods promise to be of value in studies on hypersensitivity and drug immunogenicity.

Protein drugs

The assessment of hypersensitivity potential for protein drugs involves a different strategy from that appropriate for testing low molecular weight drugs. It has long been recognized that foreign proteins are intrinsically immunogenic, generating immune responses which underlie a number of often quite serious adverse reactions in humans. However, it is an oversimplification to suggest that this is the prerogative only of overtly foreign proteins. Clinical experience indicates that specific immune responses to therapeutic proteins may be generated as a consequence of very minor structural changes and therefore the immunogenicity of human proteins for man is an important and legitimate consideration for immunotoxicology [62–64]. This is emphasized by the fact that recombinant DNA and hybridoma technologies are increasing the prospects for the use of human proteins as therapeutic agents. For protein drugs, it seems unlikely that animal studies will help predict the intrinsic immunogenicity, for man, of human proteins. A better approach might be to devote attention to protein structure analysis in relation to antigenicity as it is becoming clear that changes in secondary and tertiary structure may be detectable by biophysical techniques and these may be predictive for immunogenicity in humans. It is of interest that the same recombinant DNA and hybridoma technologies that are increasing the numbers of therapeutic protein options also offer the prospects of improved analytical procedures through which it will be possible to probe protein structure–function relationships. On the other hand, animal studies may be invaluable in determining the incidence and specificity of immune responses to extraneous proteins derived from heterologous cells or from culture medium which may be present. Preclinical immunotoxicology strategies should therefore be developed in close association with protein analysts, for both toxicologists and protein chemists have much to contribute to what is a considerable challenge.

The immunotoxicologist is concerned with three questions on drawing up test strategies. (i) What is the likely immunogenicity of the protein drug when given to humans under the circumstances dictated by clinical need? (ii) What is the specificity and affinity of antibody raised? (iii) What are the consequences of protein immunogenicity both for humans, and, equally importantly, for the validity of animal studies carried out? As in other aspects of preclinical safety clearance programmes, the immunotoxicology strategy must reflect the intended clinical use of the drug. Protein drugs may be used in acute health care in single or very few doses, as for example, the use of thrombolytic agents for the treatment of acute myocardial infarction or as replacement therapy, for example, growth hormone which may be given for very many years. Clearly, the safety assessment criteria differ. Attempts to mimic clinical use by repeat-dose animal studies may fail to provide adequate levels of reassurance because longer administration regimens may be compromised by the role of induced antibody in neutralizing administered protein and abrogating toxic responses. Equally, the studies may be irrelevant, at least for human proteins, which can be expected to be significantly less immunogenic in humans than in animals, for whom the protein represents a foreign substance. The validity of animal studies in these circumstances should be questioned and alternative approaches considered.

Immunological assessment of protein drugs includes more than consideration of intrinsic immunogenicity. Methods of production are such that the presence of impurities, contaminants and modified proteins cannot be ruled out and animal studies are needed to determine their presence and immunogenicity.

Finally, it will be necessary to consider the impact of the pharmacokinetic and pharmacodynamic properties of the protein drug on potential immunotoxicity.

Some of these issues are discussed below. This is an evolving area. No firm general recommendations can be made for immunotoxicity testing of protein drugs at this time although guidelines (see for example Table 15.5) exist [65]. Each protein—its intended clinical use, its activity and pharmacokinetics—is a unique challenge demanding an individual approach. None the less, we have tried to indicate directions for such studies. While animal

testing has an important place in the immunotoxicology of protein drugs, as indicated below, we believe that a major input to testing strategies should be that which can be derived from protein analytical studies and we anticipate that the protein chemist, and for some proteins, the molecular biologist, will be key individuals contributing to safety assessment of protein drugs.

Role of protein analytical procedures in the assessment of protein immunogenicity and immunotoxicity. The structural basis of the antigenicity of proteins has been the subject of numerous investigations since the work of Sela and colleagues [66,67], Atassi and colleagues [68,69] and Crumpton [70].

A substantial number of studies has subsequently drawn attention to structural features in proteins which may be of value in predicting antigenic determinants. It is not appropriate to give details of these studies in this chapter but it does seem likely that this approach will add to our understanding of protein immunogenicity and perhaps permit reasonably accurate predictions to be made.

A number of correlations have been made between protein structure and antigenicity. There is an association between hydrophilicity and antigenicity [71,72] which may in turn reflect the relationship between surface accessibility and the ability of the antigenic determinant to bind to antibody molecules. Correlation between antigenicity and the mobility of protein segments has also been reported [73,74], and this may well account for the fact that many antigenic determinants involve amino and carboxy terminal residues, for these are areas of high mobility and are surface-oriented [75]. These devel-

Table 15.5 Immunotoxicology of human protein drugs; recommendations of guidelines [65]

Monitor immunogenicity in test species
Induction of antibody
Pharmacokinetics of response

Monitor for immune complex formation
Immune complexes
Complexes with host macromolecules

Monitor interaction with cells of immune system

Measure release of pharmacologically active molecules

---

opments, which rely on advances in protein analytical technology and represent a specialized aspect of protein structure–function relationships, are important for consideration of the intrinsic immunogenicity of therapeutic proteins.

The question is the extent these and related approaches involving computer prediction can be used to predict immunogenicity for humans [76–78]. It would be expected that even relatively small changes in amino acid sequence or in glycosylation would have an influence on immunogenic potential [79] and thus fidelity to the natural form, especially with respect to terminal sequences, would normally be the aim for a protein therapeutic agent.

Protein analysis thus becomes a key tool in the safety evaluation of protein drugs. The main techniques available for protein structure analysis are shown in Table 15.6. During the characterization phase of the protein to be developed, it is important to gain as much information as possible and electrophoresis, protein HPLC, amino acid sequencing, tryptic mapping and probably circular dichroism would all be required [80]. For batch control purposes, full sequencing would not be necessary and reliance could be placed on electrophoretic patterns, protein HPLC, and tryptic mapping.

There is no doubt that this package of information is necessary before progression of protein drugs to humans. The overall predictive value of protein analytical studies for immunogenicity potential, however, is seriously compromised by our inability

to address the issue of protein dynamics. Even if the *N*-terminal sequence is correct, it is possible that, because of its flexibility, immunogenicity-determining changes could be introduced but not detected without recourse to protein nuclear magnetic resonance and crystallographic structure analysis. These techniques are currently outside the scope of preclinical safety evaluation procedures, as are analytical techniques to determine the glycoform of those recombinant therapeutic agents which are glycoproteins. The potential consequences of non-physiological glycosylation have been reviewed [81] and perhaps greatest concern has been expressed in terms of immunogenicity. Not only are certain oligosaccharide epitopes immunogenic but oligosaccharides may also affect the immunogenic properties of the attached polypeptide. It is certain that the rapid advances being made in this area, both in understanding the physiological significance of glycosylation and in analytical techniques, will make a contribution to predicting the immunogenicity of therapeutic glycoproteins derived by recombinant DNA technology.

Animal models. In contrast to the limited role of animal studies in predicting the intrinsic immunogenicity of human proteins for man, animal studies can be of value in determining the possible immunological complications arising from impurities or contaminants in a protein product, or of possible neo-antigens arising during processing or from chemical or physical modification procedures. Maurer and Subrahmanyam [82] for example drew attention to the influence of heat-treatment of plasma proteins in the formation of new antigenic determinants and Lundblad *et al.* [83] describe rabbit immunization experiments to determine whether pasteurization of a number of products, including factor VIII, might lead to the development of antibody to neo-antigens. Ronneberger [84] regards such studies as essential prior to clinical use of protein therapeutic agents.

A number of factors influence the outcome of an immune response. Many of these are host-determined and may involve, for example, metabolic handling, and genetic influence on isotype generation. None of these is easily amenable to preclinical study. Consideration should be given,

Table 15.6 Techniques for the structural analysis of recombinant proteins

Method	Drug development phase	
	Characterization	Control
Electrophoresis	Yes	Yes
Protein HPLC	Yes	Usually
Automated sequencing	Yes	No
Tryptic mapping	Yes	Yes
Circular dichroism	Yes	Sometimes
NMR	Sometimes	Rarely
X-ray crystallography	Rarely	No

HPLC, High performance liquid chromatography; NMR, nuclear magnetic resonance (spectroscopy).

however, to pharmacokinetic and pharmacodynamic studies in an appropriate animal species as these properties are critical, not only for therapeutic efficacy, but also for toxicity assessment. The possibility of immune complex deposition may need to be considered for protein therapeutics, especially those of long biological half-life. Equally, immunotoxicology will need to address questions which might arise due to interaction of the protein with cells of the immune and other systems causing direct damage or interfering with the production or release of biological mediators, for example, the interleukins, critical to immune function. Discussion of these problems is largely outside the remit of this chapter but they are important considerations not only for preclinical work, but also for clinical studies. It has been clear for some time that drug hypersensitivity is often misdiagnosed due to the similarity of clinical signs and symptoms between true allergy and pseudoallergic reactions which frequently share common mediators (reviewed in [85]). Examples include not only proteins, but various plasma substitutes, dextrans and polypeptides [86]. To the extent that clinical reactions are often the main trigger to immunological and mechanistic studies, it is critically important that tests are developed which permit the clinician to distinguish reactions mediated through specific immunological mechanisms from those which merely mimic these processes.

Conclusions

Some progress is being made in the development of immunotoxicology strategies to identify potential drug allergens. It will be apparent that this work is at a very preliminary stage and much validation work is required before it will be known whether any of the current approaches are useful. It is equally important to improve the accuracy of clinical diagnosis of drug allergy and to establish clear criteria for such a diagnosis. Finally, the immunotoxicologist must face the challenge of a new generation of drugs derived from recombinant DNA technology and in this task, it will be essential to marshall the skills of the protein chemist.

Thus, the immunotoxicology of drug hypersensitivity demands a multidisciplinary approach. The rewards will be not only improved risk assessment

but also improved understanding of this important group of adverse drug reactions.

References

1 Hoigné R, Stocker F, Middleton P. Epidemiology of drug allergy: drug monitoring. In: de Weck AL, Bundgaard H, eds. *Allergic Reactions to Drugs.* Berlin: Springer-Verlag, 1983:187–205.

2 Dewdney JM. Clinical diagnosis of drug allergy. In: Dean JH, Luster MI, Munson AE, Amos H, eds. *Immunotoxicology and Immunopharmacology.* New York: Raven Press, 1985:133–44.

3 Dean JH, Luster MI, Boorman GA, Lauer LD. Procedures available to examine the immunotoxicity of chemicals and drugs. *Pharmacol Rev* 1982; 34:137–48.

4 Dean JH, Murray MJ, Ward EC. Toxic responses of the immune system. In: Klassen CD, Amdur MD, Doull J, eds. *Toxicology, the Basic Science of Poisons.* New York: Macmillans, 1986:245–85.

5 Koller LD. Immunotoxicology today. *Toxicol Pathol* 1987; 15:346–51.

6 Norbury KC. Methods currently used in the pharmaceutical industry for evaluating immunotoxic effects. *Pharmacol Rev* 1982; 34:131–6.

7 Bloom JC, Thiem PA, Morgan DG. The role of conventional pathology and toxicology in evaluating the immunotoxic potential of xenobiotics. *Toxicol Pathol* 1987; 15:283–93.

8 Voss JG. The role of histopathology in assessment of immunotoxicity. In: Berlin A, Dean J, Drape MH, Smith EMB, Spreafico F, eds. *Immunotoxicology.* The Netherlands: Martinus Nijhoff, 1987:125–34.

9 Exon JH, Koller LD, Talcott PA, O'Reilly CA, Henningsen GM. Immunotoxicity testing: an economical multiple-assay approach. *Fund Appl Toxicol* 1986; 7:387–97.

10 Carrington DM, Earl HS, Sullivan TJ. Studies of human IgE to a sulfonamide determinant. *J Allergy Clin Immunol* 1987; 79:442–7.

11 Harle DG, Baldo BA, Wells JV. Drugs as allergens: detection and combining site specificities of IgE antibodies to sulfamethoxazole. *Mol Immunol* 1988; 25:1347–54.

12 Harle DG, Baldo BA, Smal MA, Fisher MM. Drugs as allergens: the molecular basis of IgE binding to thiopentone. *Int Arch Allergy Appl Immunol* 1987; 84:277–83.

13 Smal MA, Baldo BA, Harle DG. Drugs as allergens. The molecular basis of IgE binding to trimethoprim. *Allergy* 1988; 43:184–91.

14 Baldo BA, Fisher MMcD. Anaphylaxis to muscle relaxant drugs: cross-reactivity and molecular basis of binding of IgE antibodies detected by radioimmunoas-

say. *Mol Immunol* 1983; 20:1393–400.

15 Descotes J. *Immunotoxicology of Drugs and Chemicals.* Amsterdam: Elsevier Science, 1986.

16 de Weck AL, Bundgaard H, eds. *Allergic Reactions to Drugs.* Berlin:Springer-Verlag, 1983.

17 Hudson JL, Duque RE, Lovett EJ. Applications of flow cytometry in immunotoxicology. In: Dean JH, Luster MI, Munson AE, Amos H, eds. *Immunotoxicology and Immunopharmacology.* New York: Raven Press, 1985:159–78.

18 Magnusson B, Kligman AM. In: *Allergic Contact Dermatitis in the Guinea Pig. Identification of Contact Allergens.* Springfield, IL:Charles C. Thomas, 1970.

19 Maurer TH. Predictive contact allergenicity testing of drugs. *Trends Pharm Sci* 1983; 4:104–6.

20 Maurer TH, Weirich EG, Hess R. The optimization test in the guinea pig in relation to other predictive sensitization methods. *Toxicol* 1980; 15:163–71.

21 Smith H. Animal models of asthma. *Pulm Pharmacol* 1989; 2:59–74.

22 Doe JE. Animal models of sensitization via the respiratory tract. In: Gibson GG, Hubbard R, Parke DV, eds. *Immunotoxicology.* London: Academic Press, 1983:149–60.

23 Patterson R, Harris KE, Pruzansky JJ, Zeiss CR. An animal model of occupational immunologic asthma due to diphenylmethane diisocyanate, with multiple systemic immunologic responses. *J Lab Clin Med* 1982; 99:615–23.

24 Karol MH, Hauth BA, Riley EJ, Magreni CM. Dermal contact with toluene diisocyanate (TDI) produces respiratory tract hypersensitivity in guinea pigs. *Toxicol Appl Pharmacol* 1981; 58:221–30.

25 Karol MH, Stadler J, Magreni C. Immunotoxicological evaluation of the respiratory system: animal models for immediate– and delayed-onset pulmonary hypersensitivity. *Fund Appl Toxicol* 1985; 5:459–72.

26 Botham PA, Hext PM, Rattray NJ, Walsh ST, Woodcock DR. Sensitisation of guinea pigs by inhalation exposure to low molecular weight chemicals. *Toxicol Lett* 1988; 41:159–73.

27 Botham PA, Rattray NJ, Woodcock DR, Walsh ST, Hext PM. The induction of respiratory allergy in guinea pigs following intradermal injection of trimellitic anhydride: a comparison with the response to 2,4-dinitrochlorobenzene. *Toxicol Lett* 1989; 47:25–39.

28 Gleichmann H. Studies on the mechanism of drug sensitization: T-cell dependent popliteal lymph node reaction to diphenylhydantoin. *Clin Immunol Immunopathol* 1981; 18:203–11.

29 Kammüller ME, Seinen W. Structural requirements for hydantoins and 2-thiohydantoins to induce lymphoproliferative popliteal lymph node reactions in the mouse. *Int J Immunopharmacol* 1988; 10:997–1010.

30 Durdik J, Gerstein RM, Rath S, Robbins PF, Nisonoff A, Selsing E. Isotype switching by a microinjected μ immunoglobulin heavy chain gene in transgenic mice. *Proc Natl Acad Sci USA* 1989; 86:2346–50.

31 Jaenisch R. Transgenic animals. *Science* 1988; 240:1468–74.

32 *OECD Guidelines for the Testing of Chemicals. Skin Sensitization.* 1981. no.406.

33 Landsteiner K, Jacobs J. Studies on the sensitization of animals with simple chemical compounds. *J Exp Med* 1936; 64:625–39.

34 Eisen HN, Orris L, Belman S. Elicitation of delayed allergic skin reaction with haptens: dependence of elicitation on hapten combination with protein. *J Exp Med* 1952; 95:473–87.

35 Eisen HN. Hypersensitivity to simple chemicals. In: Lawrence HS, ed. *Cellular and Humoral Aspects of the Hypersensitive States.* New York: Hoeber, 1959:89–119.

36 Park BK, Coleman JW, Kitteringham NR. Drug disposition and drug hypersensitivity. *Biochem Pharmacol* 1987; 36:581–90.

37 Kristofferson A, Ahlstedt S, Svard PO. Antigens in penicillin allergy. II The influence of number of penicilloyl residues on the antigenicity of macromolecules as determined by radioimmunoassay (RIA), passive cutaneous anaphylaxis (PCA) and antibody induction. *Int Arch Allergy Appl Immunol* 1977; 55:23–8.

38 Lee D, Dewdney JM, Edwards RG. The influence of hapten density on the assay of penicilloylated proteins in fluids. *J Immunol Methods* 1985; 84:235–43.

39 Park BK, Tingle MD, Grabowski PS, Coleman JW, Kitteringham NR. Drug-protein conjugates – XI. Disposition and immunogenicity of dinitrofluorobenzene, a model compound for the investigation of drugs as haptens. *Biochem Pharmacol* 1987; 36:591–9.

40 Ahlstedt S, Kristofferson A. Immune mechanisms for induction of penicillin allergy. *Prog Allergy* 1982; 30:67.

41 Yeung JHK, Coleman JW, Park BK. Drug protein conjugates. IX. Immunogenicity of captopril-protein conjugates. *Biochem Pharmacol* 1985; 34:4005–12.

42 Parish WE. Predictive tests for occupational allergies. *Arch Toxicol* 1987; 11(suppl):177–81.

43 Pannatier A, Jenner P, Testa B, Etter JC. The skin as a drug-metabolising organ. *Drug Metab Rev* 1978; 8:319–43.

44 Kraft D. Other antibiotics. In: de Weck AL, Bundgaard H, eds. *Allergic Reactions to Drugs.* Berlin: Springer-Verlag, 1983:483–512.

45 Dewdney JM. Immunology of the antibiotics. In: Sela M, ed. *The Antigens.* New York: Academic Press, 1977:74–245.

46 Kligman AM. The identification of contact allergens by

human assay III. *J Invest Dermatol* 1966; 47:393–409.

47 Girard JP, Schwartz H. Serum haemagglutinating antibodies in streptomycin allergy. *Med Pharmacol* 1967; 17:466–74.

48 Dewdney JM. Antifungal, anthelmintic and antiprotozoal drugs. In: de Weck AL, Bundgaard H, eds. *Allergic Reactions to Drugs*. Berlin: Springer–Verlag, 1983:567–9.

49 Calnan CD. Occupational piperazine dermatitis. *Contact Derm* 1975; 1:126.

50 Foussereau J, Benezra C. Données nouvelles sur l'allergie de groupe à la pipérazine. *Bull Soc Franc Derm Syph* 1967; 76:458–61.

51 Welinder H, Hagmar L, Gustavsson C. IgE antibodies against piperazine and N-methyl-piperazine in two asthmatic subjects. *Int Arch Allergy Appl Immunol* 1986; 79:259–62.

52 Edwards RG, Dewdney JM, Dobrzanski RJ, Lee D. Immunogenicity and allergenicity studies on two beta-lactam structures, a clavam, clavulanic acid, and a carbapenem: structure activity relationships. *Int Arch Allergy Appl Immunol* 1988; 85:184–9.

53 Pfaendler HR, Gosteli J, Woodwards RB, Rihs G. Structure, reactivity and biological activity of strained bicyclic β-lactams. *J Am Chem Soc* 1981; 103:4526–31.

54 Finn MJ, Harris MA, Hunt E, Zomaya II. Studies on the hydrolysis of clavulanic acid. *J Chem Soc, Perkin Trans* I 1984:1345–9.

55 Haginaka J, Yasuda H, Uno T, Nakagawa T. Degradation of clavulanic acid in aqueous alkaline solution: isolation and structural investigation of degradation products. *Chem Pharm Bull* 1985; 33:218–44.

56 Nilsson BS. Adverse reactions in connection with zimelidine treatment—a review. *Acta Psychiatr Scand* 1983; 308 (suppl):115–19.

57 Buus Lassen J. Influences of the new 5-HT-uptake inhibitor paroxetine on hypermotility in rats produced by p-chloramphetamine and 4,-dimethyl-m-tyramine. *Psychopharmacol* 1978; 57:151–3.

58 Lund J, Lomholt B, Fabricius J, Christensen JA, Bechgaard E. Paroxetine: pharmacokinetics, tolerance and depletion of blood 5-HT in man. *Acta Pharmacol Toxicol* 1979; 44:289–95.

59 Henderson DC, Edwards RG, Weston BJ, Dewdney JM. Immunological studies on paroxetine, a novel anti-depressant drug. *Int J Immunopharmacol* 1988; 10:361–7.

60 Mulder GJ, Le CT. A rapid, simple *in vitro* screening test, using [^{3}H]glutathione and L-[^{35}S]cysteine as trapping agents, to detect reactive intermediates of xenobiotics. *Toxicol in vitro* 1988; 2:225–30.

61 Garle MJ, Fry JR. Detection of reactive metabolites *in vitro*. *Toxicol* 1989; 54:101–10.

62 Hawkins M, Horning S, Konrad M. Phase I evaluation of a synthetic mutant of beta-interferon. *Cancer Res* 1985; 45:5914–20.

63 Fineberg SE, Galloway JA, Fineberg NS, Rathbun MJ, Hufferd S. Immunogenicity of recombinant DNA human insulin. *Diabetologia* 1983; 25:465–9.

64 Westphal O. Experiences of Somatonorm in Sweden. *Acta Paediatr Scand* 1986; 325 (suppl):41–4.

65 Commission of the European Communities notes to applicants for marketing authorizations. Guidelines on the preclinical biological safety testing of medicinal products derived from biotechnology (and comparable products derived from chemical synthesis). *Tibtech* 1989; 7:13–16.

66 Sela M, Schechter B, Schechter I, Borek F. Antibodies to sequential and conformational determinants. *Cold Spring Harbor Symp Quant Biol* 1967; 32:537–45.

67 Sela M. Antigenicity: some molecular aspects. *Science* 1969; 166:1365–74.

68 Atassi MZ. Antigenic structure of myoglobin: the complete immunochemical anatomy of a protein and conclusions relating to antigenic structures of proteins. *Immunochem* 1975; 12:423–38.

69 Atassi MZ, Smith JA. A proposal for the nomenclature of antigenic sites in peptides and proteins. *Immunochem* 1978; 15:609–10.

70 Crumpton MJ. Protein antigens: the molecular bases of antigenicity and immunogenicity. In: Sela M, ed. *The Antigens*. vol. 2. New York: Academic Press, 1974:1–78.

71 Hopp TP, Woods KR. Prediction of protein antigenic determinants from amino acid sequences. *Proc Natl Acad Sci USA* 1981; 78:3824–8.

72 Kyte J, Doolittle RD. A simple method for displaying the hydropathic character of a protein. *J Mol Biol* 1982; 157:105–32.

73 Westof E, Altschuh D, Moras D, Bloomer AC, Mondragon A, Klug A, van Regenmortel MHV. Correlation between segmental mobility and the location of antigenic determinants in proteins. *Nature* 1984; 311:123–6.

74 Van Regenmortel MHV. Which structural features determine protein antigenicity? *Trends Biochem Sci* 1986; 11:36–9.

75 Thornton JM, Sibanda BL. Amino and carboxyterminal regions in globular proteins. *J Mol Biol* 1983; 167:443–60.

76 Todd PEE, East IJ, Leach SJ. The immunogenicity and antigenicity of proteins. *Trends Biochem Sci* 1982; 7:212–16.

77 Krchnak V, Mach O, Maly A. Computer prediction of potential immunogenic determinants from protein amino acid sequence. *Anal Biochem* 1987; 165:200–7.

78 Padlan EA. Quantitation of the immunogenic potential of protein antigens. *Mol Immunol* 1985; 22:1243–54.

79 Ramabhadran TV. Products from genetically engineered mammalian cells: benefits and risk factors. *Trends Biotechnol* 1987; 5:175–9.

80 Garnick RL, Solli NJ, Papa PA. The role of quality control in biotechnology: an analytical perspective. *Ann Chem* 1988; 60:2546–57.

81 Parekh RB, Dwek RA, Edge CJ, Rademacher TW. N-glycosylation and the production of recombinant glycoproteins. *Trends Biotechnol* 1989; 7:117–21.

82 Maurer PH, Subrahmanyam D. Immunological studies with plasma expanders derived from human plasma. *J Clin Invest* 1960; 39:698–705.

83 Lundblad JL, Hink JH, Ward WE, Houlihan RB, Murphy PL. The antigenic nature of heat-treated human plasma protein fractions. *Vox Sang* 1960; 5:122–37.

84 Ronneberger H. Need for additional safety assays for heat-treated plasma protein fractions. *Trends Pharm Sci* 1986;7:130–1.

85 Dukor P, Kallos P, Schlumberger HD, West GB. *PAR. Pseudo-Allergic Reaction. Involvement of Drugs and Chemicals.* New York: Karger, 1980.

86 Richer W, Hedin H. Solutions and emulsions used in intravenous infusions. In: deWeck AL, Bundgaard H, eds. *Allergic Reactions to Drugs.* Berlin:Springer-Verlag, 1983:581–615.

16
Histopathological approaches

HENK-JAN SCHUURMAN, ROEL A. DE WEGER, HENK VAN LOVEREN, MAGDA A.M. KRAJNC-FRANKEN & JOSEPH G. VOS

Introduction

In the evaluation of the toxicity of chemicals, laboratory animals are subjected to multi-dose 4-week or 3-month exposures, and their health status examined by biochemical, physiological or histopathological assessments. In such toxicity experiments, the (histo)pathological status is often the corner stone [1]. The dose levels (at least three) are between a low dose aimed to have no detectable effect and a high dose with overt toxicity. This type of toxicity testing provides a feasible basis for the assessment of immunotoxicity.

In experimental animals toxicological effects of xenobiotics on the immune system may be manifest as changes in weight and/or histology of lymphoid organs; changes in cellularity of lymphoid tissue and in numbers of peripheral blood leucocytes; changes in numbers of leucocyte subsets; impairment of immune cell function *in vivo* and *in vitro*, and finally as a decreased host resistance, i.e. an increased susceptibility to infectious agents or transplantable tumours.

It is obvious that the outcome of immunotoxicity testing of xenobiotics is intimately associated with the assay used. Nowadays an overwhelming number of tests are available to analyse the immune system for its composition and function. Moreover we encounter a still-increasing number of chemicals that require toxicological screening. It is almost impossible to assay all substances for all aspects of the altered immune system and related host defence: immunotoxicity testing has therefore to be done in a tiered approach [2]. A series of panels, flexibly composed of various immunological tests dependent on the chemical being studied, should be carried out in a hierarchical order, so that the outcome in the first panel determines the need for additional investigations and the type of investigations to be performed subsequently [3].

For the first tier screening we chose a set of general parameters of specific and non-specific host defence potential, i.e. peripheral blood leucocyte number and differential cell counts; serum immunoglobulin M (IgM), IgG, and IgA levels; cellularity of bone marrow; weight of lymphoid organs (thymus, spleen, lymph nodes); histology of lymphoid organs (thymus, spleen, lymph nodes, gut-associated lymphoid tissue, bronchus-associated lymphoid tissue), and optional cell marker analysis in immunohistochemistry and cytofluorography. The outcome of this analysis should be interpreted carefully; in particular when evaluating whether the results represent a direct action of the toxic compound on the immune system, or whether this is an indirect effect associated with, for example, undernutrition, impaired protein synthesis, stress or dysregulation by steroidal or other hormones. If there is no effect detectable in the first tier, further immunotoxicity studies are not indicated. On the other hand, the first tier screen may give a suspicion of immunotoxicity at relevant doses, that do not manifest overt toxicity in other organ systems. In this case, the immune system is a principal target of the chemical being studied, and further sequential investigations are required. (These are described in Chapter 17.)

The histology of lymphoid organs is an important parameter in the first tier. Conventional histology is done on formalin-fixed and paraffin-embedded tissue, using haematoxylin and eosin staining. This enables the pathologist to judge the changes in tissue architecture and morphology of cells in various compartments of the organ. However, gross histology and morphology may not always give sufficient information; this is underlined by the fact that cells with different functions manifest a similar morphology. In the last decades new technologies have been introduced in histology and (toxicological) pathology:

1 Electron microscopy, to study cells and tissue at the subcellular level.

2 Cell and tissue culture, to study the *in vitro* growth and characteristics of cells and tissues.

3 Histochemical methods, including enzyme histochemistry, immunohistochemistry and hybridohistochemistry (*in situ* hybridization), to study cells and the intercellular matrix for presence and location of enzymes, antigens (marker substances) and nucleotide sequences. These methods are basically the application of biochemical methods like enzyme substrate reactions, antigen–antibody reactions and DNA/RNA hybridization to tissue sections as substrate. But the change of fluid or gel as matrix to a tissue section requires special experimental conditions, and therefore merits a separate description.

These technologies have proven their value as an extension of the morphological characterization. This applies especially for complicated organ systems such as the immune system. Enzyme histochemistry and immunohistochemistry allow distinction of cell type, with an indication of its

function. To get more quantitative data, immunocytochemistry on cells harvested from disaggregated tissue is applied. Immunohistochemistry for (soluble) mediators permits assessment of the site of (local) synthesis and action. Finally, molecular biological approaches allow the demonstration of effects at the transcriptional level (mRNA). This hybridohistochemical (*in situ* hybridization) approach is especially helpful in cases where the assay for the translation protein product is not sensitive enough.

In this chapter we review some practical considerations of enzyme histochemistry, immunohistochemistry and hybridohistochemistry, as these methods are currently applied in histology and pathology, and are now in the process of being introduced in toxicity testing. These technologies may ultimately prove to be crucial for the significance of the first tier of screening in immunotoxicity assessment.

Enzyme histochemistry

A large number of enzymes can be detected using different types of detection reactions, described in standard textbooks [4–6]. Usually enzyme histochemistry is performed on frozen tissue sections, cell smears, or cytocentrifuge preparations, as most fixatives used in histology inactivate enzymes. The tissue is frozen as soon as possible after dissection to prevent autolysis which leads to the inactivation of many enzymes. Cell preparations should be dried quickly after preparation, and stored dry or frozen in sealed conditions at $-70°C$ or lower temperatures in a suitable embedding compound (e.g. Tissue-tek); prolonged storage at $-20°C$ results in reduced enzyme activity. Before analysis, frozen tissue sections or cell preparations may be mildly fixed in order to preserve morphology, e.g. in formalin/ethanol at 4°C; in 1–4% paraformaldehyde, formaldehyde (good preservation of enzyme activity) or glutaraldehyde (good preservation of tissue structure) or in formalin-macrodex (dextran).

The general principle of enzyme–histochemical reactions is that the enzyme in tissue or cells splits an appropriate substrate. One of the split-products subsequently reacts with a second reagent to yield an insoluble, coloured reaction product. The precipitate can be soluble in organic solvents and then counterstaining and embedding cannot be done in solvents like ethanol or xylene. A number of basic reactions are commonly used:

1 Metal ion precipitation, e.g. lead sulphide in the reaction between lead and an organic phosphate that is generated by phosphatase-mediated splitting of the substrate 2-glycerolphosphate, and sulphide anions.

2 Azo-dye formation: produced following the reaction between diazonium salt and α-naphthol, generated after enzymatic (phosphatase, esterase or peptidase) cleavage of a substrate containing a naphthol group).

3 Indigo reactions: indigo dyes are formed by oxidation of indoxyl groups, generated by enzymatic splitting from appropriate substrates (e.g. esterases, phosphatases, glycosidases and non-specific esterases).

4 Tetrazolium reactions: H^+ ions produced during the enzymatic process reduce tetrazolium salts to insoluble (red-coloured) formazan.

For alkaline phosphatase (AP) a combination of the indigo and tetrazolium method is frequently used. Two substrates are added to the detection reaction: 5-bromo-4-chloro-3-indodyl phosphate (BCIP) and nitro blue tetrazolium (NBT), and a double insoluble purple precipitate is formed. To demonstrate peroxidase (PO), the substrate 3,3'-diaminobenzidine (DAB) is often used. This compound forms a brown precipitate on reaction with H_2O_2 under the influence of PO. The reaction can be intensified by metal ions such as $NiCl_2$. When imidazol is added to the reaction mixture, the reaction time can be prolonged, leading to an enhanced signal-to-noise ratio. Table 16.1 lists some marker enzymes and chromogene detection reactions.

A number of substrate compounds are mutagenic, and therefore special precautions should be taken when working with these chemicals.

A number of enzyme substrate reactions are also used as markers in immunohistochemical and hybridohistochemical procedures (e.g. PO and AP). However endogenous enzyme activity may interfere with the marker enzyme. PO activity, for example, is widely present, particularly in myeloid cells and monocytes/macrophages. Even in paraffin sections of formalin-fixed material, the endogenous PO activity may interfere. AP activity occurs in granulocytes, endothelia and gut epithelia. These types of

Table 16.1 Marker enzymes and their chromogenic substrates

Enzyme	Chromogene substrate	Colour	Solubility in organic solvents	Carcinogenicity
Peroxidase (horseradish)	Benzidine	Blue	−	+
	DAB	Brown	−	±
	DAB with NiCl₂	Dark blue	−	±
	AEC	Red	+	+
	4-Chloro-1-naphthol	Blue	+	±, toxic
	p-Phenylenediamine		−	−
	with pyrocatrechol	Dark brown	−	−
	with NiCl₂	Dark blue		
Alkaline phosphatase (calf intestine)	Diazonium salts	Blue	−	+
	Diazonium salts	Red	−	+
	BCIP with NBT	Purple	+	+
Glucose oxidase	Tetrazolium salts	Red	−	+
β-Glucuronidase	Tetrazolium salts	Red	−	+
β-Galactosidase	Tetrazolium salts	Red	−	+
Di-aminopeptidase IV	Diazonium salts	Red	+	+

DAB, 3,3'-Diaminobenzidin tetrahydrochloride; AEC, 3-amino-9-ethylcarbazol; BCIP, 5-bromo-4-chloro-3-indolyl phosphate; NBT, nitro blue tetrazolium.

interference can be avoided by blocking the endogenous enzymatic activity. Endogenous PO is blocked by 1.5% H_2O_2 in (buffered) water or methanol, or with nitroferricyanide. Endogenous AP activity is blocked by 10 mmol/l levamisole treatment, but AP in gastrointestinal tissue is insensitive to this treatment, so that 20% acetic acid or 1.5% H_2O_2 and 2.5% periodic acid are used to ensure inactivation. Another way to lower endogenous enzyme activity is given by the choice of substrate and pH. For example, marker enzyme horseradish PO and endogenous tissue PO differ in activity towards the substrates 3,3'-diaminobenzidine and 3-amino-9-ethylcarbazol; horseradish PO is preferentially detected by 3-amino-9-ethylcarbazol. Working with this substrate at an optimum pH of 4.9, only horseradish PO is detected, because endogenous PO has its optimum pH with this substrate at pH 7.6. AP as marker enzyme is isolated from calf intestine and thus is insensitive to levamisole: simple addition of levamisole to the incubation mixture avoids staining of endogenous AP (except for gut specimens).

Immunohistochemistry

The basis of immunohistology is a (first-step) reaction between antigen to be visualized and its corresponding antibody [7,8]. For immunolabelling, antibodies of the IgM (molecular weight 900 kDa) and of the IgG (150 kDa) class are the most important. Species used for raising antibodies include mouse, rat, rabbit, sheep, goat and swine. Following the development of the monoclonal antibody technology, an extensive number of antibodies have become available to detect antigens both on tissue sections (immunohistochemistry) and on cells in suspension (immunocytochemistry) [9]. This also applies to the immunolabelling methods and modifications of this technology.

In indirect immunolabelling, second-step antibodies directed to the species of the first antibody are often applied, e.g. goat anti-mouse immunoglobulin (GAMIg; Fig. 16.1). Such antibodies should be carefully controlled for their reactivity towards the primary substrate (e.g. the species of the cell preparation or tissue section, illustrated in Fig. 16.1). This may differ for different substrates, e.g. a rabbit anti-mouse (RAMIg) reagent may work well for human substrates, while giving a high background on rat substrates. In this respect, the distance between the species on the phylogenetic tree is worth considering: in the example given, the background may be due to anti-rat reactivity of RAMIg, which does not recognize human antigen. When mouse

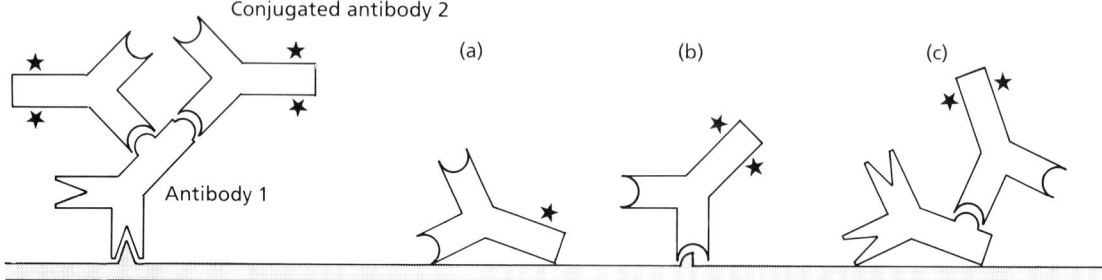

Fig. 16.1 Schematic representation of two-step indirect immunolabelling. Antibody 1 reacts to the antigen on the tissue section. The second-step incubation is performed with a conjugated antibody directed to the first one, followed by visualization of the marker on this antibody. Also shown are some possible non-specific reactions: (a) non-specific attachment of antibody 2 to the tissue section; (b) specific binding of antibody 2 to the tissue section, which shares corresponding epitopes with antibody 1; (c) non-specific attachment of antibody 1 to the section followed by specific detection in the second incubation. This non-specific binding can be prevented by (a,c) supplementing the incubation medium with non-conjugated immunoglobulin or protein before or during the incubation. Non-specific binding of type (b) can be prevented by pre-incubation with preserum or normal serum of the same species as antibody 2, or by supplementing the incubation medium with these constituents. Type b reactions can also be ascribed to natural antibodies in the serum, which occur unrelated to the antibodies to the first reagent. Proper absorption with tissue from the species of the antigen of study prevents this type of binding.

monoclonal antibodies are used in the first step it is necessary to ensure that the second antibody recognizes the various (sub)classes of mouse immunoglobulins. IgG3 is a subclass that causes problems, because it is not always recognized by anti-mouse IgG antisera. IgG3 has an electrophoretic speed significantly different from other mice IgG subclasses, and is hardly present in purified IgG that is used as an immunogen in the generation of anti-mouse IgG antisera.

Various markers or labels are used with antibodies, including fluorochromes, enzymes, and gold particles. A few examples of composite abbreviations used for conjugates are given here: MAHuKerFITC is a mouse antibody directed to human keratin (Ker) and conjugated to fluorescein isothiocyanate; RARaIgG-TRITC is a rabbit antibody directed to rat Ig of the IgG class and conjugated to tetramethyl rhodamin isothiocyanate; RAPO is a rabbit antibody against peroxidase (PO); RAMPO is a rabbit anti-mouse antibody that is conjugated with PO.

Pretreatment

Fixation of tissue is required to immobilize antigens and maintain morphology (Table 16.2). Components

Table 16.2 Fixation methods for immunohistochemistry

Methods	Use for
Freshly frozen tissue Cryostat sections, not fixed *or* fixed in methanol, ethanol, *or* acetone Freeze-dried, paraffin-embedded, section fixed in acetone Smear, touch-prepared, cytocentrifuge-preparate, not fixed *or* fixed in methanol, ethanol, *or* acetone	Extracellular antigen e.g. immunoglobulin/immune complex deposits Cell membrane antigen Tissue antigen in autoimmune diagnostics Cytoskeleton proteins, e.g. intermediate filaments
Cryostat sections of tissue fixed (perfusion, immersion) in buffered formaldehyde, or buffered *p*-benzoquinone	Peptides in endocrine cells and nerves Amines, enzymes, etc.
Freeze-dried material, followed by vapour fixation in formaldehyde, *p*-benzoquinone, or diethylpyrocarbonate, and embedded in paraffin	Intracellular water-soluble antigen, e.g. peptides in endocrine cells
Rinsing in physiological saline, ethanol fixation, paraffin embedding	Immune complex deposits and intracellular immunoglobulins
Fixation in buffered formalin, formol salt solution, sublimate formalin, Bouin's fixative, paraffin embedding, with protease treatment being optional	Intracellular antigen, peptide hormones, immunoglobulins, enzymes
Fixation in periodate–lysine–paraformaldehyde	Glycoproteins
Fixation in glutaraldehyde, glutaraldehyde formaldehyde, periodate–lysine–paraformaldehyde	Electronmicroscopic immunocytochemistry

not subject to diffusion are well demonstrated on frozen tissue sections. The main advantage of frozen tissue section investigation is the optimal preservation of the antigenic structure. The disadvantage is that the morphology is less well preserved. The tissue should be adequately frozen, preferably at $-70°C$, and well covered by tissue-embedding substance (e.g. Tissue-tek). Precautions should be taken to avoid ice crystal formation during freezing and thawing. Freeze-drying of tissues can overcome these effects. Frozen tissue sections should be air-dried for 1-3 h at room temperature or dried in a desiccator in case of high relative humidity. They may be stored until incubation at $-20°C$ or a lower temperature for longer periods, provided that the sections are wrapped to be air-tight and thawed before unpacking.

Fixation is necessary when the antigen is soluble and needs to be anchored. It varies from a slight gentle reversible precipitation by methanol, ethanol or acetone, to chemical cross-linking by formalin, paraformaldehyde or glutaraldehyde. The choice of the optimal fixative is highly dependent on the resistance of antigenicity to the denaturing fixation conditions. Thus, the balance between preservation of antigenicity and tissue structure has to be determined experimentally for each individual antigen. In this context the antibody applied should also be considered, especially with monoclonal antibodies detecting only one antigenic determinant. Epitopes on one individual antigen differ in susceptibility to denaturation by fixation, and even monoclonal antibodies have now been developed to denatured antigen. Such antibodies may even work better on fixed tissue than on frozen tissue sections. Some general outlines are presented in Table 16.2.

In immunoelectron microscopy, dehydration and plastic embedding can destroy antigenicity. Immunolabelling before embedding (pre-embedding procedure) has disadvantages, including low penetration of antibody in fresh or slightly fixed tissue sections, and poor preservation of the ultrastructural details. On the other hand, immunolabelling after embedding (post-embedding procedure) is associated with poor preservation of antigenicity. An important improvement is the cryoultramicrotomy technique, in which a compromise between preservation of ultrastructural detail and antigenicity is obtained.

Antigenic denaturation aside, antigens can be present *in situ* in a hidden configuration, e.g. peptide chains in multi-chain protein molecules and antigens in DNA chains (e.g. bromodeoxyuridine). Such antigens can be exposed by unfolding the protein molecules in the tissue section, for instance by acid urea (6 mol/l, pH 3) treatment. Because of their denaturing action some fixatives induce unfolding of protein chains. On the other hand, strong fixation may result in such extensive cross-linking that unfolding is no longer possible. In this case, acid urea treatment offers no advantage.

To demonstrate intracellular antigens in complete cells (thick tissue sections, smear- and touch-preparations, cell cultures) acetone, Triton X-100, or saponins are used to increase plasma membrane permeability to antibodies. Fixation followed by washing in a graded series of ethanol and subsequently in xylene also enhances the permeability of the cell membrane.

Immunohistochemistry requires a large number of incubations and washing steps, during which the tissue section may detach from the slide. This is obviously the case after protease treatment of the section. The detachment can be prevented by coating the slide with poly-L-lysin, agar, or Denhardt's solution (an aqueous solution of 0.2 g l^{-1} polyvinyl pyrrolidon, 0.2 g l^{-1} Ficoll 400 and 0.2 g l^{-1} bovine serum albumin). Paraffin tissue sections are usually fixed to the glass by baking. This should be done carefully, to avoid antigenic denaturation at too high a temperature; overnight drying at 37 or $56°C$ is a good procedure.

Immunolabelling methods

In the one-step (direct) method conjugated antibodies directed to the antigen of study are applied. It is a simple but relatively insensitive method. Therefore, it has a limited application, almost exclusively in immunofluorescence and for antigens present in a relatively high density in the tissue section. In two-colour immunohistochemistry the use of directly conjugated antibodies is recommended to minimalize the mutual binding of the different antibodies to each other.

In two-step indirect immunolabelling, shown in Fig. 16.1, only one conjugate is required for the second step, provided the first antibodies are from one distinct species. For example, anti-mouse antibodies for monoclonal mouse antibodies are used in the second step. The signal of the two-step method can be amplified by a third incubation with a conjugate recognizing the second antibody (three-step method). Both the three-step method with a non-conjugated second antibody and a three-step method with a conjugated second antibody are more sensitive than a two-step labelling, but may give higher background. An alternative to second antibodies is protein A, an IgG-binding protein. It is noted that not all (monoclonal mouse) antibodies have protein A-binding capacity.

The enzyme–anti-enzyme method is shown in Fig. 16.2. Originally this method was developed as an alternative to enzyme-conjugated antibodies, to prevent loss of antibody and enzyme activity by chemical conjugation. The enzyme–anti-enzyme complexes give a more intense signal than the directly conjugated second antibodies.

The immuno avidin-biotin labelling method (Fig. 16.3) utilizes the high affinity between avidin and biotin ($K = 10^{-15}$ per mol l^{-1}, considerably higher than antigen–antibody interactions with K values around 10^{-9} per mol l^{-1}). The binding is almost irreversible, up to a low pH (pH 1.5). Avidin consists of four subunits of 128 amino acids each, with a hydrophobic group in which a biotin molecule fits. The high isoelectric point (10.5) and the presence of carbohydrate groups enables avidin to bind non-specifically to glycoproteins and other tissue components, including negatively charged groups in cell membranes and nuclei. As an alternative, streptavidin has become more popular. This is a 60 kDa protein that is isolated from *Streptomyces avidinii*. It has a similar 4-subunit structure with biotin-binding places to that of avidin, but it does not contain oligosaccharides and has a neutral isoelectric point.

Immuno avidin–biotin labelling has become very popular. Biotin is easily conjugated to proteins, including protein A, antibodies, enzymes, and nucleic acids (hybridohistochemistry) and up to 150 biotin molecules can be linked to one antibody molecule. To prevent steric hindrance in avidin binding, 'spacer arms' (7-, 11-, or 16-C atoms long) can be linked to the biotin molecule. The availability of immunoavidin–biotin labelling allows performance of two-colour histochemistry, for example in combination with an enzyme–anti-enzyme antibody reaction (Fig. 16.4) or in combination with an

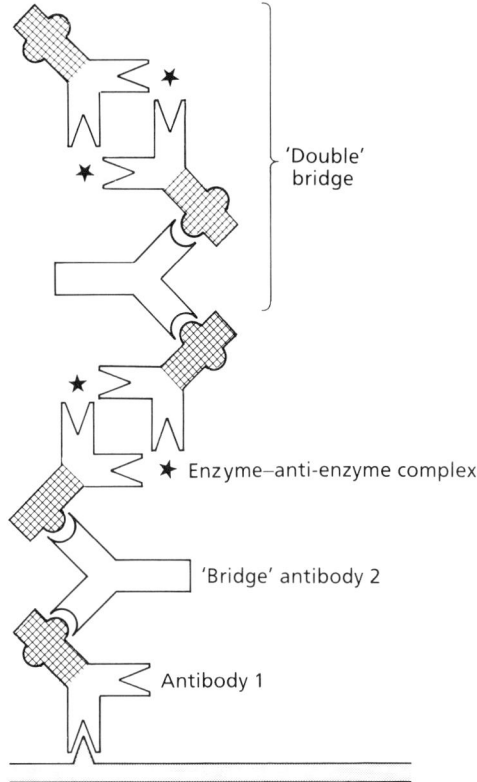

'Double' bridge

★ Enzyme–anti-enzyme complex

'Bridge' antibody 2

Antibody 1

Fig. 16.2 Enzyme–anti-enzyme immunolabelling. The antibodies in the first and third steps have the same epitopes, recognized by the 'bridge' antibody in the second step. This requirement is met by choosing the first and third antibody of the same species. The 'bridge' antibody is used in excess to generate free binding sites for binding the antibodies in the third step. An important requirement is that the 'bridge' antibody does not bind non-specifically to the tissue section. If present, this can be prevented by incubating the tissue section before with normal serum of the species of the 'bridge' antibodies. As an alternative for the 'bridge' antibody, protein A can be used: this binds the Fc fragment of IgG, so that the restriction of the same species does not apply. However, not all (monoclonal) antibodies bind protein A. Another alternative is the use of haptens conjugated to the first and third reagent, with anti-hapten antibody as the 'bridge'. This latter method is not frequently applied, but gives lower non-specific binding. The reagent in the third step is a soluble enzyme–anti-enzyme complex. Such complexes are called peroxidase–anti-peroxidase (PAP) or alkaline phosphatase–anti-alkaline phosphatase (APAAP), with designation of the species of the primary antibody to which the complex binds (e.g. mouse PAP).

The signal of the assay is intensified by repetition of the second and third incubation ('double bridge').

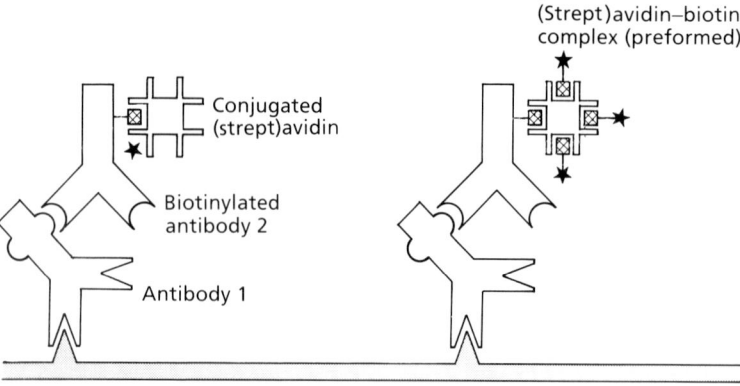

Conjugated (strept)avidin

(Strept)avidin–biotin complex (preformed)

Biotinylated antibody 2

Antibody 1

Fig. 16.3 (Strept)avidin–biotin immunolabelling. On the one hand conjugated (strept)avidin is used, e.g. with enzyme, fluorochrome or gold markers. On the other hand, for enzymes as marker, the streptavidin–biotin complex (ABC) reaction can be applied, in which streptavidin functions as a bridge between the biotinylated antibody and the biotinylated enzyme. Because of the large number of enzyme molecules that can be bound in the ABC, this technique has a high sensitivity. The figure shows indirect techniques, with biotinylated second antibodies.

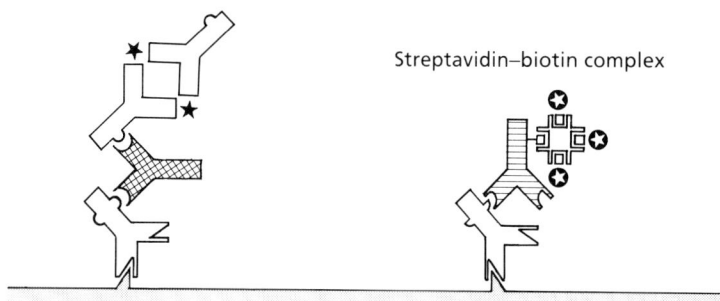

Enzyme–anti-enzyme complex

Streptavidin–biotin complex

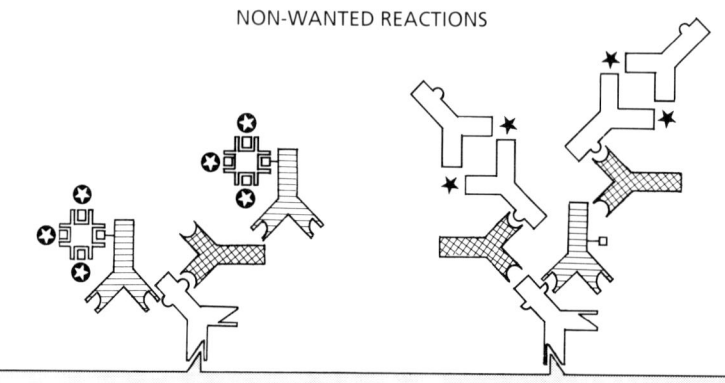

NON-WANTED REACTIONS

Fig. 16.4 Two-colour immuno-labelling with enzyme–anti-enzyme complex for the detection of one antigen, and streptavidin–biotin complex (ABC) to detect the other antigen. The first-step antibodies are from different species, and highly specific second antibodies are used. This enables a separate detection by different enzymes as marker. The incubation with the biotinylated antibody and ABC follows the enzyme–anti-enzyme antibody, but incubations can also be performed simultaneously with mixtures of second antibodies. Also shown are some examples of undesired reactions mediated by cross-reactivity of the bridge antibody in the enzyme–anti-enzyme method or the biotinylated antibody in the ABC method. The cross-reactivities shown can be due to natural antibody occurring irrespective of the specifically raised antibody, but also to the specificity of the second-layer antibody in relation to the phylogenetic distance between the species. Appropriate absorption or pre-incubation with normal serum of the species in question may reduce this undesired signal.

indirect immunoenzyme reaction. The intrinsic disadvantage of the avidin–biotin method is the endogenous presence of biotin in tissues like liver, kidney and adipose tissue. This interference can occur in frozen tissue sections but apparently does not appear in paraffin sections. With increasing sensitivity of the method this undesired signal increases. Binding to endogenous biotin can be prevented by pretreatment with (strept)avidin and biotin.

The first control in all immunolabelling procedures is the omission of antibody/immunoreagent in individual steps of the protocol. In such experiments it is preferable to replace the immunoreagent by an irrelevant one which lacks the binding characteristics (e.g. preserum; see also below).

Fluorescent markers (labels)

Fluorescent labels are small molecules which, when illuminated (excited) by light of a certain wavelength, emit light of a higher (energetically lower) wavelength (Table 16.3). The most commonly used fluorochromes are fluorescein isothiocyanate (FITC) and tetramethyl rhodamin isothiocyanate (TRITC). These two fluorochromes are often applied simultaneously in two-colour immunofluorescence, because they differ in excitation and emission wavelengths (Table 16.4; Fig. 16.5). Phycoerythrin (PE) is a fluorochrome that has a similar excitation optimum to FITC but emits red light. This means that for PE-FITC two-colour fluorescence the same wavelength is used in illumination, and separation of red and green emission signals is reached using appropriate barrier filters. Since the fluorescence signal of PE extinguishes rather fast, it is not very suitable for immunohistochemical application. However, it has found extensive applications in cell suspension analysis by cytofluorography, in which the extinguishing property does not play an important role.

The evaluation of fluorescence requires the use of a fluorescence microscope shown in Fig. 16.5. Immunofluorescence preparations are normally not counterstained, because the filter combination only allows light of certain wavelength to pass (the reader observes coloured light; Fig. 16.5), and most histochemical dyes give autofluorescence or interfere with the fluorescence signal.

The use of fluorescent markers has the important advantage of multi-colour analysis. Through the use of filter combinations several fluorescence signals can be completely separated. In photography the different fluorescence signals can be combined (there is no film transport in between different exposures). This is of great benefit in those situations where two components are found on the same place in the preparation (inclusion). As an additional marker, gold-labelling can be visualized using a filter combination in epi-luminescence. In double-labelling using enzyme markers (Fig. 16.4) the distinction between the two reaction products in either separate or mixed colours can be rather problematic, as optical separation of the colour signals is not possible using conventional microscopy.

Enzyme markers

Enzymes as marker substances have become enormously popular, especially in two- and three-step methods. The enzymes most often used are horseradish PO and AP (Table 16.1). Preparations can be counterstained allowing both histomorphologic and immunolabelling assessment. (For reaction products

Table 16.3 Fluorochromes applied in immunofluorescence

Fluorochrome	Excitation maximum (nm)	Emission maximum (nm)	Illumination/fluorescence
1-dimethyl aminonaphthalene 5-sulphonic acid (DANS)	340	525	Ultraviolet/green
4-acetamido-4'-isothiocyanato stilbene-2,2'-disulphonic acid (SITS)	350	420	Ultraviolet/blue
Fluorescein isothiocyanate (FITC)	490	525	Blue/green
Tetramethyl rhodamin isothiocyanate (TRITC)	540	570	Green/red
Phycoerythrine (PE)	490	575	Blue/orange-red

	Excitation filter (nm)	Band separation mirror (nm)	Barrier filter (nm)
FITC	Band-pass 450–490	510	Long-pass 515
FITC + TRITC*	Band-pass 450–490	510	Band-pass 520–525
TRITC	Band-pass 530–560	580	Long-pass 580

Table 16.4 Filter combinations for fluorescein isothiocyanate (FITC) and tetramethyl rhodamin isothiocyanate (TRITC) fluorescence

*This combination is used for viewing FITC in FITC/TRITC two-colour preparations, to avoid interference by TRITC fluorescence.

which are soluble in organic solvents, dissolution can be prevented by (short) post-fixation after the enzyme substrate reaction.) Haematoxylin (blue, nuclei) is often combined with a red (AEC) or brown (DAB) reaction product. In the case of a blue immunolabelling product nuclear-fast red or eosin (red, cytoplasm), and methylgreen can be used. The availability of different marker-substances and different labelling methods allows multi-colour analysis of several antigens in the preparation simultaneously (Fig. 16.4). This is especially useful when antigens are localized at different spots (exclusion).

The order of incubations and enzyme substrate reactions has to be determined for each individual application. Aspects worth considering are preservation of antigenicity of the second antigen, when immunolabelling is done after the enzyme substrate reaction for the first antigen, and possible unwanted interference of one immunolabel with another by cross-reactivity of the applied (second) antibody (illustrated in Fig. 16.4). The intrinsic disadvantage of enzymes as marker-substances is the possible presence of endogenous enzyme in the tissue section (see above).

Colloidal gold

Colloidal gold as a marker is based on the microscopic detection of gold particles in the conjugate. These gold particles are 5–10 nm large and therefore too small to be visible by light-microscopy (the resolution of light-microscopy is about 100 nm). The visualization of the particles is performed with a silver-amplification step that creates a silver deposit around the gold particle. Small-sized particles can be observed by epi-luminescence microscopy, using a fluorescence microscope with a polarizing filter combination. Polarized light is used for illumination; the gold and silver particles reflect the light, which has a

different polarization so that it can pass a polarization filter. The image read thus consists of highlighted particles on a dark background. In this way, particles up to a size of 20 nm become visible. The silver-amplification reaction is a temperature-sensitive chemical process in which silver precipitates on the gold nucleus. There is a time-limit for the amplification reaction because silver also precipitates spontaneously. The spontaneous silver precipitation occurs very slowly at the start of the amplification step, but after silver nuclei formation a visible precipitate is quickly formed. The incubation time is therefore a main factor for a good signal: noise ratio. The reaction can be followed under the light microscope.

Because other heavy metals may also function as precipitation nuclei, the glassware should be properly clean (do not use chromic acid) and adhesive substances and buffers should only be diluted with double-distilled water. Some adhesive substances such as poly-L-lysine also show non-specific labelling. When the tissue is fixed in sublimate-containing fixatives, the tissue sections should be treated with a lugol solution. Another interference in reading is through endogenous granules in the preparation. Granular dust may be present in tissues of the respiratory system or tissues (lymph nodes) associated with respiratory organs.

The advantages of the immunogold-labelling are the relative simplicity of the marker-substance; the easy way of coupling the marker substance to antibody or protein A; the sensitive detection due to the amplification by the gold-silver precipitate; the potential applications in a variety of immunolabelling methods; the possibility to keep the preparations for long times after staining, and the exact localization of antigens. Immunogold labelling is also used in immunoelectron microscopy [10]. For studies of the ultrastructure, the gold particles should be very

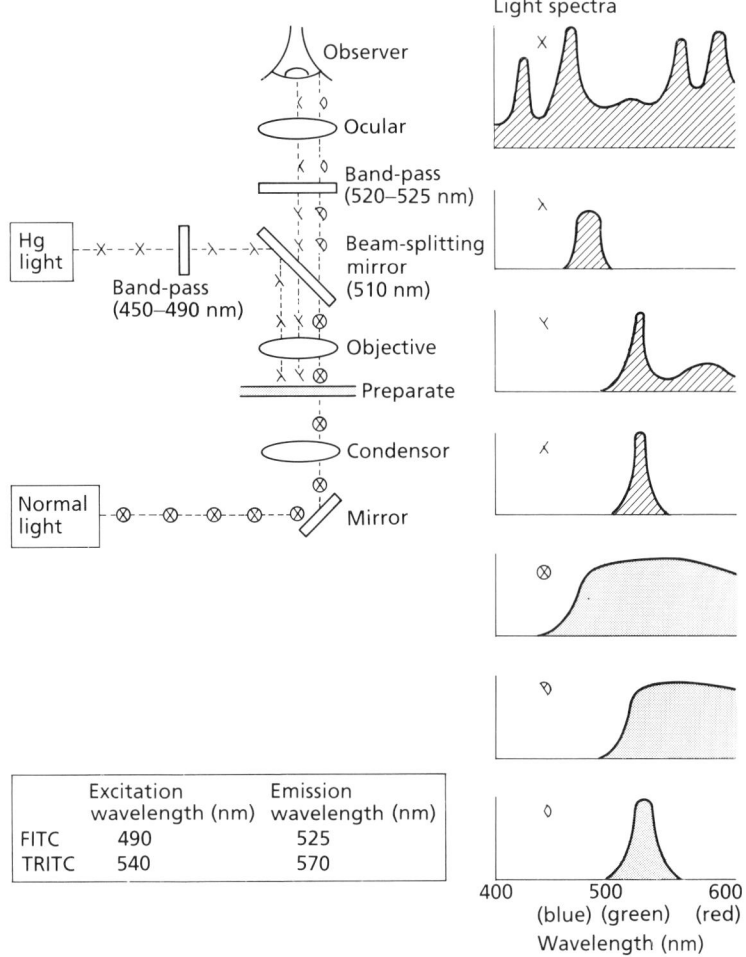

Fig. 16.5 A fluorescence microscope, with filter combination for fluorescein isothiocyanate (FITC), used in two-colour immunofluorescence combined with tetramethyl rhodamin isothiocyanate (TRITC). In the Ploem-o-pak system, the object is illuminated by the objective and the emission signal is judged by the same objective. In the filter combination (often a filter block in modern microscopes), high-energy (low-wavelength) light from the light source (high-pressure mercury lamp) at first passes the excitation filter: this transmits light in a certain wavelength area (band-pass filter), suitable for excitation of the fluorochrome. This light is then reflected by the beam-splitting mirror, which acts as a colour-separator by reflecting light from defined low-wavelength areas and transmitting light from higher wavelength areas. After excitation, the fluorochrome emits light which is of lower wavelength than the excitation light. This light is transmitted through the beam-splitting mirror, passes the barrier filter, and is then seen by the observer. In the example of FITC/TRITC two-colour immunofluorescence, TRITC is excited to some extent by the high-energy light used for FITC excitation, and emits red fluorescence. To avoid this TRITC interference, a band-pass barrier filter is used which only transmits light in the wavelength area of FITC emission. In single-colour FITC fluorescence such a barrier filter is not necessary, and mostly a long-pass filter is used (Table 16.4). The spectrum of light at different locations in the microscope is illustrated. The normal light microscopy is also drawn: in the filter combination used, the observer only sees the green light coming from the light source.

uniform in size. The use of gold particles of different size enables two-colour analysis in immunoelectron-microscopy.

Sensitivity and specificity

The combination of immunolabelling technique, marker substance, and characteristics of the conjugates (e.g. number of marker molecules per antibody molecule) are the main determinants in the sensitivity of any procedure. As a rough estimate the dilution at which the first antiserum still gives staining can be considered. Using this approach, the enzyme–anti-enzyme method and immunogold–silver labelling are about five times more sensitive than the indirect two-step immunoperoxidase, and the three-step indirect immunoperoxidase (using conjugated second and third antibodies) and the avidin-biotin method is about 10 times more sensitive. The amplified signal in indirect methods (two- or three-step) gives a higher sensitivity, but on the other hand yields aspecific signals (background, see below). The experimental protocol can be modified to obtain higher sensitivity. Usually the incubation time with antibody ranges between 30 and 60 min. An incubation time of 18 h (or even 48 h at 4°C, taking precautions to prevent dehydration) can give an amplification of 5–10 times, independent of the labelling method used. On the other hand, short-term (minutes) incubation in the microwave oven yields a higher signal:noise ratio and thereby increases the sensitivity [11].

Non-specific signals causing background occur in almost all situations. This can be based on the endogenous presence of the marker or marker-like substances, discussed above for fluorescence, enzymes, biotin, endogenous dust and residual mercury in sublimate formalin. A second source of background is the non-specific binding of conjugates (Fig. 16.1, also e.g. avidin binding). This is very dependent on the quality of the reagents. Other difficulties that may occur are summarized in Appendix I.

Quality control

Immunohistochemical procedures, by their multi-step characteristics and variable specificity of immuno-

reagents, need regular quality control. Titrations and time-block experiments are performed to determine the optimal conditions in which a maximum signal is obtained at minimum background. Aspects such as composition of incubation buffers and fixation of preparations should also be considered. It is recommended to perform (limited) chessboard experiments in which a number of parameters are varied at the same time. Control tissue should be tested regularly. This applies in particular when new batches of immunoreagents are used. The activity of the immunoreagents and other biochemicals may change in time, resulting in decreased quality of immunolabelling. Apart from these quality controls, there are a number of incidents for which the result of immunolabelling does not give the expected result. The technical reasons are summarized in Appendix I.

Hybridohistochemistry (*in situ* hybridization)

The specific detection of DNA and RNA sequences is done by binding (hybridization) complementary stretches called probes. Hybridohisto/cytochemistry uses this quality to demonstrate these gene sequences in cell smears, cytocentrifuge preparations or in tissue sections [12].

Hybridization may occur between DNA–DNA, DNA–RNA and RNA–RNA chains, provided that the base-sequence of the chains is complementary. Hybrids detecting a specific stretch can be obtained with complementary chains of 20–50 bases; in order to get strong hybrids in *in situ* hybridization, chains should be at least 200–300 complementary bases long [13–15].

Usually, probes have a length of 400–1500 bases (RNA) or base-pairs (DNA). These are prepared and multiplied (in bacteria) in vector systems like plasmids. DNA probes are directly isolated from plasmids after restriction enzyme digestion with or without subsequent size-separation from the other DNA fragments obtained. RNA probes are obtained from (DNA-)plasmids after linearization of the plasmid and transcription of DNA into RNA under the influence of RNA-polymerase; in this case the plasmid comprises a starter-site for RNA-polymerase [16–18]. (See also Chapter 19.)

Marker substance

The marker on the probe is either an internal radioactive marker (^{3}H, ^{32}P, or^{35}S) or an external one like biotin attached to the probe. In contrast to immunohistochemistry, radioactive labels are often used in hybridohistochemistry. This is because the high sensitivity required in detection of small numbers of DNA/RNA copies per cell or nucleus is more easily obtained by autoradiographic detection. Labelling is easily done by adding radioactive bases during the *in vitro* synthesis of the probe, for instance RNA synthesis from the linearized DNA-containing vector. For DNA labelling other methods are used, for which kits are commercially available. In the nick translation method small cuts (nicks) are made in intact dsDNA by DNAse I treatment. Subsequently synthesis of new DNA is started under the influence of DNA polymerase, with the incorporation of radioactive bases. The nicks are not completely repaired, and after heat-denaturation short labelled chains are obtained, which are suitable probes for *in situ* hybridization. In the random primer extension small stretches of DNA (primers) with an arbitrary nucleotide sequence are added to denatured DNA fragments or to the denatured cut plasmid in which the required DNA chain is integrated. The random primers hybridize with small complementary regions on the denatured DNA. After addition of DNA polymerase, a new complementary chain is synthesized *in vitro*, with incorporation of radioactive labelled nucleotides.

The detection after hybridization of a radioactive labelled probe is done by autoradiography. Different film types exist for different energies of the radioactive isotope in the probe. In hybridohistochemistry photographic emulsions are usually applied. After dipping the specimen in the emulsion and exposure, the film is developed. The preparations can subsequently be counterstained. The hybridization product is visible as dark grains above the tissue section. Using other film types and developers other colours of the hybridization product can be obtained. Non-specific signals come from the background of the film (especially in emulsions after longer and multiple use) and endogenous granules in the tissue section, e.g. derived from the fixative or present as granular dust (especially in respiratory organs).

The β-emitter ^{32}P is not suitable for *in situ* hybridization because its radiation energy is too high (1700 kEV), resulting in poor cellular localization of probes. ^{32}P-labelled probes have a short period of application because of their short half-life (14.3 days). In addition, in the decay of ^{32}P, breakages occur in the polynucleotide chain (decay catastrophe). The β-emitter ^{35}S is often used in *in situ* hybridization, because it provides a good cell localization (energy 167 kEV) in combination with a relatively short exposure time (days), and has a long half-life (84 days). As the ^{35}S does not combine in the chain, few breakages occur in the decay of this isotope.^{3}H is also frequently used in hybridohistochemistry. This label has a low energetic β-radiation (18 kEV), which maximally penetrates 1–3 μm in biological material. Because the radiation can only reach a short distance it provides excellent cell localization in tissue sections. The main disadvantage of tritium is its long exposure time (weeks).

Non-radioactive-labelled nucleotides have become increasingly popular in hybridohistochemistry, especially when high sensitivity is not required. Another advantage is that laboratory regulations of working with radioactive material are not applicable in this case, and these probes can be used for longer periods of time. The incorporation of the marker substance can be done in a similar way as that of radioisotopes, using marker-labelled nucleotides in *in vitro* synthesis of the probe. Often biotin-labelled nucleotides are applied. To increase its accessibility after hybridization, biotin is linked to the nucleotide by a spacer-arm. For example, an arm of 11 carbon atoms is used in Bio-11-dUTP (the most frequently used non-radioactive label), which in DNA synthesis is integrated at the site of dTTP. After *in situ* hybridization biotin is demonstrated by the avidin–biotin complex method (Fig. 16.6) or by immunohistochemistry using antibiotin antibodies. Other labelled nucleotides available are Bio-4-(d)UTP, Bio-14-ATP, Bio-17-ATP and mercury-labelled uridins Hg-(d)UTP.

When probes are available in a non-labelled form, labelling is done following methods other than *in vitro* synthesis. In most cases, new (antigenic) groups which can be demonstrated by immunohistochemical reactions are integrated by chemical changes. A

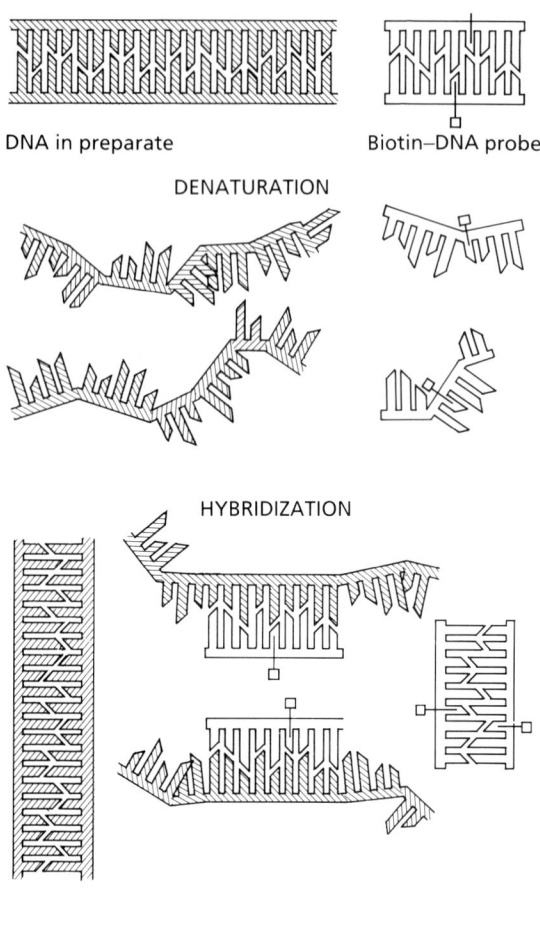

DNA in preparate

Biotin–DNA probe

DENATURATION

HYBRIDIZATION

WASHING, DETECTION

★ (Strept)avidin–biotin complex

Fig. 16.6 DNA–DNA hybridohistochemistry. The probe depicted is nine nucleotides long, but normally sequences of 400–1500 bases are used. The dsDNA stretch to be detected and the dsDNA–biotin probes are first denatured (5–10 min heating at 85–95°C in the presence of formamid) to get single strands (random-coil formation, with loss of the rigidity of the dsDNA structure). During hybridization renaturation with the formation of the original dsDNA strains occurs, but also the hybridization of probe to the dsDNA of study. Thereafter non-bound probe is washed away, and the biotin is visualized by the (strept)avidin–biotin complex reaction, followed by marker detection (usually an enzyme substrate reaction).

simple chemical modification of DNA or RNA probes is the sulphonation of probes by means of a kit (Chemiprobe). With this kit the cytosine residues in the probe are sulphonated at the carbon-6 site by sodium bisulphite. The resulting sulphon group is stabilized by substitution of the amine group at carbon-4 by a nucleophil reagent, methylhydroxylamine. The transformed cytosins are detected after *in situ* hybridization by a (monoclonal) anti-sulphon antibody, with subsequent immunolabelling. Another labelling method is the integration of the 2-acetylaminofluorene (2-AAF) group by incubation of the probe with the carcinogen *N*-acetoxy-AAF, that forms a covalent bond with guanosine residues. The linkage of this AAF group to the guanosine occurs at a position that does not interfere with the base-pairing during hybridization. The guanosine–AAF groups are detected by specific antibodies after the *in situ* hybridization reaction, with immunolabelling to visualize probe-binding.

Another example of a non-radioactive labelling method is mercuric labelling. Nucleic acids are covalently linked to mercury by incubation with mercuric acetate. After subsequent *in situ* hybridization, a sulphydryl-hapten ligand with spacer-arm is coupled to the mercury, and the haptene (e.g. trinitrophenol) can be demonstrated immunohistochemically. A non-enzyme chemical modification of probes can be obtained with photobiotin. Photobiotin consists of a light-sensitive group that is linked to biotin via a spacer-arm. During incubation of the DNA or RNA probe and irradiation with visible light a strongly reactive nitrene group from the azide group becomes activated and binds covalently to the nucleotide bases. After *in situ* hybridization, the biotin that is integrated in this way is detected by immunohistochemistry.

Procedures

A DNA–DNA *in situ* hybridization is shown in Fig. 16.6. To detect specific DNA sequences (e.g. viral DNA), both formalin-fixed paraffin-embedded tissue and freshly frozen tissue can be used. DNA can be demonstrated in fixed materials, as it is very stable (up to decades) and resistant to most fixatives. Frozen tissue section hybridohistochemistry follows the same procedure as on paraffin sections, after fixation of the section in paraformaldehyde or formalin.

Special pretreatment is required for the detection of mRNA in tissue sections. RNA is much more vulnerable to denaturation than DNA, because it exists in the single-stranded state. Moreover, RNA is susceptible to denaturation by RNAse, an enzyme which is almost ubiquitous. Therefore, all manipulations should be performed under strict RNAse-free conditions.

Another precaution is the addition of RNAse inhibitors, such as RNAsin. In most studies mRNA is demonstrated in frozen tissue, but mRNA can also be demonstrated in paraffin-embedded fixed tissue provided the tissue has not been kept for a long period. Hybridohistochemistry on frozen tissue sections requires paraformaldehyde fixation to immobilize the mRNA. For analysis on cell-smear and cytocentrifuge preparations fixation of the preparations, for instance with paraformaldehyde, is necessary.

Hybridohistochemical procedures include long incubations, and the tissues are exposed to proteolytic enzymes and high temperatures in the case of DNA detection. Slides are therefore precoated to prevent detachment of tissue sections or cell preparations, for instance with Histostick, bovine serum albumin, agar, poly-L-lysine, or Denhardt's solution (an aqueous solution of 0.2 g l^{-1} polyvinylpyrrolidon, 0.2 g l^{-1} Ficoll 400, and 0.2 g l^{-1} bovine serum albumin).

For detection of (ds) DNA, the tissue section or cell preparation is pretreated with proteolytic enzymes, in particular with proteinase K. Apart from better penetration by the probes, the proteins linked to DNA are disrupted by this enzyme, and thus the DNA can hybridize more easily. (Triton X-100 is also used.)

DNA, because of its ds configuration, can only hybridize to the probe after denaturation, which is obtained by 5–10 min heating at 85–95°C in the presence of formamid. Formamid inhibits the renaturation reaction. Often the labelled (DNA) probe is added to the mixture during denaturation (Fig. 16.6). The incubation mixture of the hybridization comprises the probe (about 0.1 μg) in de-ionized formamid (50%), sodium dextran sulphate (10%), sodium chloride (0.15 mol l^{-1})/sodium citrate (0.015 mol l^{-1}); buffer (SSC) 2 ×, and herring sperm DNA (1 mg ml^{-1}). To minimize its volume, the reaction is performed under a cover-slide in humid conditions.

Depending on the protocol a pre-hybridization step is performed with the hybridization mixture without probe, to reduce further the non-specific binding. After hybridization (8–16 h at 37°C) washing is performed. Variation in washing conditions not only affects the non-specific binding but also the extent to which the probe binds DNA or RNA molecules that are not complementary to the probe. In case of high binding strength (high complementarity between probe and DNA to be detected), the probe remains attached under stringent washing conditions (high temperature, low saline concentration, high formamid concentration). Hybridization products with low complementarity are detached under such conditions (Fig. 16.7). When the washing is performed under non-stringent conditions (low temperature, high saline concentration, low formamid concentration) the probe remains bound to complementary DNA or RNA molecules that permit only a partial hybridization, but under such conditions non-specific binding is higher. Thus, the quality of the probe is crucial in the signal:noise ratio: when using a probe of low binding strength stringent washing cannot be done and more background arises (Fig. 16.7). Background non-specific binding of RNA probes to the section can be prevented by RNAse-treatment after hybridization. This is an advantage of using RNA over DNA probes. After washing, detection with autoradiographic or immunohistochemical techniques is employed.

An important control is the *in situ* hybridization of a labelled (non-reactive) control probe. When the plasmid plus insert are used without prior separation, the labelled plasmid (without insert) can be used as control DNA. When only the labelled insert is used as the probe, an arbitrary unrelated stretch of labelled DNA can be used as a control.

In essence, the principles for DNA detection also apply for the detection of mRNA in cells or tissue sections. As stated earlier, for the detection of mRNA, RNAse-free conditions should be carefully controlled (see also Chapter 19). The mRNA *in situ* hybridization reaction can be controlled by using a probe in the sense orientation. This stems from the fact that only one strand, in the non-sense orientation, is transcribed from dsDNA in mRNA. Thus mRNA is in the sense orientation, which is detected by a non-sense probe. The probe in sense orientation is therefore an appropriate non-hybridizing control probe.

Concluding remarks: application in immunotoxicity testing

Enzyme histochemistry has the advantage that its costs are low. Specific applications in histology of the immune system are the detection of T lymphocytes by di-aminopeptidase IV activity, and macrophages by non-specific esterase activity. The scarce availability of antibodies with specificity for macrophages in all differentiation/maturation stages renders non-specific esterase as a general marker for macrophages. This analysis is relevant, for example, in degenerative/necrotic processes, where activated macrophages can accumulate. For tissue sections, non-specific esterase activity of epithelial and fatty cells may interfere when reading the results. Adenosine triphosphatase activity is a good marker for Langerhans cells in the skin. In peripheral lymphoid tissue B lymphocytes show adenosine triphosphatase activity, but here the activity of stromal components largely interferes with the results. For this reason enzyme histochemistry is often performed on touch

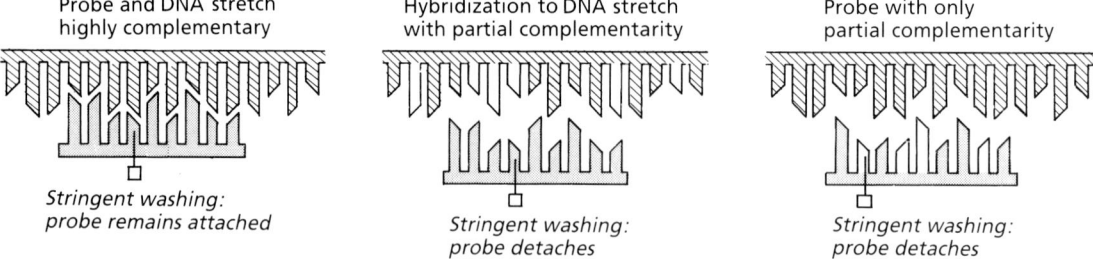

Fig. 16.7 Stringency of washing in relation to binding strength of a probe. Under stringent washing conditions (high temperature, low salt concentration, high formamid concentration) probes with high binding strength due to high complementarity or to high numbers of guanosine–cytosine interactions remain attached, whereas probes with low binding strength due to non-specific binding or binding to a stretch with partial complementarity become detached.

Table 16.5 Enzyme histochemical features of reticulum cells in lymphoid tissue

Cell type	Lysozyme	NSE	Acid phosphatase	Alkaline phosphatase	5′NT	ATPase
Histiocytic	+	+ / + +	+ / + +	−	−	+ / −
Follicular dendritic	−	+	+ / −	−	+	−
Interdigitating	−	(+)	+	−	−	+
Fibroblastic	−	−	(+)	+	−	−
Endothelial	−	− / ±	− / ±	− / +	+	+

NSE, non-specific esterase; 5′NT, 5′-nucleotidase; ATPase, adenosine triphosphatase.
−, no staining; ±, weak staining; (+), occasional staining; + and + +, staining and increased intensity of staining.

preparations, in which the matrix components are not present. Various types of stromal cells in lymphoid tissue can easily be distinguished by enzyme histochemistry (Table 16.5).

The application of enzyme histochemistry in cell typing has been replaced to a large extent by immunohistochemical methods. This is due to a larger number of specific reagents available for immunological phenotyping (Appendix II).

Immunohistochemistry can be applied in immunotoxicology in two ways. First, for screening immunotoxic effects the method can be applied to describe toxic damage to lymphoid organs in the first tier screen. Appendix II lists antibodies to various types of cells in lymphoid organs of humans, mice and rats. Some of these antibodies have been clustered in so-called clusters of differentiation (CD). These CD have been proposed during international workshops [19–22] on human leucocyte differentiation antigens; each CD comprises monoclonal antibodies to different epitopes of an antigen. The clustering is based on multi-centre analysis including quantitative data from cytofluorographic analysis on populations of normal and malignant leucocytes; molecular weight of the corresponding antigen determined by immunoprecipitation, and immunohistochemical data. For a number of clusters immunohistochemistry showed variable staining patterns by individual antibodies. This indicates the different specificity of antibodies in a given CD, visible by binding cross-reacting epitopes in tissue sections, that are not present in leucocyte subsets. The CD nomenclature has been adapted for antibodies reacting to leucocyte subsets in other species including mouse and rat [23].

Second, immunohistochemistry is helpful in elucidating the immunopathological mechanism of toxic compounds. Examples come from the autoimmune or immune complex-mediated destruction of target organs, induced by toxicological or pharmaceutic substances like drugs [24]. The role of immune complexes or autoantibodies in toxicological processes is established by the demonstration of immunoglobulins and complement components at the site of inflammation.

Hybridohistochemistry finds its application particularly in the investigation of viral infections. In this case a number of viral DNA copies are present in one cell, sufficient to be detected. The analysis of DNA sequences in describing the individual's immune status is irrelevant in hybridohistochemistry as the number of copies of endogenous DNA stretches is too low. It is, however, very useful in detecting rearranged genes, for instance immunoglobulin genes and T-cell receptor genes, using Southern blotting procedures. Also chromosomal damage in genetic toxicology (gene breakage, point mutations) can be detected using such procedures. These aspects are outside the scope of the present chapter. The detection of cellular genes provides little information on the activity of the cell. The demonstration of cellular genes has relevance for the localization of these genes at the chromosomal level. With the help of *in situ* hybridization it became possible to demonstrate gene localization on chromosomes in chromosome preparations.

The detection of mRNA is a different topic, because it gives information on gene expression. Cells actively synthesizing proteins have normally a number of mRNA molecules in their cytoplasm, enabling the detection by hybridohistochemistry. This is especially relevant when the translation product, i.e. the protein synthesized, is present in too low quantities to be detected by immunohistochemistry, or when antibodies to the protein are not available. Examples are found in the field of cytokines (interleukins or growth factors), mediators involved in the regulation of immune reactions. For some special cases protocols are now available to demonstrate mRNA and protein product on the same tissue section. mRNA hybrido-histochemistry provides information on the mere capacity of a particular cell type to synthesize protein, thus the steps in between transcription and protein excretion. It does not present any information on the site where the excreted product exerts its function. Nonetheless, mRNA detection is expected to become increasingly important in the area of genetic toxicology, where the effect of toxic compounds on gene expression is studied.

Appendix I Trouble-shooting

Uniform background staining
Enzymes: time of enzyme substrate reaction too long
Immunogold: silver-enhancement step too long
Immunogold: control media and glassware for metal ions
Immunogold: mercury not removed after sublimate formaldehyde fixation
Section dried out during one of the incubation steps
Dilution of primary or secondary antibody too low (control by omission of antibody or by different dilutions)
Sections have not been sufficiently rinsed
Incorrect normal serum used for pre-incubation (e.g. normal rabbit serum (NRS) for sections of human material)

Part of the section gives background staining
Part of section dried out
Enzymes: reaction product solubilized in embedding medium and diffused in section

Part of the section not stained
Deparaffination incomplete
Part of section dried out

No staining for all antibodies, using different incubations
Enzymes: control substrate–chromogene solutions (concentration, pH)
Control second or third step
Incorrect normal serum used in diluent (e.g. NRS for swine anti-rabbit peroxidase conjugate, SwARPO)
Enzymes: reaction product solubilized during dehydration (ethanol, xylene) or in embedding fluid
Fluorescence: embedding in incorrect medium; control salt concentration and pH

No staining for some antibodies
If required, enzyme digestion has not been performed
Peroxidase: blocking done for endogenous peroxidase activity, which partly inactivates antigens or antigenic activity

Section has had too much heat during attachment or drying
Antibody too dilute
Antibody used after expiration date, or denatured by freeze–thawing

Endogenous enzyme activity
Peroxidase: H_2O_2 methanol step not performed properly
Alkaline phosphatase: levamisole concentration in chromogene–substrate mixture too low

Sections detach from glass
Use gelatine and agar solution for attachment of sections
Use glassware with coating
Let sections dry well (preferably overnight at 56°C)
Frozen tissue sections: tissue has been fixed before freezing

Foggy nuclear contours
Sections dried out (especially for frozen tissue sections)
Haematoxylin dye solution not satisfactory

Staining pattern not interpretable
Incorrect first antibody applied

Aspecific dye precipitation (enzymes)
Substrate–chromogene solution not filtered before use
Antibodies not centrifuged before use (denaturation due to long use, *or* freeze–thawing too often)

Intensity of staining too weak
Activity of antibodies and/or other reagents diminished
Time in dye reaction too short
Incorrect dilution or incubation time for one antibody
Too much buffer on section before application of antibodies
Fluorescence: microscope lamp too old
Fluorescence: filter blocks too old and less transmissible

Appendix II Some relevant monoclonal antibodies to leucocytes and stromal cells applied in lymphoid tissue section analysis

CD	Mol.wt	Human	Mouse	Rat	Reactivity
To T cells					
1	gp45,12	OKT6	Ly-38		Lymphocytes in thymus cortex, Langerhans cells in skin, interdigitating cells
2	gp50	a-Leu-5 OKT11	Ly-37	MRC OX-34	All T cells in thymus and peripheral lymphoid organs, subset macrophages (rat), sheep erythrocyte receptor, ligand for LFA-3 (CD58) in cell–cell contact
3	gp19,29	a-Leu-4 OKT3	(Not commercially available)		T cells in thymus medulla and peripheral lymphoid organs (T-cell receptor-associated, cytoplasmic in precursor T cells in thymus)
4	gp65	a-Leu-3 OKT4	Ly-4, L3T4	MRC OX-35 (ER2) W3/25	Lymphocytes in thymus cortex, about 66% of T cells in peripheral lymphoid organs, subset macrophages (T helper/inducer and T delayed-type-hypersensitivity phenotype, MHC class II binding, receptor for human immunodeficiency virus)
5	gp56-62	a-Leu-1	Ly-1, Lyt-1	MRC OX-19	Lymphocytes in thymus cortex (faint), all T cells in thymus medulla and peripheral lymphoid tissue, subset B cells
6	gp120	Tu33			T cells in thymus medulla and peripheral lymphoid organs
7	gp41	WT1 a-Leu-9			Prethymic T cell precursors, all T cells in thymus and peripheral lymphoid organs
8	gp32-33	a-Leu-2 OKT8	Ly-2/3, Lyt-2/3	MRC OX-8	Lymphocytes in thymus cortex, about 33% of T cells in peripheral lymphoid organs, splenic sinusoids (T suppressor/cytotoxic phenotype, NK cells)
		WT31 T α F1 T β F1		(F073) (HIS42)	T-cell receptor α/β chain; mature T cells in thymus medulla and peripheral T lymphoid tissue

Continued

Appendix II *continued*

CD	Mol.wt	Human	Mouse	Rat	Reactivity
8	gp32–33	TCRδ1 δTCS1	(Not commercially available)		T-cell receptor τ/δ chain
	p95			W3/13 (HIS17)	(Pro)-thymocytes, T cells, plasma cells, cells in bone marrow, polymorphonuclear granulocytes, brain cells
	p41–55			MRC OX-44	Pro-thymocytes, medullary thymocytes, T and B cells
	p41,47			MRC OX-2	Thymocytes, dendritic cells, B cells, brain cells
			Ly-24, PgP-1		All non-T leucocytes, pro-thymocytes, memory T cells
	p25–30		Thy-1	(ER4) MRC OX-7	T lymphocytes, epithelial cells, fibroblasts, neurons, stem cells (T-cell activation molecule)
			Thy-2		Thymocytes
MHC class I		(Various antibodies to polymorphic and non-polymorphic epitopes)			All nucleated cells, including leucocytes and stromal cells: for T cells absent on thymus cortex cells (Hu)

To B cells

CD	Mol.wt	Human	Mouse	Rat	Reactivity
19	gp95	a-Leu-12 B4			B cells in germinal centres and mantles, follicular dendritic cells
20	p35	B1	Ly-44		B cells in germinal centres and mantles, follicular dendritic cells
21	gp140	B2, BL13			B cells in germinal centres and mantles (faint), follicular dendritic cells (C3d receptor CR2, receptor for Epstein–Barr virus
22	gp35	a-Leu-14 To 15			B cells in germinal centres and mantles, cytoplasmic in precursor B cells
23	p45	Tu 1 a-Leu-20	Ly-42		Some B cells in germinal centres and mantles, subset of follicular dendritic cells (IgE-Fc receptor, associatedwith cell activation)

Appendix II *continued*

CD	Mol.wt	Human	Mouse	Rat	Reactivity
37	gp40–45	BL14			B cells in germinal centres and mantles
38	gp45	OKT10 a-Leu-17			Lymphocytes in thymus cortex, cells in germinal centres, plasma cells (immature lymphoid cells, activated cells, plasma cells)
w75	p53?	LN1, OKB4			B cells in germinal centre, in corona (faint), macrophages, epithelium
	p200			(HIS14)	All B cells, including TdT-precursors
	p200			(HIS22)	All B cells in corona, pre-B cells
	p200			(HIS24)	All peripheral B cells except cells in marginal zone, pre-B cells
MHC Class II		(Various antibodies to polymorphic and non-polymorphic epitopes)			B lymphocytes, activated T cells, monocytes/macrophages, interdigitating cells, Langerhans cells, epithelia, endothelia
Anti-immunoglobulin					B cells (surface), plasma cells (cytoplasmic)
Monocytes/macrophages, myeloid cells					
13	p130–150	MY7			Aminopeptidase N; monocytes, granulocytes, dendritic reticulum cells
15	p170–190	a-Leu-M1			Lacto-N-fucose pentaosyl; granulocytes, monocytes
68		Ki-M6,Ki-M7			Macrophages (specific)
	p160		F4/80		Monocytes, macrophages
	p32		Mac-2		Thioglycollate-elicited peritoneal macrophages
68	p92–110		Mac-3		Peritoneal macrophages
				ED1	Monocytes, macrophages
				ED2	Subset macrophages (F4/80 like)

Continued

Appendix II *continued*

CD	Mol.wt	Human	Mouse	Rat	Reactivity
				ED3	Subset macrophages, restricted, negative in thymus
				MRC OX-41	Macrophages, granulocytes, dendritic cells
NK cells					
16	p50–70	a-Leu-11			IgG-FcRIII (low affinity, complexed IgG); NK cells, subset of T cells, neutrophilic granulocytes, activated macrophages
56	p220/135	a-Leu-19			NK cells, monocytes, neuroectodermal cells
57	p110	a-Leu-7			NK cells, subset T cells, some B cells, monocytes
			A-asialo-GM1		NK cells, stromal components
Follicular dendritic cells		Ki-M4, DRC-1		ED5, ED6 MRC OX-2	Follicular dendritic cells
Epithelial cells (thymus)		Anti-keratins			Epithelium
		Anti-EMA			Epithelial membrane antigen
	TE-3, (MR3, MR6)		(ER-TR4)	(HIS38)	Thymus cortex epithelium
	TE-4, (MR19), RFD4		(ER-TR5)	(HIS39)	Thymus subcapsular/medullary epithelium
Complement receptors					
11b	p160	Mac-1	Ly-40	MRC OX-42	C3biR (CR3); macrophages, a-Leu-15 granulocytes, CD^{5+}-B cells
21	gp140	B2,BL13			B cells in germinal centres and mantles (faint), follicular dendritic cells (C3d receptor CR2, receptor for Epstein–Barr virus
35	p220	To 5			C3b receptor (CR1). Follicular dendritic cells, macrophages, B cells in corona (faint), renal glomerular epithelium

Appendix II *continued*

CD	Mol.wt	Human	Mouse	Rat	Reactivity
IgG-Fc receptors					
64	p75	32.2			IgG-FcRI (high affinity, monomeric IgG); monocytes
16	p50-70	a-Leu-11			IgG-FcRIII (low affinity, complexed IgG); NK cells, subset of T cells, neutrophilic granulocytes, activated macrophages
w32	gp140	2E1,CIKM5	Ly-17		IgG-FcRII (low affinity, complexed IgG); B cells, myeloid cells, macrophages
CD11–CD18 family					
11a	p180	LFA-1	Ly-15		Leucocyte function-associated antigen 1 involved in cell adhesion; T and B cells, myeloid cells, NK cells, erythroid and myeloid stem cells; ligand for ICAM-1 (CD54)
11b	p160	Mac-1	Ly-40	MRC OX-42	C3biR (CR3); macrophages, a-Leu-15 granulocytes, CD5$^+$-B cells
11c	p150	a-Leu-M5			CR4; monocytes macrophages, granulocytes (faint), activated lymphocytes
18	p95	BL5			β-chain of CD11 antigens: all lymphocytes
	p160–95			ED7,ED8	CD11–CD18 molecule
Others					
Terminal deoxynucleotidyl transferase (TdT)					Immature (lymphoid) cells in bone marrow and thymuscortex (nuclear staining)
25	p55	Tac, IL2-R	Ly-43	MRC OX-39	Interleukin-2 receptor; activated lymphocytes at scattered location in thymus cortex and T-cell areas in peripheral lymphoid organs

Continued

Appendix II *continued*

CD	Mol.wt	Human	Mouse	Rat	Reactivity
26	p120	134-2C2			Di-peptidyl peptidase IV; (activated) T cells
71	p180–90	B3/25		MRC OX-26	Transferrin receptor; proliferating cells in germinal centres, some cells in thymus and T-cell areas in peripheral lymphoid organs; stromal cells
		Ki-67			Cells in late G1, S, M, G2 phase; proliferating cells in germinal centres, some cells in thymus and T-cell areas in peripheral lymphoid organs
44	p65-85	(Hermes-1)			Lymphocyte homing receptor; T cells, small-sized B cells
			MEL14		Lymphocyte homing receptor; recirculating T and B cells
45	p180–210	T29/33		MRC OX-1	Common leucocyte antigen; all leucocytes
45R	p190,220	a-Leu-18 MB1, MT2	Ly-5, B220	MRC OX-22 MRC OX-32	Common leucocyte antigen: all B and subset T cells
45RO	p190,220	UCHL1			Common leucocyte antigen: T cells in immature and memory stage

Antibodies within brackets are not commercially available. CD, Clusters of differentiation; MHC, major histocompatibility complex; NK, natural killer. Some companies providing monoclonal reagents: Becton Dickinson, Mountain View, CA, USA; Behringwerke, Marburg/Lahn, Germany; Biotest, Dreieich, Germany; Boehringer Mannheim, Mannheim, Germany; Coulter Immunology, Hialeah, FL, USA; Dakopatts, Glostrup, Denmark; Hybritech, La Jolla, CA, USA; Immunotech, Marseille, France; Ortho Diagnostic Systems, Raritan, NJ, USA; Sera-Lab, Crawley Down, Sussex, UK; Serotec, Oxford, UK; T cell Sciences, Cambridge, MA, USA.

Acknowledgements

The text of this chapter is based in part on a course in modern histochemistry developed in the Division for Histochemistry and Electron Microscopy, University Hospital, Utrecht, in collaboration with the School for Higher Laboratory Technicians, Utrecht, The Netherlands. Collaborators in this course were C van Basten, R Broekhuizen, P Compier-Spies, M van Blokland, P Roholl and A J Van Houte.

References

1 Vos JG. The role of histopathology in assessment of immunotoxicity. In: Berlin A, Dean J, Draper MH, Smith EMB, Spreafico F, eds. *Immunotoxicology.* Dordrecht: Martinus Nijhoff, 1987:125–34.

2 Vos JG. Screening and function tests to detect immune suppression in toxicity studies. In: Sharma RP, ed. *Immunotoxicologic Considerations in Toxicology.* Boca Raton: CRC Press, 1977:109–22.

3 Van Loveren H, Vos JG. Immunotoxicologic considerations: a practical approach to immunotoxicity testing in the rat. In: Dayan AD, Paine AS, eds. *Advances in Applied Toxicology.* London: Taylor & Francis, 1989:143–64.

4 Lodja Z, Gossrau R, Schieber TH. *Enzyme-Histochemical Methods.* Berlin: Springer-Verlag, 1976.

5 Lodja Z, Gossrau R, Schieber TH. *Enzyme Histochemistry. A Laboratory Manual.* Berlin: Springer-Verlag, 1979.

6 Pearse AGE. *Histochemistry, Theoretical and Applied.* 4th edn. vol. 1: *Preparative and Optical Technology;* vol. 2: *Analytical Technology.* Edinburgh: Churchill Livingstone, 1985.

7 Bullock GR, Petrusz P (eds). *Techniques in Immunocytochemistry.* vol. 1, 1982; vol. 2, 1986; vol. 3, 1985; vol. 4, 1990. London: Academic Press.

8 Polak JM, Van Noorden S (eds). *Immunocytochemistry: Modern Methods and Applications.* 2nd edn. Bristol: Wright, 1987.

9 *Linscott Directory of Immunological and Biological Reagents.* 7th edn. Mill Valley, California: 1990.

10 Polak JM, Varndell IM. *Immunolabeling for Electron Microscopy.* Amsterdam: Elsevier, 1984.

11 Boon ME, Kok LP. *Microwave Cookbook of Pathology.* Leiden: Coulomb Press Leyden, 1987.

12 Hames BD, Higgins SJ. *Nucleic Acid Hybridization; A Practical Approach.* Oxford: IRL Press, 1985.

13 Polak JM, McGee JO'D, eds. *In situ Hybridization. Principles and Practice.* Oxford: Oxford University Press, 1990.

14 Old RW, Primrose SB. *Principles of Gene Manipulation.* 4th edn. Oxford: Blackwell, 1988.

15 Watson JD, Tooze J, Kurtz DT. *Recombinant DNA, A Short Course.* New York: Scientific American Books, 1983.

16 Davis LG, Dibner MD, Battey JF. *Basic Methods in Molecular Biology.* Amsterdam: Elsevier, 1986.

17 Maniatis T, Fritsh EF, Sambrook J. *Molecular Cloning: A Laboratory Manual.* 2nd edn. New York: Cold Spring Harbor Laboratory, 1988.

18 Zyskind JW, Bernstein SI. *Recombinant DNA Laboratory Manual.* London: Academic Press, 1989.

19 Bernard A, Boumsell L, Dausset J, Milstein C, Schlossman SF (eds). *Leucocyte Typing. Human Leucocyte Differentiation Antigens Detected by Monoclonal Antibodies.* Berlin: Springer Verlag, 1984.

20 Knapp W, Dörken B, Gillas WR *et al.* eds *Leucocyte Typing IV White Cell Differentiation Antigens.* Oxford: Oxford University Press, 1989.

21 McMichael AJ, Beverley PCL, Cobbold S *et al.* eds. *Leucocyte Typing III.* Oxford: Oxford University Press, 1987.

22 Reinherz EL, Haynes BF, Nadler LM, Bernstein ID (eds). *Leucocyte Typing II* (3 vols). New York: Springer Verlag, 1986.

23 Holmes KL, Morse III HC. Murine hematopoietic cell surface antigen expression. *Immunol Today* 1988; 9:344–50.

24 Kammuller ME, Bloksma N, Seinen W (eds). *Autoimmunity and Toxicology. Immune Disregulation Induced by Drugs and Chemicals.* Amsterdam: Elsevier, 1989.

17
Specific immune function assays

KIMBER L. WHITE, JR

Introduction

During the last decade, the development of functional assays for evaluation of the immune system has grown at an enormous rate. Although numerous assays are available for evaluating virtually all components of the immune system, very few have been successfully adapted for use in evaluating the immune response in a toxicological manner. In the adaptation of an immunological assay for use in a toxicological setting, the assay must fulfil requirements often not considered from an immunological perspective. The assay must be able to accommodate individual animals from multiple dose levels with sufficient numbers in each group to obtain appropriate statistical analysis. Furthermore, the assay should be reproducible across laboratories, relatively simple to perform and the results obtained must be interpretable. With the development of various monoclonal antibodies to cell-surface markers, significant advances have been made in identifying cell populations and the developmental and maturational status of various cell types. While cell markers are of enormous value in identifying cell types, they in themselves cannot replace measurement of the functional ability of the cells to respond to antigens or other stimulatory signals.

Several approaches describing methods for evaluating the immune system as a target for toxicity have been published [1–8]. Use of multiple assays in a single animal has also been proposed [9]. While the mouse has been the predominant species of choice in the past, other species, including the rat, guinea pig, chicken, fish, and monkey, are being used to evaluate the immunotoxicity of xenobiotics [10,11]. A considerable effort has been made in the last several years to establish functional assays which produce interpretable data useful for immunotoxicological assessment. In 1988, Luster and colleagues [3] published the results of the National Toxicology Program (NTP) interlaboratory study, whose purpose was to show that selected immunological assays were validated in the mouse. In conducting this validation process, four different laboratories evaluated multiple test compounds using the same methodology. Prior to evaluating the test compounds, the immunological methods selected were standardized and optimized by the various laboratories.

The outcome of these studies was the identification of selected assays which were both reproducible and interpretable. The assays were divided into two tiers where the first tier focused primarily on end-line assays. The second tier assays were more comprehensive in nature, providing in-depth mechanistic information regarding the effect of the test agent on the immune system. In addition to functional assays, immunological assays included in the tier approach were enumeration of cell types, including T and B cells, resident peritoneal cells, and various stem cells of the bone marrow. Selected toxicological studies were also included in the tier approach in order to provide a background of data by which the immunological findings could be interpreted in the light of effects on other target organs. These standard toxicological studies include changes in body weight, selected organ weights, selected haematological parameters and selected serum chemistries. This intralaboratory validation study demonstrated that reproducible results could be obtained within and between laboratories.

In this chapter, the functional assays used in the NTP approach for assisting the immunotoxic potential of a xenobiotic will be described, as will some of the potential problems and pitfalls associated with conducting the assays. Additionally, other functional assays routinely used in our laboratory to evaluate immune function will be discussed.

Assessment of humoral immunity

Three primary assays are utilized for routine evaluation of humoral immunity. These include the antibody-forming cell response to the T-dependent antigen sheep erythrocytes, the proliferative response to the B-cell mitogen lipopolysaccharide (LPS) and enumeration of B cells in the spleen, which technically is not a functional assay.

Measurement of the ability of mice to mount an antibody response to sheep erythrocytes represents one of the most useful indicators of immunocompetence. Most xenobiotics which decrease this response will alter host resistance to one or more of the microbial or tumour models. In our laboratory, several antigens were investigated for use and the sheep erythrocyte was selected as the antigen for initial evaluation of immunocompetence. Other antigens are used for mechanistic or confirmatory studies. Developmental studies performed have shown that the effect of a xenobiotic on antibody-forming cell (AFC) response to sheep erythrocytes was at least as sensitive an indicator as the T-independent antigens evaluated.

Several points must be considered in conducting the T-dependent antibody-forming cell response to sheep erythrocytes. The source and age of sheep cells can dramatically affect the magnitude of the response observed. We have observed that the antigenicity of erythrocytes from various sheep can differ significantly. Furthermore, sheep cells should be used within 2 weeks of drawing the blood for the best response. In order to optimize the response, each laboratory should conduct an antigen concentration response study with the sheep red blood cells (SRBC) they intend to use. With very high concentrations of SRBC, a decrease in the AFC response is observed. The administration of 2×10^8 SRBC gives us the optimum response with B6C3F1 mice. However, this is not necessarily optimum for other strains of mice. Thus, each laboratory must optimize the response depending on the strain and species of the animal model they are using. Routinely, the peak response of the AFC response is observed on day 4 after antigen administration. Although measurement of the response on days 3, 4, and 5 would show changes in drug-induced temporal kinetics of the response, only one xenobiotic from over 30 examined over the last 7 years has shown a change in temporal kinetics.

The most important factor in carrying out the AFC assay is the route of administration. Our experience has shown that administration of the antigen by the intravenous route is by far the preferred method. Intravenous administration of SRBCs via the lateral tail veins is easily accomplished if the animals are warmed slightly by placing them in empty cages on heating pads set for low intensity. The tail veins can be further dilated by wiping the tail with gauze dipped in warm water just prior to injection. While intraperitoneal administration may be considered by some to be easier, even with the most technically competent individual there is always the possibility of a missed injection.

Furthermore, with intraperitoneal injections there tends to be a small number of animals which do not respond to the antigen challenge. This is not the case with intravenous administration. The number of non-responders following intraperitoneal injections may represent missed injections or lack of sufficient antigen reaching the spleen due to peritoneal macrophage activity. Peritoneal administration is particularly undesirable if the test agent has been administered by the interperitoneal route, since inflammatory cells may be present at the site, and thus alter antigen distribution.

While the SRBC antigen has been the antigen of primary use, other antigens can also be employed. For in-depth or mechanistic studies, the use of T-independent antigens such as dinitrophenyl-Ficoll (DNP-Ficoll) or trinitrophenyl-lipopolysaccha-ride (TNP-LPS) can be used to determine which cell types are being affected by exposure to a xenobiotic [12]. While the enumeration of antigen-specific antibody-forming cells detected by plaque formation [13] is the most often used method for assessing the humoral response to SRBC, other methods also exist. The enzyme-linked immunospot (ELISPOT) and the filter immuno-plaque assay (FIPA) are two other methods for detecting antibody-forming cells [14,15]. Alternative methods for measuring humoral immunity include measuring haemoglobin released from a fixed number of SRBC target cells or measuring the release of a radiolabelled material from a target cell with a haemolytic antibody isotope release (HAIR) assay [16]. Measurement of antibody produced using enzyme-linked immunosorbent assay (ELISA) techniques are also being used [17]. However, to interpret ELISA data properly, sample values must be compared to a standard curve. Due to the curvilinear nature of most ELISA assays [18], reporting data only in terms of absorbance values can lead to erroneous conclusions.

Measurement of the spleen IgM and IgG antibody response to the T-dependent antigen, SRBC

In our laboratory, the primary IgM and IgG responses to SRBC are enumerated using a modified haemolytic plaque assay [13]. In a standard 14-day immunotoxicological study, mice are treated daily with the vehicle or the appropriate doses of the test article. Animals are sensitized with 2×10^8 SRBC administered intravenously on day 11 for evaluation of IgM response or on day 10 for evaluation of the primary IgG response of the exposure period. Separate groups of animals are used to evaluate the IgM response, which peaks on day 4 after immunization and the IgG primary response which peaks 1 day later. On day 15, 1 day after the last exposure to the test article, animals are sacrificed, and spleen cells are prepared by mincing the spleen in 3 ml of balanced salt solution (BSS) medium between two frosted microscope slides. After washing, an aliquot of cells (100 μl) is added to a test tube containing guinea pig complement (25 μl), SRBC (25 μl) and 350 μl of a warm agar solution, 0.5% bacto-agar, containing 0.05% diethylaminoethyl-dextran (DEAE-dextran). After thoroughly mixing, the test tube mixture is plated on to a plastic petri dish and covered with a microscope cover slip. The petri dishes are then incubated at 37°C for 3 h. Routinely, at least two dilutions of the spleen cells are used to ensure that the number of AFCs are in a range which can be accurately counted. The plaques which developed are counted using a Bellco plaque viewer. Cell counts are performed on the 3-ml sample and the number of nucleated cells present in the spleen is determined. The humoral immunity data are expressed as specific activity (AFC/10^6 spleen cells) and AFC per spleen. Measurement of the number of IgG AFC is conducted in a similar manner except that an appropriate dilution of rabbit anti-mouse IgG antibody is added to the complement to facilitate the development of the IgG plaques.

The number of IgG AFCs is calculated by counting the number of plaques which developed in the presence of the rabbit anti-mouse IgG antibody (total AFCs) minus the number of IgM plaques which were developed without anti-IgG antibody. As with the IgM AFC, the data are expressed as specific activity (IgG AFC/10^6 spleen cells) and IgG AFC per spleen. Of the numerous compounds we have evaluated over the years, none has shown a selective target for the primary IgG response.

As shown in Fig. 17.1, the AFC response gives remarkably consistent results. The values in the figure represent the mean ± s.e. for control animals from studies conducted in our laboratory using the female B6C3F1 mouse.

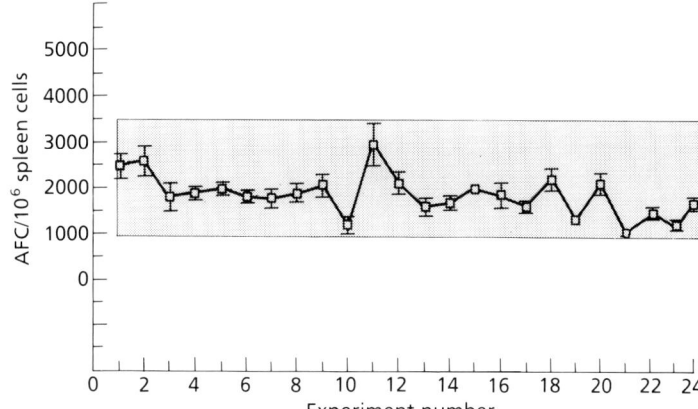

Fig. 17.1 Control values for AFC/10⁶ spleen cells in female B6C3F1 mice. The numbers represent the mean ± s.e. derived from eight mice per experiment. The number of experiments over approximately a 20-month period is shown on the *X* axis.

An example of representative AFC data is shown in Fig. 17.2. In this study, B6C3F1 mice were exposed daily to corn oil (vehicle), technical-grade pentachlorophenol (PCP), or 'pure' pentachlorophenol (PCP EC-7), which had been purified to reduce manufacturing contaminants. An additional group received no treatment. As can be seen, the technical-grade PCP produced a dose-dependent suppression of the IgM antibody response when evaluated as AFC/10⁶ spleen cells. The primary IgG antibody response was also suppressed at the high dose of technical-grade PCP. Animals receiving 'pure' PCP had responses which were not significantly different from either vehicle or untreated mice. Thus, the immunosuppression resulting from exposure to technical-grade PCP resulted from the contaminants present in the material.

Spleen cell response to bacterial LPS

The lymphocyte proliferative response assay to both B- and T-cell mitogens developed in our laboratory is a modification of the previously reported methods [19,20]. Blastogenesis and proliferation are an inte-

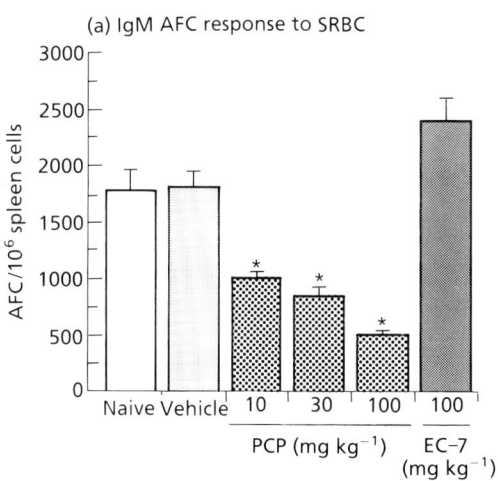

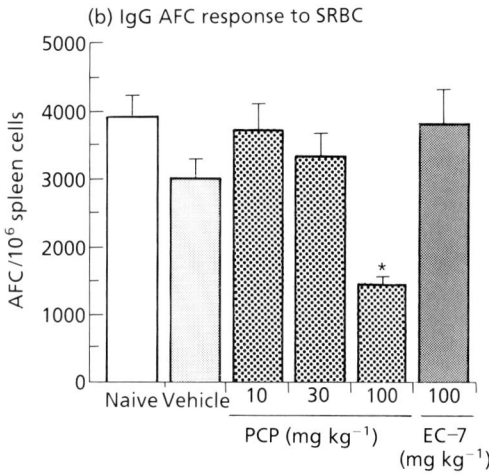

Fig. 17.2 Example of a study assessing humoral immunity. Female B6C3F1 mice were exposed for 14 days to corn oil vehicle, technical-grade pentachlorophenol (PCP), 'pure' PCP (EC-7) or were untreated. The AFC response to SRBC was evaluated on day 4 for IgM and Day 5 for IgG. Values represent the mean ± s.e. from eight animals per group. *Statistically significant difference from vehicle control at $P \leqslant 0.05$.

gral part of B-cell maturation to an immunoglobulin-producing cell. The LPS from *Salmonella typhosa* 0901 is used to evaluate the ability of a xenobiotic to alter the response of B lymphocytes to undergo blastogenesis and proliferation. Several LPS preparations were initially examined for ability to induce blastogenesis and proliferation. *S. typhosa* 0901 has been found to be a reproducible mitogen in our studies. Evaluation of the B-cell response to LPS is usually conducted on the same cell preparation used for performing the T-cell mitogens response to concanavalin A (Con A) and phytohaemagglutinin (PHA). Routinely, for NTP studies mice are exposed to the xenobiotic for a 14-day period. Twenty-four hours after the last exposure, the spleens are removed and single-cell suspensions prepared in BSS using sterilized glass slides. After washing, cells are counted and appropriately diluted in RPMI-1640 media containing 5–10% serum, such that 2×10^5 cells are put into each well of a micro-titre plate containing the appropriate concentration of LPS. We have found that the maximum length of time for which the cells can be out of the animal and not incubating with mitogen is about 3 h. Cells are incubated for 3 days at 37°C under 5% CO_2 and during the last 18 h of incubation 3.7×10^4 Bq ^{3}H-thymidine is present in the cultures.

Cells are harvested and counted in a liquid scintillation counter and the data are expressed as c.p.m. per culture. The micro-titre plates are prepared within 1 week of assay and maintained at -80°C until used. Developmental studies should be carried out to optimize the mitogen assays for the appropriate cell number per well and the day of peak response. The optimal cell concentration in our laboratory was found to be 2×10^5 and the response peaks on day 3. In running all of our mitogen assays, multiple concentrations of each mitogen are used to ensure that an optimal concentration has been included. We routinely use 10 and 100 μg ml^{-1} as two of our concentrations of LPS. We have found that the optimal mitogen concentration varies from lot to lot of mice. An example of the type of data one can obtain from mitogen studies is shown in Table 17.1. In this study, female B6C3F1 mice were exposed by oral gavage to nitrobenzene or the corn oil vehicle daily for 14 days. On day 15, spleen cells were prepared as described above and the lympho-cyte proliferation response to LPS, Con A and PHA was evaluated.

Serum immunoglobulin levels

Our experience in the NTP has shown that measurement of basal serum immunoglobulin levels was of minimum value as a predictor of immunotoxic compounds. The basal immunoglobulin levels are useful in providing a history of antigen stimulation of the animals but, for short duration studies due to the half-life of the immunoglobulins, they were found not to represent a sensitive indicator of an altered immune system. For example, studies in our laboratory have shown that mice exposed to benzo(a)pyrene at doses which significantly decreased the AFC response to SRBC had no effect on basal serum IgM, immunoglobulin levels. Basal immunoglobulin levels are no longer included in the NTP evaluation panel. Others have reported that, for the rat, basal immunoglobulin levels can be a sensitive indicator of immunotoxicity [21].

Assessment of cell-mediated immunity

While there are many assays capable of assessing cell-mediated immunity, four assays have been selected for routine use in the NTP approach to evaluating the immunotoxic potential of a xenobiotic. These include: the mixed leucocyte response (MLR); spleen lymphocyte response to the T-lymphocyte mitogen Con A; the cytotoxic T-lymphocyte assay (CTL), and the delayed hypersensitivity response (DHR) to keyhole limpet haemocyanin (KLH). In addition to these functional assays, enumeration of T lymphocytes in the spleen, including T subsets, is routinely conducted.

Mixed leucocyte culture response

The response of spleen cells from xenobiotic-exposed mice to an allogenic spleen cell has been one of the most sensitive indicators of effects on cell-mediated immunity of any of the assays we have evaluated. In order to conduct the assay in a toxicological mode, we have modified procedures previously reported [22]. In our assay, DBA/2 spleen cells are used as the allogenic (stimulator) cell for

Table 17.1 Effect of nitrobenzene on the lymphocyte proliferation response in female B6C3F1 mice exposed to nitrobenzene daily for 14 days

Mitogen	Concentration ($\mu g\ ml^{-1}$)	Vehicle ($n = 7$)	Nitrobenzene (mg kg^{-1})			Dose–response
			30 ($n = 8$)	100 ($n = 7$)	300 ($n = 7$)	
Concanavalin A	0.5	16136 ± 2186	15076 ± 3277	10105 ± 3277	8138 ± 1804	$P < 0.01$
	0.1	46950 ± 5104	54172 ± 4910	$19468 \pm 3290^{**}$	$24577 \pm 2845^{**}$	$P < 0.01$
	5.0	106152 ± 10326	106813 ± 7148	$48885 \pm 4204^{**}$	$59602 \pm 5189^{**}$	$P < 0.01$
	10.0	37351 ± 3745	44491 ± 6939	$16540 \pm 1836^{**}$	32166 ± 5210	$P < 0.05$
Phytohaemagglutinin	0.1	4923 ± 499	$10899 \pm 1180^{**}$	$2584 \pm 403^{*}$	$2414 \pm 494^{*}$	$P < 0.01$
	0.5	69234 ± 5297	81569 ± 4465	$37832 \pm 3785^{**}$	54241 ± 5349	$P < 0.05$
	1.0	62350 ± 4075	65783 ± 5295	$35208 \pm 3529^{*}$	$43712 \pm 3421^{*}$	$P < 0.01$
	5.0	2994 ± 252	3664 ± 525	2956 ± 395	$4667 \pm 477^{*}$	$P < 0.05$
Lipopolysaccharide	10	9271 ± 1049	9270 ± 1645	7544 ± 846	7838 ± 927	NS
	100	17919 ± 1607	15826 ± 2911	13438 ± 1173	15735 ± 3128	NS
Media		293 ± 139	332 ± 62	$801 \pm 208^{*}$	$1625 \pm 748^{*}$	$P < 0.01$
Spleen cell no. $\times 10^7$		14.5 ± 0.9	13.0 ± 0.7	$25.0 \pm 1.5^{**}$	$23.1 \pm 1.1^{*}$	$P < 0.01$

Female B6C3F1 mice were gavaged with corn oil or nitrobenzene daily for 14 days. On day 15, mice were sacrificed and spleen cell suspensions cultured (2×10^5 cells/culture) with concanavalin A, phytohaemagglutinin, lipopolysaccharide or medium alone in the presence of 5% human AB serum. Cultures were pulsed with 3.7×10^4 Bq ^{3}H-thymidine after 24 h and harvested after 48 h. Values represent the mean c.p.m. $\pm$ S.E. derived from the number of animals indicated. The data were evaluated using an analysis of variance. When significant differences occurred, treatment groups were compared to vehicle control using a Dunnett's t-test. Values significantly different from vehicle control at the $P < 0.05$ level are indicated by *, while those significantly different at the $P < 0.01$ level are noted by **. The Jonckheere's test was used to test for dose-dependence among the vehicle and treatment groups.

B6C3F1 (responder) mice. Spleen cells from the DBA/2 mice are usually prepared first since they are treated with mitomycin C to render them incapable of proliferation and require repeated washing to ensure removal of any residual mitomycin C.

Spleens from the DBA/2 mice are collected using aseptic techniques and placed in sterile BSS. Spleen cell suspensions are prepared by pressing the spleens between frosted glass slides which have first been autoclaved. Cells are washed, adjusted to 2×10^7 cells ml^{-1} and incubated for 45 min with mitomycin C (50 $\mu g\ ml^{-1}$) at 37°C. The mitomycin-treated cells are washed at least four times and adjusted to a final concentration of 4×10^6 cells ml^{-1} in RPMI-1640 with 10% foetal calf serum. In lieu of mitomycin C treatment, stimulator cells can be irradiated if the laboratory has this capability. Cells from the responder mice are collected in a similar fashion and

are adjusted to a concentration of 1×10^6 cells ml^{-1} in RPMI-1640 with 10% foetal calf serum. Spleen cells are added to each well of a U-bottom plate at a concentration of 1×10^5 cells per well. The stimulator cells are added (4×10^5 cells per well) to give a 4 : 1 stimulator: responder ratio. The ratio of stimulator to responder cells is a parameter which needs to be optimized in each laboratory conducting the assay. The U-bottom plates are centrifuged at 400 r.p.m. for 5 min at 4°C to improve cell–cell contact and the plates are then incubated at 37°C in 5% CO_2. In our assay, the peak response occurred on day 5, but the time of peak response also needs to be established for each laboratory. During the last 18–24 h of culture, 3.7×10^4 Bq of ^{3}H-thymidine is added to each well. Cells from each well are collected with a cell-harvester and counted in a scintillation counter.

There are also two control groups which should be run with each experiment. The stimulator cells, after mitomycin C, are incubated with a single concentration of Con A to ensure that their ability to proliferate has been inhibited. Conversely, the responder cells are also incubated with Con A to ensure that they are capable of proliferation. The data from the control animals and those receiving treatment are usually presented as the c.p.m. of the responder cells alone and the c.p.m. of the responders + stimulator cells. Another method of presenting the MLR data is to express the data as a stimulation index. In the published literature, stimulation indexes have been calculated in various manners. In our laboratory, we calculated the stimulation index by dividing the c.p.m. of the responder + stimulator cells by the c.p.m. of the responder cells alone for each individual animal. Figure 17.3 shows historical control data for this assay in female B6C3F1 mice. As indicated earlier, this assay has been very useful in detecting xenobiotics that affect cell-mediated immunity. A good correlation was observed between the suppression of this assay and increased susceptibility to host resistance models, i.e. *Listeria* and PYB6 sarcoma, for which cell-mediated immunity is known to play a major role in the host defence [3].

Spleen cell response to Con A

The response of spleen cells to the T lymphocyte mitogen, Con A, provides an evaluation of the ability of T lymphocytes to undergo blastogenesis and proliferation. The spleen cells used for this assay are prepared in an identical manner as those used for the mitogen response to LPS, described in the humoral immunity section. Routinely, the same spleen cell preparation is used to evaluate the response to both B- and T-cell mitogens in the same experiment. We have found this to be an efficient way to conduct the assay, since the mitogens can be prepared, placed in the plates prior to the day of assay and stored frozen without losing their ability to stimulate spleen cells. For evaluating the Con A response, four concentrations of the mitogen are used. Three micro-titre wells, i.e. triplicate cultures, are used for each mitogen concentration for each individual animal. As with the B-cell mitogen LPS, the optimal concentration for Con A can vary between groups of mice; thus, multiple concentrations of the Con A are employed. We use 0.5, 1.0, 5.0 and 10 μg per well of Con A to ensure that an optimal concentration has been included. For the T-cell mitogens, there is a pronounced bell-shaped curve with the optimal concentration usually being 1.0 or 5.0 μg for Con A. Another mitogen often used to evaluate the proliferation and blastogenesis of T cells is PHA. The concentrations of this mitogen used in our laboratory are 0.1, 0.5, 1, and 5 μg per well and the peak response is usually observed with the 0.5 or 1.0 μg per well concentration. As with most of the mitogen assays, the peak day of response should be established for each mitogen by the laboratory undertaking the assay. The end-point of these assays is the incorporation of ^{3}H-thymidine

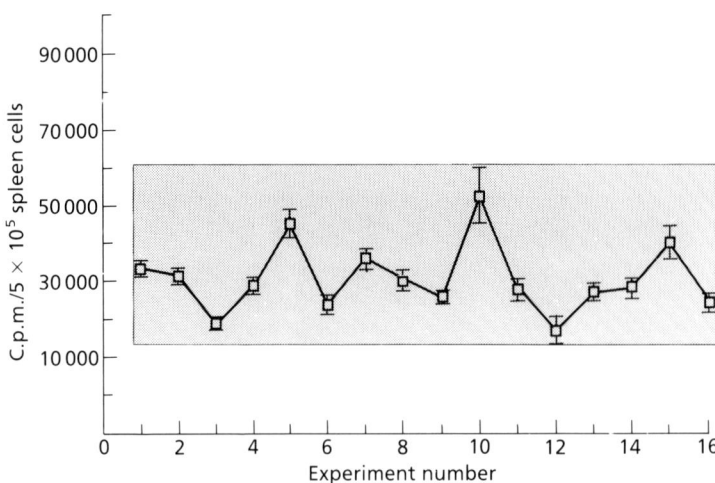

Fig. 17.3 Control values for spleen mixed leucocyte response (MLR) in female B6C3F1 mice. The numbers represent the mean ± s.e. derived from eight mice per experiment. The number of experiments over approximately a 20-month period is shown on the X axis.

into the proliferating cells and the data are usually expressed as c.p.m. per culture. An example of the type of data obtained from the T-cell mitogens is shown in Table 17.1.

Cytotoxic T-lymphocyte assay

This assay measures the ability of the spleen cells to recognize allogenic cells, proliferate, and differentiate into mature cells which are capable of identifying and lysing the foreign cell. In our laboratory, measurement of the lysed cell is via a ^{51}Cr release. Our *in vitro* CTL assay has been adapted from one previously reported [23].

One day after the final exposure to the test article, animals are sacrificed and spleens are removed under sterile conditions. A single-cell suspension is prepared using frosted microscope slides, as described in earlier assays. The suspension of splenocytes from control and treated mice is washed once with phosphate-buffered saline (PBS). Cell concentrations are adjusted to 4×10^7 total cells in 19.5 ml of sensitization medium and added to a 25-cm^2 tissue culture flask. The sensitization medium is Eagle's minimal essential medium (E-MEM) supplemented with 10% foetal calf serum, 25 mmol l^{-1} HEPES, 1 mmol l^{-1} L-glutamine, 50 μg ml^{-1} gentamicin and 1×10^{-5} mmol l^{-1} 2-mercaptoethanol.

P815 mastocytoma cells are used as the sensitizer cells for this assay. These cells are grown in culture and during their log phase of growth they are harvested and treated with mitomycin C, 50 μg per 2×10^7 cells. The sensitizer cells are added to each flask in a volume of 0.5 ml to yield a final responder: sensitizer ratio of 50:1. The cultures are incubated in an upright position for 5 days at 37°C in 5% CO$_2$. One flask is used for each animal. Following the sensitization phase, cultured spleen cells are harvested by gentle agitation, decanting and rinsing the flask with PBS. The cells are washed once with PBS and resuspended in E-MEM medium for determination of cytotoxic T cell activity. The P815 cells, which are also used for the target cells, are cultivated in Dulbecco's modified minimal essential medium with 10% foetal calf serum and are labelled with ^{51}Cr (1.85×10^6 Bq ^{51}Cr as sodium chromate per 2×10^7 cells) for 60 min at 37°C. The cells are washed twice with PBS, allowed to remain at room temperature for 30 min, and washed twice with E-MEM. One hundred μl of labelled target cells (2×10^4 cells per well) is co-cultured in duplicate with 100 μl of graded numbers of splenic effector cells in U-bottom micro-titre culture plates to yield a serial half-dilution of effector: target ratios from 25:1 to 0.75:1. After a 4-h incubation at 37°C and 5% CO$_2$, the plates are centrifuged for 10 min and 100 μl of supernatant from each well is removed and counted in a γ-spectrophotometer. The labelled target cells in the presence of E-MEM medium and 0.1% Triton X-100 serve as the spontaneous and maximum ^{51}Cr release controls, respectively. The data are expressed as percentage of specific release as a function of effector:target ratio. Data can also be expressed in terms of lytic units, where the lytic unit is defined as the number of splenocytes required to kill 50% of the target cells.

It is important to note that the CTL assay described above measures only the actions of the drug on the afferent arm of the response, since the responder cells are removed from the treated animal and stimulated *in vitro* with the allogenic cell. Our developmental studies have demonstrated that a good CTL response *in vivo* requires a proliferating antigen. This creates unique problems if the assay is to be used in an immunotoxicology mode. For example, if the CTL response is depressed by the test compound, *in vivo* sensitization with a proliferating antigen, such as tumour cells, fungi, or bacteria, could result in a progressive disease state which would make quantitation of cytotoxic T-cell activity difficult.

Delayed hypersensitivity response

One of the reasons the AFC assay has been so successful in identifying compounds which modulate the immune response is that the assay is holistic in nature. The animals are treated with the test compound *in vivo* and are sensitized *in vivo* with SRBC. On the day of peak response, cells are evaluated for their ability to produce antibody in an *in vitro* assay which usually lasts no more than 4 h after the spleens are removed from the animal. This is in contrast to assays such as the mitogen response, MLR, and CTL where spleen cells remain in culture for as much as 5 days after being removed from the animals. As a result, an immunomodulatory effect produced by a xenobiotic may be lost with this extended period of time in culture.

One approach to circumvent this problem is to use a holistic assay capable of measuring cell-mediated immunity. In our laboratory, we have evaluated several assays to measure a DHR. Our current DHR assay utilizes KLH as the sensitizing antigen [24]. This assay is a modification of the method of Lefford [25] which quantitates the influx of labelled monocytes into the site undergoing a DHR. In studies where the test compound is administered for a 14-day exposure period, animals are induced with KLH (100 μg) via a subcutaneous injection in the central portion of the back between the shoulders on the first day of dosing. On day 8 of exposure, a second inducing injection is made, as previously described. On day 14 of exposure, mononuclear cells are labelled *in vivo* by administering 7.4×10^4 Bq ^{125}I-5-iododeoxyuridine (IUdR) per mouse by intravenous injection. The specific activity of the IUdR used in these studies is 8.14×10^{10} Bq mmol^{-1}. On day 15, the day following the final exposure, animals are challenged in the central portion of the left ear with an intradermal injection of KLH (30 μg).

Twenty-four hours after challenge, animals are sacrificed and a central portion of each ear is removed with a punch-borer. Each ear biopsy is counted in a γ-counter. The results are expressed as a stimulation index, which represents the counts in the challenged ear divided by the counts in the unchallenged ear, after correcting for non-specific monocyte influx. In this manner, each animal serves as its own control. The non-specific monocyte influx is calculated from a group of animals which receives only the intradermal injection of KLH and not the two inducing injections.

Our earlier methods for measurement of the DHR response [7] had utilized SRBC as the sensitizing antigen. SRBC were injected into the foot-pad following the procedure originally established [26] and foot-pad swelling was quantitated by measuring the extravasation of ^{125}I-human serum albumin into the oedematous area produced by the DHR. This assay was subsequently replaced by the DHR response to KLH when it was observed that measurements of DHR responses that used the SRBC antigen may have a significant antibody component contributing to the response observed. This is illustrated in Fig. 17.4.

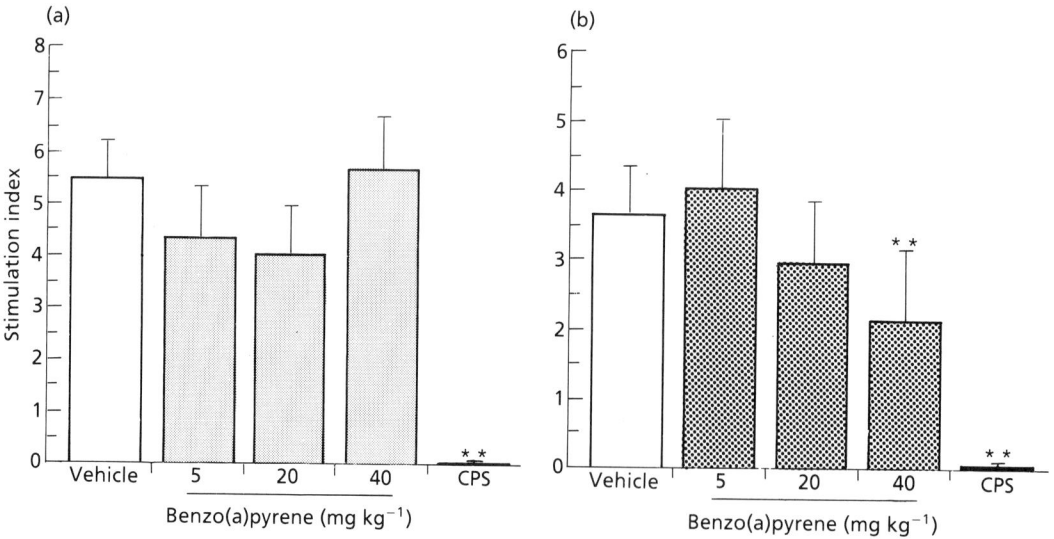

Fig. 17.4 Comparison of the delayed hypersensitivity (DHR) response to keyhole limpet haemocyanin (KLH) and sheep erythrocytes. Animals were exposed to corn oil vehicle or benzo(a)pyrene for 14 days, or cyclophosphamide (50 mg kg^{-1}) during the last 4 days of the treatment regimen. Values represent the mean $\pm$ s.e. from eight animals per group. **Statistically significant difference from vehicle control at $P \leqslant 0.01$.

Studies in our laboratory and others [27] have shown that benzo(a)pyrene (BAP) had no effect on cell-mediated immune functions in adult mice. However, when the DHR response was evaluated in BAP-treated mice, a decrease in DHR was observed, which corresponded with the decrease seen in the AFC response to SRBC. When animals treated in the identical manner were evaluated using the KLH antigen, no decrease in cell-mediated immunity was observed. The lack of effect on the KLH-DHR was consistent with the failure of BAP to affect other cell-mediated immune functions. Other antigens, such as heat-aggregated bovine serum albumin, have also been utilized to produce DHR responses used in immunotoxicological testing [17].

The DHR to KLH is an assay which requires numerous immunological components to function properly to produce the DHR. Among these are antigen recognition, cell proliferation, production of lymphokines, and the recruitment of inflammatory cells capable of releasing substances that produce immunologically mediated inflammation. Since a multitude of immunologically competent cells are required to function in concert, the DHR response to KLH represents a useful assay for a holistic evaluation of cell-mediated immunity.

Assessment of innate immunity

Innate immunity or non-specific immunity encompasses those immunological functions which do not require prior exposure to a specific antigen [28]. As with the other components of the immune system, numerous assays are available to assess the potential action of xenobiotics on non-specific immunity. Assays which have been selected for use by the NTP include natural killer cell activity and evaluation of macrophage function. Two additional assays routinely used in our laboratory to evaluate the complement system, a major component of innate immunity, are the determination of serum total haemolytic activity (CH50) and the levels of complement component C3 present in mouse serum [29].

Natural killer cell activity

Natural killer cells are thought to play a key role in non-specific immunity. It is currently believed that natural killer cells possess innate cytotoxicity against a variety of tumour cells. These cells play an important role in deterring neoplasia by controlling tumour growth as well as metastatic dissemination [30]. For many xenobiotics, results from the *in vitro* natural killer cell assay will correlate with the results from the *in vivo* B16F10 melanoma tumour model [3]. Natural killer cells are also reported to have activity against various bacteria including *Listeria monocytogenes*. In evaluating natural killer cell activity, an *in vitro* cytotoxicity assay is conducted which utilizes the YAC-1 cell line as the target cell. YAC-1 are labelled with ^{51}Cr and the desired effector:target ratios are established with splenic natural killer cells which are used as the effector cells in this assay [31].

For NTP studies, this assay is routinely conducted 24 h after the last xenobiotic exposure. Following sacrifice of the animal, spleens are removed and weighed. Single-cell suspensions from individual spleens are prepared aseptically. Following centrifugation, the pellet is resuspended in RPMI-1640 supplemented with 10% foetal calf serum. The cell suspension is adjusted to three concentrations—10^7, 5×10^6, and 2.5×10^6 cells ml^{-1}, to obtain effector-to-target ratios of 100:1, 50:1, and 25:1. The target cells, YAC-1 cells, are maintained in a stock culture and are adjusted to a concentration of 10^7 cells ml^{-1}. These cells are labelled by incubation with 7.4×10^6 Bq of ^{51}Cr for 90 min in a 37°C water bath with frequent agitation. Following the incubation, the cells are washed three times in BSS plus 25 mmol l^{-1} HEPES, counted, and adjusted to 10^5 cells ml^{-1}. The maximum release is determined by adding 0.1 ml of the 10^5 YAC-1 cells ml^{-1} and 0.1 ml 2.0 mol l^{-1} HCl to each of 12 replicate wells on a 96-well microtitre plate. The spontaneous release is determined by adding 0.1 ml of medium to 12 replicate cultures containing the targets. The target cells, 0.1 ml of the 10^5 YAC-1 cells ml^{-1}, are added to each well. The effector cells from each animal are then added (0.1 ml) to each of four replicate wells of targets cells at each effector concentration. The plates are incubated for 4 h at 37°C at 5% CO_2. Following the incubation, the plates are centrifuged for 10 min, and 0.1 ml of the supernatant is removed from each well and counted. After correcting for spontaneous release, the percentage of cytotoxicity at each effector concentration is determined for each treatment group and compared to the comparable values for the control mice.

One of the major factors affecting this assay is controlling the amount of spontaneous release occurring. In a standard 4-h incubation period, the spontaneous release should be below 10%. Among the factors affecting the spontaneous release are the condition of the YAC-1 cells, age of the ^{51}Cr used in the labelling, and the presence of an appropriate foetal calf serum in the medium during the labelling procedure. Each of these items can affect the labelling of the YAC-1 cells, resulting in high spontaneous release and an unusable assay. An example of the type of data obtained in the assay is shown in Fig. 17.5. In this study, female B6C3F1 mice were administered 2,4-diaminotoluene by gavage for 14 days, and on day 15 natural killer cell activity was evaluated as described above. Exposure to 2,4-diaminotoluene produced a dose-dependent decrease in natural killer cell activity, which was significant for each of the effector: target ratios for the two higher doses.

Macrophage assays. Over the last several years numerous macrophage function assays have been evaluated in our laboratory and in the other NTP laboratories. While some assays initially appeared to be useful, with time it became apparent that as part of an immunotoxicological testing panel, they were of little value in that they did not give reproducible results or they failed to correlate with other macrophage parameters. An example of one such assay no longer utilized is the evaluation of ectoenzyme levels [32]. Currently, the phagocytic ability of macrophages and the ability of the peritoneal macrophages to be activated to a tumoricidal state are being used as assays to assess macrophage function. These functional assays are used in conjunction with peritoneal macrophage cell number and differential cell count to provide information on this component of innate immunity. When an *in vivo* assessment of the fixed macrophages of the reticuloendothelial system is necessary, the functional activity of the reticuloendothelial system can be measured in the whole animal [33].

Two assays are used to measure functional phagocytic capacity of macrophages. The first evaluates non-immune-mediated phagocytes by measuring the uptake of latex covaspheres. The second assay measures immune-mediated phagocytes, since the target cell is first opsonized and phagocytosis is mediated by the Fc receptor on the macrophages. Both adherence of target cells to the macrophage and the subsequent phagocytosis are quantitated in this assay [34].

Macrophage phagocytosis of fluorescent covaspheres

Animals are sacrificed using a procedure which does not result in bleeding into the peritoneal cavity and macrophages are obtained from the peritoneal cavity by lavage. Hank's balanced salt solution (HBSS; 8 ml) is injected into the peritoneum and the peritoneal cells are loosened by shaking the mouse by the tail. Peritoneal cells are collected, centrifuged, and resuspended in RPMI with 10% foetal calf serum at a concentration of 5×10^5 cells ml^{-1}. To each chamber of a Lab-Tek tissue culture slide, 2.5×10^5 macrophages are added in a volume of 0.5 ml. The slides are then incubated for 2 h at 37°C in a 5% CO_2 incubator to allow cells to adhere. The medium is removed and replaced with 0.5 ml of fresh medium, containing 75 μl of a 1:100 dilution of

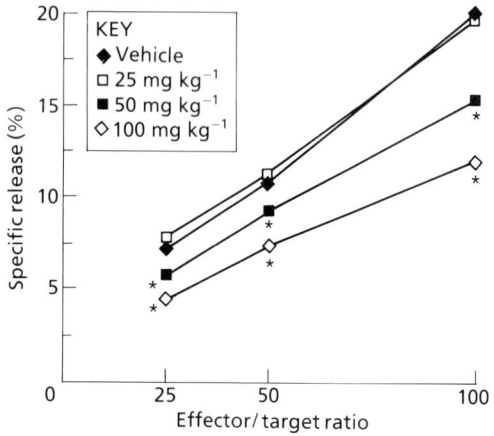

Fig. 17.5 Example of a study assessing innate immunity. Natural killer cell activity was evaluated in female B6C3F1 mice exposed for 14 days to vehicle (distilled water) or 2, 4-diaminotoluene. Values represent the mean ± s.e. derived from eight mice per group. *Statistically significant difference from vehicle control at $P \leqslant 0.05$.

fluorescent latex covaspheres (0.98 μ in diameter) in PBS. The macrophages are incubated with the covaspheres for 24 h at 37°C in a 5% CO_2 incubator on a rocker platform. The slides are then washed three times with PBS, fixed in methanol for 30 s, immersed in methylene chloride for 30–60 s, and read on a fluorescent microscope. Macrophages with more than five latex particles are counted as positive for phagocytosis. Data are expressed as a percentage of phagocytosis, which is calculated as the ratio of the number of macrophages with five covaspheres/ total number of macrophages counted. By immersing the slides in methylene chloride, the covaspheres which have not been phagocytized are dissolved, and thus one can easily quantitate phagocytized fluorescent latex particles [35].

Macrophage phagocytosis of chicken erythrocytes

Macrophage phagocytic capacity, involving an immunologically mediated (Fc receptor) response, is measured using chicken erythrocytes. As described above, cells of the peritoneal cavity are removed by lavage. The peritoneal exudate cells from four mice from the same treatment group are usually pooled to obtain the necessary number of cells. Cells are adjusted to 2×10^6 cells ml^{-1} and 0.5 ml of the cell suspension is added to each well of a 24-well tissue culture plate. The plates are then incubated for 2–3 h at 37°C in a 5% CO_2 incubator to allow adherence of the peritoneal exudate cells. Chicken erythrocytes are labelled with ^{51}Cr by incubating 5×10^8 pelleted cells with 7.4×10^6 Bq at 37°C for 30 min. The peritoneal exudate cells are washed twice to remove non-adhering cells and 400 μl of media containing a maximum subagglutinating dilution of the antisera is added to each well. The labelled chicken erythrocytes are washed to remove any ^{51}Cr not taken up by the cells and 100 μl of the labelled cells is added to each well. Plates are incubated by rocking for 1 h at 37°C in a 5% CO_2 incubator. Following the incubation, each well is washed to remove unbound chicken erythrocytes, and an ammonium chloride solution is added to lyse adhered chicken erythrocytes. The supernatant from each well is removed and counted to determine adherence of chicken erythrocytes to the macrophages.

Next, 0.1 N NaOH is added to lyse the macrophages and phagocytized chicken erythrocytes. This lysate is removed and counted to determine the amount of phagocytosis which has occurred. Three to six wells per treatment group of peritoneal exudate cells which do not receive the ^{51}Cr chicken erythrocytes are lysed with Triton-X 100 (0.05%) and the lysate used to evaluate DNA content [36]. The data are expressed as adherence c.p.m., phagocytized c.p.m., and as the specific activity for adherence and phagocytosis. Specific activity is determined by dividing the number of adhered or phagocytized c.p.m., respectively, by the DNA per well. It is necessary to express the data in terms of specific activity since compounds which affect the macrophages' ability to adhere to the 24-well tissue plates will significantly alter the results obtained. Originally, protein determinations were used to establish the number of macrophages adhering to the culture plates; however, we have found that DNA content was less affected by exposure to xenobiotics, and thus, was better suited to determine specific activity.

Macrophage-activating factor (MAF) assay

The activation of macrophages to inhibit tumour growth and to kill tumour cells represents one of the highest activation states achievable by macrophages. Gamma-interferon, in the presence of a small amount of LPS, is now known to be a lymphokine which activates macrophages to a tumoricidal level. If exposure to a xenobiotic blocked the ability of γ-interferon to activate the macrophage to a tumoricidal state, then the xenobiotic has the potential to affect innate immunity adversely. Conversely, exposure to xenobiotics may activate macrophages to a more tumoricidal state, and thus augment the innate ability of these cells to kill tumour cells. The MAF assay is used to evaluate a xenobiotic's effect on macrophage activation.

In this assay, peritoneal cells are collected from individual animals as described for the phagocytosis assays. They are first centrifuged and adjusted to 5×10^5 cells ml^{-1} in RPMI-1640 containing 10% foetal calf serum. Cells are pipetted into 96-well plates, 200 μl per well, and allowed to adhere for 2 h at 37°C in a 5% CO_2 incubator. Following incubation, the wells are washed twice with PBS to remove any non-adhering cells. Gamma-interferon, 10 units ml^{-1} including 10 ng LPS per ml, is added to the adhered cells and allowed to incubate for 4 h under the same conditions. Plates are then washed twice with HBSS and 200 μl of B16F10 tumour cells (5×10^4 ml^{-1}) is added to each well. The macrophages are then incubated with the tumour cells for 48 h at 37°C in 5% CO_2, during which time the tumour cells adhere to culture plates. Plates are washed three times with PBS and stained with 0.5% crystal violet, 70% methanol. The amount of staining is measured using an ELISA reader at 600 nm and the amount of stain is correlated with the number of tumour cells remaining after incubation with the macrophages. In addition to the macrophages which are treated with the γ-interferon, untreated macrophages from each animal are also evaluated to determine if exposure to the xenobiotic activated the macrophage to a more tumoricidal state.

While many other assays are available for evaluating the status of macrophages, our experience has indicated that at present most are too labour-intensive or lack the reproducibility and interpretability needed for use in a toxicology mode.

Host resistance challenge studies

Host resistance studies represent one of the recognized approaches for assaying the effects of xenobiotics on the immune system. Bradley and Morahan [37] have provided an excellent summary, with extensive references, of infectious models used to assess changes in host resistance to environmental chemicals. While host resistance studies do not represent the panacea for immunotoxicological testing purported by some, when carried out correctly they are useful in evaluating the immunotoxic potential of a xenobiotic and also provide insight as to the mechanism through which a compound is acting. For example, host resistance to the bacterial pathogen *Streptococcus pneumoniae* is mediated primarily by the complement system, polymorphonuclear leucocytes (PMNs) and, in the latter stages of the infection, the development of antigen-specific antibody [38]. Early deaths following challenge with this organism, i.e. less than 24 h after challenge, can be directly related to effects on the complement system. Animals which succumb during the intermediate time of the 7-day infection period can be shown to be the result of decreased PMNs, while deaths late in the disease process can result from effects on the production of antibody.

Shown in Table 17.2 are some of the organisms which we have evaluated for their potential use as models for host resistance. Those which are included in the NTP approach are indicated with an asterisk. Additionally, the murine acquired immune deficiency syndrome (AIDS) virus (MuLPBM5) is currently being utilized for evaluation of potential AIDS drugs.

One of the problems associated with the use of host resistance models is that there is no one model which can be used to measure overall immunocompetence. An example of the problems associated with using a single host resistance assay to evaluate the immunotoxicity of a test compound is illustrated

Table 17.2 Organisms evaluated for use in host resistance models

Viruses
Encephalomyocarditis virus
Herpes simplex virus type 2
Influenza virus (strain A_2/Taiwan/64)
Murine acquired immune deficiency syndrome virus (MuLPBM5)

Bacteria
*Streptococcus pneumoniae**
*Listeria monocytogenes**
Escherichia coli
Corynebacterium parvum
Pseudomonas aeruginosa

Parasites
Naegleria foleri
*Plasmodium berghei**
*Plasmodium yoelii**

Yeast and fungi
Candida albicans
Cryptococcus neoformans

Tumour models
B16F10 Melanoma*
PYB6 Fibrosarcoma*

*Included in the National Toxicology Program's approach.

below. The bacterial, viral, and tumour studies were conducted in our laboratory and plasmodium parasitaemia studies were carried out by our colleagues [39]. The host resistance studies were conducted using two bacteria, two viruses, two parasites, and one tumour model. Four concentrations of the pathogen were used in all studies, except the plasmodium parasitaemia studies, where a single challenge level was utilized. Three doses of the xenobiotic, benzo(a)pyrene, were used. Benzo(a)pyrene was administered subcutaneously for 14 days to female B6C3F1 mice, and the pathogen was administered 1 day after the last exposure. Benzo(a)pyrene has immunosuppressive activity which has been reported by our laboratory as well as others [27,40]. Benzo(e)pyrene, the non-carcinogenic congener of benzo(a)pyrene, which has been shown not to be immunosuppressive [27,41], was included in all but the parasite studies. Benzo(e)pyrene did not change host resistance to any of the pathogens tested. Similarly, a positive control which was used for all but the parasite studies produced a decrease in host resistance to each of the pathogens. A summary of the host resistance to the five pathogens in benzopyrene exposed animals is shown in Table 17.3. The results of these host resistance models clearly show the diversity in the response to a potent immunosuppressive agent. Four of the models (herpes simplex type 2, *Streptococcus pneumoniae, Plasmodium yoelii,* and B16F10 melanoma) showed dose-dependent reduction in host resistance. One of the models *(Listeria monocytogenes)* showed an increase in host resistance, and two models (influenza A_2 and *Plasmodium berghei*) showed no change in host resistance.

In carrying out host resistance studies, several factors related to both the pathogen and the animal host must be considered. Depending on the host resistance model selected, the age and sex of the animals can have a significant impact on the results. Similarly, an inappropriate route of exposure or pathogen burden can produce results which are uninterpretable. Again, returning to the *Streptococcus pneumoniae* model as an example, we have found that administration of the organism by the intravenous route will result in no animal deaths, while the same challenge level administered intraperitoneally will produce 100% mortality. The decreased mortality with intravenous administration may result from increased phagocytosis by the fixed macrophages of the reticuloendothelial system. Similarly, male animals are much more susceptible to this organism than females. A challenge level which will produce 100% mortality in B6C3F1 males is not lethal in B6C3F1 females. This is particularly interesting in the light of the fact that male mice of this

Table 17.3 Summary of host resistance studies of female B6C3F1 mice exposed to benzo(a)pyrene

Challenge model	Pathogen	Benzo(a)pyrene
Bacterial	*Listeria monocytogenes*	Increase
	Streptococcus pneumoniae	Decrease
Viral	Herpes simplex type 2	Decrease
	Influenza A_2	No change
Parasite	*Plasmodium yoelii*	Decrease
	Plasmodium berghei	No change
Tumour	B16F10 Melanoma	Decrease

Benzo(a)pyrene, benzo(e)pyrene, or a positive control was administered to mice. Benzo(a)pyrene and benzo(e)pyrene were administered subcutaneously daily for 14 days. The pathogen challenge was administered 1 day after the last exposure. The positive control for *Listeria monocytogenes,* herpes simplex 2, influenza A_2, and B16F10 melanoma was cyclophosphamide. The positive control for *Streptococcus pneumoniae* was cobra venom. Plasmodium studies were conducted without positive controls. Benzo(e)pyrene had no effect on any host resistance models, while the positive control used in each study decreased host resistance.

strain have higher serum complement haemolytic activity than do females.

For best statistical analysis, at least 12 animals per treatment group should be used and to obtain various degrees of lethality, at least three challenge levels should be employed. Ideally, the challenge levels selected should result in approximately 20% mortality in the vehicle control animals of the low challenge group and between 75 and 100% in the high challenge group. If the test compound has immunoenhancement activity, then protection should be observed at the high challenge levels. If the test compound decreases host resistance, an increased number of deaths would be expected at lower challenge levels compared to the appropriate control. If too high a challenge level is administered, one will not be able to detect decreased host resistance due to high mortality in both control and treatment groups. Whenever possible, a positive control compound specific for the respective pathogen should be included. While cyclophosphamide is often used as a positive control for numerous organisms [3], the proper dose and time of exposure are critical in using the drug in this capacity. When the mechanism of host defence of the pathogen is well understood, a more selective positive control agent can be utilized. Cobra venom factor, administrated parenterally at a dose of 100 anticomplementary $u\ kg^{-1}$ 1 day before challenge with *Streptococcus pneumoniae*, is an excellent positive control due to its decomplementary activity. Statistical analysis of mortality data is usually evaluated both as the number of animals succumbing to the pathogen and the time and rate at which deaths occur.

Discussed below are three examples of host resistance models which have found wide acceptance in evaluating immunotoxicity of xenobiotics. In addition to detailing the assay procedure, examples of how these models can be used with different compounds are given.

Change in host resistance to Streptococcus pneumoniae

The *Streptococcus pneumoniae* model has been one of our most sensitive indicators for detecting changes in host resistance. As indicated before, host resistance to this Gram-positive cocci is multi-faceted with several immune defence mechanisms participating in the protection from this organism. The first line of defence is the complement system. Activation of the complement system can result in direct lysis of certain strains of *Streptococcus pneumoniae*. Other strains, resistant to lysis, become opsinized as a result of complement component C3 being deposited on their surface, which facilitates phagocytosis by PMNs and macrophages. In the later stages of the infection, antigen-specific antibody plays a major role in controlling the infection. *Streptococcus pneumoniae* represents an excellent model for evaluating immunotoxicity since it elicits multiple immune components which participate in the host resistance, each of which can be a potential target site for an adverse effect of a xenobiotic.

In our laboratory, stock preparations of *Streptococcus pneumoniae* (ATCC 6314) are maintained at $-70°C$ in defibrinated rabbit blood. A 5 μl aliquot of the stock preparation is used to inoculate 50 ml of brain–heart infusion broth, which is incubated overnight at $37°C$. The turbidity of the overnight culture is determined, using the Abbott bichromatic analyser and diluted with fresh brain–heart infusion broth to yield an absorbance difference (Ad) of 0.020–0.025. The turbidity of the subculture is monitored periodically and, when the optical density reaches an Ad of 0.080, the subculture is rapidly cooled in an ice bath and diluted to the desired inoculum level. The turbidity of each inoculum is checked in the analyser and adjustments are made to obtain the preselected Ad levels. Routinely, 1 day after the last exposure, female mice are challenged intraperitoneally with 0.2 ml of the *Streptococcus pneumoniae* inoculum. Three inocula, each at a different concentration, are prepared to give a range of lethality. A sample of each inoculum is serially diluted and plated on blood agar plates to determine the number of colony-forming units administered to the animals. Due to the rapid onset of the infection, mortality observations are recorded twice daily for the 7-day mortality period.

Shown in Fig. 17.6 are the results from a representative *Streptococcus pneumoniae* study. Female B6C3F1 mice were exposed daily for 14 days to the corn oil vehicle, 1,2,3,6,7,8-hexachlorodibenzo-*p*-dioxin (HCDD); or 2,3,7,8-tetrachlorodibenzo-*p*-dioxin (TCDD) by oral gavage. On day 15, the day

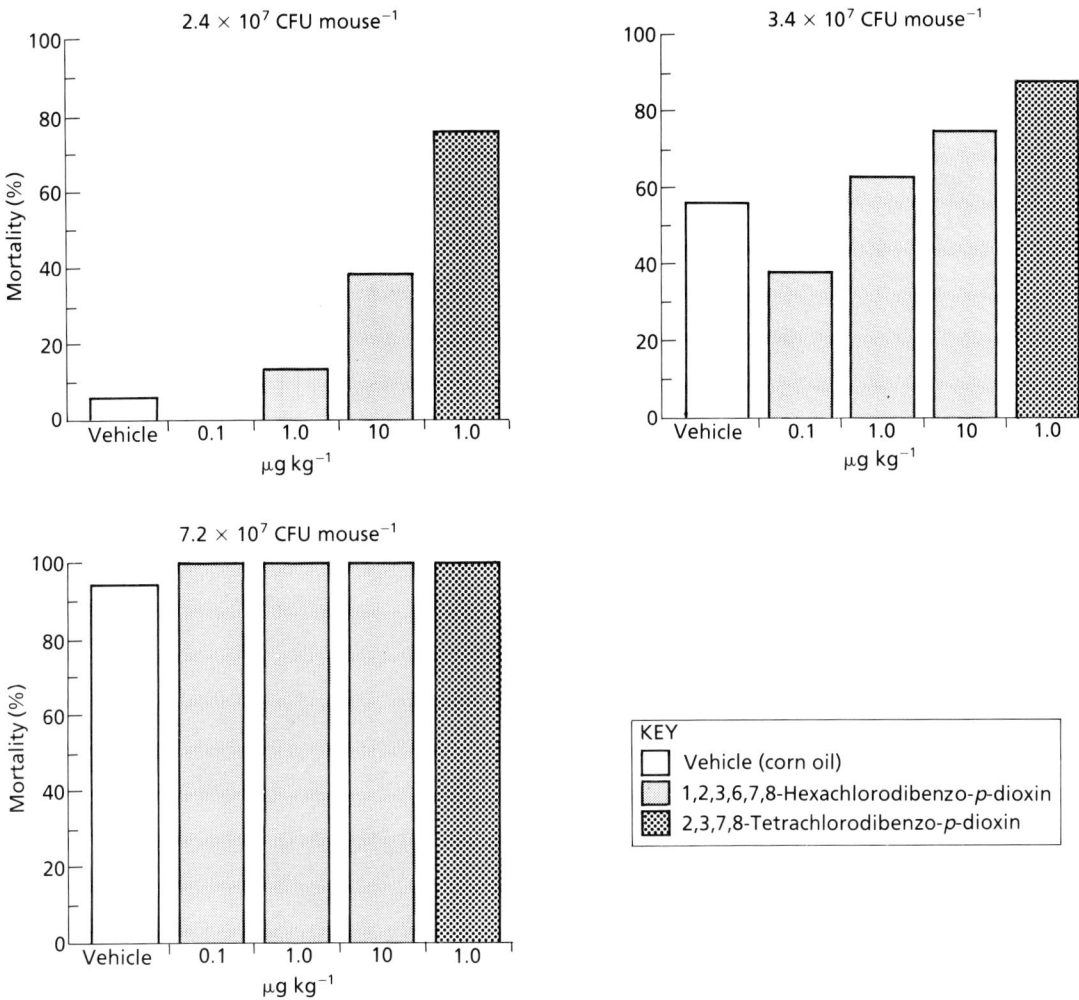

Fig. 17.6 Host resistance study with *Streptococcus pneumoniae*. Female B6C3F1 mice were exposed to corn oil vehicle, 1,2,3,6,7,8-hexachlorodibenzo-*p*-dioxin or 2,3,7,8-tetrachlorodibenzo-*p*-dioxin, for 14 days. On day 15 they were challenged with *Streptococcus pneumoniae*. Mortality was measured over a 7-day period. Adapted from [33].

following the last exposure, animals were administered one of three challenge levels of *Streptococcus pneumoniae* by intraperitoneal injection. Animals were monitored twice daily for mortality for 7 days. At the two lower challenge levels, a dose-related increase in mortality was observed in animals which had been exposed to HCDD. A statistically significant increase in mortality was observed in the animals which had been exposed to both HCDD and TCDD. Due to the high level of mortality in all groups receiving the 7.2×10^7 colony-forming units/mouse inoculum, no treatment effect could be observed.

Change in host resistance to Listeria monocytogenes

Listeria monocytogenes is a Gram-positive bacterium which has been widely used as a host resistance model. The pathogenesis and the role of the immune response in limiting infection have been well established [42,43]. Recovery from infection depends on the phagocytosis of the organism by macrophages and the subsequent activation of the macrophage to a bactericidal state following interaction with sensitized T lymphocytes. Fixed macrophages of the reticuloendothelium system also play a major role in the initial inactivation of *Listeria monocytogenes*. Interference with either phagocytosis of the organism by fixed or mobile macrophages or the interaction between T cells and macrophages can result in decreased host resistance and eventually death of the host. This assay has been shown to be extremely reproducible when the organism is administered by the intravenous route. It is an excellent model for assessing competence of macrophages and T lymphocytes. Both mortality and bacterial colony counts, particularly of the spleen and liver, the major site of the bacterium replication, can be used to assess host resistance.

Listeria monocytogenes is prepared as previously described [44]. Strain 19303 was used in the study described below. The stock preparation was prepared and maintained as frozen aliquots, stored at $-70°C$. The stock contained approximately 10^8 colony-forming units per ml. Serial dilution in sterile saline was made to obtain the desired challenge level. Dilutions of the inocula were maintained on ice. Twenty-four hours after the last exposure, mice were challenged intravenously at one of three challenge levels of *Listeria monocytogenes*. All animals were injected within 1 h of preparing the proper challenge level. The number of viable bacteria inoculated at each challenge level was enumerated by plating a sample of the inocula and counting the number of colony-forming units per plate. Animal mortality was recorded daily for 14 days.

As shown in Fig. 17.7, B6C3F1 mice which were exposed to *m*-nitrotoluene (600 mg kg^{-1}) for 14 days had a significantly decreased host resistance to *Listeria monocytogenes*. This is dramatically illustrated by the increase in mortality of the treated animals compared to the vehicle at the two higher challenge levels. All animals exposed to *m*-nitrotoluene died following challenge with the *Listeria monocytogenes* while only 13 and 58% of the vehicle animals succumbed to the pathogen at the middle and high challenge levels.

Change in host resistance to B16F10 melanoma

The tumour challenge model we have found to be most useful in assessing the immunotoxic potential of a test compound is the artificial metastasis model

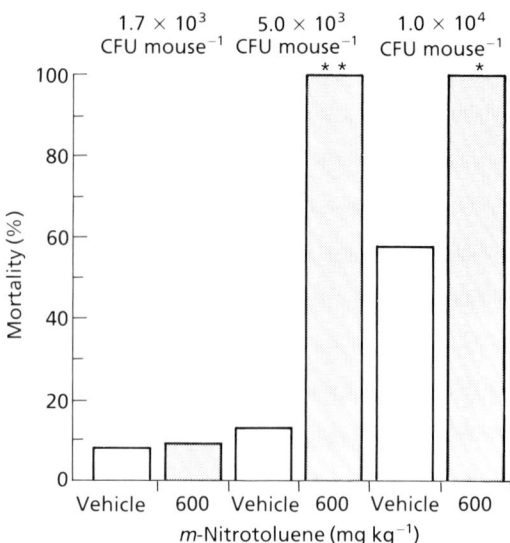

Fig. 17.7 Host resistance study with *Listeria monocytogenes*. Female B6C3F1 mice were exposed to corn oil vehicle, or *m*-nitrotoluene for 14 days. On day 15 they were challenged with *Listeria monocytogenes*. Mortality was measured over a 14-day period.

using the B16F10 melanoma. This model was developed from the work of Fiedler *et al.* [45].

For this assay, the B16F10 tumour cells are usually grown in culture flasks. Just prior to challenge, cells are trypsonized and a single cell suspension is prepared at the desired concentration. Routinely, concentrations between 1×10^5 and 5×10^5 cells ml^{-1} are utilized as the challenge levels. Animals are injected intravenously with the tumour cells in a volume of 0.2 ml. One day prior to sacrifice, mice are pulsed intraperitoneally with 0.2 ml of 10^{-6} mol l^{-1} 5-fluorodeoxyuridine, followed 30 min later with 7.4×10^4 Bq ^{125}iododeoxyuridine administered by the intravenous route. On the following day, animals are sacrificed, lungs removed, and placed in Bouin's solution.

Two parameters are used to assess tumour burden. One is the measurement of DNA synthesis in the lung of mice bearing tumours. The background DNA synthesis of mice without tumours is extremely low and the detectable DNA synthesis rate is a result of the tumour presence. The fixed lungs are then placed in test-tubes and counted in a γ-counter. A second assessment of tumour burden is the enumeration of the tumour nodules following fix-ation in Bouin's solution. The black nodules of the B16F10 tumour on the yellow background of the fixed lung tissue allows for enumeration of up to 200–250 nodules on the surface of the lungs. To ensure that the number of tumours in the lung are countable, sentinel mice, which have received the highest challenge level, are periodically evaluated to determine the number of tumour nodules which have developed. Starting on days 10–12 after tu-mour cells are injected, sentinel mice are sacrificed and the number of nodules present is determined. The day of sacrifice for the study is selected to ensure the number of nodules are in the countable range. As shown in Fig. 17.8, there is good corre-lation between enumerated tumour nodules and radioactivity present in the lungs. If too large a tumour challenge is used, or if the animals are sacrificed at a time when the tumour nodules have become too numerous to count, then the results of the study can still be determined using the radio-assay data.

Figure 17.9 shows typical results from a B16F10 melanoma study. Female B6C3F1 mice were ex-posed to gallium arsenide by a single intratracheal administration. Fourteen days after exposure, ani-mals were injected intravenously with 2×10^5 tu-mour cells. Fourteen days after tumour challenge—

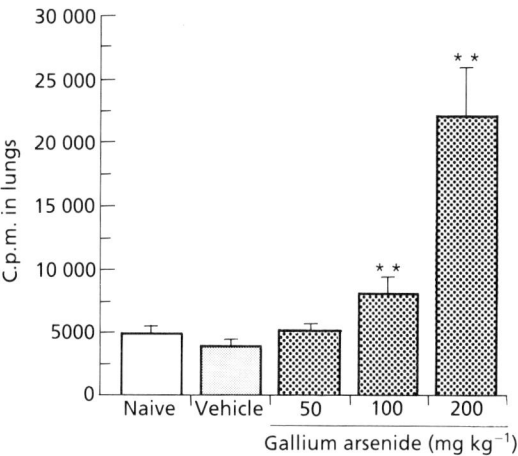

Fig. 17.9 Change in host resistance to B16F10 melanoma. Female B6C3F1 mice were untreated or exposed by a single intratracheal instillation to gallium arsenide or vehicle (0.05% (v/v) Tween 80). Animals received 2×10^5 tumour cells by intravenous injection 14 days after exposure and lungs were radioassayed 14 days after injection of tumour cells. Values represent the mean ± s.e. from eight animals per group. **Statistically significant difference from vehicle control at $P \leqslant 0.01$.

the optimum time for this study based on the results of the sentinel mice—animals were sacrificed, tu-mour nodules enumerated visually, and then lungs were radioassayed. In animals receiving gallium arsenide at doses greater than 100 mg kg^{-1}, a significant increase in tumour burden was observed. Naive, vehicle-treated mice, and animals which received 50 mg kg^{-1} gallium arsenide had similar tumour burdens.

In conclusion, it has been our experience in conducting immunotoxicological evaluation of nu-merous xenobiotics over the last 12 years that the most sensitive and reproducible indicators of an altered immune system are the functional assays.

Acknowledgements

The author thanks Dr Albert Munson, Ms J. Ann McCay and the other members of the Medical College of Virginia/Virginia Commonwealth Univer-sity Immunotoxicology Program who developed the functional assay described in this chapter and were responsible for the data presented. He also thanks Ms G. Price for clerical assistance.

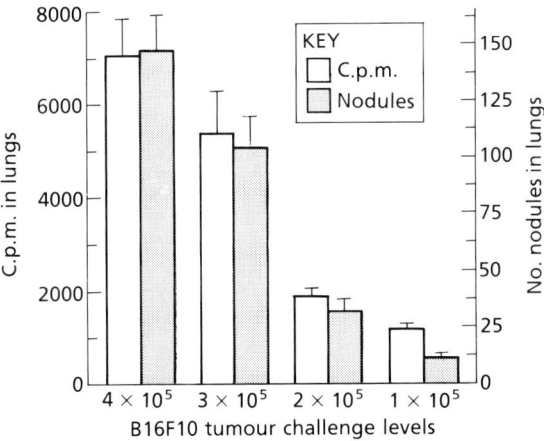

Fig. 17.8 Comparison of c.p.m. per lungs and nodules per lungs from animals receiving increasing numbers of B16F10 tumour cells. Values represent the mean ± s.e. from eight animals per group.

References

1 Dean JH, Murray MJ, Ward EC. Toxic responses of the immune system. In: Klaassen CD, Amdur MO, Doull J, eds. *The Basic Science of Poisons*. New York: Mac-Millan, 1986:245–85.

2 Dean JH, Cornacoff JB, Rosenthal GJ, Luster MI. Immune system: evaluation of injury. In: Hayes AW ed. *Principles and Methods of Toxicology*. 2nd edn. New York: Raven Press, 1989:741–60.

3 Luster MI, Munson AE, Thomas P, Holsapple MP, Fenters J, White KL Jr, Lauer LD, Dean JH. Development of testing battery to assess chemical-induced immunotoxicity. *Fund Appl Toxicol* 1988; 10:2–19.

4 Munson AE, Sanders VM Douglas KA, Sain LE, Kauffmann BM, White KL Jr. *In vivo* assessment of immunotoxicity. *Environ Hlth Persp* 1982; 43:41–52.

5 Norbury KE. Immunotoxicological evaluation: an overview. *J Am Coll Toxicol* 1985; 4:279–90.

6 Trizio D, Basketter DA, Botham PA, Graepel PH, Lambre CI, Magda SJ, Pal TM, Riley AJ, Ronneberger H, Van Sittert NJ, Bontinck WJ. Identification of immunotoxic effects of chemicals and assessment of their relevance to man. *Fund Chem Toxicol* 1988; 26:527–39.

7 White KL Jr, Sanders VM, Barnes DW, Shopp GM Jr, Munson AE. Immunotoxicological investigations in the mouse: general approach and methods. *Drug Chem Toxicol* 1985; 8:299–331.

8 Yoshida S, Golub MS, Gershwin EG. Immunological aspects of toxicology: premises not promises. *Reg Toxicol Pharmacol* 1989; 9:56–80.

9 Exon JH, Koller LD, Henningsen GM, Osborne CA. Multiple immunoassay in a single animal: a practical approach to immunotoxicologic testing. *Fund Appl Toxicol* 1984; 4:278–83.

10 Sharma RP. *Immunologic Consideration in Toxicology*. Boca Raton: CRC Press, 1981:1.

11 Baecher-Steppan L, Nakaue HS, Matsumoto M, Gainer JH, Kerkvliet NI. The broiler chicken as a model for immunotoxicity assessment. 1. Standardization of *in vitro* immunological assays. *Fund Appl Toxicol* 1989; 12:773–86.

12 Kerkvliet NI, Brauner JA. Mechanisms of 1,2,3,4,6,7,8- hepachlorodibenzo-p-dioxin (HpCDD)-induced humoral immune suppression: evidence of primary defects in T-cell regulation. *Toxicol Appl Pharmacol* 1987; 87:18–31.

13 Jerne NK, Nordin AA. Plaque formation in agar by single antibody-producing cells. *Science* 1963; 140:405.

14 Czerkinsky C, Andersson G, Ekre H, Nilsson L, Klareskog L, Ouchterlony O. Reverse ELISPOT assay for clonal analysis of cytokine production. I. Enumeration of gamma-interferon-secreting cells. *J Immunol Methods* 1888; 110:29–36.

15 Moller SA, Borrebaeck CAK. A filter immuno-plaque assay for the detection of antibody-secreting cells *in vitro*. *J Immunol Methods* 1985; 79:195–204.

16 Kerkvliet NI, Baecher-Steppan L, Claycomb AT, Craig AM, Sheggeby GG. Immunotoxicity of technical pentachlorophenol (PCP-T): depressed humoral immune responses to T-dependent and T-independent antigen stimulation on PCP-T exposed mice. *Fund Appl Toxicol* 1982; 2:90–9.

17 Koller LD, Exon JH, Moore SA. Evaluation of ELISA for detecting *in vivo* chemical immunomodulation. *J Toxicol Environ Hlth* 1983; 11:15–22.

18 Kemeny DM, Challacombe SJ. *ELISA and Other Solid Phase Immunoassays. Theoretical and Practical Aspects*. New York: John Wiley, 1988.

19 Janossy G, Greaves MF. Lymphocyte activation. I. Response of T and B lymphocytes to phytomitogens. *Clin Exp Immunol* 1971; 9:483–98.

20 Janossy G, Greaves MF. Lymphocyte activation. II. Discriminating stimulation of lymphocyte subpopulations by phytomitogens and heterologous antilymphocyte sera. *Clin Exp Immunol* 1972; 10:525–36.

21 Vos JG, De Klerk A, Krajne EI, Kruizinga W, Van Ommen B, Rozing J. Toxicity of bis(tri-n-butyltin) oxide on the rat. II. Suppression of thymus-dependent immune response and of parameters of non-specific resistance after short-term exposure. *Toxicol Appl Pharmacol* 1984; 75:387–408.

22 Thorpe PE, Knight SC. Microplate culture of mouse lymph node cells. I. Quantitation of responses to allogeneic lymphocytes endotoxin and phytomitogens. *J Immunol Methods* 1974; 5:387–404.

23 House RV, Lauer LD, Murray MJ, Dean JH. Suppression of T helper cell function in mice following exposure to the carcinogen 7,12-dimethylbenz[a] anthracene and its restoration by interleukin-2. *Int J Immunopharmacol* 1987; 9:89–97.

24 Holsapple MP, Page DG, Bick PH, Shopp GM. Characterization of the delayed hypersensitivity response to a protein antigen in the mouse – I. Kinetics of reactivity and sensitivity to classical immunosuppressants. *Int J Immunopharmacol* 1984; 6: 399–405.

25 Lefford MJ. The measurement of tuberculin hypersensitivity in rats. *Int Arch Allergy* 1974; 47:570–85.

26 Paranjpe MS, Boone CW. Delayed hypersensitivity to simian virus 40 tumor cells in BALB/c mice demonstrated by a radioisotopic footpad assay. *J Natl Cancer Inst* 1972; 48:563–6.

27 Dean JH, Luster MI, Boorman GA, Lauer LD, Leubke RW, Lawson L. Selective immunosuppression resulting from exposure to the carcinogenic congener of benzopyrene in B6C3F1 mice. *Clin Exp Immunol* 1983; 53:199–206.

28 Roitt I, Brostoff J, Male D. *Immunology.* New York: CV Mosby, 1985.

29 White KL Jr, Lysy HH, McCay JA, Anderson AC. Modulation of serum complement levels following exposure to polychlorinated dibenzo-p-dioxins. *Toxicol Appl Pharmacol* 1986; 84:209–19.

30 Herberman RB. Immunologic mechanisms of host resistance to tumors. In: Dean JH, Luster MI, Munson AE, Amos H, eds. *Immunotoxicology and Immunopharmacology.* New York: Raven Press, 1985:69–77.

31 Reynolds CW, Herberman RB. *In vitro* augmentation of rat natural killer (NK) cell activity. *J Immunol* 1981; 126:1581–5.

32 Morahan PS, Edelson PJ, Gass K. Changes in macrophage ectoenzymes associated with anti-tumor activity. *J Immunol* 1980; 125:1312–21.

33 White KL Jr, Krasula RW, Munson AE, Holsapple MP. Effects of hydroxyethylstarch (HESPAN˜R), a plasma expander, on the functional activity of the reticuloendothelial system. Comparison with human serum albumin and pyran copolymer. *Drug Chem Toxicol* 1986; 9:305–22.

34 Holsapple MP, White KL Jr, McCay JA, Bradley SG, Munson AE. An immunotoxicological evaluation of 4, 4'-thiobis-(6-t-butyl-m-cresol) in female B6C3F1 mice. *Fund Appl Toxicol* 1988; 10:701–16.

35 Burleson GR, Fuller LB, Menache MG, Graham JA. Poly(I): poly(C)-enhanced alveolar and peritoneal macrophage phagocytosis: quantification by a new method utilizing fluorescent beads. *Proc Soc Exp Biol Med* 1987; 184:468–76.

36 Labara C, Paigen K. A simple, rapid, and sensitive DNA assay procedure. *Ann Biochem* 1980; 102:344.

37 Bradley SG, Morahan PS. Approaches to assessing host resistance. *Environ Hlth Persp* 1982; 43:61–9.

38 Winkelstein JA. The role of complement in the host's defense against *Streptococcus pneumoniae. Rev Infect Dis* 1981; 3:289–97.

39 Fouant MM, Bradley SG. Effects of benzo(a)pyrene on host resistance to *Plasmodium yoelii* and *P. berghei* in B6C3F1 mice *Toxicologist* 1987; 7:224.

40 Myers MJ, Schook LB, Bick PH. Mechanisms of benzo(a)pyrene-induced modulation of antigen presentation. *J Pharmacol Exp Ther* 1987; 242:399–404.

41 White KL Jr, Lysy HH, Holsapple MP. Immunosuppression by polycyclic aromatic hydrocarbons: a structure–activity relationship in B6C3F1 and DBA/2 mice. *Immunopharmacol* 1985; 9:155–64.

42 North RJ. Importance of thymus derived lymphocytes in cell mediated immunity to infection. *Cell Immunol* 1973; 7:166–76.

43 Mackawess GB. Cellular immunity. In: Van Furth R, ed. *Mononuclear Phagocytes.* Oxford: Blackwell Press, 1970:461–4.

44 Morahan PS, Klykken PC, Smith SH, Harris LS, Munson AE. Effects of cannabinoids on host resistance to *Listeria monocytogenes* and herpes simplex virus. *Infect Immun* 1979; 23:670–4.

45 Fiedler IJ, Gersten DM, Hart IR. The biology of cancer invasion and metastases. *Adv Cancer Res* 1978; 28:149–250.

18

Integrating *in vitro* systems with animal models in mechanistic studies of immunotoxic agents

DANIEL WIERDA & WILLIAM F. GREENLEE

Introduction

The immune system is a tightly regulated network of lymphoid organs and dispersed cell populations responsible for the maintenance of host resistance to foreign materials. Major functional populations of immunocompetent cells include T and B lymphocytes which mediate cell and humoral immune responses, respectively. A variety of environmental chemicals and pharmaceutical agents have been found to alter host immunocompetence [1]. Although numerous studies of the interactions of chemicals with the immune system have been carried out, most have been largely descriptive accounts of chemical-induced changes in T- and B-lymphocyte function as assessed by standard immunological assays. With the development of contemporary cell and molecular biology, greater opportunities have become available for immunotoxicologists to study in detail the actions of chemicals on specific immune system target cells.

There is strong evidence that treatment with therapeutic agents, as well as exposure to drugs of abuse, alter immune function in humans (reviewed in [2]). In contrast, there are relatively few well documented reports linking exposure to environmental chemicals to impaired immune function resulting in an adverse health outcome (reviewed in [3]), even though in animal models it can be shown that environmental chemicals produce adverse effects on the immune system in a dose-dependent manner. A principal reason for this dilemma lies in the very nature of the immune system—a complex network with different components possessing overlapping functions or reserve capacity. A second reason is the lack of understanding about mechanisms responsible for chemical-induced immunotoxicity.

The intent of this chapter is not to present an inclusive account of all immunotoxicology research being carried out, but rather to focus on some specific examples in which *in vitro* model systems have been developed to gain knowledge of the mechanisms responsible for immunotoxic responses observed in animals. Integration of knowledge at the molecular and cellular level with animal data can be used in conjunction with a quantitative description of the relationship of exposure to tissue dose to provide an improved assessment of the potential human health risks associated with exposure to immunotoxic chemicals.

Determinants of target cell specificity

Role of biotransformation

Biotransformation of xenobiotics occurs predominantly in the liver and is influenced by multiple factors including the physicochemical properties of the given agent, and genetic and sex-specific differences in pharmacokinetics and metabolism [4]. Hepatic biotransformation is involved in the production of immunotoxic metabolites for many therapeutic or environmental xenobiotics such as azathioprine, cyclophosphamide, benzene, and polycyclic aromatic hydrocarbons, to name a few. However, almost all tissues have some capability for metabolizing and detoxifying xenobiotics and there is now evidence indicating that biotransformation in specific immune system target tissues such as the spleen or bone marrow is required for the immunotoxicity of some chemicals.

Hepatic biotransformation. Hepatic biotransformation appears to be a necessary condition for immunotoxicity following exposure to diethylnitrosamine. In *in vitro* studies with mouse spleen cells, diethylnitrosamine and cyclophosphamide suppressed the generation of antibody-producing cells to antigens only in spleen cell cultures containing hepatocytes [5,6]. Microsomal fractions of liver homogenates supplemented with an NADPH-generating system do not catalyse the formation of immunotoxic metabolites [7], suggesting a difference in the microsomal fraction-dependent metabolism of diethylnitrosamine in comparison with intact hepatocytes [8]. It was also noted in these studies that cell-to-cell contact was necessary between hepatocytes and splenocytes for immunotoxicity to occur as separation of these cells reversed the suppression of antibody responses by diethylnitrosamine [8].

Benzene is a solvent that is biotransformed *in vivo* to putative myelotoxic, haematotoxic, and leukaemogenic metabolites [9]. Evidence supporting the involvement of hepatic biotransformation came from studies demonstrating that the severity of benzene-induced myelotoxicity could be decreased by partial hepatectomy [10]. Although the formation of reactive benzene metabolites in the liver which in turn enter the circulation to act on immune system target tissues was not readily accepted [11], a number of studies have reported on the specific uptake of primary benzene metabolites by bone marrow and other immune system cells (reviewed in [12]). The accumulation of these metabolites appears to be associated at least in part with subsequent toxicity; however, there is also evidence (discussed in the following section) for bone marrow-dependent metabolism of benzene.

Target cell biotransformation. Biotransformation by immune system target cells appears to be an important factor contributing to the immunotoxicity associated with certain aromatic compounds. Okano and co-workers [13] reported that human monocytes and lymphocytes metabolize benzo(a)pyrene via cytochrome P450 mixed-function oxidases to at least eight polyhydroxy metabolites. The profile of metabolites produced is cell-specific, can be altered by exposure to mixed-function oxidase inducers such as benzanthracene, and displays interindividual variability. The addition of α-naphthaflavone, a cytochrome P-450 inhibitor, to spleen cell cultures ameliorates benzo(a)pyrene immunotoxicity [14]. This effect correlates with an increased recovery of unmetabolized, radiolabelled benzo(a)pyrene extracted from culture supernatants previously treated with α-naphthaflavone. Taken together these observations support the direct involvement of immune system target cells in the biotransformation of benzo(a)pyrene to immunotoxic metabolites. Observed differences in susceptibility to benzo(a)pyrene-induced immunotoxicity may be attributable in part to specific mixed-function oxidase activities expressed in a given immune system target cell.

The myelotoxicity of benzene has been postulated to result from the metabolism of the parent compound by bone marrow target cells. This hypothesis is supported by the demonstration of the appearance of benzene metabolites in an isolated bone marrow preparation exposed directly to benzene [15]. Bone marrow macrophages and neutrophils contain significant levels of peroxidase enzymes, such as myeloperoxidase and prostaglandin synthetase, which can readily oxidize phenolic benzene metabolites and generate reactive quinones [16–18]. The presence of myeloperoxidase activity in macrophages and neutrophils may account for the apparent selective toxicity of hydroquinone to these cells, as contrasted with the relative insensitivity of bone marrow stromal fibroblasts which do not have detectable myeloperoxidase activity [18,19]. Prostaglandin synthetase activity was implicated in the reduction in bone marrow cellularity caused by benzene, by demonstrating that the administration of indomethacin, an inhibitor of the cyclo-oxygenase component of prostaglandin synthetase, prior to benzene exposure ameliorates benzene toxicity in mice [20,21]. Similar effects were observed in mice pretreated with other cyclo-oxygenase inhibitors such as aspirin, and meclofenamate [21]. Prostaglandin E_2 had previously been shown to be inhibitory to bone marrow myelopoiesis [22].

It was initially hypothesized that an increase in bone marrow prostaglandin E_2 in benzene-treated mice was due to the generation of hydroquinone from benzene. However, it was observed that *in vitro*, whereas indomethacin pretreatment had a positive effect on granulocyte/monocyte colony forming units in culture (GM-CFU-C) growth in stromal cell co-cultures exposed to hydroquinone, levels of prostaglandin E_2 were not significantly decreased in comparison with control cultures [20]. These results suggested that the expression of benzene toxicity could not be attributed solely to increased prostaglandin production stimulated by hydroquinone. Additional support for this conclusion was provided by Pirozzi and co-workers [21], who demonstrated that indomethacin could not ameliorate the decrease in bone marrow cellularity caused by the simultaneous administration of phenol and hydroquinone to mice, although indomethacin significantly reduced bone marrow prostaglandin E_2 production. These observations suggest that indomethacin may positively modulate haemopoiesis independent of lowering marrow prostaglandin levels. Leukotriene levels in bone marrow may actually increase due to increased availability of arachidonic acid (via inhibition of cyclo-oxygenase) which is subsequently metabolized by cellular lipoxygenases [23]. Several studies have provided support for a direct role for leukotrienes in the growth and development of bone marrow myeloid and lymphoid cells [24,25].

Hydroquinone has been shown to have additional effects on bone marrow macrophages via local biotransformation by myeloperoxidase. In culture, bone marrow macrophages, but not bone marrow fibroblasts, metabolize hydroquinone to 1,4-benzoquinone which covalently binds to cellular macromolecules [18,19]. This effect is partly responsible for the selective inhibition of macrophage regulation of haemopoiesis, as discussed later in this chapter. In contrast, stromal fibroblast function remains unaffected by concentrations of hydroquinone that are toxic to bone marrow macrophages. The resistance of stromal fibroblasts to hydroquinone appears to be due to the absence of detectable myeloperoxidase activity and the presence of high levels of DT-diaphorase, an enzyme which reduces quinones to benzoquinones, and thereby serves as a protective, or detoxification enzyme in the case of hydroquinone exposure [18,26,27]. A hypothesis for how these observations relate to a unified theory of benzene myelotoxicity is presented later in this chapter.

Biochemical mechanisms

Reactivity with thiol proteins on microtubules. Protein–thiol modification by xenobiotics has been implicated as a potential mechanism responsible for immunotoxicity. Support for this mechanism has been obtained from investigations comparing the effects of known, thiol-reactive compounds on lymphocyte activation with those caused by agents deemed to have immunotoxic activity. For example, *N*-ethylmaleimide, a known membrane-penetrating alkylating agent with specificity for thiol groups, inhibits lymphocyte agglutination and mitogenesis *in vitro* at the same concentrations (10^{-5} mol l^{-1}) at which hydroquinone inhibits lymphocyte mitogenesis [28,29]. Quinones are capable of reversibly modifying protein thiol groups by forming disulphide cross-linkages or mixed disulphides with other proteins [30]. Pfeifer and Irons [28] proposed that the quinone metabolites of benzene, which inhibit lymphocyte mitogenesis at 10^{-6}–10^{-5} mol l^{-1} concentrations, do so by altering thiol groups important for cellular microtubule assembly. This conclusion was based on results showing that hydroquinone inhibits microtubule self-assembly and tubulin–colchicine binding activity *in vitro*, possibly by interfering with guanosine triphosphate binding to sulphydryl groups on tubulin [31].

A similar mechanism has been proposed to account in part for the reduction in cell-mediated immunity caused by oestrogen compounds [32,33]. The catechol oestrogen, 2-OH oestrone, is a major metabolite of 17-β oestradiol which is believed to be oxidized to reactive quinone intermediates. 17-β Oestradiol and its metabolites can either inhibit or enhance macrophage-mediated cytotoxicity depending upon whether macrophages are treated prior to or after activation with supernatant from concanavalin A-activated spleen cell cultures [34]. Further studies have suggested that oestrogens modulate early membrane events associated with lymphocyte activation. This conclusion is derived from observations that oestrogen metabolites inhibit phytohaemagglutinin (PHA)-induced lymphocyte mitogenesis coincident with a reduction in the degree of PHA-induced agglutination [35]. This effect is similar to the reduction in PHA-induced agglutination and mitogenesis which occurs in lymphocyte cultures after exposure to non-cytotoxic concentrations of hydroquinone (< 4 μmol l^{-1} [28,29]).

Overall, the results of these studies suggested that thiol-reactive compounds disrupt microtubule function and thereby inhibit lectin-induced agglutination and mitogenesis. However, some thiol-reactive chemicals are immunotoxic but do not affect microtubules. For example, iodoacetic acid (100 μmol l^{-1}) effectively inhibits lymphocyte blastogenesis, but does not affect lectin-induced agglutination, nor does it inhibit microtubule assembly [36]. Therefore, other sulphydryl-dependent processes which are important for lymphocyte activation must also be targets for thiol-reactive chemicals.

Reactivity with cellular thiol proteins. Studies carried out by Lawrence and co-workers have focused on the different biochemical reactivity of immunotoxic, sulphydryl-modifying compounds based on the heterogeneity which exists among cellular sulphydryl constituents [37–39]. By assessing the effect of a series of *N*-ethylmaleimide analogues on T-lymphocyte responsiveness to PHA, it was determined that only non-polar maleimides blocked early activation events [38]. Furthermore, *N*-ethylmaleimide apparently reacts with only 12% of

cellular thiols, but this is sufficient to inhibit lymphocyte mitogenesis. These results suggest that specific thiols in non-polar regions of certain proteins are important for the induction of mitogenesis.

This point becomes more apparent when one considers that four structurally unrelated, thiol-modifying compounds (copper sulphate/O-phenanthroline complex, *N*-ethylmaleimide, D,L-buthionine-S,R-sulphoxime and hydrogen peroxide) all produce similar effects on splenic lymphocytes: specifically, an increase in mitogenesis at low concentrations, but an inhibition of mitogenesis at high concentrations [37]. These effects resemble those reported to occur in lymphocyte cultures exposed to microtubule-disrupting quinones [28]. With the exception of *N*-ethylmaleimide, each of these chemicals exerts heterogeneous effects on cellular thiols other than those on microtubules [37]. Moreover, these studies were the first to show that lipopolysaccharide-induced mitogenesis is consistently more sensitive to these agents than is concanavalin A-induced mitogenesis. This difference between T- and B-cell responsiveness cannot be explained by differences in total thiols as the amount of protein and non-protein thiols in T and B populations is similar. The reason for the increased sensitivity of B cells to these agents is unknown. In attempting to sort out a common denominator to account for thiol dependence, it was concluded that cell surface thiols are critical for mitogen responsiveness in murine cells. This was based primarily on observations that the copper sulphate/O-phenanthroline complex had little effect on total thiol content but is known to oxidize membrane thiols, and of the four compounds tested, it was the most effective inhibitor of mitogenesis [37].

Studies with *N*-ethylmaleimide and its effects on concanavalin A-induced agglutination, interleukin-2 (IL-2) production and receptor expression in human peripheral blood mononuclear cells indicate that some thiol-reactive agents exert a broad spectrum of effects on lymphocyte activation. Production of IL-2 and the expression of IL-2 receptors is inhibited at concentrations of *N*-ethylmaleimide (2–4 μmol l^{-1}) that have no effect on lectin-induced agglutination [39]. The authors concluded that microtubule disruption is not necessarily required to prevent lymphocyte activation. Indeed, there is some disagreement as to whether or not lectin agglutination is necessarily mediated by microtubules [40,41]. An alternative to the microtubule disruption hypothesis is the consideration that *N*-ethylmaleimide and related sulphydryl reagents alter thiols involved in signal transduction events such as calcium influx or protein kinase C activity [39]. To understand whether this hypothesis also applies to benzene metabolites and oestrogens requires further research. It is likely, given the heterogeneity of thiol proteins in all cells and the chemical diversity of each toxicant, that the manifestation of toxicity occurs as a result of alteration in a combination of thiol-dependent events.

Phosphoinositide signal transduction. Cationic amphiphilic drugs induce a phospholipidosis disorder in animals or humans characterized by lamellar-type inclusions in peripheral blood lymphocytes [42,43]. In addition to the morphological changes observed in lymphocytes following exposure to this class of drugs, it has also been shown that certain cationic amphiphilic drugs inhibit the functional responses of lymphocytes [44,45]. Mice treated with chlorphentermine *in vivo* display reduced delayed hypersensitivity responses to oxazalone and generate fewer antibodies against sheep red blood cell antigens than controls. In addition, mouse splenic and human peripheral blood lymphocytes, exposed to subtherapeutic concentrations of chlorphentermine *in vitro*, demonstrate a significantly depressed mitogenic response to concanavalin A [44].

Chlorphentermine inhibits lymphocyte blastogenesis only if added before or at the same time as mitogen. The observed kinetics for the inhibitory activity of chlorphentermine suggested that this drug was acting on early stages of mitogen-dependent lymphocyte activation. This hypothesis is supported by the finding that chlorphentermine does not alter lectin-induced agglutination of mouse splenic lymphocytes, indicating that the drug must be inhibiting a step in the activation pathway subsequent to the binding of mitogen to lymphocyte membranes.

Many early biochemical events are associated with lymphocyte activation. These include changes in cellular permeability of monovalent cations [46], changes in intracellular cyclic nucleotide levels [47], activation of membrane methyltransferases [48],

activation of the phosphatidylinositol pathway [49] and cellular depolarization [50]. Because other studies indirectly suggested that cationic amphiphilic drugs alter membrane phospholipids [45], it was hypothesized that chlorphentermine may alter signal transduction by interfering with the phosphatidylinositol pathway [51]. Activation of this pathway by antigen or lectin leads to the hydrolysis of phosphatidylinositol in the lymphocyte plasma membrane by phospholipase C to yield inositol triphosphates and diacylglycerol as products [52]. Inositol phosphates, by increasing intracellular calcium, and diacylglycerol, by activating protein kinase C, act as second messengers (Fig. 18.1).

Sauers and co-workers [53] determined that chlorphentermine (10^{-5} mol 1^{-1}) significantly depresses mitogen-induced formation of inositol in mouse splenic lymphocytes. Phospholipase C activity in cellular homogenates is also inhibited by 0.2–1.0 mmol 1^{-1} concentrations of chlorphentermine. These results suggested that inhibition of lymphocyte function was associated with an impaired phosphatidylinositol signal transduction pathway. Moreover, it was demonstrated that a combination of the calcium ionophore A23187 (10^{-6} mol 1^{-1}) and the phorbol ester mezerein (10^{-7} mol 1^{-1}) prevent the inhibition of lymphocyte blastogenesis by low doses of chlorphentermine (10^{-7}–10^{-6} mol 1^{-1}) [53]. Purportedly, A231287 and mezerein induce mitogenesis via a phosphatidylinositol-independent pathway [54–56]; thus, the association of chlorphentermine-dependent suppression of lymphocyte mitogenesis with inhibition of phospholipase C activity [57] is not ruled out.

Based on these results, it was hypothesized that chlorphentermine apparently binds to phosphatidylinositol or other phospholipids in the membrane and may do so by displacing calcium [51]. Bound drug would then render phosphatidylinositol resistant to hydrolysis by phospholipase C. A lack of phosphatidylinositol hydrolysis would prevent the formation of inositol phosphates and diacylglycerol, as well as prevent lymphocyte activation. However, it is also apparent that at higher concentrations (> 10^{-6} mol 1^{-1}) chlorphentermine exerts multiple effects, as evidenced by the inability of A23187 and mezerein to prevent the drug-induced decrease in mitogenesis [53].

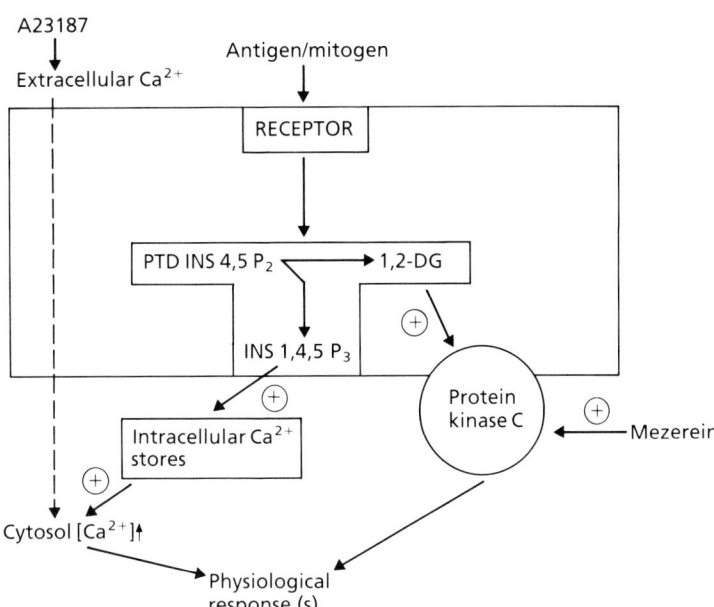

Fig. 18.1 The phosphatidylinositol pathway. Activation of this pathway by antigen or mitogen leads to the hydrolysis of phosphatidylinositol bisphosphate (PTD INS 4,5 P_2) by phospholipase C to yield inositol trisphosphate (INS 1,4,5 P_3) and diacylglycerol (1,2-DG). These products act as second messengers and continue lymphocyte blastogenesis. Inositol trisphosphate functions to release intracellular stores of calcium. The calcium ionophore A23187 can mimic this response. Diacylglycerol and the tumour promoter, meqerein, can act to activate directly protein kinase C. Reprinted with permission from [53].

Mechanisms of toxicity—haemopoietic cells

Cellular interactions during haemopoiesis

Exposure to xenobiotics which inhibit bone marrow haemopoiesis can result in immunosuppression in the host. A competent immune response to foreign antigens requires the recruitment of newly formed B and T lymphocytes in conjunction with co-operation from accessory cells. Bone marrow is the source of these cells, in humans producing more than 200 billion red cells and 10 billion white cells each day. Myelotoxic xenobiotics compromise the generation of an immune response by inhibiting lymphopoiesis or myelopoiesis. Thus, the bone marrow represents an important target site for immunotoxic responses associated with exposure to many xenobiotics in which the parent compound or metabolites can achieve critical biologically active concentrations in this tissue.

Bone marrow macrophages

Initial studies in mice given diethylnitrosamine (5 mg kg^{-1}) demonstrated paradoxical effects on the immune system. Despite a decrease in cell-mediated immune responses after diethylnitrosamine expo-

sure, treated mice were more resistant to B16F10 melanoma than were control mice [58,59]. Concomitantly, immature and mature peripheral blood monocytes and neutrophils were increased in treated mice. The bone marrow of treated mice contained greater numbers of macrophage progenitors as assessed by colony-forming units in soft agar (CFU-M), but fewer bone marrow cells in the S-phase as well as fewer Ia$^+$ cells. These results were interpreted as evidence that diethylnitrosamine alters the growth and differentiation of bone marrow macrophages. Because macrophages are necessary for cell-mediated immune responses, it was reasoned that a shift in the percentage of mature macrophages in the bone marrow and blood was somehow related to a concomitant decrease in T cell function [60]. In contrast, the increase in mature macrophages was hypothesized to be beneficial from the standpoint of cytotoxicity of B16F10 tumour cells [60].

The actions of diethylnitrosamine appear to involve a change in regulatory processes in the bone marrow. Failure of stem cells to respond appropriately to growth factors was ruled out after determining that diethylnitrosamine does not reduce the frequency of bone marrow stem cells (colony forming unit-stem cells; CFU-S) in treated mice and does not alter the number of bone marrow CFUmegakaryocyte (CFU-Meg) generated *in vitro* in response to interleukin-3 [60]. Instead, diethylnitrosamine was observed to alter membrane transferrin receptor expression in peritoneal exudate cells and bone marrow-derived macrophages [61]. Because transferrin receptors possibly reflect macrophage activation, these results suggested that diethylnitrosamine alters the normal maturation of precursor macrophages. Further analysis showed that diethylnitrosamine increases bone marrow CFU-granulocyte macrophage (CFU-GM) and CFU-M in mice [62]. However, stimulation of cell proliferation in bone marrow cultures indicated decreased responsiveness to macrophage colony-stimulating factor (M-CSF), but not to IL-3 or granulocyte macrophage colony-stimulating factor (GM-CSF), to which activity was actually enhanced. If myeloid progenitors acquire receptors for colony-stimulating activity in a hierarchical fashion (IL-3 > GM-CSF > M-CSF), then it appears that diethylnitrosamine affects the responsiveness of macrophage precursors at the M-CSF receptor stage. However, this effect could also be accounted for by a reduction in M-CSF production. This proved to be the case, when it was determined that M-CSF activity was significantly reduced in the sera from mice exposed to diethylnitrosamine when compared with activity in control sera [62].

How then could one account for an increase in macrophages observed in earlier studies if diethylnitrosamine reduced circulating M-CSF activity *in vivo*? The answer was obtained in experiments showing that another macrophage growth factor, GM-CSF, was detectable only in the sera of mice treated with diethylnitrosamine, but not in control sera [63]. Thus, a decrease in circulating M-CSF activity was offset by a compensatory increase in circulating GM-CSF activity. The source of this growth activity was hypothesized to be liver tissue, based on the idea that this organ is the principal target organ of toxicity for diethylnitrosamine and, more importantly, based on studies showing that neither diethylnitrosamine nor its metabolites affect myelopoiesis *in vitro*, except when cells are in direct contact with hepatocytes [8]. Using messenger RNA phenotyping procedures, GM-CSF transcripts were detected in the livers of diethylnitrosamine-exposed mice [64]. However, GM-CSF transcripts were also found in livers of control animals and information about differences in levels of transcripts between these two groups is lacking. Another caveat that must be considered in these studies is that a decrease in sera M-CSF activity may simply reflect an increased utilization of this factor by the greater numbers of macrophages present in diethylnitrosamine-exposed animals.

Indirect effects of tissue cytokines on haemopoiesis

The above studies also illustrate an important concept that has not yet been formally addressed in immunotoxicology studies: specifically, that bone marrow lymphopoiesis and myelopoiesis may be altered via release of regulatory molecules following damage to peripheral organs. Studies conducted by Osmond and co-workers [65–67] provide support for such a mechanism. They established that bone marrow B lymphopoiesis *in vivo* is amplified by an increased load of external environmental antigens and that cells within the spleen are partly responsible for this effect. Using adoptive transfer procedures, it was shown that spleen cells from mice previously injected with sheep red blood cells stimulated increased proliferation among bone marrow pre-B cells [67]. This effect could be abolished if spleen donors were injected with silica, which pointed to the involvement of splenic macrophages [66]. It was also noted that stromal elements of the spleen were probably responsible as spleen fragments were more effective than spleen cells alone [66]. The nature of the putative growth factors released from the spleen have not been reported, but given that macrophages may be mediating this effect, IL-1 would be a strong candidate for one of the factors.

Further studies are warranted to determine whether liver tissue may also influence bone marrow haemopoiesis. Damage to the liver from exposure to xenobiotics such as diethylnitrosamine could conceivably stimulate the synthesis of cytokines during the hepatic repair process. Foetal liver certainly has this capacity during embryogenesis when it functions as a haemopoietic organ [68]. Experiments incorporating the adoptive transfer of liver tissue from animals exposed to xenobiotics may provide an appropriate model to address this intriguing question.

Bone marrow stromal cells

Bone marrow stromal cells function as an essential component of haemopoiesis by providing a supporting matrix for developing precursor cells and by releasing cytokines involved in the regulation of haemopoiesis [68,69]. Stromal cells include osteoblasts, pre-osteoblasts, fibroblasts and reticular cells, endothelial cells, adipocytes and macrophages [70]. The importance of stromal cells was first highlighted by demonstrating that in ectopically implanted bone marrow, haemopoiesis is reconstituted only after the stroma has developed [71]. Moreover, long-term bone marrow cultures (LTBMC), which contain an intact adherent layer of stromal cells, have provided evidence that microenvironmental influences regulate myeloid and lymphoid development [72]. Cytotoxic drugs can damage stromal cells and indirectly affect haemopoiesis, including lymphopoiesis and myelopoiesis, by interfering in the interactions between bone marrow stromal cells and progenitor cells. A classic example of such a drug effect is busulphan which induces long-term damage to the microenvironment, manifested by a reduction in stem cells [73].

Stromal-dependent myelopoiesis

Environmental xenobiotics are also potentially toxic to stromal cells. Experimentally benzene will alter bone marrow stromal cell function and inhibit stromal cell-dependent haemopoiesis in culture [20,74–77]. Benzene metabolites, hydroquinone and benzoquinone, consistently inhibit *in vitro* stromal cell colony growth along with the ability of these cells to support granulocyte/monocyte colony formation in soft agar co-cultures [76]. Exposure of mice to benzene or phenol, at concentrations which do not alter stromal colony growth, is sufficient to inhibit growth of stromal cell-dependent granulocyte–monocyte colony-forming cells [77]. These results support the hypothesis that damaged stromal cells are a significant factor in the aetiology of benzene-induced myelotoxicity.

It is apparent in these experiments that benzene or its metabolites did not affect adherent stromal fibroblasts and macrophages equally. To address this point, independent populations of stromal fibro-

blasts and bone marrow-derived macrophages were evaluated for selective sensitivity to hydroquinone *in vitro* [78]. These experiments indicated that macrophages were specific targets of hydroquinone toxicity. Addition of $0.1–10\ \mu\text{mol}\ l^{-1}$ hydroquinone for 48 h to a stromal fibroblast cell line, derived from LTBMC, had no effect on their ability to support granulocyte–monocyte colony formation in soft agar co-culture. In contrast, the addition of bone marrow macrophages, previously pulsed with non-cytotoxic concentrations of hydroquinone, reduced granulocyte–monocyte colony formation in co-cultures [78]. This indicated that stromal fibroblast secretion of colony-stimulating activity was unaffected by hydroquinone, whereas macrophage regulation of stromal cell function was altered to the extent of suppressing colony-stimulating activity in co-cultures. These results supported previous studies that indicated that benzene metabolites inhibit mouse peritoneal macrophage function [79]. Macrophages cultured with non-cytotoxic concentrations of benzene metabolites, including hydroquinone, selectively inhibit one or more macrophage functions required for effective host defences *in vivo*. Both hydroquinone and benzoquinone significantly inhibited hydrogen peroxide release following zymosan stimulation and interferon-γ induced tumour cytolysis activity [79].

Further investigations revealed that hydroquinone treatment of bone marrow macrophages *in vitro* for 12 h with $0.1–1\ \mu\text{mol}\ l^{-1}$ hydroquinone also reduced the quantity of IL-1 activity in culture supernatant following induction of secretion by lipopolysaccharide (LPS) activation [79]. Macrophage membrane-associated IL-1 activity was also decreased with $1\ \mu\text{mol}\ l^{-1}$ hydroquinone. The significance of this effect in relation to regulation of myelopoiesis and lymphopoiesis is discussed in the following section. The sensitivity of macrophages to hydroquinone *in vitro* is apparently due to peroxidase-dependent biotransformation of hydroquinone to benzoquinone, as discussed above.

Stromal-dependent lymphopoiesis

Lymphocytopenia is one of the earliest indicators of toxicity in individuals exposed to significant concentrations of benzene [12]. This effect may be due in part to the apparent sensitivity of B lymphopoiesis to benzene or to benzene metabolites [80–83]. Administration of benzene to mice (100 mg kg^{-1} day^{-1}) for 4 days induced a significant (four- to sixfold) increase in bone marrow pre-B cells and a twofold reduction in surface immunoglobulin-positive B cells [82]. Pre-B cells are the earliest recognizable cells belonging to the B-cell lineage in the bone marrow. These cells are detected phenotypically by the expression of μ heavy chain of immunoglobulin M (IgM) without detectable light chain expression. Pre-B cells differentiate from a proliferating pool of progenitor cells and within 12 h can mature into B cells through the process of gene rearrangement and the expression of immunoglobulin light chains. This entire process is influenced by cytokines released from bone marrow stromal cells and other accessory cells.

A similar effect occurred in bone marrow cultures exposed to hydroquinone. A dose-dependent arrest in B lymphopoiesis was observed after a 1-h exposure to 0.1 μmol l^{-1} hydroquinone [84]. To determine if hydroquinone was acting on pre-B cells or on the stromal cells, B-lymphocyte-depleted bone marrow cell suspensions or stromal cells were pulsed with hydroquinone for 1 h and then co-cultured in various combinations. Co-cultures of control B-lymphocyte-depleted bone marrow cells with hydroquinone-treated stromal cells contained normal or slightly increased number of pre-B cells, but a reduced content of B lymphocytes. In contrast, co-cultures of hydroquinone-treated pre-B cells with control stromal cells produced normal numbers of B lymphocytes. Taken together, these findings suggest that hydroquinone inhibits the maturation of pre-B cells.

Studies carried out with conditioned medium indicated that hydroquinone inhibited the stromal cell production of a factor (or factors) required for the maturation of pre-B cells. Partial purification of bone marrow stromal cell-conditioned medium by high performance liquid chromatography and gel filtration yielded a protein with a molecular weight of approximately 17 kDa with B lymphopoietic activity [85]. The B lymphopoietic activity contained in this purified fraction could be neutralized by a monoclonal antibody to IL-4, but not by an anti-IL-1 antibody, suggesting that the B-

lymphopoietic factor produced by the stromal cells was IL-4. This hypothesis was supported by experiments indicating that a human recombinant IL-4 mimicked the actions of stromal cell-conditioned medium on B lymphopoiesis in stromal cell-depleted bone marrow cultures. The recombinant IL-4 also reversed the pre-B cell maturation arrest in hydroquinone-treated cultures, suggesting that hydroquinone was inhibiting either the production or release of IL-4 by the bone marrow stromal cells.

A stromal cell line SCL-173 was derived from LTBMC and was selected on the basis of constitutive production of IL-4 [85]. Conditioned medium from SCL-173 cells treated with hydroquinone supported B lymphopoiesis, suggesting that hydroquinone was not altering IL-4 production by stromal fibroblasts. Previous studies had shown that bone marrow-derived macrophages produce IL-1 which in turn stimulates stromal fibroblasts to produce IL-4. This observation, coupled with the results obtained with the hydroquinone-treated stromal fibroblasts, suggested that hydroquinone may be inhibiting the production of IL-1 by bone marrow macrophages (Fig. 18.2).

As noted above, treatment of macrophages with hydroquinone decreases IL-1 secretion in response to LPS stimulation [79]. A second stromal fibroblast cell line, SCL-160, which does not produce IL-4 constitutively, but can be induced to produce IL-4 by the addition of recombinant IL-1 or in the presence of bone marrow macrophages, was unaffected by exposure to hydroquinone [85]. However, the SCL-160 line could not be induced by macrophages previously pulsed with hydroquinone. These findings corroborated the observations in SCL-173 cells and supported the hypothesis that hydroquinone acts directly on stromal macrophages to inhibit the IL-1 mediated production of IL-4 by the stromal fibroblasts. The mechanism responsible for this effect is unknown; however, SK&F 86002, an anti-inflammatory drug, has also been observed to inhibit monocyte IL-1 production [103]. The mechanism for its effect is also unknown but at least three possible sites of action have been suggested: transcription, translation or post-translational events. These sites could also be targets for hydroquinone activity on IL-1 production in bone marrow macrophages and further research should be directed

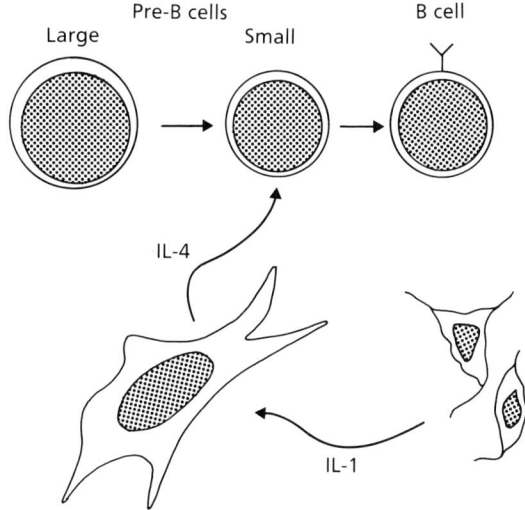

Fig. 18.2 Model depicting postulated bone marrow stromal cell regulation of pre-B cell maturation. Experimental results suggest that hydroquinone treatment reduces the amount of soluble IL-1 released from bone marrow-derived macrophages. This results in reduced IL-4 production by fibroblastic stromal cells. IL-4 is required for maturation of pre-B cells to B cells and a failure of IL-1 release results in a maturation arrest at the pre-B-cell stage. Adapted with permission from [85].

toward understanding how hydroquinone may alter the synthesis and processing of IL-1 in these cells.

Collectively, the information currently available about the myelotoxic mechanism of action of benzene and its metabolites allows for the formulation of a hypothetical model encompassing the various interactions of bone marrow physiology with these toxicants (Fig. 18.3). Foremost is the notion that hepatic metabolism of benzene is important for the expression of benzene cytotoxicity to bone marrow cells, especially at high benzene exposure levels. Many studies have shown that high concentrations of individual metabolites, or combinations of metabolites, are intrinsically cytotoxic to all haemopoietic cell lineages. However, at low exposure levels, either acutely or chronically, more subtle changes are apparently involved which appear to depend on further local or cellular metabolism of the intermediates initially produced by the liver as well as unmetabolized benzene which readily reaches the bone marrow. A portion of this metabolism occurs

via macrophages by both a cyclo-oxygenase and a myeloperoxidase-dependent process. A number of factors will influence the outcome of this metabolism, including the level of metabolites in the marrow and collective effects on regulatory cells in the haemopoietic microenvironment during exposure to benzene or its metabolites.

Mechanisms of toxicity—immune cells

Specificity of immunotoxicants

Many immunosuppressive xenobiotics are highly specific for certain immune system target cells. In order to evaluate the determinants for this specificity, a number of approaches are utilized which rely principally on *in vitro* studies with purified cells belonging to specific lineages. Some examples of these methods can be found in those studies listed in Table 18.1. Selective toxicity is usually established by a detailed characterization *in vitro* of how each xenobiotic affects cell phenotype, as determined by the immunofluorescent profile of cell-specific markers, in conjunction with different functional parameters, including cytokine production, response to cytokines, alteration in cell growth and maturation as well as changes in specific immune responses. By combining this information with results from animal studies, the potential for selective immunosuppression can be ascertained for individual xenobiotics or their reactive metabolites.

Anthraquinones

An example of such an *in vivo/in vitro* approach is provided by recent studies which examined the toxicity of a substituted anthracycline compound, 1, 4-bis[(2-aminoethyl)amino]5, 8-dihydroxy-9, 10-anthracenenedione dihydrochloride (AEAD) to cytotoxic T lymphocytes [86,108]. It was initially determined that neither IL-1 nor IL-2 production was affected by AEAD in cultures of adherent peritoneal cells or spleen cells, respectively. Both of these cytokines are required for the activation and growth of cytotoxic T cells. Further experiments indicated that the responsiveness of thymocytes to IL-1 or of cytotoxic T lymphocyte-2 (CTL-2) cells to IL-2 was also unaffected by AEAD at 1×10^{-5}

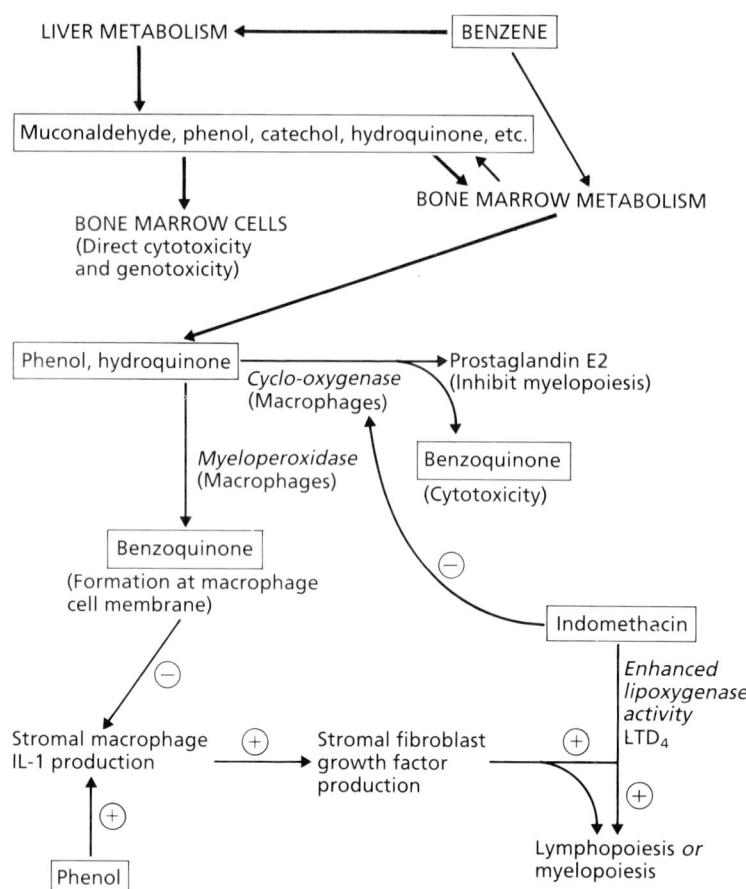

Fig. 18.3 Hypothetical model depicting the activity of benzene and its metabolites on bone marrow haemopoiesis. It is postulated that hepatic metabolism generates benzene metabolites which localize in the bone marrow. These metabolites, as well as some unmetabolized benzene, may act directly on cells in the bone marrow or may undergo further biotransformation via peroxidase-dependent mechanisms.

$\times 10^{-3}$ µg ml^{-1}. However, the addition of exogenous IL-1 or IL-2 to CTL induction cultures treated with AEAD failed to reconstitute CTL activation. Moreover, AEAD treatment did not alter the relative populations of helper or suppressor T cells.

Taken together, these results indicated that AEAD was affecting cytotoxic T lymphocytes at the progenitor cell level. This hypothesis was further supported by the finding that neither spleen cells treated with AEAD nor thymocytes from AEAD-treated mice could support the activation or differentiation of CTL progenitors into functional cytotoxic T lymphocytes. Subsequent animal studies further supported this conclusion. AEAD, at doses which inhibit cytotoxic T-lymphocyte function, fails to alter antibody responses or natural killer cell function [86].

Cyclosporin

Another xenobiotic that affects T-cytotoxic lymphocytes is cyclosporin (C$_s$A). Cyclosporin inhibits the activation of cytotoxic T lymphocytes, but spares the activation and amplification of suppressor T lymphocytes [87,88,109]. Mechanistic studies have shown that this effect is due to pleiotropic effects of C$_s$A, including inhibition of IL-2 production (in contrast to AEAD) and inhibition of antigen presentation by monocytes/macrophages. However, it is important to consider C$_s$A-induced immunosuppression in terms of dosage-related activity. As pointed out by Hess and co-workers [88], IL-2 production and cytotoxic T-lymphocyte induction are very sensitive to C$_s$A (10–50 ng), whereas suppressor cell activation and IL-2-dependent proliferation is very resistant (> 1000 ng ml^{-1}). The mechanism respon-

Table 18.1 Partial list of xenobiotics with selectivity toward immune cells

Xenobiotic	Primary effect	Secondary effect	Reference
Anthraquinones	CTL		[86,87]
Cyclosporin	T_h cells, CTL		[88,89]
Deoxycorformycin	NK		[90]
Diethylstilboestrol	Macrophages	T cells	[91]
Dimethylbenzcanthracene	T_h cells	CTL	[92–94]
Heptachlorodibenzo-*p*-dioxin	T_h cells	B cells	[95]
Hydroquinone	Macrophages	B cells	[79,84]
Lead	Macrophages	T cells B cells	[96–98]
Manganese	NK cells		[99,100]
Methotrexate	B cells		[101]
Phorbols	NK cells		[102]
SKF 860022	Macrophages		[103]
Tetrachlorodibenzo-*p*-dioxin	Epithelial cells B cells	T cells	[104–107]

CTL, Cytotoxic T lymphocytes; T_h, T helper; NK, natural killer.

sible for C_sA activity is apparently related to the binding of C_sA to intracellular proteins [109–111]. Two major binding proteins are cytophilin and calmodulin. The function of cytophilin is unknown but is postulated to have kinase activity. Calmodulin is required for further activation of intracellular enzymes within lymphocytes and for progression of lymphocytes through the cell cycle and gene expression. A role for these proteins in C_sA immunosuppression is supported by observations that C_sA activity is potentiated by calcium channel blockers and competitively inhibited by calmodulin inhibitors [88].

However, there are still many unanswered questions regarding C_sA's mechanism of action. For example, it has been observed that cellular resistance and sensitivity are inversely correlated with the binding of C_sA to T lymphocytes [88]. That is, the IL-2-producing helper T cells and cytotoxic T lymphocytes, which are most sensitive to C_sA, take up the least amount of C_sA. On the other hand, some B-cell subsets (distinguished by responsiveness to

T-independent or T-dependent antigens) are resistant to C_sA but contain relatively high amounts of C_sA. The reason for this inverse relationship between accumulation and suppressive activity is not known and is complicated by the observation that cyclophilin content is much higher in resistant cells that in sensitive cytotoxic T lymphocytes or IL-2-producing helper T cells [112,113].

These studies illustrate the concept that certain xenobiotics can exert selective activity on different immune cells by pleiotropic mechanisms operating at the cellular or subcellular level. Specific biochemical events that have been implicated in immunotoxity include inhibition or alteration of gene expression, lymphokine production, signal transduction, and enzyme activity and are discussed in detail below.

2,3,7,8-Tetrachlorodibenzo-p-dioxin (TCDD)

Effects on terminal B-cell maturation. Studies in animal models and in human and animal cells in culture indicate that TCDD acts on selected cell targets within the immune system to produce a spectrum of age-dependent lesions: thymus atrophy and suppressed cell-mediated immunity (CMI) in young animals [114] and suppressed humoral immunity in adult animals [115]. The observed actions of TCDD on immune system target cells appear to be initiated by binding to a specific intracellular receptor protein (designated the TCDD or *Ah* receptor) [116].

In adult mice, TCDD appears to exert its principal immunosuppressive effects on B-lineage cells [104,116,117]. Experimental data indicate that TCDD inhibits the terminal maturation of B cells into antibody-producing cells following stimulation with anti-Ig [118]. Cross-linking of surface Ig on B cells induces an increase in phosphoinositol which can be assessed by intracellular accumulation of ^{3}H-inositol phosphate (Fig. 18.1). TCDD exposure ($1-10$ nmol l^{-1}), in contrast to chlorphentermine as described above, did not significantly alter the normal accumulation of inositol phosphate in stimulated cells. Neither did TCDD alter B cell transition from G_o to S or surface Ia expression. However, a definite temporal relationship was observed relative to inhibition of antibody synthesis in that TCDD was most effective when added at the initiation of culture rather than 2 or 3 days later [118].

Other experiments have detected an early increase in the phosphorylation of membrane proteins in B cells exposed to TCDD [105]. It was initially believed that, similar to TCDD-induced protein kinase C activity in hepatocytes [119], the increase was due to enhanced protein kinase C activity. This was ruled out, however, when it was determined that protein kinase C activity remained unaltered and TCDD did not alter the ability of phorbol 12-myristate-13-acetate to increase protein kinase C activity. Instead, evidence pointed toward tyrosine-specific kinase activity as a target enzyme for TCDD. Tyrosine-protein kinases appear to function in the regulation of cellular growth and development [120,121]. TCDD exposure not only increased tyrosine-specific phosphorylation of membrane proteins, but did so only in B cells from *Ah*-responsive mice [105]. These results have led to speculation about *Ah*-receptor control of cellular maturation

processes. However, as pointed out by Clark and co-workers [105], no direct evidence yet exists implicating tyrosine kinase activity and antibody inhibition. Further studies will be required to address this question.

Interestingly, these studies suggest a novel hypothesis: TCDD could alter the response of B lymphocytes to regulatory molecules or cytokines which are required for normal growth and development of B-lineage cells. Many of the tyrosine-protein kinases are transmembrane receptors for cytokines and growth factors. For example, recent studies have shown that the Lck and lck genes encode for tyrosine-protein kinase activity and are associated with haemopoietic cells, primarily those of the myeloid or lymphoid lineages, respectively [122–124]. Expression of these genes in granulocytic and monocytic leukaemia cells increases after the cells have been experimentally induced to differentiate. If these kinases are involved in the pathway that transmits signals to genes regulating B-cell phenotype expression, then TCDD may interfere with a tyrosine-protein kinase that interacts with a receptor for a B-cell cytokine. This could result in inhibition of terminal B-cell maturation, as observed in cultures following TCDD exposure. Alternatively, the interaction of TCDD could simply involve a decrease in cytokine binding to a tyrosine-protein kinase-encoded receptor, as suggested by Umbreit and Gallo [125]. One candidate cytokine receptor that immediately comes to mind is the IL-4 receptor. TCDD is most effective when present early in lymphocyte cultures and IL-4 is one of the earliest factors required temporarily during B-cell activation induced by anti-Ig stimulation [126]. Moreover, a recent study reports the appearance of a novel plasma-membrane phosphoprotein in resting B cells exposed to recombinant IL-4 [127].

Effects on T-cell maturation. In young animals exposure to TCDD results in thymic atrophy. *In vitro* model systems have been developed to identify and study target cell populations in murine thymus and to assess the potential toxicity of TCDD to human thymus. The data obtained from these models indicate that TCDD can act directly on thymic epithelial cells to suppress thymus-dependent maturation of T-lymphocyte precursors.

The clinical significance of the observations made in the *in vitro* model systems to humans has not been established.

T-lymphocyte precursors originate from the bone marrow and traffic to both cortical and medullary regions of the thymus where maturation of the precursors (designated within the thymus as thymocytes) occurs by a multi-stage process dependent on cell–cell contact between thymocytes and the thymic reticulum and on humoral factors produced by medullary thymic epithelial (TE) cells [128]. Several phenotypic changes mark the various stages of thymocyte maturation. These include differential expression of membrane antigens, decreased sensitivity to corticosteroids, and enhanced responsiveness to mitogens [128–130].

To identify target cell populations for TCDD in the thymus, a reconstituted thymus system was developed using tissues from inbred mice [106,130]. Thymocytes were co-cultured with syngeneic confluent monolayers of primary TE cells (Fig. 18.4). Initial studies were carried out using cells isolated from the thymuses of an inbred mouse strain previously shown to be sensitive to TCDD-induced thymic atrophy. TCDD acted directly on TE monolayers to alter maturation of co-cultured syngeneic thymocytes, as judged by decreased thymocyte responsiveness to the mitogens concanavalin A and PHA (Fig. 18.5). The dose-dependence and structure–activity relationship of the actions of TCDD and other structurally similar compounds on TE cells indicated involvement of the TCDD receptor.

The studies described above using thymus cell populations from mice were extended to the human thymus [131]. Human TE lines were established from thymuses removed from children undergoing corrective cardiac surgery. All human TE lines examined were shown to support thymocyte maturation and to possess the TCDD receptor protein [132], as had been observed previously in TE cells established from mouse thymus. Both the induction of cytochrome P450 mono-oxygenase activity (a biochemical marker for TCDD responsiveness) and immunosuppressive responses elicited by TCDD in the human TE cells were mediated by the TCDD receptor.

Further characterization of these TCDD receptor-mediated responses in several strains of human TE cells indicated significant interstrain differences in cytochrome P450 inducibility, which did not appear to correlate directly with the measured concentrations of the cytosolic TCDD receptor, and differences in the sensitivity and magnitude of TCDD-dependent immunosuppressive and induction responses [131]. Taken together, these observations on the actions of TCDD in the *in vitro* human thymus system suggest that this tissue is a potential target for TCDD and structurally similar homologues. However, for these human target cells, measurement of the levels of the TCDD receptor or of a well characterized marker response to TCDD does not appear to provide accurate quantitative assessment of susceptibility to TCDD-dependent immunosuppressive actions.

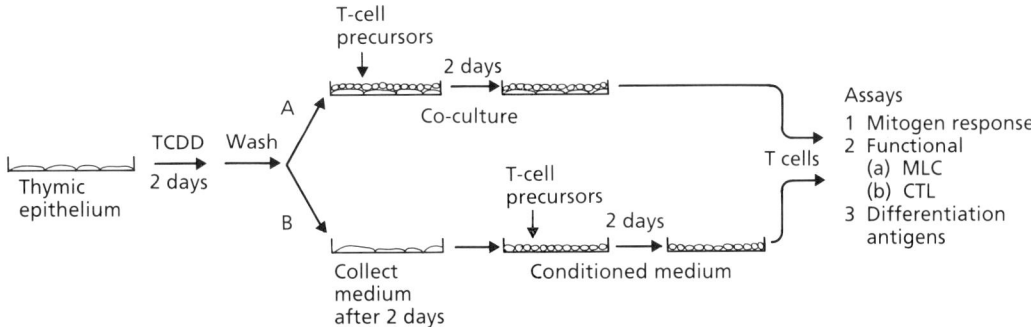

Fig. 18.4 Schematic representation of the experimental procedures used for the thymic epithelium co-culture and conditioned medium-dependent maturation of T-lymphocyte precursors.

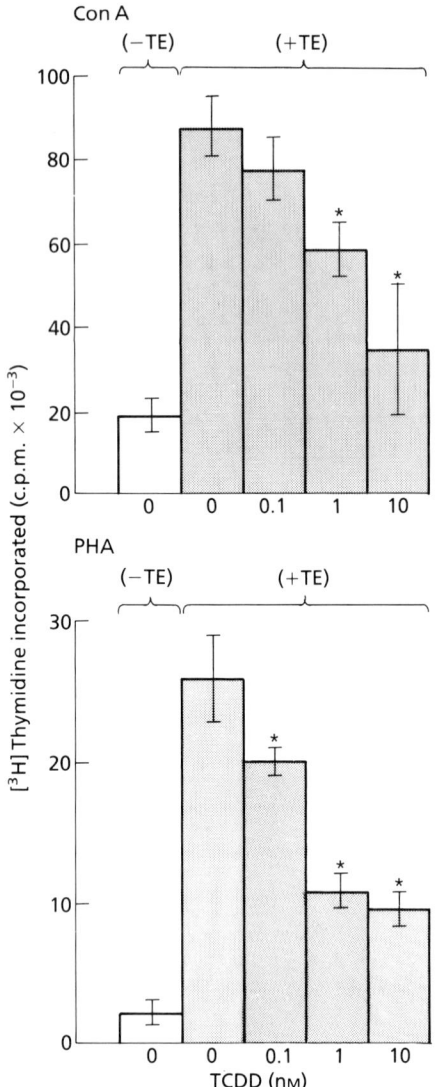

Fig. 18.5 Lymphoproliferative responses of thymocytes from C57BL/6 mice co-cultivated on 2,3,7,8-tetrachlorodibenzo-*p*-dioxin (TCDD)-treated syngeneic thymic epithelial (TE) monolayers. Each bar represents the mean ± S.D. of four determinations. *Value significantly different ($P < 0.05$) from the DMSO-treated co-culture control. Reprinted with permission from [106].

Although the studies described above provide evidence for the direct action of TCDD on TE target cells, actions on this cell population alone most likely do not account fully for the thymic atrophy and suppressed cell immunity observed in TCDD-treated animals. McConkey *et al.* [133], have reported that TCDD can kill immature thymocytes by enhancing calcium-mediated endonuclease activation. Presumably this is a result of TCDD-dependent increase in the intracellular calcium concentration. Fine *et al.* [134] have demonstrated that TCDD can act directly on lymphocyte stem cell populations in animals exposed perinatally. Taken together the observations in animal and in *in vitro* model systems indicate that TCDD potentially can act at at least three target cells to suppress host cellular immunocompetence.

Conclusions

Studies carried out in animal model systems have shown that many chemicals have the potential to alter immune function, resulting in either hypersensitivity responses in organs such as the skin or lung, or in immunosuppression with an associated increase in host susceptibility to infectious agents. Of the two responses, immunosuppression offers the greatest challenge, particularly with regard to understanding the clinical significance of partial inhibition of a measured immune system parameter. Given the large functional reserve of the immune system, can one assume that a 10–20% suppression in a measured immune system parameter is likely to result in an adverse health outcome? This question is best addressed by detailed study of the mechanisms by which a chemical (or reactive metabolite) alters immune function.

The immune system is a tightly regulated network of lymphoid organs and dispersed cell populations present in circulating blood and interstitial tissue spaces. Given the complex nature of the interactions of the various lymphoid and non-lymphoid cell populations, studies of the mechanisms of action of immunotoxic agents would be difficult to carry out in animal models alone. In this chapter several examples were presented in which *in vitro* model systems were developed and used in conjunction with animal models to gain insight into the mechanisms of action of several known immunotoxic compounds. It is important to note that an understanding of the mechanisms by which a chemical can alter immune function must be coupled with a quantitative description of tissue dosimetry, specifically, the linking of tissue dose to exposure. Integration of data obtained in animals with studies at the cell and molecular level can be used in combination with available epidemiological data to develop biological-based mechanistic models to support human risk assessment.

References

1 Vos JG. Immune suppression as related to toxicology. *CRC Crit Rev Toxicol* 1977; 5:67–101.

2 Dean JH, Murray MJ, Ward EC. Toxic responses of the immune system. *Casarett and Doull's Toxicology. The Basic Science of Poisons.* New York, NY: Macmillan, 1986:245–85.

3 Luster MF, Wierda D, Rosenthal GJ. Environmentally related disorders of the hematologic and immunc systems. *Environmental Medicine.* Philadelphia, PA: W.B. Saunders, 1990.

4 Sipes IG, Gandolfi AJ. Biotransformation of toxicants. *Casarett and Doull's Toxicology. The Basic Science of Poisons.* New York, NY: Macmillan, 1986:64–98.

5 Kim D, Yang KH, Johnson KW, Holsapple MP. Suppression of *in vitro* antibody production by cyclophosphamide and dimethylnitrosoamine in mixed cultures of mouse primary hepatocytes and mouse splenocytes. *Toxicol Appl Pharmacol* 1987; 87:32–42.

6 Kaminiski NE, Jordan SD, Page D, Kim BS, Holsapple MP. Suppression of humoral immune responses by dialkylnitrosamines: structure–activity measurements. *Fund Appl Toxicol* 1989; 12:321–32.

7 Holsapple MP, Tucker AN, McNerney PJ, White KL. Effects of N-nitrosodimethylamine on humoral immunity. *J Pharmacol Exp Ther* 1984; 229:493–500.

8 Johnson KW, Kim D, Munson AE, Holsapple MP. Dependence on intact cells for the *in vitro* activation of dimethylnitrosamine to an immunosuppressive form. *Mut Res* 1987; 182:211–21.

9 Irons RD, Greenlee WF, Wierda D, Bus JS. Relationship between benzene metabolism and toxicity: a proposed mechanism for the formation of reactive intermediates from polyphenol metabolites. In: Snyder R, Parke DV, Kocis JJ, Jollow CJ, Gibson CG, Witmer CM, eds. *Biological Reactive Intermediates.* 11. New York: Plenum Press, 1982:229–43.

10 Sammett D, Lee EW, Kocisis JJ, Snyder R. Partial hepatectomy reduces both metabolism and toxicity of benzene. *J Toxicol Environ Hlth* 1979; 5:785–92.

11 Mitchell JR. Mechanisms of benzene-induced aplastic anemia. *Fed Am Soc Exp Biol* 1971; 30:A561.

12 Goldstein BD. Benzene toxicity. *Occ Med* 1988; 3:541–54.

13 Okano P, Miller HN, Robinson RC, Gelboin HV. Comparison of benzo(a)pyrene and (-)-trans-7,8-dihydroxy-7,8-dihydrobenzo(a)pyrene metabolism in human blood. *Cancer Res* 1979; 39:3184–93.

14 Kawabata TT, White JKL. Suppression of the *in vitro* humoral immune response of mouse splenocytes by benzo(a)pyrene metabolites and inhibition of benzo(a)pyrene-induced immunosuppression by alpha-naphthoflavone. *Cancer Res* 1987; 47:2317–22.

15 Irons RD, Dent JG, Baker TS, Rickert DE. Benzene is metabolized and covalently bound in bone marrow *in situ. Chem-Biol Interact* 1980; 30:214–45.

16 Smart RC, Zannoni VG. DT-diaphorase and peroxidase influence on the covalent binding of the metabolites of phenol, the major metabolite of benzene. *Mol Pharmacol* 1984; 26:105–11.

17 Sawahata T, Neal RA. Biotransformation of phenol to hydroquinone and catechol by rat liver microsomes. *Mol Pharmacol* 1983; 23:453–60.

18 Thomas DJ, Sadlere A, Subrahmanyam VV, Siegel D, Reasor MJ, Wierda D, Ross D. Bone marrow stromal cell bioactivation and detoxification of the benzene metabolite hydroquinone: comparison of macrophage JS and fibroblastoid cells. *Mol Pharmacol* 1990; 37:255–62.

19 Schlosser MJ, Kalf GF. Metabolic activation of hydroquinone by macrophage peroxidase. *Chem-Biol Interact* 1989; in press.

20 Gaido KW, Wierda D. Suppression of bone marrow stromal cell function by benzene and hydroquinone is ameliorated by indomethacin. *Toxicol Appl Pharmacol* 1987; 89:378–90.

21 Pirozzi SJ, Schlosser MJ, Kalf GF. Prevention of benzene-induced myelotoxicity and prostaglandin synthesis in bone marrow of mice by inhibitors of prostaglandin H synthase. *Immunopharmacol* 1989; 18:39–55.

22 Kurland JI, Broxmeyer LM, Pelus LM, Bockman RS, Moore MAS. Role for monocyte-macrophage–derived colony-stimulating factor and prostaglandin E in the positive and negative control of myeloid stem cell proliferation. *Blood* 1978; 52:388–407.

23 Piper PJ. Pharmacology of leukotrienes. *Br Med Bull* 1978; 39:255-9.

24 Vore SJ, Eling TE, Danilowicz RM, Tucker AN, Luster MI. Regulation of murine hematopoiesis by arachidonic acid metabolites. *Int J Immunopharmacol* 1989; 11:435–42.

25 Miller AM, Weiner RS, Ziboh VA. Evidence for the role of leukotrienes C4 and D4 as essential intermediates in CSF-stimulated human myeloid colony formation. *Exp Hematol* 1986; 14:760–5.

26 Ross D, Siegel D, Gibson NW, Pacheco D, Thomas DJ, Reasor M, Wierda D. (Submitted). Activation and

deactivation of quinones catalyzed by DT-diaphorase. Evidence for bioreductive activation of diaziquone (AZQ) in human tumour cells and detoxification of benzene metabolites in bone marrow stroma. *Free Rad Res Commun.* 1990; 8:373–81.

27 Twerdok LE, Trush MA. Quinone reductase as a determinant of stromal cell susceptibility to hydroquinone. *Toxicol* 1989; 9:A1159.

28 Pfeifer RW, Irons RD. Inhibition of lectin-stimulated lymphocyte agglutination and mitogenesis by hydroquinone: reactivity with intracellular sulfhydryl groups. *Exp Mol Pathol* 1981; 35:189–98.

29 Irons RD, Neptun DA, Pfeifer RW. Inhibition of lymphocyte transformation and microtubule assembly by quinone metabolites of benzene: evidence for a common mechanism. *J Reticuloendothel Soc* 1981; 30:359–72.

30 Boobis AR, Fawthrop DJ, Davies DS. Mechanisms of cell death. *Trends Pharmacol* 1989; 10:275–80.

31 Irons RD, Neptun DA. Effects of the principal hydroxy-metabolites of benzene on microtubule polymerization. *Arch Toxicol* 1980; 45:297–305.

32 Luster MI, Boorman GA, Korach KS, Dieter MP, Hong L. Mechanisms of estrogen-induced myelotoxicity: evidence of thymic regulation. *Int J Immunopharmacol* 1984; 6:287–97.

33 Luster MI, Pfeifer RW, Tucker AN. The immunotoxicity of natural and environmental estrogens. In: Dean JH, Luster MI, Munson AE, Amos H, eds. *Immunotoxicology and Immunopharmacology.* New York: Raven Press, 1985:315–26.

34 Pfeifer RW, Patterson RM. Modulation of lymphokine–induced macrophage activation by estrogen metabolites. *J Immunopharmacol* 1985; 7:247–63.

35 Pfeifer RW, Patterson RM. Modulation of lectin-stimulated lymphocyte agglutination and mitogenesis by estrogen metabolites: effects on early events of lymphocyte activation. *Arch Toxicol* 1986; 58:157–64.

36 Si ECC, Pfeifer RW, Yim GKW. Iodoacetic acid and related sulfhydryl reagents fail to inhibit cell-cell communication: mechanisms of immunotoxicity in vitro. *Toxicol* 1987; 44:73–89.

37 Duncan DD, Lawrence DA. Four sulfhydryl-modifying compounds cause different structural damage but similar functional damage in murine lymphocytes. *Chem Biol Interact* 1988; 68:137–52.

38 Freed B, Mozayeni B, Lawrence DA, Wallach FR, Lempert N. Differential inhibition of human T-lymphocyte activation by maleimide probes. *Cell Immunol* 1986; 101:181–94.

39 Freed BM, Lempert N, Lawrence DA. The inhibitory effects of N-ethylmaleimide, colchicine and ctyochalasins on human T–cell functions. *Int J Immunopharmacol* 1989; 11:459–65.

40 Loor F. Lectin-induced lymphocyte agglutination. An active cellular process? *Exp Cell Res* 1973; 82:415–25.

41 Edelman GM. Surface modulation in cell recognition and cell growth. *Science* 1976; 192:218–26.

42 Reasor MJ. Drug-induced lipidosis and the alveolar macrophage. *Toxicol* 1981; 20:1–33.

43 Dake MD, Madison JM, Montgomery CK, Shellito JE, Bainton DF. Electron microscopic demonstration of lysomal inclusion bodies in lung, liver, lymph nodes, and blood leukocytes of patients with amiodarone pulmonary toxicity. *Am J Med* 1985; 78:506–12.

44 Sauers LJ, Wierda D, Walker ER, Reasor MJ. Chlorphentermine-induced alterations in the response of human lymphocytes to mitogens. *Biochem Pharmacol* 1986; 35:3651–4.

45 Sauers LJ, Wierda D, Walker ER, Reasor MJ. Morphological and functional changes in mouse splenic lymphocytes following *in vivo* and *in vitro* exposure to chlorphentermine. *J Immunopharmacol* 1986; 8:611–31.

46 Quastel MB, Kaplan JG. Early stimulation of potassium uptake in lymphocytes stimulated with PHA. *Exp Cell Res* 1970; 63:230–3.

47 Coffey RA, Hadden EM, Hadden JW. Evidence for cyclic GMP and calcium mediation of lymphocyte activation by mitogens. *J Immunol* 1977; 119:1387–94.

48 Waxdal MJ. Membrane methylation and other early biochemical reactions in the mitogenic action of lymphocytes. *Advances in Immunopharmacology.* Oxford: Pergamon Press, 1983:75–9.

49 Abdel-Latif AA. Calcium-mobilizing receptors, phosphoinositides and the generation of second messengers. *Pharmacol Rev* 1974; 38:227.

50 Tsein RY, Pozzan T, Rink TJ. T cell mitogens cause early changes in cytoplasmic free calcium and membrane potential in lymphocytes. *Nature* 1982; 295:68–71.

51 Sauers LJ. *The immunotoxicity of cationic amphiphilic drugs.* Doctoral dissertation. West Virginia University, Morgantown, WV, 1986.

52 Hasegawa-Sasaki H, Sasaki T. Phytomitogen-induced stimulation of synthesis *de novo* of phosphatidyl inositol, phosphatidic acid and diacylglycerol in rat and human lymphocytes. *Biochem Biophys Acta* 1981; 666:252–8.

53 Sauers LJ, Wierda D, Reasor MJ. Chlorphentermine suppresses the phosphatidylinositol pathway in concanavalin A-activated mouse splenic lymphocytes. *Immunopharmacol Immunotoxicol* 1988; 10:1–19.

54 Guy GR, Gordon BJ, Michell RH, Brown G. A combination of calcium ionophore and 12-0-tetradeconyl-13-acetate (TPA) simulates the growth of purified resting B cells. *Scand J Immunol* 1985; 22:591–6.

55 Mastro AM, Smith MC. Calcium-dependent activation of lymphocytes by ionophore, A23187 and phorbol ester tumor promoter. *J Cell Physiol* 1983; 116:51.

56 Truneh A, Albert F, Golstein P, Schmitt-Verhulst A. Early steps of lymphocyte activation bypassed by synergy between calcium ionophores and phorbal ester. *Nature* 1985; 313:318–20.

57 Allan D, Michell RH. Phosphatidylinositol cleavage by the soluble fraction from lymphocytes. *Biochem J* 1974; 1142:591–7.

58 Duke SS, Schook LB, Holsapple MP. Effects of N-nitrodimethylamine on tumor susceptibility. *J Leuk Biol* 1985; 37:383–94.

59 Holsapple MP, Bick PH, Duke SS. Effects of N-nitrosodimethylamine on cell-mediated immunity. *J Leuk Biol* 1985; 37:367–81.

60 Myers MJ, Pullen JK, Schook LB. Alteration of macrophage differentiation into accessory and effector cells from exposure to dimcthylnitrosamine in vivo. *Immunopharmacol* 1986; 12:105–15.

61 Myers MJ, Dickens CS, Schook LB. Alteration of macrophage anti-tumor activity and transferrin receptor expression by exposure to dimethylnitrosamine *in vivo*. *Immunopharmacol* 1987; 13:195–205.

62 Myers MJ, Schook LB. Modification of macrophage differentiation: dimethylnitrosamine induced alteration in the responses towards the regulatory signals controlling myelopoiesis. *Int J Immunopharmacol* 1987; 9:817–25.

63 Myers MJ, Hanafin WP, Schook LB. Augmented macrophage PGE_2 production following exposure to dimethylnitrosamine *in vivo*: relevance to suppressed T cell responses. *Immunopharmacol* 1989; 18:115–24.

64 Myers MJ, Witsell AL, Schook LB. Induction of serum colony-stimulating activity following diemethylnitrosamine exposure: effects on macrophage differentiation. *Immunopharmacol* 1989; 18:125–34.

65 Fulop GM, Osmond DG. Regulation of bone marrow lymphocyte production III. Increased production of B and non-B lymphocytes after administering systemic antigens. *Cell Immunol* 1983; 75:80–90.

66 Pietrangeli CE, Osmond DG. Regulation of B-lymphocyte production in the bone marrow: role of macrophages and the spleen in mediating responses to exogenous agents. *Cell-Immunol* 1985; 94:147–58.

67 Pietrangeli CE, Osmond DG. Regulation of B-lymphocyte production in the bone marrow: mediation of the effects of exogenous stimulants by adoptively transferred spleen cells. *Cell Immunol* 1987; 107:348–57.

68 Landreth KS, Kincade PW. Mammalian B lymphocyte precursors. *Dev Comp Immunol* 1984; 8:773–90.

69 Lichtman MA. The ultrastructure of the hemopoietic environment of the marrow: a review. *Exp Hematol* 1981; 9:391–410.

70 Allen TD, Dexter TM. The essential cells of the hemopoietic microenvironment. *Exp Hematol* 1984; 12:517–21.

71 Owen M. Marrow stromal stem cells. *J Cell Sci* 1988; 10 (suppl):63–76

72 Tavassoli M, Crosby WH. Transplantation of marrow to extramedullary sites. *Science* 1968; 161:54–6.

73 Johnson A, Dorshkind K. Stromal cells in myeloid and lymphoid long-term bone marrow cultures can support multiple hemopoietic lineages and modulate their production of hemopoietic growth factors. *Blood* 1986; 68:1348.

74 Gale RP. Myelosuppressive effects of antineoplastic chemotherapy. In: Testa NG, Gale RP, eds. *Hematopoiesis. Long-term Effects of Chemotherapy and Radiation.* New York: Marcel Dekker, 1988: 63–74.

75 Harigaya K, Miller ME, Cronkite EP, Drew RT. The detection of in vivo hematotoxicity of benzene by in vitro liquid bone marrow cultures. *Toxicol Appl Pharmacol* 1981; 60:346–53.

76 Garnett HM, Cronkite EP, Drew RT. Effect of *in vivo* exposure to benzene on the characteristics of bone marrow adherent cells. *Leuk Res* 1983; 7:803–10.

77 Gaido K, Wierda D. *In vitro* effects of benzene metabolites on mouse bone marrow stromal cells. *Toxicol Appl Pharmacol* 1984; 76:45–55.

78 Gaido KW, Wierda D. Modulation of stromal cell function in DBA/2J and B6C3F1 mice exposed to benzene or phenol. *Toxicol Appl Pharmacol* 1985; 81:469–75.

79 Thomas DJ, Reasor MJ, Wierda D. Macrophage regulation of myelopoiesis is altered by exposure to the benzene metabolite hydroquinone. *Toxicol Appl Pharmacol* 1989; 97:440–53.

80 Lewis JG, Odom B, Adams DO. Toxic effects of benzene and benzene metabolites on mononuclear phagocytes. *Toxicol Appl Pharmacol* 1988; 92:246–54.

81 Wierda D, Irons RD. Hydroquinone and catechol reduce the frequency of progenitor B lymphocytes in mouse spleen and bone marrow. *Immunopharmacol* 1982; 4:41–54.

82 King AG, Landreth KS, Wierda D. Hydroquinone inhibits bone marrow pre-B cell maturation *in vitro*. *Mol Pharmacol* 1987; 32:807–12.

83 Wierda D, King AG, Luebvke RW, Reasor MJ, Smialowicz RJ. Perinatal immunotoxicity of benzene toward mouse B cell development. *J Am Coll Toxicol* 1989; 8:981–96.

84 King AG, Wierda D, Landreth KS. Bone marrow stromal cell regulation of B lymphopoiesis. I. The role of macrophages, IL-1 and IL-4 in pre-B cell maturation. *J Immunol* 1988; 141:2016–26.

85 King AG, Landreth KS, Wierda D. Bone marrow

stromal cell regulation of B-lymphopoiesis. II. Mechanisms of hydroquinone inhibition of pre-B cell maturation. *J Pharmacol Exp Ther* 1989; 250:582–90.

86 House RV, Dean JH. Target cell specificity of immunosuppression in murine lymphocytes exposed to 1, 4-Bis[(2-aminoethyl)amino]-5, 8-Dihydroxy-9, 10-anthracenedione dihydrochloride (AEAD). *Int J Immunopharmacol* 1989; 11:85–93.

87 House RV, Lauer LD, Thurmond LM, Cornacoff JB, Dean JH. Selective immunosuppression following exposure to a novel anthraquinone, 2,4-bis[(2-aminoethyl)amino]-5, 8-dihydroxy-9, 10-anthracenedione dihydrochloride (AEAD). *Int J Immunopharmacol* 1989; 11:95-101.

88 Hess AD, Tutschka PJ, Pu Z, Santos GW. Effect of cyclosporin A on human lymphocyte responses in vitro. IV. Production of T cell stimulatory growth factors and development of responsiveness to these growth factors in CsA-treated primary MLR cultures. *J Immunol* 1982; 128:360–7.

89 Borel JG, Feurer C, Gubler U, Stahelin H. Biological effects of cyclosporin A: a new antilymphocyte agent. *Agents Actions* 1976; 6:468–75.

90 Luebke RW, Lawson LD, Rogers RR, Riddle MM, Rowe DG, Smialowicz RJ. Selective immunotoxic effects in mice treated with adenosine deaminase inhibitor 2-deoxycoformycin. *Immunopharmacol* 1987; 13:25–35.

91 Dean JH, Lauer LD, Murray MJ, Luster MI, Neptune D, Adams DO. Functions of mononuclear phagocytes in mice exposed to diethylstilbestrol: a model of aberrant macrophage development. *Cell Immunol* 1986; 102:315–22.

92 Burchel SW, Hadley WM, Barton SL, Fincher RH, Lauer LD, Dean JH. Persistent suppression of humoral immunity produced by 7,12-dimethylbenz(a)anthracene(DMBA) in B6C3F1 mice: correlation with changes in spleen cell surface markers detected by flow cytometry. *Int J Immunopharmacol* 1988; 10: 369–76.

93 House RV, Lauer LD, Murray MJ, Dean JH. Suppression of T- helper cell function in mice following exposure to the carcinogen 7,12-dimethylbenz(a)anthracene and its restoration by interleukin-2. *Int J Immunopharmacol* 1987; 9:89–97.

94 House RV, Pallardy MJ, Dean JH. Suppression of murine cytotoxic T-lymphocyte induction following exposure to 7,12-dimethylbenz(a)anthracene: dysfunction of antigen recognition. *Int J Immunopharmacol* 1989; 11:207–15.

95 Kerkvliet NF, Brauner JA. Mechanisms of 1,2,3,4,6,7,8-heptachlorodibenzo-p-dioxin (HpCDD)-induced humoral immune suppression: evidence of primary defect in T-cell regulation. *Toxicol Appl Pharmacol* 1987; 87:18–31.

96 Blakley BR, Archer DL. The effect of lead acetate on the immune response in mice. *Toxicol Appl Pharmacol* 1981; 61:18–26.

97 Kowolenko M, Tracy L, Mudzinski S, Lawrence DA. Effect of lead on macrophage function. *J Leuk Biol* 1988; 43:357–64.

98 Kowolenko M, Tracy L, Lawrence DA. Lead-induced alterations of *in vitro* bone marrow cell responses to colony stimulating factor-1. *J Leuk Biol* 1989; 45:198–206.

99 Smialowicz RJ, Luebke RW, Rogers RR, Riddle MM, Rowe DG. Manganese chloride enhances natural cell-mediated immune effector cell function: effects on macrophages. *Immunopharmacol* 1985; 9:1–11.

100 Smialowicz RJ, Riddle MM, Rogers RR, Luebke RW, Burleson GR. Enhancement of natural killer cell activity and interferon production by manganese in young mice. *J Immunopharmacol* 1988; 10:93–107.

101 Rosenthal GJ, Weigand GW, Germolec DR, Blank JA, Luster MI. Suppression of B cell function by methotrexate and trimetrexate. Evidence for inhibition of purine biosynthesis as a major mechanism of action. *J Immunol* 1988; 141:410–16.

102 Updyke LW, Chuthaputtii A, Pfeifer R, Yim GKW. Modulation of natural killer activity by 12-0-tetradeconylphorbol-13-acetate and benzoyl peroxide in phorbol ester-sensitive (SENCAR) and resistant (B6C3F1) mice. *Carcinogenesis* 1988; 9:1943–51.

103 Lee JC, Griswold DE, Votta B, Hanna N. Inhibition of monocyte IL-1 production by the anti-inflammatory compound, SK&F 86002. *Int J Immunopharmacol* 1988; 10:835–43.

104 Tucker AN, Vore SJ, Luster MI. Suppression of B cell differentiation by 2,3,7,8-tetrachlorodibenzo-p-dioxin (TCDD). *Mol Pharmacol* 1985; 29:372–7.

105 Luster MI, Germolec DR, Clark G, Wiegand G, Rosenthal GJ. Selective effects of 2,3,7,8-tetrachlorodibenzo-p-dioxin and corticosteroid on *in vitro* lymphocyte maturation. *J Immunol* 1988; 140: 928–35.

106 Greenlee WF, Dold KM, Irons RD, Osborne R. Evidence for direct action of 2,3,7,8-tetrachlorodibenzo-p-dioxin (TCDD) on thymic epithelium. *Toxicol Appl Pharmacol* 1985; 19:112–20.

107 Kramer CM, Johnson KW, Dooley RK, Holsapple MP. 2,3,7,8-Tetrachlorodibenzo-p-dioxin (TCDD) enhances antibody production and protein kinase activity in murine B cells. *Biochem Biophys Res Comm* 1987; 145:25–33.

108 Luster MI, Bland JA. Molecular and cellular basis of chemically induced immunotoxicity. *Annu Rev Pharmacol Toxicol* 1987; 27:23–49.

109 Hess AD, Esa AH, Colombani PM. Mechanisms of

action of cyclosporine: effect on cells in the immune system and on subcellular events in T cell activation. *Transplant Proc* 1988; 20(suppl 2):29–40.

110 Drugge RJ, Handschumacher RE. Cyclosporine-mechanism of action. *Transplant Proc* 1988; 20(suppl 2):301–9.

111 Colombani PM, Robb A, Hess AD. Cyclosporin A binding to calmodulin: a possible site of action on T lymphocytes. *Science* 1985; 228:337–9.

112 Handschumacher RE, Harding MW, Rice J. Cyclophilin: a specific cytosolic binding protein for cyclosporin A. *Science* 1984; 226:544–7.

113 Koletsky AJ, Harding MW, Handschumacher RE. Cyclophilin: distribution and variant properties in normal and neoplastic tissues. *J Immunol* 1986; 137:1054–9.

114 Vos JG, Moore JA. Suppression of cellular immunity in rats and mice by maternal treatment with 2,3,7,8-tetrachlorodibenzo-*p*-dioxin. *Int Arch Allergy Appl Immunol* 1974; 47:777–94.

115 Vecchi A, Mantovani A, Sironi M, Luini W, Cairo M, Garattini S. Effect of acute exposure to 2,3,7,8-tetrachlorodibenzo-*p*-dioxin. *Chem-Biol Interact* 1980; 30:337–42.

116 Poland A, Glover E. 2,3,7,8-Tetrachlorodibenzo-*p*-dioxin: segregation of toxicity with the Ah locus. *Mol Pharmacol* 1980; 17:86–94.

117 Holsapple MP, McNerney P, Barnes D, White K. Suppression of humoral antibody production by exposure to 1,2,3,6,7,8-hexachlorobenzo-*p*-dioxin. *J Pharmacol Exp Ther* 1984; 231:518–26.

118 Holsapple M, McNerney P, Barnes D, White K. Suppression of humoral antibody production to 1,2,3,6,7,8-hexachlorobenzo-*p*-dioxin. *J. Pharmacol Exp Ther* 1985; 231:518–26.

119 Clark GC, Blank JA, Germolec DR, Luster MI. 2,3,7,8-Tetrachlorodibenzo-p-dioxin (TCDD) stimulates protein phosphorylation and tyrosine kinase activity in B lymphocytes. *Mol Pharmacol* 1991; in press.

120 Bombick DW, Madukar BV, Brewster DW, Matsumura F. TCDD (2,3,7,8-tetrachloro-dibenza-*p*-dioxin) causes increases in protein kinases particularly protein kinase C in hepatic plasma membrane of the rat and guinea pig. *Biophys Res Commun* 1985; 127:296–302.

121 Hunter T, Cooper JA. Protein-tyrosine kinases. *Annu Rev Biochem* 1985; 54:897–931.

122 Gee CE, Griffin J, Sastre L, Miller LJ, Springer TA, Piwnica-Worms H, Roberts TM. Differentiation of myeloid cells is accompanied by increased levels of pp60 c-src protein and kinase activity. *P N A S* 1986; 83:5131–5.

123 Marth JD, Peet R, Krebs EG, Perlumutter RM. A lymphocyte-specific protein-tyrosine kinase gene is rearranged and overexpressed in the murine T cell lymphoma LSTRA. *Cell* 1985; 43:393–404.

124 Quintrell N, Lebo R, Varmus H, Bishop MJ, Pettenati MJ, Lebeau MM, Diaz MO, Rowley JD. Identification of a human gene (HCK) that encodes a protein-tyrosine kinase and is expressed in hemopoietic cells. *Mol Cell Biol* 1987; 7:2267–75.

125 Umbreit TH, Gallo MA. Physiological implications of estrogen receptor modulation by 2,3,7,8-tetrachloro-dibenzo-dioxin (TCDD). *Rev Biochem Toxicol* 1987; 8:1–35.

126 Kishimoto T, Hirano T. Molecular regulation of B lymphocyte response. *Adv Immunol* 1988; 6:485–512.

127 McGarvie GM, Cushley W. Appearance of a novel plasma-membrane phosphoprotein following culture of resting murine B-lymphocytes with recombinant inter-leukin 4. *Immunol Lett* 1989; 22:221–6.

128 Haynes BF. The human thymic microenvironment. *Adv Immunol* 1984; 36:87–142.

129 Stutman O. Intrathymic and extrathymic T-cell maturation. *Immunol Rev* 1978; 42:138–84.

130 Kruisbeck AM. Thymic factors and T cell maturation *in vitro*: a comparison of the effects of thymic epithelial cultures with thymic extracts and thymic dependent serum factors. *Thymus* 1979; 1:163–85.

131 Cook JC, Dold KM, Greenlee WF. An *in vitro* model for studying the toxicity of 2,3,7,8-tetrachlorodibenzo-*p*-dioxin to human thymus. *Toxicol Appl Pharmacol* 1987; 89:256–68.

132 Cook JC, Greenlee WF. Characterization of a specific binding protein for 2,3,7,8-tetrachlorodibenzo-*p*-dioxin in human thymic epithelial cells. *Mol Pharmacol* 1989; 35:713–19.

133 McConkey DJ, Hartzell P, Duddy SK, Hakansson H, Orrenius S. 2,3,7,8-Tetrachlorodibenzo-p-dioxin kills immature thymocytes by Ca^{2+}-mediated endonuclease activation. *Science* 1988; 242:256–9.

134 Fine JS, Gasiewicz TA, Silverstone AE. Lymphocyte stem cell alterations following perinatal exposure to 2,3,7,8-tetrachlorodibenzo-*p*-dioxin. *Mol Pharmacol* 1989; 35:18–25.

19

Molecular immunotoxicology

CLIVE MEREDITH

Introduction

There is a growing conviction among toxicologists that the discipline of immunotoxicology will have an increasingly important role to play in the risk assessment of pharmaceutical and industrial chemicals in the 1990s and beyond. This chapter presents a personal view of the emergence of the subdiscipline of molecular immunotoxicology. Why do we need yet another subdiscipline when there is already a confusion of other techniques available to the toxicologist? The question is self-explanatory. Molecular immunotoxicology represents an attempt to introduce modern technology to the analysis of a highly complex system such that the contemporary requirements of immunotoxicology are matched by contemporary techniques. In order fully to comprehend the necessity for such an approach it is first necessary briefly to review the current standing of conventional immunotoxicology.

The driving force behind the emergence of immunotoxicology as a mainstream discipline is increased public awareness of the potential of exogenous agents to alter immune function. Largely as a result of the worldwide acquired immune deficiency syndrome (AIDS) epidemic, the public increasingly understands the consequences of impaired immune function, characterized in AIDS patients by an increased susceptibility to bacterial, fungal and viral infections and certain forms of cancer. Whilst it is not legitimate directly to compare the effects of the AIDS virus with the effects of immunotoxic drugs or chemicals, it is worth emphasizing that the ultimate lethality of AIDS is not directly attributable to the viral infection but is a secondary effect resulting from chronically impaired immune function. As immunotoxicologists it is this impairment of immune function which we seek to characterize in relation to exposure to putative immunomodulatory drugs and chemicals.

Our essential hypothesis is that human exposure to environmental or chemical agents can in some cases exert a toxic effect on the immune system causing its dysfunction. In some cases the manifestations of this dysfunction may be primary, such as in autoallergic disease. Mainly, however, the consequences are likely to be secondary, in that impairment of immune function leads to an increased susceptibility to infection and perhaps to certain forms of cancer. Because epidemiological evidence is almost impossible to obtain, given the diversity of human behaviour and a very high background incidence, it is impossible at this stage accurately to assess the scale of the problem.

Through the natural process of democracy, increased public concern leads the regulators and legislators to require that appropriate tests should be performed to establish the safety of new drugs and chemicals before they are approved for general use. However, to date there has been remarkably little requirement for the submission of immunotoxicity data for new product licences, and there has certainly been no attempt to legislate retrospectively, i.e. to require existing products to be evaluated for immunotoxic hazard. It is tempting, and traditional, to attribute blame for the failure to include appropriate tests on the regulatory authorities, for lack of will, and on manufacturers, for purely economic reasons. However, it is the opinion of this contributor that a third group are equally to blame— immunotoxicologists themselves. The essential problem is that there is a lack of concordance between groups of scientists involved in immunotoxicology as to which tests would be most appropriate to assess and predict the immunotoxicity of any given group of compounds. This is in large part due to a situation where conventional toxicologists favour the rat as their test animal whereas immunologists use the mouse. Indeed, in the USA the National Toxicology Program has selected a number of assays for use in B6C3F1 mice (see also Chapter 17). Although there has been some recent progress by groups of scientists attempting to design tiered testing structures and to perform interlaboratory validations in the rat (as reported at several recent workshops) it is not unreasonable to suggest that if 30 immunotoxicology laboratories throughout the world were asked to produce a test battery to predict the immunotoxic potential of a group of chemicals, the net result would be 30 different protocols! If immunotoxicologists cannot at present agree among themselves then the pressure on regulators and manufacturers to introduce meaningful tests is much alleviated.

This lack of concordance between different laboratories stems from the diverse nature of the immune system itself. Unfortunately, it is not represented by a single discrete organ within the body but comprises a number of organs with incompletely defined roles, e.g. spleen, thymus, bone marrow and a diverse array of peripheral circulating and tissue-specific cells which interact via a network of communicative and effector molecules of labyrinthine complexity. Thus, unlike the liver for example, which is amenable to analysis by pathology, enzymology or biochemistry, the immune system cannot

easily be dissected and subjected to classic toxicological analysis.

Although some pathology can be performed, much reliance is placed on immune function tests which assess the ability of discrete components of the system to participate in defined immunological/immunochemical reactions. Alternatively, emphasis is placed on the host-resistance assay, where groups of animals are exposed to the test chemical and subsequently infected with high titres of pathogenic bacteria or viruses. Apart from considerable concerns over the ethics of this type of animal experiment, host-resistance analysis has many parallels with the largely redundant median lethal dose (LD_{50}) test; any arguments valid against that assay can be invoked against the host-resistance assay.

Clearly, if immunotoxicology is to play a significant role in the safety evaluation of drugs and chemicals, it is important that it can offer tests which are sensitive, specific and reproducible. In this laboratory, our ongoing research programme is attempting to establish such tests by the application of molecular biological techniques to the analysis of immune cell populations. It is beyond dispute that molecular analysis of the modulation of gene expression is a very powerful technique. However, it is the manner in which this technology is harnessed and applied to problems in immunotoxicology which will determine its value not only as a potential immunotoxicological screening system but also to give insight into the biochemical mechanisms which underlie immunotoxic effects. It is not the purpose of this essay to claim that this sub-discipline, which we term molecular immunotoxicology is a panacea for all the failings of conventional immunotoxicity studies; we do propose, however, that it has an immediate contribution to make and that that contribution will become increasingly more important as *in vitro* studies gain acceptance in testing protocols.

The basis of molecular immunotoxicology

In order fully to appreciate the potential value of the application of molecular biological techniques to immunotoxicological problems, it is necessary to summarize certain fundamental concepts. Firstly, we must consider the flow of information in the cell:

$$DNA \rightarrow RNA \rightarrow protein$$

DNA contains all the relevant information, within the genetic sequence, to ensure not only the replication and propagation of that information to successive generations, but also to ensure the correct phenotypic expression of that information for any particular generation. That expression is mediated by RNA, particularly the messenger RNA (mRNA) species, which takes a copy of that information from nucleus to cytoplasm where it is able to direct the synthesis of polypeptides or proteins at discrete cytoplasmic factories called ribosomes. It is the expression of these proteins, particularly after they have undergone post-translational processing, which gives a cell its unique biochemical and structural characteristics.

Thus we can analyse three different types of macromolecule to determine expression or altered expression within a cell. If we analyse DNA and the intricate control systems within that DNA we are essentially studying what a cell is programmed to perform. If we study polypeptides or proteins, we can identify those events which have occurred as a result of programming or as a result of change in environment, perhaps in response to external stimuli. This can be an important analytical tool in our repertoire. However, we feel that the most direct form of analysis is the expression of mRNA species within the cell. Since most mRNA species are relatively short-lived, existing only for the purpose of conveying information from nucleus to cytoplasm, the analysis of mRNA can pinpoint precisely what a cell is doing at any point in time and how it is responding to external stimuli. We will therefore focus our attention, for the remainder of this chapter, on the analysis of mRNA expression in immune cell populations and its application in testing drugs and chemicals for their immunomodulatory potential.

Molecular immunotoxicology has been extremely fortunate in that a considerable proportion of the efforts in molecular biology over the last decade have been directed toward a better understanding of the immune system. This has resulted in a large number of immunoregulatory cytokines and growth factors being cloned at both complementary DNA (cDNA) and genomic level, most often in mouse or in human. As molecular immunotoxicologists we are the beneficiaries of a great deal of this industry since

cDNA clones or probes make ideal reagents with which to study gene expression at the mRNA level and thus to assess modulation of this expression in response to various stimuli. Because of the origins of these cDNA clones, we are generally restricted to test systems originating from mouse or human cells; in general this is most appropriate since conventional immunology is best understood in the mouse. This approach is slightly at odds with conventional toxicologists who favour the rat as their test species. There are some situations where cDNA probes will cross-hybridize, e.g. we have successfully used murine interleukin-1 (IL-1) probes on rat mRNA (there is 83% homology in predicted amino acid sequence [1] for IL-1α whereas for others, e.g. IL-3, there appears to be a lack of homology between species [2].

Analysis of modulated mRNA expression can be applied to at least three situations which are relevant to immunotoxicological testing. Firstly, the analysis can be conducted on *in vivo* exposed animals; tissues such as spleen, thymus and lymph glands can be removed and gross analysis for specific mRNAs can be conducted. Secondly, analysis can be performed on *ex vivo* material; tissue or cells taken from exposed animals can be stimulated or manipulated *in vitro* to determine the effects of pre-exposure *in vivo* on the ability of cells to generate characteristic patterns of mRNA expression. Finally, analysis can be performed exclusively *in vitro*, where defined cell populations, e.g. alveolar or peritoneal macrophages, can be pre-incubated with test compound before stimulation and expression analysis. In certain cases, it is possible that well defined cell lines can be used instead of primary cultures. In this laboratory, all three types of analysis have been successfully performed with good correlations between responses *in vivo* and *in vitro*. This is particularly satisfying in view of our ultimate objective which is the development of validated *in vitro* screening systems.

Techniques of molecular immunotoxicology

This section introduces the essential experimental techniques used in molecular immunotoxicology and has deliberate emphasis on the analysis of mRNA expression in cell cultures since we feel this to be the most important aspect of this discipline. It is not intended to be comprehensive, nor does it provide detailed protocols; for that the reader is directed toward any of the popular cloning manuals, e.g. that by Maniatis *et al.* [3], recently re-issued as a three-volume set [4] or the *Guide to Molecular Cloning Techniques* (issued as a full volume of *Methods in Enzymology* [5]). Rather, the intention is to outline the most important stages to this technique and to provide notes based on personal experience where appropriate. It is trusted that this will be of particular value to researchers wishing to enter this field.

In terms of overall strategy, this molecular immunotoxicological analysis is relatively straightforward. From cells or tissue exposed to test compound, RNA is extracted, purified and immobilized on a membrane support. Bound mRNA species are detected using probes derived from cDNA or oligonucleotides; these probes are radiolabelled or coupled to enzyme-substrate detection systems. After stringent washing to reduce background and eliminate non-specific binding, the membrane is subjected to autoradiography or other detection systems, whence the presence of specific mRNAs can be confirmed and semi-quantitative analysis performed by densitometry. That, in a nutshell, summarizes the essentials of the technique (Fig. 19.1); the following sections will concentrate on experimental details pertinent to each step.

EXPOSURE TO TEST COMPOUND

For animal experiments, the preferred model is the inbred mouse, for reasons stated earlier regarding background knowledge and availability of probes. If rats are employed, normally because the study has to dovetail with conventional toxicological analysis, then a number of preliminary experiments are necessary to determine the suitability of any murine or human probes for cross-hybridization. Age and sex of the test animal are important considerations since there is ample evidence that the nature of the cytokine response varies with age [6]. In this laboratory, we routinely use female mice and our specifications are for either the 4–6 or 6–8-week age range. The route of administration is dependent on the nature of the compound but there are some caveats, for example, intraperitoneal dosing often results in irritation and infiltration into the peritoneum; this might subsequently affect macrophage harvest from this site. Cells or tissue selected for analysis may depend on previous indications of toxic effect; in this laboratory we have on occasions taken spleen (whole and isolated splenocytes), thymus, lymph nodes (e.g. popliteal, mesenteric), macrophages (alveolar and peritoneal) and peripheral blood cells (both lymphocyte and monocyte fractions).

For *ex vivo* experiments, a similar range of cell types can be isolated. The object of the exercise is then to manipulate these cells *in vitro* and to determine whether known patterns of gene expression in response to *in vitro* stimulation are altered by prior exposure *in vivo*, e.g. lipopolysaccharide stimulation of macrophages/monocytes, mitogenic stimulation of lymphocytes. In certain respects, this type of analysis is highly appropriate since the *in vivo*

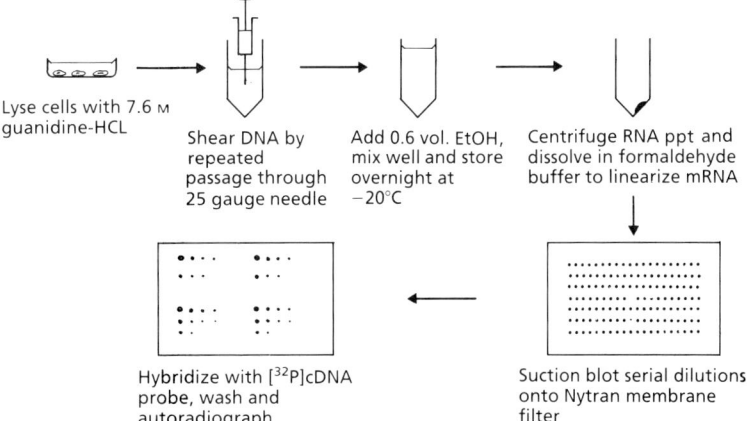

Fig. 19.1 Summary of molecular immunotoxicology analysis using the mRNA dot-blotting technique as performed in our laboratory.

Lyse cells with 7.6 M guanidine-HCL

Shear DNA by repeated passage through 25 gauge needle

Add 0.6 vol. EtOH, mix well and store overnight at −20°C

Centrifuge RNA ppt and dissolve in formaldehyde buffer to linearize mRNA

Suction blot serial dilutions onto Nytran membrane filter

Hybridize with [^{32}P]cDNA probe, wash and autoradiograph exposure takes into account any peculiarities of metabolism or pharmacokinetics pertinent to the test compound, whereas *in vitro* stimulation is highly sensitive and easily manipulable. However, in terms of developing rapid screening systems, it is less attractive since it makes use of extensive animal experimentation which is politically and economically undesirable in contemporary toxicology.

More appropriate to the needs of toxicology today, and in the future, are *in vitro* exposure systems. The development of these systems has formed the focus of work in the laboratory over the past few years. One immediate criticism that is made of *in vitro* systems is that they neglect the influence of metabolism. However, there are several answers to this criticism. Many of the compounds which are putative immunomodulatory agents are either not metabolized, e.g. heavy metals, or else the metabolites are well documented, e.g. aflatoxin. In fact, any compound which has undergone extensive toxicological evaluation will likely have documented metabolites, in many cases isolated or synthesized. It is also possible to provide a crude mimic of metabolism by pre-incubating test compounds with liver extracts. For example, in studies *in vitro* on the immunotoxicity of malathion, the metabolite O, O, S-trimethylphosphorothioate was generated by pre-incubation with a post-mitochondrial supernatant from Aroclor-induced rat liver [7].

The *in vitro* systems which we have chosen to study most closely are primary cultures of murine peritoneal macrophages and splenocytes. These cell populations are obtained following relatively trivial procedures and are amenable to short-term culture. Macrophage yields are increased by harvesting peritoneal exudate 4 days after an intraperitoneal injection of sterile 1.5% thioglycollate. We find no differences between the responses of elicited and non-elicited macrophages. Providing that viable cultures can be maintained it is possible to establish *in vitro* exposure systems using cells from many tissues relevant to the immune system, e.g. lymph node, skin.

Although small numbers of animals have to be sacrificed to provide cells for primary culture, it is likely in future that suitable cell-lines can be employed e.g. P388D1, the mouse monocyte/macrophage line, thus further reducing the necessity

for use of laboratory animals. Also, since it is possible to work with cell fractions from peripheral blood, there is a direct opportunity to work with human cells; this approach has many attractions since the ultimate objective of toxicological assessment is to relate hazard to human exposure. Finally, it is possible that human cell lines might be employed; there are, however, a large number of comparative and validatory experiments required before this possibility becomes reality.

EXTRACTION OF RNA FROM CELLS AND TISSUES

This is probably the most critical stage in the experiment and one which, if not performed correctly, will result in a waste of time and resources. The essential problem is that mRNA species are very short-lived, not by virtue of chemical instability, but because they are highly susceptible to attack by ribonuclease. *In vivo*, the resulting short half-life of mRNA is probably a deliberate mechanism to control expression; this is to our advantage since it affords us a view of cellular activity via a very narrow time-window. However, the disadvantage is that unless this endogenous ribonuclease activity is controlled then a substantial proportion of mRNA can be degraded during the extraction process. Even when purified, mRNA is not safe since it can be attacked by exogenous ribonuclease from the operator or from dirty equipment. Ribonuclease is a particularly persistent enzyme and has the unusual property of spontaneous reactivation following denaturation [8]. It is therefore extremely important to follow some simple rules when preparing to isolate RNA. This laboratory is fortunate in having a dedicated facility with restricted access for RNA work; at the very least a laboratory bench should be set aside and kept scrupulously clean with supplies of glassware and pipettes which are exclusively for use in RNA work. The following notes are routinely supplied by us to collaborating laboratories involved in RNA extraction.

General comment

Use the best sterile facilities available, wear gloves and facemask if manipulating on the open bench. Guanidine hydrochloride will take care of the endogenous ribonuclease; the onus is on you to prevent subsequent contamination by exogenous ribonuclease. Chief sources are dirty glassware, contaminated solutions, fingers and respiratory aerosols.

Preliminary work

1 Bake all glassware for 3 h at 250°C (it is preferable to use virgin glassware).
2 Autoclave all plastic-ware.
3 Treat a supply of water with diethylpyrocarbonate (DEPC) 0.1% v/v; add carefully to filtered de-ionized water with mixing and leave with stirring in a fume-hood overnight. Autoclave the treated water in pre-baked glass bottles and store tightly capped.

Solutions required

95% ethanol prepared in DEPC-treated water. Store at $-20°C$. Guanidine hydrochloride lysis solution is prepared in DEPC-treated water.

7.6 mol l^{-1} guanidine hydrochloride
0.1 mol l^{-1} potassium acetate
10 mmol l^{-1} dithiothreitol (DTT), pH 5.0

Warm the solution to dissolve the guanidine hydrochloride, add DTT last. Store this solution tightly capped at room temperature for no longer than a month. It is permissible to prepare stocks of guanidine hydrochloride and to add DTT fresh when required.

For further information, the reader is referred to an excellent short chapter in the *Methods in Enzymology* series [9]; this should be considered compulsory reading for anyone entering the field.

In our experience, the most effective technique for minimizing ribonuclease activity is vigorously to disrupt cells or tissue in the presence of guanidinium salts. Guanidine thiocyanate (4 mol l^{-1}) is more effective than 7.5 mol l^{-1} guanidine hydrochloride [10], presumably due to the additional chaotropic effect of the thiocyanate ion, but in our hands guanidine hydrochloride is adequate for cell monolayers. Techniques which do not use guanidinium salts, e.g. cytoplasmic dot-hybridization [11], or inclusion of vanadyl complexes [12] have proved inadequate in our hands, particularly with macrophage cultures which appear to have a high endogenous ribonuclease activity.

The following is an abbreviated account of the way in which we extract RNA from adherent macrophage cultures and is a modification to an existing method [13].

Guanidine buffer (0.5 ml) (7.6 mol l^{-1} guanidine hydrochloride, 0.1 mol l^{-1} potassium acetate, 10 mmol l^{-1} dithiothreitol, pH 5.0) is added to the adherent macrophage layer on the plates, swirled gently and incubated for 5 min. The plates are rinsed with a further 0.5 ml of guanidine buffer which is pooled with the original lysate. DNA in the lysate is sheared by repeated passage through a 25 gauge needle and 0.6 vol of 95% EtOH is added with vigorous mixing. Following overnight storage at $-20°C$, the specifically precipitated RNA is recovered by centrifugation at 13 000 g for 20 min. The pellet is washed in 90% ethanol and dried *in vacuo* for 10 min.

This single ethanolic precipitation appears to be adequate for part-purifying RNA for dot-blotting and it is also possible to perform Northern-blot analysis on these samples [14], although the quality of Northern blots is improved if contaminating protein is removed by organic extraction. Further purification of mRNA species from total RNA, e.g. for *in vitro* translation or cDNA synthesis, requires chromatography on oligo-dT cellulose or poly-U-sepharose [15] but is not considered advantageous for multiple sample screening. The ethanolic precipitate of RNA appears to be stable at $-20°C$ for several weeks.

For Northern-blot analysis, total RNA is dissolved in an appropriate buffer (e.g. for formaldehyde gels: 57% formamide, 7.6% formaldehyde, 0.04 mmol l^{-1} morpholinopropanesulphonic acid, 10 mmol l^{-1} sodium acetate, 1 mmol l^{-1} ethylenediamine-tetra-acetic acid) at 70°C for 10 min. For dot-blot analysis we routinely dissolve total RNA in 8.4% formaldehyde, 6.7 × standard saline citrate at 65°C for 20 min. Samples or aliquots of samples can be snap-frozen and stored at $-70°C$ or below pending analysis, but should be re-heated to 65°C briefly before use.

The choice between dot-blotting and Northern-blotting depends on the nature of the experiment. Northern-blotting, where samples are size-fractionated prior to blotting, has the advantage that confirmation is made that mRNA species are full-length and that the signals are not from spurious sources. However, only a limited number of samples can be co-processed and the sensitivity is not as great as dot- or slot-blotting. Our view is that every investigation should begin with a series of Northern blots to check on technique and specificity of hybridization; once satisfied, it is legitimate to use dot-blots to facilitate rapid multiple sample analysis. Dot-blotting involves direct transfer of sample to membrane (formerly nitrocellulose but now more often charge-modified nylon) which is usually achieved using an 8 × 12-well manifold. At least one dilution of the samples is usually blotted to check quantitation of probe binding. The use of multiple channel pipettes is strongly recommended when performing multiple manipulations.

Much debate is centred on the most appropriate membranes to use. Unfortunately, different membranes vary in their binding capacities, particularly with respect to background binding of certain probes. We recommend that at least two types of membranes are used in preliminary experiments; in this laboratory successful results have been obtained using a combination of Nytran (Schleicher & Schuell) and GeneScreen Plus (Dupont), for up to 20 different probes. We strongly suggest that manufacturers' instructions are adhered to.

Following incubation of samples on the membrane (we routinely allow 20 min), solvent is drawn through the membrane by application of a vacuum to the cassette and the membrane is air-dried. In some cases it is helpful to bake the membrane at 80°C in order to maximize covalent binding of macromolecules. Alternatively, a carefully calibrated exposure to ultraviolet light can achieve similar or better results [16]. Dried membranes can be sealed in plastic film and stored for several weeks in the dark.

PREPARATION OF LABELLED PROBES

There are numerous ways to generate labelled probes; the most widely used and the one which will be discussed in technical detail here is the incorporation of ^{32}P (normally as α-^{32}P dCTP) into cDNA sequences. Alternatives include the synthesis of labelled RNA transcripts from expression vectors [17], or the use of commercially available chemically modified bases (e.g. biotinylated) with subsequent detection using enzyme-substrate-linked antibodies. We have no direct experience of non-isotopic methods but it is unlikely that their sensitivity equals that of ^{32}P-labelled probes. Their advantage stems from safety considerations and from the fact that it is not necessary regularly to prepare fresh radiolabelled probes. One other alternative is the use of labelled oligonucleotide probes; these are short synthetic molecules (up to about 40 nucleotides) specifically complementary to the mRNA of interest. A well equipped molecular biology laboratory will have facilities for design and synthesis of appropriate oligonucleotide probes but the beginner in this field is unlikely to have such equipment. Coupled with the fact that labelled oligonucleotide probes are intrinsically less sensitive than cDNAs (since they are usually end-labelled only), their application seems limited. However they do have a role to play in this commercial world. Given that interlaboratory donation of cDNAs is at the discretion of those groups who originally cloned and published the sequence, there are some instances where commercial decision can interfere with free transfer of technology. In this case, oligonucleotide probes represent an alternative to re-cloning the appropriate cDNA. Design and radiolabelling techniques for oligonucleotides are reviewed in cloning manuals [18].

In this laboratory we normally use ^{32}P-labelled cDNA probes since we have been the fortunate recipients of gifts of cDNAs from various research and commercial laboratories. Plasmids bearing cDNAs are amplified in suitable host–vector systems [3], and cDNAs excised from flanking plasmid using appropriate endonucleases. DNA is purified by simple agarose gel electrophoresis. There are a number of techniques for radiolabelling cDNA probes: the method we routinely employ is based on the random hexanucleotide priming reaction [19] and the incorporation of α-^{32}P dCTP, except that we do not normally extract the electrophoretically separated DNA from agarose. The reaction with Klenow fragment is therefore performed at the higher temperature of 37°C, above the gelling temperature of LMP agarose. Specific activities of the labelled probes range from 5×10^8–10^9 c.p.m. μg^{-1}. It is assumed throughout that prospective researchers will have appropriate radioisotope handling and disposal facilities.

HYBRIDIZATION

It is strongly recommended that initial experiments are conducted using hybridization conditions, as suggested by the membrane manufacturers. Some protocols demand the use of a separate pre-hybridization step; others simply add an excess of denatured DNA (to saturate non-specific binding sites) to the hybridization solution. In the presence of 50% formamide, hybridization is normally performed at 42°C whereas in aqueous solution the temperature is considerably higher. Dextran sulphate is incorporated in some recipes to promote formation of the hybrid.

For oligonucleotide probes, the hybridization temperature has to be calculated or empirically determined and is normally about 5°C below the calculated T_m of the hybrid [18]. In all cases it is necessary to denature cDNA probes by heating to 95°C briefly before addition to hybridization solutions. Reactions can be performed in small volumes in sealed plastic bags, or in larger volumes in sandwich boxes on a shaking incubator or in roller bottles in a hybridization oven. The latter two techniques have been successfully used in this laboratory, largely because we invariably produce far more labelled probe than is immediately needed and are not restricted to small hybridization volumes to maintain effective probe concentration. The use of roller bottles on an oven rotisserie (Hybaid) requires more manipulations but is undoubtedly safer for the operator.

POST-HYBRIDIZATION ANALYSIS

It is almost inevitable that a substantial quantity of labelled probe will be non-specifically bound to the RNA or to the membrane following hybridization. This can be removed using a series of washes; again the instructions of the manufacturers of the particular nylon membrane should be heeded. The final, most stringent, wash normally uses a 0.1 × standard saline citrate solution at a temperature up to 65°C. This assumes that the probes are perfect hybrids for the mRNA samples; for non-perfect hybrids either the temperature of the wash can be lowered or the stringency can be lowered (i.e. increase the salt concentration). It is often necessary to accept less-than-perfect backgrounds when using probes which are not perfect hybrids.

Following washing, blots can be manually scanned with a Geiger counter, to check that the majority of label has been removed, and sealed in plastic bags or plastic film. Blots should always be bagged up whilst still damp since this will facilitate subsequent re-processing if, for example, it is desired to strip the first probe from the membrane and use a second one. In fact, this process can be repeated 5–6 times before the signal noise ratio becomes unacceptable. Sealed blots are then autoradiographed by exposure to X-ray film using intensifying screens at – 70°C. For a full discussion of autoradiography the reader is referred to an article by Bonner [20]. Usually an overnight exposure is sufficient to determine whether background levels are acceptable and to make an estimate of the required exposure time, remembering that ^{32}P has a half-life of only 14 days.

Although the developed autoradiograph usually gives a very good visual image of the relative abundance of mRNAs between samples, it is also possible to provide a semi-quantitative analysis by densitometry. There are certain limitations to this procedure, for example, the response of film to radioactivity only approximates to linearity from optical density 0.2–1.0 and the assumption is made that probe-binding is directly proportional to the quantity of mRNA on the membrane. The way forward in this area is illustrated by the recent work of Smith *et al.* [21] who, by including on their blots cytokine mRNA standards derived from cDNAs cloned into expression vectors, have eliminated the need for assumption of linearity.

Applications of molecular immunotoxicology

The combination of classical genetics and contemporary molecular biology has revealed a wealth of information about the organization and regulation of the immune system at the molecular level. A great deal is known about the expression of immunoglobulin genes [22], T-cell antigen receptor genes [23] and the major histocompatibility complex antigen genes [24]. However, as molecular immunotoxicologists seeking to develop and exploit common markers for use in screening systems *in vitro*, there is almost too much information available, and the presence of large pools of genetic information which generate diversity by subtle rearrangement seems an unlikely starting point for development of such markers. Our interest has therefore focused on the expression of the series of secreted polypeptides which underpin and maintain normal immune function and control the development of the immune response. These molecules, collectively termed cytokines, are the subject of another contribution to this volume (see Chapter 2). This section will focus on how the analysis of modulation of cytokine mRNA expression in defined immune systems can provide important information on the immunomodulatory effects of drugs and chemicals and can form the basis of an *in vitro* screening system.

From Chapter 2 it is clear that all cytokines are important, but that some are more important than others. For example, IL-1 and IL-2 appear to be involved in a variety of intercellular communication and can be considered as central to the development of the immune response, whereas others appear to have more specialized roles, e.g. IL-5 in the development of eosinophilia in parasitic infection. In developing *in vitro* screening systems we have sought to analyse expression of those cytokines upon which the immune response is pivotal, although in certain cases analysis of certain more peripheral cytokines may be indicated. For reasons stated earlier, it is preferable to develop this cytokine expression analysis using murine cells.

In order to characterize any test system, it is necessary to select model compounds to define the response. Unfortunately there are very few chemicals which have clearly defined immunotoxic properties and it was necessary to employ pharmaceutical agents with intended immunomodulatory effects, namely Biostim (RU41740), a bacterial glycoprotein extract with immunopotentiating properties and cyclosporin A, an immunosuppressant. At the molecular level, the mode of action of cyclosporin A is well understood, resulting in inhibition of transcription of IL-2 gene [25] by a mechanism involving the inhibition of binding of lymphocyte-specific factors to the IL-2 enhancer [26]. Biostim is less well understood but appears to involve increased IL-1

release as measured by functional assay [27].

The challenge then was for these effects to be clearly demonstrable in our *in vitro* screening system. We chose to examine the effects of test chemicals on peritoneal macrophages in culture and on the ability of cultured splenocytes to participate in a mixed lymphocyte reaction. For technical details the reader is referred to recent publications from this laboratory [14, 28] but the following essentially summarizes our findings.

Murine C3H-strain peritoneal macrophages were isolated and incubated with test compounds (1 pg ml^{-1}–100 μg ml^{-1} Biostim, 1–1000 ng ml^{-1} cyclosporin A) for periods of 3 or 24 h. Reaction to allogenic determinants (C57/B1 stimulator cells versus C3H responders) were assessed by incubating splenic lymphocytes with test compound for periods of 24 or 48 h: ^{3}H-thymidine incorporation was used to give an index of cellular proliferation. mRNA was extracted from cell lysates using a modification to a standard procedure. Northern and dot-blot samples of mRNA purified from cell lysates were hybridized with ^{32}P-cDNA probes for the cytokines IL-1α, IL-1β, tumour necrosis factor-α (TNF-α), IL-6, IL-2 and IL-2 receptor; α-actin was used as a control. Blots were stringently washed, autoradiographed and quantified by scanning video densitometry.

Initial results showed that isolated peritoneal macrophages displayed transient expression of cytokine mRNAs as a result of adherence to plastic culture dishes; overnight incubation (18 h) allowed them to become essentially quiescent with respect to cytokine expression and enhanced the sensitivity of the assays. Biostim had no effect on the turnover of α-actin in macrophages but dramatically elevated IL-1α, IL-1β, TNF-α and IL-6 mRNA transcripts at levels as low as 1–10 pg ml^{-1}. The expression was transient, peaking after 2–3 h exposure and declining rapidly after 8 h. Only transcripts for IL-1β mRNA were detectable after 24 h. Cyclosporin A had no effect on IL-1 expression in mixed lymphocyte reactions, but dramatically reduced the expression of IL-2 mRNA at both 24 and 48 h, presenting levels as low as 10% of the control at concentrations of 100 and 1000 ng ml^{-1} at 48 h. IL-2 receptor mRNA expression was less affected (80% of control).

Other immunomodulatory compounds are thought to act via a broadly similar modulation of cytokines such as IL-1, TNF and IL-2. For example, IL-1 production can be inhibited by tetrandrine [29]; a variety of quinolones can inhibit both IL-1 and TNF [30]. FK565 and FK156 appear to induce an enhanced release of IL-1 from lipopolysaccharide-stimulated macrophages, whereas both compounds inhibit the release of IL-2 from concanavalin A-induced splenocytes [31]. Fluorinated 4-quinolones have recently been shown to induce a hyperproduction of IL-2 [32]. To date, none of these effects has been documented at the molecular level and these compounds may represent ideal reagents to characterize further our *in vitro* system.

One line of criticism which has been levelled at this type of *in vitro* analysis is that not all immunotoxic compounds exert their effects by direct modulation of expression of a few key cytokines. However, this is to miss the point; the value of these *in vitro* systems does not simply lie in analysing the molecular mechanisms of cytokine modulation by immunopharmacological agents. Since cytokine expression is essential for the development of immune responses both *in vivo* and *in vitro*, it is possible to establish patterns of expression for *in vitro* models of immune activation, e.g. macrophage stimulation by lipopolysaccharide, mitogen/alloantigen stimulation of lymphocyte cultures. The effect of test chemicals on these characteristic patterns of cytokine expression can then be monitored following *in vivo* or *in vitro* exposure. Under these conditions, analysis of cytokine and related mRNAs becomes a semi-quantitative marker of immunotoxicity. We have applied this type of analysis to the compounds azathioprine and tributyltin and we can demonstrate inhibition of the expression of mRNAs for IL-2 and IL-2 receptor in mixed lymphocyte cultures en route to the development of cytotoxic T cells. The use of a highly specific probe for cytotoxic T cells, based on the DNA sequence for a serine esterase unique to this cell population [33], allows confirmation of the ultimate development or failure of development of functional cytotoxic lymphocytes. The inclusion of determination of expression of a high-turnover housekeeping gene such as actin or a metabolic gene allows discrimination between those compounds which exert a selective immunotoxicity and compounds which act via a non-specific cytotoxic mechanism.

On the basis of our experience in the field of molecular immunotoxicity, we would propose the following simple experiments for the investigation of the immunomodulatory potential of a drug or chemical.

1 Ability to induce expression of monokine mRNAs, e.g. IL-1α/β, IL-6, TNFα in cultured macrophages.

2 Ability to modulate expression of these monokine mRNAs in lipopolysaccharide-stimulated cultured macrophages.

3 Ability to induce expression of lymphokine mRNAs, e.g. IL-2, IL-4, IL-2 receptor, IL-6 in cultured splenocytes.

4 Ability to modulate expression of those lymphokine mRNAs in cultured splenocytes stimulated with alloantigen or mitogen. Analysis of mRNAs specific to cytotoxic T cells (proteases or lipases [34]).

5 Analysis of total cytokine mRNA levels in selected cells or tissues, e.g. spleen, thymus, lymph node, alveolar/peritoneal macrophages following *in vivo* exposure.

6 Analysis of *ex vivo* cells as in points 2 and 4, above.

This structure is liable to modification as the amount of data available expands and indicates priorities to be evaluated; there may also be specialized assays which merit inclusion in a preliminary screen. At present however it represents a framework within which pertinent information can be obtained and which can point the way to other more specific experiments.

Future applications and techniques

Clearly it is important to identify areas on which this technology is likely to have impact and to attempt to foresee the applications of current technical developments. In terms of pharmaceutical compounds, it is likely that researchers whose drugs are targeted toward the immune system already have this sort of technology on board. However, there is a very large number of pharmaceutical compounds on the market or in development whose effects on the immune system are poorly understood. As stated at the beginning of this chapter, this reflects almost non-existent legislation and is a situation which is likely to change within the next decade.

There are tremendous economic benefits of a

simple, sensitive, reproducible screening system for determining immunomodulatory potential and, should legislation ever become retrospective, there might be little alternative given the escalating costs of conventional animal experimentation.

In terms of industrial and environmental chemicals there are also remarkably few sound immunotoxicological data available; this can be illustrated by reference to a class of compounds such as pesticides, briefly reviewed in other chapters.

Pesticides comprise a group of chemical agents which require very careful toxicological evaluation but in an important reference work on immunotoxicological data, Descotes [39] stated that 'generally speaking, the influence if any of pesticides on the immune response has been nearly totally ignored despite obvious health implications'. This reference work cites such data as is available for a few organochlorines, including dichlorodiphenyltrichloroethane, 10 organophosphates, two carbamates, four pyrethroids and four fungicides, including hexachlorobenzene and pentachlorophenol. The data available are patchy and include a spectrum of immune function assays which often reveal conflicting or unclear results.

Clearly, in view of increasing public awareness of the consequences of impaired immune function, it is important that screening assays should be developed to assess the immunotoxic potential of chemicals such as pesticides to which the public may be exposed via food, occupation or environment. Pesticides, in particular, are coming under increasing scrutiny by the public and pressure groups. It is impractical to carry out major toxicological re-testing of all pesticides for immunotoxicity, so it is likely that economic and political pressure will dictate that a significant proportion of screening tests for immunotoxicity be performed *in vitro*, with a consequent reduction in the number and severity of laboratory animal experiments. Although there are a number of *in vivo* tests available, e.g. the host-resistance assay, they are often technically intricate, expensive and difficult to interpret. Controversy also surrounds the use of host-resistance assays, which in their crudest form are not dissimilar to the LD_{50} assay. We would propose that the type of *in vitro* screening system described in this chapter might be of great value in assessing the immunotoxic

potential of pesticides.

It was the thesis at the outset of this chapter that public pressure was the driving force behind the current discussion on how to conduct immunotoxicological testing sensibly. The onus is now on the scientist to propose sensitive and specific testing protocols and on the legislator to ensure that they are properly validated, relevant tests. It is their response which will determine whether the contemporary technology described here remains a tool of the research scientist or becomes incorporated into mainstream toxicology.

This chapter concludes with a brief discussion of other techniques which are likely to play an important role in the development of molecular immunotoxicology. *In situ* hybridization (covered in detail in Chapter 16) is a powerful technique which attempts to marry the talents of the histochemist and the molecular biologist. Although considered by many to be a technically intricate technique which does not always transfer well between laboratories, there have been some impressive demonstrations of modulation of mRNA expression at the single-cell level, e.g. for IL-1 and TNF [35], and for fibronectin [36] in isolated macrophage populations. The capacity to correlate specific mRNA expression to histochemically defined cell type has almost unlimited potential, particularly in relation to the immune system with its diversity of cell types and subpopulations.

The polymerase chain reaction (PCR) is another technique which has great potential in molecular immunotoxicology. The technology described in this chapter relies on the availability of relatively large numbers of cells, typically about 10^5 for monokine mRNAs from activated macrophages and up to 10^7 for cytokine receptor mRNAs in lymphocytes. In theory, PCR technology can be applied to the single cell where isolated mRNA molecules can be used as a template for cDNA synthesis and, in the presence of appropriate oligonucleotide primers and the heat-stable Taq polymerase, millions of copies of the sequence can be generated within a few hours. Clearly this technique is attractive when only small numbers of cells are available for analysis. However there are a number of pitfalls and precautions to working with and interpreting PCR technology; these have recently been comprehensively reviewed [37]. Not least of these difficulties, from the point of view of altered gene expression, is that relative quantitation between samples can prove inaccurate since minute discrepancies in original sample preparation are magnified over the 30 or more amplification cycles required. However, a novel solution has recently been developed which employs a competitor DNA fragment within each reaction vial; the competitor cDNA differs from the unknown DNA only by possession of a small intron [38]. Relative product yield can therefore be determined by densitometric scanning of the higher molecular weight product on stained gels. Using this technique reliable quantitation is claimed for numbers as low as 200 cells. The successful development of exploitation of this potent technique will therefore be of immense benefit to the molecular immunotoxicologist by offering an analytical capacity unrestrained by low cell numbers or by low abundance of mRNAs.

The opinions stated here are entirely personal and do not necessarily reflect the views of host or sponsoring organizations.

Acknowledgements

Research in this laboratory is supported by the Commission of European Communities (No. BAP 0272) and by the UK Ministry of Agriculture, Fisheries and Food.

References

1 Nishida T, Nishino N, Takano M, Sekiguchi Y, Kawai K, Mizuno K, Nakai S, Masui Y, Hirai Y. Molecular cloning and expression of rat interleukin-1α cDNA. *J Biochem (Jpn)* 1989; 105:351–7.

2 Yang Y-C, Clarletta AB, Temple PA, Chung MP, Kovacic S, Witek-Giannotti JS, Leary AC, Kriz R, Donahue RE, Wong GG, Clark SC. Human IL-3 (multi-CSF) identification by expression cloning of a novel hematopoietic growth factor related to murine IL-3. *Cell* 1986; 47:3–10.

3 Maniatis T, Fritsch EF, Sambrook J. *Molecular Cloning. A Laboratory Manual.* Cold Spring Harbor, NY: Cold Spring Harbor Laboratory Press. 1982.

4 Sambrook J, Fritsch EF, Maniatis T. *Molecular Cloning. A Laboratory Manual.* 2nd ed. Cold Spring Harbor, NY: Cold Spring Harbor Laboratory Press. 1989.

5 Berger SL, Kimmel AR, eds. Guide to molecular cloning techniques. 1987; 152.

6 Li DD, Chien Y-K, Gu M-Z, Richardson A, Cheung

HT. The age-related decline in interleukin-3 expression in mice. *Life Sci* 1988; 43:1215–22.

7 Rodgers KE, Grayson MH, Imamura T, Devens BH. *In vitro* effects of malathion and O,O,S-trimethyl phosphorothioate on cytotoxic T-lymphocyte responses. *Pest Biochem Physiol* 1985; 24:260–6.

8 Sela M, Anfinsen CB, Harrington WF. The correlation of ribonuclease activity with specific aspects of tertiary structure. *Biochim Biophys Acta* 1957; 26:502–12.

9 Blumberg DD. Creating a ribonuclease-free environment. *Methods Enzymol* 1987; 152:20–4.

10 MacDonald RJ, Swift GH, Przybyla AE, Chirgwin JM. Isolation of RNA using guanidinium salts. *Methods Enzymol* 1987; 152:219–27.

11 White BA, Bancroft FC. Cytoplasmic dot hybridisation. *J Biol Chem* 1982; 257:8569–72.

12 Berger SL. Isolation of cytoplasmic RNA: ribonucleoside–vanadyl complexes. *Methods Enzymol* 1987; 152: 227–34.

13 Cheley S, Anderson R. A reproducible micro-analytical method for the detection of specific RNA sequences by dot-blot hybridisation. *Anal Biochem* 1984; 137:15–19.

14 Meredith C, Scott MP, Pekelharing H, Miller K. The effect of Biostim (RU 41740) on the expression of cytokine mRNA in murine peritoneal macrophages *in vitro*. *Toxicol Letts* 1990; 53:327–37.

15 Jacobson A. Purification and fractionation of poly(A)† RNA. *Methods Enzymol* 1987; 152:254–61.

16 Church GM, Gilbert W. Genomic sequencing. *Proc Natl Acad Sci USA* 1984; 81:1991–5.

17 Melton DA, Krieg PA, Rebagliata MR, Maniatis T, Zinn K, Green MR. Efficient *in vitro* synthesis of biologically active RNA and RNA hybridisation probes from plasmids containing a bacteriophage SP6 promoter. *Nucl Acids Res* 1984; 18:7035–56.

18 Wallace RB, Miyada CG. Oligonucleotide probes for the screening of recombinant DNA libraries. *Methods Enzymol* 1987; 152:432–42.

19 Feinberg AP, Vogelstein B. A technique for radiolabelling DNA restriction endonuclease fragments to high specific activity. *Anal Biochem* 1983; 132:6–13.

20 Bonner WM. Autoradiograms: ^{35}S and ^{32}P. *Methods Enzymol* 1987; 152:55–61.

21 Smith MF, Kueppers FR, Young PR, Lee JC. A rapid and quantitative method for the determination of interleukin-1α and β mRNA expression in human monocytes and macrophages. *J Immunol Methods* 1989; 118:265–72.

22 Blackwell TK, Alt FW. Immunoglobulin genes. In: Hames BD, Glover DM, eds. *Molecular Immunology.* Oxford: IRL Press, 1988:1–60.

23 Davis MM. T cell antigen receptor genes. In: Hames B D, Glover DM, eds. *Molecular Immunology.* Oxford: IRL Press, 1988:61–79.

24 Guillemot F, Auffray C, Orr HT, Strominger JL. MHC antigen genes. In: Hames BD, Glover DM, eds. *Molecular Immunology.* Oxford: IRL Press, 1988:81–143.

25 Granelli-Piperno A. Lymphokine gene expression *in vivo* is inhibited by cyclosporin A. *J Exp Med* 1990; 171:533–44.

26 Randak C, Brabletz T, Hergenrother M, Sobotta I, Serfling E. Cyclosporin A suppresses the expression of the interleukin 2 gene by inhibiting the binding of lymphocyte-specific factors to the IL-2 enhancer. *Embo J* 1990; 9:2529–36.

27 Sozzani S, D'Alessandro F, Capsoni F, Luini W, Barcellini W, Guidi G, Spreafico F. *In vitro* modulation of human monocyte functions by RU 41740 (Biostim). *Int J Immunopharmacol* 1988; 10:93–102.

28 Meredith C, Scott MP, Miller K. Immunotoxicology screening *in vitro:* modulation of expression of immunoregulatory genes. *Human Toxicol* 1989; 8;411–12.

29 Seow WK, Ferrante A, Si-Ying L, Thong YH. Suppression of human monocyte interleukin-1 production by the plant alkaloid tetrandrine. *Clin Exp Immunol* 1989; 75:47–51.

30 Bailly S, Fay M, Roche Y, Gougerot-Pocidalo MA. Effects of quinolones on tumour necrosis factor production by human monocytes. *Int J Immunopharmacol* 1990; 12:31–6.

31 Ahmed K, Turk JL. Effect of anticancer agents neothramycin, aclacinomycin, FK-565 and FK-156 on the release of interleukin-2 and interleukin-1 *in vitro*. *Cancer Immunol Immunother* 1989; 28:87–92.

32 Riesback K, Andersson J, Gullberg M, Forsgren A. Fluorinated 4-quinolones induce hyperproduction of interleukin 2. *Proc Natl Acad Sci USA* 1989; 86:2809–13.

33 Lobe CG, Finlay BB, Paranchych W, Paetkau VH, Bleackley RC. Novel serine proteases encoded by two cytotoxic T lymphocyte-specific genes. *Science* 1986; 232:858–61.

34 Grusby MJ, Nabavi N, Wong H, Dick RF, Bluestone JA, Scholtz MC, Glimcher LH. Cloning of an interleukin-4 inducible gene from cytotoxic T lymphocytes and its identification as a lipase. *Cell* 1990; 60:451–9.

35 Remick DG, Scales WE, May MA, Spengler M, Nguyen D, Kunkel SL. *In situ* hybridization analysis of macrophage-derived tumour necrosis factor and interleukin-1 mRNA. *Lab Invest* 1988; 59:809–16.

36 Adachi K, Yamauchi K, Bernaudin JF, Fouret P, Ferrans, VJ, Crystal RG. Evaluation of fibronectin gene expression by *in situ* hybridisation. *Am J Pathol* 1988; 133:193–203.

37 Wright PA, Wynford-Thomas D. The polymerase chain reaction: miracle or mirage? A critical review of its uses and limitations in diagnosis and research. *J Pathol* 1990; 162:99–117.

38 Gilliland G, Perrin S, Blanchard K, Bunn HF. Analysis of cytokine mRNA and DNA: detection and quantitation by competitive polymerase chain reaction. *Proc Natl Acad Sci USA* 1990; 87:2725–9.

39 Descotes J. *Immunotoxicology of Drugs and Chemicals.* Oxford: Elsevier, 1986:314–32.

Part V

20
Concluding remarks

KLARA MILLER & JOHN L. TURK

The subject of immunotoxicology covers both the effects of agents stimulating the immune system and those that depress the immune response. Amongst the stimulating effects that have been covered are those of small molecules acting as haptens. Molecules of larger molecular weight can act as antigens in their own right. Molecules that depress the immune response may act directly as immunosuppressive agents on the T- and B-cell response. On the other hand, they might stimulate the suppressor arm of the immune response rather than its effector mechanisms. This latter area has as yet been insufficiently investigated. Other chemical agents that are immunosuppressive may act by allowing the proliferation of biological agents such as retroviruses that could be the final pathway to depression of the immune response. This is also a field which needs further study.

Another approach which is under development is the direct effect of toxic agents on the non-specific mediators of the immune response. Examples of this are the direct effect of metals and mineral dusts on the complement cascade. A further area that is receiving an increasing amount of attention is the action of a number of agents on cytokine production. Cytokines are now accepted as important regulatory molecules involved in lymphocyte proliferation and macrophage activation. They also act on other cells involved both in the immune response and in the pathogenic processes.

The genetic constitution of an individual is particularly important in determining how the immune response reacts to any potential toxic agent. Although there have been some animal studies along these lines, these have been strictly limited and they relate only to the allergic and autoimmune responses. Studies at the human level are limited by the large population that would need to be surveyed and by the current inability to characterize all the genetic factors that might be involved. Epidemiology is of limited value in assessing small differences in susceptibility.

It should also be remembered that dose–response relationships for immune effects are different from those that occur in non-immunologically mediated toxic effects. It is important to take this into account when designing laboratory-based or clinical studies. In an immunological study one may well get an effect at a low dose and fail to get a similar effect at a medium or high dose. A high dose may induce tolerance, whereas the low dose might sensitize.

In the human situation, one must not ignore the role of socioeconomic factors, nutrition and age. Both young children and the aged may prove more susceptible under certain circumstances to the toxic action of agents on the immune system. Babies have a different profile of immunoglobulin synthesis than do older children. Young children who are malnourished and have recently had measles infection will have a double reason to be immunosuppressed and thus are more susceptible to further insults to their immune system by chemical agents.

The continuous low-level exposure of the immune system to chemical agents increasingly present in the environment must lead to greater concern in the future. So far, much information is available only from studies in which individuals have been exposed to large doses over a relatively short period of time.

359

More studies are necessary on the effects of low-level exposure over longer periods of time on defined populations of both experimental animals and people. In these studies, as exposure would be to low concentrations of toxic agents, observations should be made on an increased number of individuals. Alteration in the immune system could be reflected in an increased susceptibility to infection. Evidence in humans is, by its very nature, hard to come by and might be apparent only in longitudinal studies. These would be difficult to design and carry out. Although the role of the immune system in cancer surveillance has as yet been poorly defined, the findings from patients treated with immunosuppressive agents and those treated with human immunodeficiency virus infection indicate that a connection exists. Thus, one should be aware of the possibility that low-level exposure to toxic agents that lead to a disturbance of normal immunological homeostatic mechanisms, might in turn lead to a risk of cancer development, especially if the individual is exposed in addition to a low-level carcinogen.

We conclude by suggesting that toxic agents acting on the immune system may be only part of a series of multi-factorial effects leading to the development of disease. Thus, immunotoxicological testing remains an important part of risk assessment.

Index

Page numbers in *italics* refer to figures and tables.